The Immune Consequences of Trauma, Shock and Sepsis - Mechanisms and Therapeutic Approaches

Volume 2/1

E. Faist, A. E. Baue, F. W. Schildberg (Eds.)

The Immune Consequences of Trauma, Shock and Sepsis - Mechanisms and Therapeutic Approaches

Volume 2/1

MOF, MODS and SIRS
Concepts, Clinical Correlates and Therapy

PABST SCIENCE PUBLISHERS
Lengerich, Berlin, Düsseldorf, Leipzig,
Riga, Scottsdale (USA), Wien, Zagreb

Library of Congress Cataloging-in-Publication Data

**The Immune Consequences of Trauma, Shock and Sepsis -
Mechanisms and Therapeutic Approaches.** Volume 2/1 / E. Faist ... (Eds.). -
Lengerich ; Berlin ; Düsseldorf ; Riga ; Scottsdale (USA) ; Wien ;
Zagreb : Pabst Science Publishers 1996
   ISBN 3-928057-76-6
NE: Faist, Eugen ... [Eds.]

This work is subject to copyright. All rights are reserved, whether the whole or part of the material is concerned, specifically the rights of translation, reprinting, reuse of illustrations, recitation, broadcasting, reproduction on microfilms or in other ways, and storage in data banks. The use of registered names, trademarks, etc. in this publication does not imply, even in the absence of a specific statement, that such names are exempt from the relevant protective laws and regulations and therefore free for general use.
The authors and the publisher of this volume have taken care that the information and recommendations contained herein are accurate and compatible with the standards generally accepted at the time of publication. Nevertheless, it is difficult to ensure that all the information given is entirely accurate for all circumstances. The publisher disclaims any liability, loss, or damage incurred as a consequence, directly or indirectly, of the use and application of any of the contents of this volume.

Editors:
E. Faist, M.D., Prof. of Surgery
Clinic Grosshadern, Ludwig-Maximilians-University, Dept. of Surgery,
Marchioninistr. 15, D-81377 Munich, Germany, Phone: 49-89-7095-3441/2461,
Telefax: 49-89-7095-2460

A. E. Baue, M.D., Prof. of Surgery
St. Louis University, Medical Center, 3635 Vista Ave. at Grand Blvd., P. O. Box 15250,
St. Louis, MO 63110-0250, USA, Phone: 001-314-577-8372, Telefax: 001-314-771-1945

F. W. Schildberg, M.D., Prof. of Surgery
Clinic Grosshadern, Ludwig-Maximilians-University, Dept. of Surgery,
Marchioninistr. 15, D-81377 Munich, Germany, Phone: 49-89-7095-2790,
Telefax: 49-89-7095-8893

© 1996
Pabst Science Publishers
D-49525 Lengerich
Telefax: 49-5484-550
E-mail: pabst.publishers@t-online.de

Editorial Office:
Robert Borenic, Evi Gerstmeyr,
Visnja Kabalin-Borenic

Printing: krips repro meppel

ISBN 3-928057-76-6

MOF, MODS and SIRS - Volume II, 1 and II, 2: Concepts, Clinical Correlates and Therapy

These two volumes contain the program of the Third International Congress on the Immune Consequences of Trauma, Shock and Sepsis - Mechanisms and Therapeutic Approaches. The Congress took place in Munich, Germany from March, 2-5 1994 under the title used at the two previous Congresses, held in 1988 and 1991. This provides continuity and historical background for the immense changes currently taking place in the science of injury and patient care. However, the evolution in science and the rapid advances in knowledge presented in the proceedings of this Congress require a very different title. Thus, Volume I is dedicated to basic mechanisms, inflammation and tissue injury, whereas Volumes II, 1 and II, 2 are devoted to concepts, clinical correlates and therapy. Part one presents the basic approach to the problems of injury, sepsis, illness and operations. It contains information which is crucial for surgeons who wish to advance their knowledge in this field, and for other medical professionals in the fields of intensive care, emergency medicine and other clinical areas. Volume two is predominantly devoted to the clinical and therapeutical aspects of MOF, MODS and SIRS. However, our colleagues from the basic sciences have also greatly contributed to this part. Thus, all parts, basic and clinical, compose a whole that is of interest to all of us involved in caring for the ill. For those who attended and/or participated at the congress in Munich in March 1994, these proceedings will provide an accurate record of what took place there and the advances reported in our understanding of injury, inflammation and organ failure. To those who could not attend, these volumes will help to remain on the leading edge of patient care and research presented in Munich.

Multiple organ failure (MOF) is the ultimate complication of trauma, illness and intensive or critical care. Thus, it is a problem of ICU patients after multiple system injury accompanied with shock, after operation, infection, severe inflammatory disease, low cardiac output, organ transplantation and its complications or other. Organ failure is usually a remote result of an original problem, such as peritonitis, which can lead to heart, liver and kidney failure. A large number of descriptions, classifications and scoring systems for organ failures that were presented will not be mentioned here. For our purposes it suffices to say that there is organ failure when it is necessary to support organ function. Ventilatory failure along with circulatory instability, which are most evident, are common initial symptoms of MOF. They are normally followed by hepatic and renal failure, coagulation problems and failure of the gut and central nervous, musculoskeletal, immune, and metabolic systems failure. Sophisticated techniques of monitoring and organ support have allowed the development of MOF in patients who would have previously died. However, when MOF develops morbidity and mortality remain high.

A new system of terminology has now been recommended focusing on organ dysfunction rather than on organ failure during critical illness. The definition of multiple organ dysfunction syndrome (MODS) is "the presence of altered organ function in acutely ill patients such that homeostasis cannot be maintained without intervention." Organ dysfunctions for each organ system are being defined. The systemic inflammatory response syndrome (SIRS) has been proposed to take the place of what was previously called sepsis or the sepsis syndrome. SIRS is defined as manifestations of two or more of the following conditions: temperature >38°C or < 36°C; heart rate > 90 beats/min, respiratory rate > 20 breaths/min or $PaCO_2$ less than torr (< 4.3 kPa); WBC > 12.000 cells/mm^3 or > 10% immature (band) forms. How these various terms will be used in the future remains to be seen. Certainly there is considerable interest in how we describe the effects of remote organ dysfunction or failure and the inflammatory response in sick patients.

Volumes II, 1 and II, 2 are dedicated to clinical concepts, correlations and therapy. It begins with a definition of the clinical syndrome of MODS or MOF, the reasons for their development, methods of severity measurements, and other aspects of MOF and MODS that remain a major cause of death in many injured and sick patients. Specific organ dysfunctions and their mechanisms and changes are reviewed. Extensive work on the immune response to injury, its means of diagnosis, and their molecular aspects provide an interesting number of papers dedicated to exploring the clinical aspects of these syndromes further.

The question of whether the systemic mediator response in injury and sepsis is well-regulated or dysregulated is an important consideration. Both sides of the issue are examined in detail. Indicators and predictors of the development of MOF, MODS and SIRS come from a number of sources.

The problem of peritonitis and its biologic basis present exciting new avenues of therapy. Inflammatory lung injury or ARDS are reviewed, providing important information on development mechanisms and strategies for counter-regulation. Acute pancreatitis, its biologic aspects and potential future therapy are presented in detail, as are infections in organ transplantation, which strongly affect prolonged function and survival during immunosuppression in patients with transplanted organs.

The vast amount of information about mediators and their importance in disease is impressive. It has raised our hopes of a magic bullet that might be used to alter or block an excessive inflammatory response. However, it has not been found. Why not? Our science is powerful, but our therapy still weak. A number of clinical trials were reported at this Congress, including the "sue" of monoclonal antibodies to endotoxin, monoclonal antibodies to TNF, IL-1 receptor antagonists, soluble receptors to TNF and other approaches. When these agents were evaluated in prospective randomized trials in sick or septic patients, results were not positive, and the question is "why not?". So far our highly promising expectation of a magic bullet to deal with inflammation, injury and infection has not yielded satisfactory results. The design, methodology and interpretation of clinical trials in shock and sepsis were reviewed in detail. The possibility of using only high risk patients, multiple therapeutic agents, patients with the same disease process are appropriate alternatives for future studies.

Modern aspects of antimicrobial therapy in critically ill patients are reviewed in detail along with the treatment of perioperative anemia. An exciting aspect of current molecular biology is the use of hemopoietic growth factors and study of their impact on host defense systems. Their clinical significance is being evaluated with considerable excitement. The relationship of nutrition and immune function is also an important aspect and considerable new information is available. The entire subject of immunonutrition is reviewed in great detail. Growth hormone has been used in a number of clinical situations with positive results, which is presented in a number of reports. The relationship of immune suppression, the possibility of modulating the immune response and of modulating the inflammatory response is the subject of several papers, all of which have a potential clinical impact. Anti-endotoxin interventions were studied in detail, especially the possibility of a more specific interference with the effects of endotoxin. Immunotherapy for sepsis has come forward as an important part of potential therapy. Finally, better approaches in wound healing, acceleration of the healing process and better burn wound coverage form an inspiring area of scientific development using growth factors and other biologic substances. Even though there is no single magic bullet for injured, septic and sick patients, nor is there likely to be one, there are a number of promising and specific therapeutic approaches that are useful now and will become increasingly helpful in the future.

Munich, August 1996 *Prof. E. Faist*
Prof. A. E. Baue
Prof. F. W. Schildberg

Contents

Section 1:
MODS/MOF - The Clinical Syndrome

Arthur E. Baue
Prologue: The Concept of Limits and Emergence of Multiple Organ Failure 20

D.E. Fry
Genesis of Multiple System Organ Failure 32

J. C. Marshall
SEPSIS, SIRS, and MODS: Consensus, Controversy, and Challenge 41

J. R. Le Gall
Development, Validation and Use of the SAPS II Model for Early Severe Sepsis . . . 51

J.H. Siegel, D. Rixen, A. Abu-Salih, M. Bertolini, F. Panagakos, N. Espina
Physiologic State Classification and Bayesian Probability Analysis as a
Technique for Stratification of Severity and Prediction of Outcome in Human
Post-traumatic Sepsis and ARDS 58

A.E. Baue
Epilogue - Toward a Consensus 73

Section 2:
Mechanistic and Biochemical Profiles of Specific
Organ Dysfunction/Failure

J. Cervós-Navarro
Pathogenic Mechanisms of Brain Failure 84

J.-L. Vincent, G. Friedman
Definition of Cardiovascular Dysfunction/Failure 99

P. Boekstegers, K. Werdan
Challenges of the Concept of Supranormal Oxygen Delivery in Patients
with Sepsis: Evidence Against Tissue Hypoxia but for Impaired Oxygen
Metabolism in Sepsis 105

A.E. Barber, W.J. Millikan, H. Illner, L. Montalvo, L. Griffith, G.T. Shires
Hemorrhagic Shock Severely Impairs Liver Function 115

E.A. Deitch, N. Cruz
Mechanisms of Gut Barrier Failure 120

E.E. Moore, F.A. Moore, R.J. Franciose, F.J. Kim
Postischemic Gut Serves as a Priming Bed for Circulating Neutrophils
That Provoke Multiple Organ Failure 132

Section 3:
Spectrum of Immuno- and Molecular Diagnostics

D. Fuchs, A. Gruber, C. Murr, G. Reibnegger, H. Wachter
Use of Neopterin for the Monitoring of Cell-Mediated Immune Response In Vivo . . 144

G.P. Tilz, E. Faist, F. Schreiber, U. Demel, D. Demel, H. Becker, J. Schafhalter,
H. Wachter, L. Kenner, D. Fuchs
Interleukin-2 Receptor as a Useful Tool for Diagnosis and Treatment of
Autoimmune, Infectious and Malignant Diseases in Clinical Medicine
and Immunopathology: Comparison with Other Markers of Immune Activation
and Therapeutical Consequences 151

H.Denz
Soluble Tumor Necrosis Factor Receptors 155

C. Bohuon, M. Assicot
Procalcitonin: A New Innovative Marker for Sepsis and Very Severe
Inflammatory Diseases 158

S.Stöve, H.Hartmann, A.Klos, W.Bautsch, J.Köhl
Early Diagnosis of Sepsis by Rapid Measurement of C3a/C3 Plasma Levels 162

T.J. Novitsky
Endotoxin: Does Its Detection Provide Diagnostic Benefit? 171

F. Stüber, F.U. Schade, J. Schröder, F. Bokelmann, M. Petersen, J. Seifert
Acute-Phase Proteins in SIRS 183

A. Gaitzsch, R. Lefering, D. Weber, S. Sauerland, M.L. Dangel, D. Rixen, P. Fink
Early Recognition of Sepsis Using IL-6, TNF, Elastase, and CRP 187

Å. Lasson, J. Göransson, K. Jönsson
Acute-Phase Response Predicts Complications After Trauma Better than
Protease Inhibitors or Collagen Precursor 192

U. Lehmann, M. Oellerich, G. Regel, D. Pape
Lidocaine Metabolite Formation: An Indicator of MOF After Multiple Trauma 199

J. Pincemail, J.O. Defraigne, C. Franssen, O. Detry, D. Serteyn, G. Hartstein,
M. Meurisse, M. Lamy, M. Limet
Assessment of Free Radical Production by Electron Spin Resonance Spectroscopy
During the Ischemia-Reperfusion Phenomenon: From Animal Models to Clinical
Investigation 203

C.W. Schweinfest, M.W. Graber, X.-K. Zhang, P.G. Vanek, D.K. Watson
Gene Cloning I: Preparation of DNA Libraries 215

D.K. Watson, P.G. Vanek, X.-K. Zhang, M.W. Graber, C.W. Schweinfest
Gene Cloning II: Screening and Sequencing of Genes 229

Section 4:
Regulation and Dysregulation of the Systemic Mediator Response in Injury and Sepsis

J.W. Holaday, C.A., Nacy, E.A. Neugebauer
Alphabet Soup: An Analysis of Mediators of Sepsis 244

B.A. Pruitt, Jr., D.G. Burleson, A.C. Drost, W.G. Cioffi, A.D. Mason, Jr.
Humoral Manifestations of Regulation and Dysregulation of the
Systemic Mediator Response in Injury and Sepsis 248

M. Miyashita, M. Onda, K. Sasajima, T. Matsutani, Y. Akiya, K. Okawa,
H. Maruyama, T. Nakamura, K. Furukawa, K. Yamashita
Humoral Mediators in Surgical Stress and Multiple Organ Failure 256

J. Shelby, W.W. Ku, H. C. Nielson
Neurohormone and Neuropeptide Regulation of the
Posttraumatic Immune Response 262

Ch.-F. Wolf, A. Brinkmann, D. Berger, E. Kneitinger, H. Wiedeck, R. Wennauer,
M.Büchler, M. Georgieff, A. Grünert, W.D. Seeling
Endocrine Responses to Mesenteric Traction During Major Abdominal Surgery . . . 272

S. Dimmeler, E. Neugebauer, A. Lechleuthner
Histamine in Septic/Endotoxic Shock 277

J.K. Horn, G.A. Hamon, R.H. Mulloy, C. Birkenmaier
Immune Complexes: Mediators of Sepsis and Immune Dysfunction 282

Section 5:
Indicators and Crucial Functional Mechanisms for the Development of MODS/MOF and SIRS

A.E. Baue
Shock, Tissue Damage and Immune Dysfunction: Blood Flow Mediated
or Persistent Inflammatory Cascade 294

M.L. Rodrick, J.A. Mannick
Human Volunteer Endotoxin Studies: A Useful Approach for the
Understanding of Immunologic and Inflammatory Pathways 307

B.J. Rowlands, M.I. Halliday, W.B.D. Clements, J.A. Kennedy
Experimental and Clinical Aspects of Sepsis Associated with Obstructive Jaundice . 317

M. Grotz, G. Regel, A. Dwenger, H.-C. Pape, C. Hainer, R. Vaske, H. Tscherne
Standardized Sheep Model for Multiple Organ Failure (MOF)
After Severe Trauma 325

M. Ogawa, S. Ikei, H. Sameshima, K. Sakamoto, J. Yamashita
Increased Cytokine Release in Severe Acute Pancreatitis Is Closely
Related to the Development of Organ Failure 332

M. Gawaz, S. Fateh-Moghadam, G. Pilz, H.-J. Gurland, K. Werdan
Severity of Multiple Organ Failure but not of Sepsis Correlates with
Irreversible Platelet Degranulation 338

G. Sganga, G. Gangeri, D. Gui, M. Castagneto
Oxidative Stress and Antioxidants in Clinical Sepsis 344

T. Hase, T. Tani, H. Oka, T. Yokota, M. Kodama, H. Kimura, I. Tooyama
Expression of c-fos Protein in Brain and Endotoxin Levels in Plama
Following Occlusion of Superior Mesenteric Artery of Rat 353

A. Brinkmann, Ch.-F. Wolf, E. Kneitinger, D. Berger, M. Rockemann, M. Büchler,
H. Wiedeck, W.Seeling, M.Georgieff
Acute Hypoxemia Due to Prostacyclin Release During Major Abdominal Surgery . . 359

J.G. Gallucci, J.V. Quinn, D. Woolley, G. Seidel, G.J. Slotman
Prostacyclin Mediates Increased Oxygen Consumption and Arterial
Hypoxemia, Preserves Cardiac Index, and Prevents Platelet Aggregation
During Graded Bacteremia 365

K. Hirata, T. Ohmura, H. Yamaguchi, T. Matsuno, K. Yamashiro, T. Katsuramaki,
M. Mukaiya, X.A. Ming, R. Denno
Significance of Sinusoidal Lining Cells and of Humoral Factors on
Hepatocytic Function Following Sepsis and Major Surgery 370

Section 6:
Mechanisms of Inflammatory Lung Injury and Strategies for Counterregulation

R. Rabinovici, L.F. Neville, G. Feuerstein
New Concepts in Septic ARDS: Initiation by Synergism Between
Nontoxic Doses of Lipopolysaccharide and Platelet-Activating Factor 386

A. Dwenger, M. Grotz, H.-C. Pape, C. Hainer, G. Schweitzer, G. Regel
Neutrophil Function and Lung Injury in a Standardized Sheep Model
of Multiple Organ Failure 395

A. Catania, D. McCoy, K. Carnes, A. Macaluso, G. Ceriani, J. Biltz, J.M. Lipton
Anti-inflammatory Effects of the Neuropeptide a-Melanocyte
Stimulating Hormone in Systemic Inflammation 400

H.-C. Pape, A. Dwenger, D. Remmers, G. Regel
Unreamed Femoral Nailing Reduces Lung Function Impairment and
Increased Inflammatory Response in Polytrauma Patients 403

K. Sakamoto, H. Arakawa, T. Ishiko, S. Mita, M. Ogawa
Evidence for Involvement of IL-8 in Lung Injury after Esophagectomy 407

H. Gerlach, M. Gerlach, T. Kerner, C. Heid, S. Seiler, D. Keh, K.J. Fulke, J. Falke
Ischemia/Hypoxia-Induced Cell Damage Mediated by Enhanced
Receptor-Ligand Interaction of Tumor Necrosis Factor-α (TNF) 412

T. Koch, H.P. Duncker, J. Fisahn, F. Lutz, and H. Neuhof
Pathomechanisms and Therapeutic Aspects of Pseudomonas Aeruginosa
Cytotoxin-Induced Pulmonary Microvascular Injury: Studies on Isolated
Perfused Rabbit Lungs 417

R. Rossaint, H. Gerlach, R. Kuhlen, K. Falke
Inhaled Nitric Oxide in Acute Lung Injury 427

J. Schilling, R. Bürki, H. Joller, M. Lachat, D. Gyurech, S. Geroulanos
Effect of Nitric Oxide Synthase Inhibitors on Pulmonary Shunt Volume
and Cytokines in Human Septic Shock 434

R. Rossaint, D. Pappert, K. Lewandowski, K. Falke
Extracorporeal Lung Support in Severe ARDS 437

Section 7:
Peritonitis - The Biological Basis for Treatment

O.D. Rotstein
Microbial Synergy in Intraabdominal Infections 448

D.L. Dunn
Host Defenses of the Peritoneal Cavity 456

P. Kinnaert
Regulation of Intraabdominal Inflammation: The Cellular Aspect 462

E.H. Farthmann, U. Schöffel
Generalized Response in Secondary Peritonitis 467

H.Wacha, Ch. Ohmann L.M. Reichert, and the SIS-E Peritonitis Study Group
Scores in Peritonitis and Their Limitations 473

A. Hunsicker, W. Kullich, W. Weissenhofer, D. Lorenz, J. Petermann,
K. Boden, H. Rokos
Correlations Between Endotoxin, γ-Interferon, Biopterin and Serum
Phospholipase A_2 Activities During Lethal Gram-Negative Sepsis in Rats 485

K.-P. Reimund, F. Weitzel, W. Lorenz, I. Celik, M. Kurnatowski, W. Mannheim,
A. Heiske, K. Neumann, B. Greger, M. Bartscherer, M. Rothmund
Granulocyte-Colony-Stimulating Factor Prophylaxis and Treatment in
Postoperative Peritonitis: Animal Experiments and a Successful Case Report 493

D. Moch, B. Schröppel, M.H. Schoenberg, H.-J. Schulz, B.-E. Hedlund
U.B. Brückner
Protective Effects of Hydroxyethyl Starch-Deferoxamine in Early Sepsis 504

Section 8:
Acute pancreatitis - Biology and Therapeutic Consequences

C. Niederau, R. Lüthen, J.W. Heise, H. Becker
Biochemical Pattern, Systemic Complications, and
Outcome in Acute Pancreatitis 510

D. Closa, L. Fernández-Cruz, J. Roselló-Catafau, M. Bardaj, E. Gelpí
Oxygen Free Radicals and Acute Pancreatitis 531

J. Baas, N. Senninger, H. Elser, F. Willeke, R. Langer, C. Herfarth
The Effect of Biliary Obstruction on the Phagocytic Function of the
Reticuloendothelial System in the Opossum Model 539

S. Kopprasch, H. Kühne, T. Zimmermann, A. Dörfler, H.-E. Schröder, K. Ludwig
Effect of Sodium Selenite in Combination with Aprotinin on Inflammatory
Plasma Markers During Acute Pancreatitis 543

S. Pierrakakis, P. Karydakis, N. Economou, A. Ninos, G. Antsaklis
The Effects of Toxemia on the Cascade Systems of Patients with
Acute Pancreatitis 548

R. Függer, P. Götzinger, T. Sautner, H. Andel, G. Huemer
ICU Treatment of Patients with Acute Necrotizing Pancreatitis 551

W. Uhl, M.W. Büchler
Surgical Treatment of Necrotizing Pancreatitis 557

Section 9:
Infections in Transplantation: Epidemiology, Prevention and Treatment

H. Einsele, H. Hebart, U. Schumacher
Epidemiology of Infections After Bone Marrow Transplantation 566

*A. Michalopoulos, V. Kadas, A. Anthi, E. Papadakis, J. Kriaras, G. Tzelepis,
S. Geroulanos*
Infections in Lung - Transplant Recipients 572

E.E. Etheredge, L.M. Flint
Fungal Infections Following Solid-Organ Transplantation 579

W. Weimar, H.J. Metselaar, A.H.M.M. Balk
Cytomegalovirus Prophylaxis by Passive Immunization in High-Risk
Kidney and Heart Transplant Recipients 587

V.A. Morrison, B.A. Peterson, D.L. Dunn
Posttransplant Lymphoproliferative Disorders: Pathogenesis Presentation,
and Approaches to Therapy 592

F. Stöblen, G. Blumhardt, W.-O. Bechstein, P. Neuhaus
Impact of Selective Decontamination of the Digestive Tract for Infecion
Prophylaxis in Orthotopic Liver Transplantation: Incidence and Outcome
of Infections Within 90 Days After Transplantation 603

Section 10:
Design, Methodology and Interpretation of Clinical Trials in Shock and Sepsis

A.E. Baue
Causality of Disease - the Problems of Animal Studies and Clinical Results 612

G. Pilz, S. Kääb, E. Kreuzer, K. Werdan
Comparison of Criteria for Early Sepsis Classification (Elebute Score, SIRS) in
Postcardiac Surgical Patients 623

W. Lorenz, H. Sitter, F. Weitzel
Consensus-Assisted Development of a Study Protocol for Sepsis:
Discussion Forum, Protocol Chart and a Formalized Method for
Clinical Algorithms 631

M. Koller, W. Lorenz
Threats to Double-Blinding in Sepsis Trials: Role of Expectancies
Toward Treatment Outcome 640

C.Z. Margolis
Clinical Algorithms in Sepsis Trials 646

M. Evans
Organisational Problems Peculiar to Multicentre Trials 649

C.H. Shatney, P. Peduzzi
End Point Selection, Sample Size, Interim Monitoring, and Final Data Analysis
in Multicenter Clinical Trials in Sepsis 654

List of Contributors 660

Index 665

Section 1:

MODS/MOF - The Clinical Syndrome

Prologue:
The Concept of Limits and Emergence of Multiple Organ Failure

Arthur E. Baue

"A chain is only as strong as its weakest links. When links are strengthened where the chain has broken previously, new weak spots appear simply because the chain holds to test them. The obvious weak link in the severely wounded in this war [World War II] was the kidney." [1]

Introduction

Throughout the short history of modern medicine - whether one begins with surgeons such as Ambros Paré, John Hunter and Theodor Billroth or physicians such as Semmelweiss or Sir William Osler - there have been limits to our capability. Limits were imposed by pain requiring the development of anesthesia, by hemorrhage and fluid loss requiring hemostasis and intravenous fluids, infection requiring hand washing, antisepsis and then asepsis, and finally antibiotics. These challenge us to develop the technical resources and biologic understanding to go beyond our existing capability. This striving by the practitioner, academician, or investigator to extend the limits of medicine is part not only of our heritage but of our responsibility to our patients and the profession. Certainly, there are limits in the treatment of many diseases, with extirpation of cancer and bypass grafts for atherosclerotic occlusions serving as prime examples. There are limits or weak links also in our overall capability to care for patients after severe injury, major life-threatening operations, or catastrophic illnesses which may require operations for treatment and in patients with significant chronic illnesses who face any of these problems.

History of Organ Failure

At any given time in recent surgical and/or medical history, one or another single, limiting organ system has stood out as the primary factor in producing morbidity and mortality after injury. I use the generic meaning of "injury," which includes both trauma (accidental trauma) and an operation (planned trauma in the operating room). At the beginning of World War II the cardiovascular system and shock were the major problems. Patients who died after injury or operation frequently died of circulatory failure or inadequacy or shock. As our knowledge of the concepts and problems of hypovolemic shock and volume replacement developed, the treatment of shock greatly improved. Hemodynamic studies eliminated the mystique of wound shock. Fluid resuscitation and volume replacement eliminated shock as the single most important limiting factor or system contributing to morbidity and mortality after injury.

By the end of World War II and through the Korean conflict, the kidneys became the limiting organ system. The US Army Surgical Research Unit in Korea used the term "post-traumatic renal insufficiency" to describe a condition that occurred 20 - 30 times more commonly in Korea than it did later in the Vietnam conflict [2]. The Army team demonstrated that the most common cause of delayed death in patients who had been successfully resuscitated from severe injury was acute renal failure. At that time it developed in 1 in 200 seriously injured patients with a mortality rate close to 90%. Rush (personal communication), who was part of the research team in Korea, indicated that this was the time when sodium retention was recognized as part of the biologic response to injury. Surgeons hesitated to give sodium solutions in any great quantity to injured and postoperative patients because these fluids would be retained. Thus injured and operated patients were given blood and plasma, but they were not given sufficient fluid and electrolyte solutions, particularly sodium ions. In other words, they were kept dry. Shires and his group [3] developed the concept that injured and operated patients needed larger volumes of intravenous water and sodium and particularly lactated Ringer's solution. This and the recognition of the problem of post-traumatic renal insufficiency led to better support of this organ system. As our understanding of the factors producing renal insufficiency developed, the problem was often prevented by rapid fluid resuscitation, supporting the kidney by improving renal blood flow and promoting adequate urine output. Also, renal failure could be treated more adequately when it did occur.

As the circulation and renal function received better support after injury, a new problem came into focus and that was pulmonary failure. During the Vietnam War this was called "post-traumatic pulmonary insufficiency" [4]. Soon the lungs also became the limiting organ system after injury in civilian practice as well. None of the four volumes of reports and papers by the U.S. Army Surgical Research Team in Korea mentioned the lungs - they were not a problem at that time [5]. Did pulmonary failure then develop because of better resuscitation and support of the cardiovascular and renal systems, or because aggressive and perhaps, on occasion, excessive fluid resuscitation jeopardized the lungs? Probably both of these problems occurred. Both adequate (not excessive) fluid resuscitation after injury and recognition of the lung as a limiting organ system after injury have since contributed to more frequent prevention of respiratory failure. When we cannot prevent respiratory failure, often we can treat it much more satisfactorily. Today, the mortality caused solely by ventilatory failure should be fairly low. Thus post-traumatic pulmonary insufficiency was no longer the single most important or limiting organ system after injury.

Along with this, the artificial kidney was developed. Primitive ventilators were improved so that long-term ventilatory support could be provided with safety. Monitoring capability and intensive care units which began in the early 1960s have also contributed greatly to the support of sick individuals who previously would have died. The next limiting organ system that appeared was not a single organ, but the complex of multiple organ failure (MOF). Morbidity and death after operation or injury still occur from various complications such as thromboembolism, acute vascular occlusions or infarction, shock, post-traumatic renal failure, post-traumatic pulmonary failure, sepsis, peritonitis, and other complications. However, we can often successfully treat each of these problems occurring by itself. Renal failure associated with sepsis and respiratory or hepatic failure still has a grave prognosis, but renal failure itself is no longer the critical event. The incidence of renal failure in the injured in Vietnam was only 0.1% - 0.2%, but the mortality of those whose kidneys failed was high (63% - 77%) because of associated injuries and sepsis rather than renal failure per se. The research efforts by the Armed Forces during times of armed conflict have contributed greatly to our current understanding of injuries in young, otherwise normal individuals. We are now recognizing liver problems (hepatomegaly and jaundice) with trauma or sepsis more frequently (post-traumatic hepatic insufficiency). Likewise, the gastrointestinal tract, which heretofore we thought waited quietly and innocently during starvation and sepsis, is now recognized as causing problems by bleeding or perforation, translocation of organisms, altered permeability, overgrowth of organisms, or altered immune function. The occurrence of these problems of organ failure in combination or in sequence often exceeds the limits of our present capabilities for supporting and providing for survival of such patients. This led to the development of the concept of multiple organ failure. First, however, it is necessary to review the history of remote organ failure or failure of an organ unrelated to the primary problem in that patient.

Remote Organ Failure

Many have contributed to our knowledge of remote organ failure. Finding the origins of ideas is as difficult as recognizing all the contributors. In 1963, Burke et al. [6] described high-output respiratory failure in patients with peritonitis, most of whom died eventually of renal failure. Skillman et al. [7] found a high mortality in patients with peritonitis who developed respiratory failure as did Clowes et al. [8] and Border et al. [9]. Siegel et al. [10] described myocardial failure with sepsis. Skillman et al. described respiratory failure, hypotension, sepsis and jaundice which led to lethal hemorrhage from stress ulcerations. Horowitz et al. [12] found that sepsis was the factor that most jeopardized the lungs after injury. Fulton and Jones [13] concluded from 399 patients with major illness/injury that respiratory failure frequently followed sepsis. Vito et al. [14] described acute respiratory insufficiency occurring as the initial change with sepsis elsewhere. Tilney et al. [15] used the term "sequential systems failure" for patients with renal failure after repair of ruptured abdominal aortic aneurysms. I then reviewed our experiences after injury and operation and suggested that multiple, progressive or sequential systems or organ failure was a syndrome to be reckoned with in the 1970s [16].
The background for this idea came from Dr. Churchill, our chief at the Massachusetts General Hospital, who wrote about his experiences during World War II in *Surgeon to Soldiers* [1]. Although this book was published in 1972, it recounted clearly some of the many lessons learned during World War II about war wounds, injury, and the care of injured and operated patients. When I read Professor Churchill's book in 1972, the concept of "weak links in the chain" fascinated me. At that time, we were developing a cardiac surgical program in St. Louis at the Jewish Hospital of St. Louis and the Washington University School of Medicine. The capability to support failed organs had been developed, but the concept of remote organ failure had not yet developed fully. Low cardiac output was a frequent postoperative problem and the intraaortic balloon pump was just being developed.
I decided to review the autopsy reports on our patients who died after a prolonged period of resuscitation and support in our intensive care units. Review of these reports and of the

problems detailed within them began to suggest a pattern of problems in various organs remote from the primary site of injury or pathologic condition. For example, in a patient who, following a colon resection, had anastomotic breakdown with peritonitis and died after 6 weeks of progressive difficulty, the following were among the findings at autopsy: pulmonary congestion and edema; focal organizing pneumonia; thrombi in the renal glomerular capillaries with acute tubular necrosis in a stage of early healing; icterus; massive acute, noninflammatory hepatic necrosis; multiple infarcts of the spleen; and autolysis of the adrenal glands. Thus, this patient, although dying essentially of peritonitis, had the findings of multiple organ failure including evidence of failure of the lungs, liver, kidneys, and adrenal glands.

In a patient who died after a prolonged period of support for hemorrhagic pancreatitis, the autopsy findings indicated generalized jaundice, pleural fluid, aspiration pneumonia, acute tubular necrosis, extensive necrosis of the liver, and ulcerations of the gut. A third example was a patient with autopsy findings of necrotizing bacterial arteritis, interstitial pulmonary edema with hyaline membranes, acute renal failure in a stage of healing, massive acute centrilobular necrosis of the liver, and passive congestion of the spleen. This patient died about 1 1/2 months after an aortic and mitral valve replacement for valvular heart disease, and had continuous low cardiac output after operation. Again, however, the final pathologic manifestations were those of MOF. Thus, these three patients had very different initial diseases, (peritonitis, inflammation and low cardiac output) but the final problem and syndrome were very similar. This, in combination with Professor Churchill's weak links concept, led me to contemplate and try to define the problem.

Eiseman et al. [17] then wrote about "multiple organ failure," especially with liver failure. Polk et al. [18] found that remote organ failure often signaled occult intra-abdominal infection. Fry et al. [19] emphasized the role of uncontrolled infection in organ failure. Border et al. [20] described metabolic alterations with MOF and used the term multiple-systems organ failure (MSOF). Other early contributors to our knowledge of MOF include Faist [21,22], Trunkey and Miller [23], Marshall and Dimick [24], Cassone [25], Carrico et al. [26], and Maier [27]. Goris et al. [28] provided evidence from the animal and clinical laboratory for inflammation being a major factor in the development of MOF.

The expressions MOF or MSOF were used commonly throughout the world. Cerra coined the terms "post-traumatic septic syndrome" and "hypermetabolism organ failure complex" [29], and Border et al. [30] used the expression "gut origin septic states" to indicate important current aspects of the generic problem of organ failure and death. Other terms include acute organ-system failure, multiple organ injury syndrome, post-traumatic multi-system organ failure and post-traumatic organ system infection syndrome (PTOSIS) [31]. I believe the term "multiple organ failure" is clean, neat and says it all. The many terms suggested for the problems of organ failure and difficulty are shown in Table 1.

Definitions of MOF

A number of investigators have proposed definitions of MOF including what is considered failure of each specific organ, and how it should be documented. Some have also developed scoring systems for organ failure so that a composite score can be provided. The number of proposals and the first authors are shown in Table 2. These are very similar and it would be very straightforward to develop common definitions of organ failure and a scoring system for that, if everyone would agree.

Table 1: Terms Used to Describe the Effects of Severe Injury, Overwhelming Inflammation, and Infection

MOF, MOSF, or sequential systems or MSOF, SIRS, MODS - multiple, progressive, or sequential systems or organ failure	Severe generalized autoinflammatory response (Goris)
	Whole body inflammation (Goris)
Cooperative, concentrated destruction	Polytrauma schlussel
Angry macrophages (Maier)	Leaky gut
Sepsis-peripheral vascular failure	Gastrointestinal tract - the undrained abscess of MOF (motor of MOF) (Meakins)
Gut-origin septic states (Border)	Multi-organ instability (Baue)
Malignant intravascular inflammation	Malignant systemic inflammation
Hyperemic hypoxia (Cerra)	Biologic cyanide capsule (Michie, Wilmore)
Septic hypermetabolic state (Cerra)	Septic syndrome (Bone)
Hypermetabolism organ failure complex (Cerra)	Horror autotoxicus (Ehrlich-Baue)
Multiple organ injury syndrome (Hyers)	Fatal expression of uncontrolled sepsis (Fry)
Remote organ failure (Polk)	Acute organ system failure (Knaus)
Post-traumatic septic syndrome	Favorably primed-good SIRS (Moore)
Sindrome de insuficiencia multiple de organos y systemas (Bumaschny)	Adversely primed-bad SIRS (Moore)
One hit-two hit (Faist, Meakins)	Post-traumatic multisystem organ failure (Demling)
Post-traumatic organ-system infection syndrome (PTOSIS) (Baue)	Post-traumatic host defense failure syndrome (Siegel)

When more than one system or organ cannot support its activities spontaneously, MOF is present. Exact definitions of organ failures are shown in Table 3 as adapted from Knaus et al. [32] and in Table 4 as adapted from Goris et al. [28]. Failure of the *ventilatory system* is defined as the need for assisted ventilation to maintain adequate gas exchange, including

Table 2: Definitions in the literature of organ failure and MOF

Definitions of organ failure	Definitions and scoring of MOF
Faist and Baue - J Trauma 1984 [21]	Saffle et al. - Crit Care Med 1993 [47]
Knaus et al. - Ann Surg 1985 [32]	Marshall et al. - Arch Surg 1988 [48]
Fry et al. - Arch Surg 1980 [19]	Hebert et al. - Chest 1993 [49]
Norton - Am J Surg 1985 [37]	Goris et al. - Arch Surg 1985 [28]
Pine et al. - Arch Surg 1983 [26]	Kollef - JAMA 1993 [50]
Carrico et al. - Arch Surg 1986 [26]	
Bihari et al. - N Engl J Med [39]	
Roukonen et al. - Crit Care Med 1990 [40]	
Bell et al. - Ann Int Med 1983 [41]	
Dorinsky et al. - Clin Chest Med 1990 [42]	
Darling et al. - Can J Surg 1988 [43]	
Manship et al. - Am J Surg 1984 [44]	
Dobb (Royal Perth Hospital) - Int Care World 1991 [45]	
Rubin et al. - J Clin Inv 1990 [46]	

Table 3: Definitions of organ failure as proposed by Knaus (modified from [32])

Definitions of organ system failure

If the patient had one or more of the following during a 24-h hour period (regardless of other values), organ system failure existed on that day:
1. Cardiovascular failure (presence of *one or more* of the following):
    a) Heart rate ≤54 beats/min
    b) Mean arterial blood pressure ≤49 mmHg
    c) Occurrence of ventricular tachycardia and/or ventricular fibrillation
    d) Serum pH ≤7.24 with a $PaCO_2$ of ≤49 mmHg
2. Respiratory failure (presence of *one or more* of the following):
    a) Respiratory rate ≤5 or ≥49 breaths/min
    b) $PaCO_2$ ≥50 mmHg
    c) $AaDO_2$ ≥350 mmHg ($AaDO_2 = 713\ FIO_2 - PaCO_2 - PaO_2$)
    d) Dependent on ventilator on the 4th day of organ system failure, e.g., *not* applicable for the initial 72 h of organ system failure
3. Renal failure (presence of one or more of the following)[a]:
    a) Urine output ≤479 ml/24 h or ≤159 ml/8 h
    b) Serum blood urea nitrogen ≥100 mg/dl
    c) Serum creatinine ≥3.5 mg/dl
4. Hematologic failure (presence of *one or more* of the following):
    a) White blood cell count ≤1000/mm^3
    b) Platelets ≤20000/mm^3
    c) Hematocrit ≤20%
5. Neurologic failure
    Glasgow Coma Score ≤6 (in absence of sedation at any one point in day)
    Glasgow Coma Score: sum of best eye-opening, best verbal, and best motor responses.
    Scoring of responses as follows (points):
        Eye - open: spontaneously (4), to verbal command (3), to pain (2), no response (1)
        Motor - obeys verbal command (6); response to painful stimuli; localizes pain (5); flexion-withdrawal (4); decorticate rigidity (3); decerebrate rigidity (2); no response (1); movement without any control (4)
        Verbal - oriented and converses (5); disoriented and converses (4); inappropriate words (3); incomprehensible sounds (2); no response (1). If intubated use clinical judgement for verbal responses as follows: patient generally unresponsive (1); patient's ability to converse in question (3); patient appears able to converse (5)

eliminating carbon dioxide and oxygenation. *Cardiovascular system* failure is hypotension, low or marginal cardiac output, or, in general terms an inadequate circulation that requires pharmacologic and/or mechanical circulatory assistance. *Renal failure* is the inability of the kidneys to regulate volume and electrolytes and remove waste products. The definition of *hepatic failure* is inexact at present but includes an elevated bilirubin level, elevated hepatic enzyme levels, and the end stage, which is hepatic coma. *Coagulation system* failure includes diffuse intravascular coagulation on one hand, or primary bleeding problems on the other. *Gastrointestinal failure* is the inability of the gut to function and maintain nutrition by oral intake, gastrointestinal bleeding that becomes life threatening, perforation from acute or

Table 4: Definitions of organ failure as proposed by Goris (modified from [28])

Definitions of organ failure
Several classifications of organ failure have been described. Based on these systems, a scoring method was developed for each organ failure with severity grading of 0 as not present, 1 as moderate, and 2 as severe. The following criteria were also established for specific organ failures: 1. For pulmonary failure, 0 signified no mechanical ventilation; 1, mechanical ventilation with a positive end-expiratory pressure of 10 cm H_2O or less and a fraction of inspired oxygen (FIO_2) of 0.4 or less; and 2, mechanical ventilation with a positive end-expiratory pressure greater than 10 cm H_2O and/or FIO_2 freater than 0.4.   2. For cardiac failure, 0 signified normal blood pressure with no vasoactive substances necessary; 1, periods with hypotension necessitating manipulations, such as volume loading, to keep blood pressure above 100 mmHg, dopamine hydrochloride infusion of 10 g/kg/min or less, or nitroglycerin of 20 g/min or less; and 2, periods with hypotension below 100 mmHg, and/or dopamine hydrochloride greater than 10 g/kg/min, and/or nitroglycerin greater than 20 g/min.   3. For renal failure, 0 signified serum creatinine less than 2 mg/dl; 1, serum creatinine of 2 mg/dl or greater; and 2, hemodialysis or peritoneal dialysis necessary.   4. For hepatic failure, 0 signified a level of serum glutamic-oxaloacetic transaminase (SGOT) less than 25 units/l and a total bilirubin level less than 2 mg/dl; 1, bilirubin of 2 mg/dl or greater and less than 6 mg/dl or SGOT of 25 units/l or greater and less than 50 units/l; and 2, bilirubin of 6 mg/dl or greater or SGOT of 50 units/l or greater.   5. For hematologic failure, 0 signified normal counts of thrombocytes and leukocytes; 1, a thrombocyte count less than 50×10^9/l and/or leukocyte count of 30×10^6/l or greater and less than 60×10^6/l; and 2 hemorrhagic diathesis or a leukocyte count less than 2.5×10^6/l or of 60×10^6/l or greater.   6. For gastrointestinal tract failure, 0 signified normal functioning; 1, acalculous cholecystitis or stress ulcer; and 2, bleeding from stress ulcer necessitating transfusion of more than 2 units blood/24 h.   7. For central nervous system failure, 0 signified normal functioning; 1, clearly diminished responsiveness; and 2, severely disturbed responsiveness and/or diffuse neuropathy.

stress ulceration, translocation of bacteria, and altered immune function. Failure of the *metabolic and musculoskeletal systems* is a twofold problem: (1) failure to provide for protein synthesis and prevent the central metabolic alterations of catabolism and (2) catabolism of skeletal muscle, with loss of strength producing problems with ventilation, ambulation, decubitus ulcers, and others. Failure of the *immune system* is exemplified by the development of sepsis that is unexpected or difficult to control or that cannot be eliminated. Failure of the *central nervous system* is defined as a decreased or depressed sensorium or coma. Injury to the central nervous system, however, frequently becomes the limiting factor that prevents survival. Not included in Knaus' definitions were the GI tract and liver. Sample definitions used by many are shown in Table 5. Whether several organs fail progressively, sequentially, or all at once depends on the severity of the insult and the individual's preinjury or preoperative state.

Several organs failing together may cause death because of certain specific relationships. Simultaneous renal and ventilatory failure is potentially lethal because, as renal failure occurs or

Table 5: Sample definitions of MOF

GI failure	Bleeding - 2 or more units blood/24 h
	Acalculous cholecystitis
	Enterocolitis, pancreatitis
	Inability to take in orally
Liver failure	Bilirubin >3.0 mg% for 48 h
	GLDH > 10 mu/ml
	SGOT > 25 units/L
	Encephalopathy

is diagnosed, we usually use large fluid loads in its treatment. Such overcompensation overloads the lungs, and perhaps only peritoneal dialysis or hemodialysis can get rid of this fluid immediately. Another difficult combination is ventilatory and metabolic failure. Weaning a patient from a ventilator who is catabolic with decreased muscular strength may be difficult or impossible because he or she cannot breathe spontaneously. One such example is the patient with end-stage valvular heart disease and cardiac cachexia, for whom we can replace the cardiac valve and provide good cardiovascular function, but in whom muscle mass loss is so great that spontaneous ventilation is impossible and complications eventually occur. Renal failure in a patient with a ruptured aneurysm is particularly lethal because of shock, problems with cross-clamping the aorta, arteriosclerotic embolization, and vascular disease of the kidney. Some patients with this problem now survive, particularly if we can prevent all complications (especially sepsis) while they undergo a prolonged period of anuria, oliguria and dialysis. Cardiac failure and ventilatory failure occurring together are a difficult problem because the treatment of ventilatory failure (including high levels of positive end-expiratory pressure) may alter cardiac output and adversely influence cardiac function. Finally, the combination of peritonitis with organ failure - whether ventilatory failure, cardiovascular instability, hepatic problems, or renal failure - is common and often lethal unless the primary problem of peritonitis can be controlled.

The central nervous system remains a major limitation after accidental injury. Baker at the San Francisco General Hospital [33], Faist et al. [21, 22] at the University of Munich, and Baker and our group at Yale [34] documented that primary central nervous system problems are the cause of death in 50% of patients dying after accidental injury. This finding is consistent in all experiences and provides a major challenge in preventing injury and caring for the injured. Patients with primary central nervous system injury may die of the central nervous system injury itself, or multiple organ problems may develop. Nonetheless, the central nervous system remains the major single limiting organ system after injury. The recognition of multiple or sequential systems or organ failure as a current problem has prompted study of how some of these sequences or simultaneous events occur and how they might be prevented.

Five clinical characteristics are involved in producing the sequences of problems and events of MOF:

1. The patient who has suffered a severe metabolic insult, an injury, an operation, or both. A major operation or multiple systems injury in an otherwise normal individual can set the stage for MOF.
2. Clinical or technical errors may occur that escape recognition initially, such as continued bleeding, inadequate wound closure, a difficult anastomosis that leaks, a collection in the chest or the peritoneal cavity, or massive bacterial contamination.

3. Infection, especially peritonitis or pneumonia, is often the underlying problem, either initiating the sequence of organ failure or developing concurrently as one or more organs fail.
4. Severe inflammation, particularly when associated with tissue necrosis, may produce or activate mediators that depress the circulation and alter organ function.
5. An individual with functional limitations in one or more organs before operation or injury is more susceptible to MOF than is an otherwise normal individual. Patients with vascular occlusive disease, chronic obstructive lung disease, hepatic damage, immunosuppression from various disease processes or organ transplantation, or cardiac diseases are especially susceptible.

A common thread in all these problems is altered circulation, reduced blood flow, inadequate tissue perfusion, and ischemia.

Concept of Limits and Prevention

Multiple organ failure is not only a current problem but also a concept in the care and study of injured patients. This concept holds that, at any point in time, limitations in postoperative and sick patients can be defined. By defining our limitations we can overcome them, improving the care of the injured and often preventing MOF. This concept provides a framework for clinical problem solving that should be an important activity for all physicians whether working individually or collectively. Observation of one's own limitations, limitations within a hospital, and the limits set by the patient's problems challenge everyone to do better the next time.

Although we must strive to provide better means of support for organs that have failed - especially the long-term support of failed kidneys, lungs, and the circulation - the primary approach I wish to emphasize is preventing multiple systems failure during the initial phase of treatment, operation, or injury. A preventive attack on this problem requires increased understanding in four areas: (1) defining and recognizing the problem; (2) identifying the setting in which these problems occur and the types of disease processes, abnormalities, and sequences that produce the problem; (3) determining the relationships among the various systems that can lead to the domino effect of one system triggering problems in another; and (4) ensuring that the currently available methods to support organs and systems prevent failure of individual organs or do not trigger problems and failure in other systems. Thus the concept of limits includes defining our present biologic, scientific, technical, and personal limits and trying to exceed them. I hope readers will increase their personal limits by developing further and contributing to the biologic and scientific limits with which we work. To achieve this, one must have a clear understanding of all that is involved in the care of intensive care unit patients. A more extensive review of this is found in my book *Multiple Organ Failure: Patient Care and Prevention* [35] and in my chapter "Historical Perspective" in Dr. Ed Deitch's book [36].

Now there is a proposal for a new set of terminologies and definitions - MODS and SIRS. I have written previously about these recommendations [31]. Will they be helpful in the study and care of patients? A fresh look at old problems is always good. These proposals have already made a contribution by getting us to review and rethink where we are and what we are doing. This is always a healthy phenomenon. Our speakers in this session will review these proposals and the evidence for them as we strive for consensus.

References

1. Churchill ED (1972) Surgeon to soldiers. Lippincott, Philadelphia
2. U.S. Army. (1955) Post-traumatic renal insufficiency. Army Medical Service Graduate School, Walter Reed Army Medical Center, Washington (Battle casualties in Korea - studies of the surgical research team, vol 4)
3. Shires GT, Canizaro DC, Carrico CJ (1979) Shock. In: Schwartz SJ (ed.) Textbook of surgery. McGraw-Hill Book, New York
4. Moore FD, Lyons JH, Pierce EF Jr, Morgan AP, Drinker PA, MacArthur JD, Mannin GJ (1969) Post-traumatic respiratory insufficiency. Saunders, Philadelphia
5. US Army (1955) Battle casualties in Korea - studies of the surgical research team, vols 1-4. Brooke Army Medical Center and Army Medical Service Graduate School, Walter Reed Army Medical Center, Washington
6. Burke JF, Pontoppidan H, Welch CE (1963) High output respiratory failure: an important cause of the intestine. Ann Surg 142:739
7. Skillman JJ, Bushnell LS, Hedley-Whyte J (1969) Peritonitis and respiratory failure after abdominal operations. Ann Surg 170:122
8. Clowes GHA Jr, Zuschneid W, Turner M, Blackburn G, Rubin J, Toala P, Green G (1968) Observations on the pathogenesis of the pneumonitis associated with severe infections in other parts of the body. Ann Surg 167:630
9. Border JR, Tibbets JC, Schenk WG (1968) Hypoxic hyperventilation and acute respiratory failure in the severely stressed patient: massive pulmonary arteriovenous shunts? Surgery 64:710
10. Siegel JH, Greenspan M, DelGuercio LRM (1967) Abnormal vascular tone, defective oxygen transport and myocardial failure in human septic shock. Ann Surg 165:504
11. Skillman JJ, Bushnell LS, Goldman H, Silen W (1969) Respiratory failure, hypotension, sepsis and jaundice. Am J Surg 117:523
12. Horowitz JH, Carricol J and Shires T (1974) Pulmonary response to major injury. Arch Surg 108:349
13. Fulton RL, Jones CE (1975) The etiology of post-traumatic pulmonary insufficiency in man. Rev Surg 32:84
14. Vito L, Dennis RC, Weisel RD et al. (1974) Sepsis presenting as acute respiratory insufficiency. Surg Gynecol Obstet 138:896
15. Tilney NL, Bailey GL, Morgan AP (1973) Sequential system failure after rupture of abdominal aortic aneurysms: an unsolved problem in postoperative care. Ann Surg 178:117
16. Baue AE (1975) Multiple, progressive, or sequential systems failure: a syndrome of the 1970s. Arch Surg 110:779
17. Eiseman B, Beart R, Norton L (1977) Multiple organ failure. Surg Gynecol Obstet 144:323
18. Polk HC Jr, Shields CL (1977) Remote organ failure: a valid sign of occult intra-abdominal infection. Surgery 81:310
19. Fry DE, Pearlstein L, Fulton RL, Polk HC Jr (1980) Multiple system organ failure. Arch Surg 115:136

20. Border JR, Chenier R, McMenamy RH, LaDuca J, Seibel R, Birkhahn R, Yu L (1976) Multiple systems organ failure: muscle fuel deficit with visceral protein malnutrition. Surg Clin North Am 56:1147
21. Faist E, Baue AE, Dittmer H, Heberer G (1983) Multiple organ failure in polytrauma patients. J Trauma 23:775
22. Faist E, Heberer G, Baue AE (1983) Das Mehrorganversagen beim polytraumatisierten Patienten. Krankenhausarzt 56:1
23. Trunkey DD, Miller CL (1982) Multiple organ failure and sepsis. In: Najarian JS, Delaney JP (eds.) Emergency surgery. Year Book Medical Publishers, Chicago, pp. 273-285
24. Marshall WG Jr, Dimick AR (1983) The natural history of major burns with multiple subsystem failure. J Trauma 23:102
25. Cassone E (1983) Clinical and laboratory signs of multiple organ failure. Infecti Surg 2:857-862
26. Carrico CJ, Meakins JL, Marshall JC et al. (1986) Multiple-organ-failure syndrome. Arch Surg 121:196
27. Maier RV (1986) Multisystem organ failure. Arch Surg 121:204
28. Goris RJA, te Boekhorst TPA, Nuytinck JKS (1985) Multiple organ failure: generalized autodestructive inflammation? Arch Surg 120:1109
29. Cerra FB (1987) The hypermetabolism organ failure complex. World J Surg 11:173
30. Border JR, Hassett J, LaDuca J et al. (1987) The gut origin septic states in blunt multiple trauma (ISS = 40) in the ICU. Ann Surg 206:417
31. Baue AE (1993) What's in a name? An acronym or a response? Am J Surg 165:299
32. Knaus WA, Draper EA, Wagner DP et al. (1985) Prognosis in acute organ system failure. Ann Surg 202:685
33. Baker CC, Oppenheimer L, Stephens B et al. (1980) Epidemiology of trauma deaths. Am J Surg 140:144
34. Baker CC, Degutis LE, DeSantis JG et al. (1985) Impact of a trauma service on trauma care in a university hospital. Am J Surg 149:453
35. Baue AE (1990) Multiple organ failure: patient care and prevention. Mosby-Year Book, St Louis
36. Baue AE (1990) Historical perspective. In: Deitch E (ed) Multiple organ failure. Thieme, New York
37. Norton LW (1985) Does drainage of intraabdominal pus reverse multiple organ failure? Am J Surg 149: 347-350
38. Pine RW, Wertz MJ, Lennard ES, Dellinger EP, Carrico CJ, Minshew BH (1983) Determinants of organ malfunction or death in patients with intraabdominal sepsis. Arch Surg 118: 242-249
39. Bihari D, Smithies M, Gimson A, Tinker J (1987) The effects of vasodilation with prostacyclin on oxygen delivery and uptake in critically ill patients. N Engl J Med 317: 397-403
40. Ruokenen E, Takala J, Kari A, Alhava E (1991) Septic shock and multiple organ failure. Crit Care Med 19: 1146-1151
41. Bell RC, Coalson JJ, Smith JD, Johanson WG (1983) Multiple organ system failure and infection in adult respiratory distress. Ann Intern Med 99: 293-298
42. Dorinsky PM, Gadek JE (1990) Multiple organ failure. Clin Chest Med 11: 581-591
43. Darling GE, Duff JH, Mustard RA, Finley RJ (1988) Multiorgan failure in critically ill patients. Canad J Surg 31: 172-176
44. Manship L, McMillin RD, Brown JI (1984) The influence of sepsis and multisystem and organ failure on mortality in surgical intensive care unit. Am Surg 50: 94-101

45. Dobb GJ (1991) Multiple organ failure - "Words mean what I say they mean." Intensive Care World 8: 157-159
46. Rubin DB, Wiener-Kronish JP, Murray JF, Green DR, Turner J, Luce JM, Montgomery AB, Marks JD, Matthay MA (1990) Elevated von Willebrand factor antigen is an early plasma predictor of acute lung injury in nonpulmonary sepsis syndrome. J Clin Invest 86: 474-480
47. Saffle JR, Sullivan JJ, Tuohig GM, Larson CM (1993) Multiple organ failure in patients with thermal injury. Crit Care Med 21: 1673-1683
48. Marshall JC, Christou NV, Horn R, Meakins JL (1988) The microbiology of multiple organ failure. Arch Surg 123: 309-315
49. Hebert PC, Drummond AJ, Singer J, Bernard GR, Russell JA (1993) A simple multiple system organ failure scoring system predicts mortality of patients who have sepsis syndrome. Chest 104: 230-235
50. Kollef MN (1993) Ventilator-associated pneumonia. JAMA 270: 1965

Genesis of Multiple System Organ Failure

D.E. Fry

Introduction

Multiple system organ failure (MSOF) has been a frequently identified pattern of death in patients who have sustained severe traumatic injury or are critically ill regardless of the cause [1-4]. MSOF has been identified as the sequential or simultaneous failure of critical organ functions in the severely ill intensive care unit patient [5-7]. The principal organs that have been involved in this syndrome include the lung, liver and kidney. Stress-associated gastritis has similarly been an associated failed system that is part of the syndrome. Cardiac dysfunction, loss of metabolic and endocrine regulation, and neurologic failure have been considered to also be potential components of MSOF. The failure of these functional and anatomically different organ systems in a close temporal relationship has led many authors to hypothesize that a common mechanism may account for MSOF. The identification of clinical correlations will hopefully lead to definition of the disease mechanisms. Better definition of the mechanisms of MSOF will hopefully lead to more effective treatments.

Association of Multiple System Organ Failure with the Septic Response

Several clinical variables were initially associated with MSOF. Since organ failure complexes were initially identified among the many military casualties of this century, MSOF was associated with blood loss and hemorrhagic shock. "Shock lung," "shock liver," and oligemic renal failure were common clinical terms used to describe the relationship of shock and hemorrhage with MSOF. Systemic hypoxemia, massive resuscitation, multiple organ injury, long bone fractures, central nervous system injury, and protein-calorie malnutrition were likewise all associated. Perhaps uncontrolled infection, more than any other one variable, received the greatest attention as the clinical event which was a prodrome to MSOF. We studied a large number of patients who underwent emergency surgical procedures in an attempt to define which clinical variables had the strongest correlation with the development of MSOF [1]. Specific criteria were arbitrarily developed to define pulmonary failure, liver failure, renal failure, and stress-associated gastrointestinal bleeding (Table 1). Organ failure was identified as occurring in a specific pattern among these patients. Among this group of patients, we defined failure of two or more organ systems as representing MSOF. This study identified MSOF occurring in 38 (7%) patients (Table 2). The mortality rate for these patients with MSOF was 74%. Amount the organ systems which were studied, renal failure appeared to have the greatest impact upon patients survival.

The emergence of MSOF appeared to follow a prototype pattern. Pulmonary failure was consistently the first event to be identified among these patients (Fig. 1). Hepatic failure and stress gastrointestinal bleeding then occurred subsequently. Kidney function appeared to be the most resilient among these patients and was noted to fail last; but as noted above, when renal failure emerged it was most predictive of a fatal outcome.

Table 1: Definitions employed in four major studies on the epidemiology of MSOF [1-4]

Pulmonary failure	Five or more consecutive days of ventilator support at an FiO_2 of 0.4 or greater. These criteria were used to identify the truly hypoxic patient in need of pulmonary support while excluding patients with transient hypoxia readily responsive to short-term management.
Hepatic failure	The presence of both hyperbilirubinemia greater than 2.0 mg/dl and increases of serum glutamic-oxaloacetic transaminase (SGOT) and lactic dehydrogenase (LDH) to levels greater than twice normal. The inclusion of enzyme data was designed to exclude transient hyperbilirubinemia that might be associated with retroperitoneal hematoma, pelvic fracture, or potential icterus from an incompatible unit of blood.
Gastrointestinal failure	Upper gastrointestinal hemorrhage from documented or presumed stress-associated acute gastric ulceration. Bleeding that was endoscopically documented from acute gastric lesions was also considered as evidence of failure. During the early phases of these clinical studies, endoscopy was not routinely performed for all acute gastrointestinal bleeding. In these latter patients, need for greater than two units blood transfusion was required to classify a patient in this category when the presumption was bleeding secondary to stress ulceration.
Renal failure	An elevation of serum creatinine to a level greater than 2.0 mg/dl. Because polyuric renal failure is not an infrequent complication in multiple trauma patients, daily or hourly urine output was thought not to be a reliable criterion for renal dysfunction.

Table 2: Mortality rate among emergency surgical patients when stratified by the number of organ systems that failed[a]

Number of failed organ systems	Number of patients	Number of deaths
One	46	14 (30%)
Two	20	12 (60%)
Three	13	11 (85%)
Four	5	5 (100%)
Multiple (two or more)	38	28 (74%)

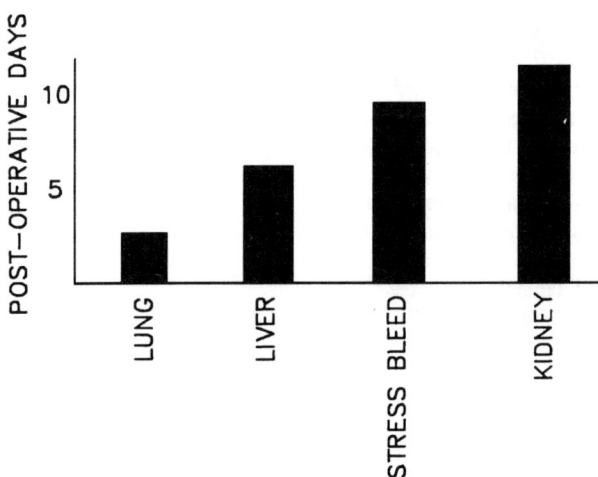

Fig. 1: The temporal sequence of individual organ system failures in emergency surgical

Statistical associations with the clinical events in these patients initially demonstrated numerous variables to have an association with the development of MSOF. Shock, large volume resuscitation, blood transfusion, multiple system injury, and severe infection were all statistically associated with MSOF (Table 3). It was notable that 34 of 38 MSOF patients fulfilled the criteria of uncontrolled infection that we used in this study. Because of this strong apparent association, we noted that deletion of the septic cohort of patients from the overall study resulted in none of the other variables being statistically valid in the non-septic patient population. However, when the cohorts of patients for those apparently valid other variables were deleted, infection remained strongly associated with the emergence of MSOF.

Table 3: Statistically significant variables which were associated with the development of MSOF in emergency surgical patients [1]

Variable	Number of patients	Number of MSOF	p
Hypovolemic shock	67	16	<0.01
Massive blood therapy	32	9	<0.01
Massive crystalloid therapy	35	10	<0.01
Chest injury	113	14	<0.01
Septicemia	123	34	<0.01

Another important relationship in the MSOF patients was with clinical septic shock. Transient episodes of shock secondary to infection were commonly seen among these MSOF patients. Supportive care seemed to be effective in the correction of the hypotensive events. The occurrence of these transient hypotensive events with the MSOF patients further reinforced the apparent relationship of MSOF with uncontrolled infection. It seemed that support technology was able to rescue the patients from the septic shock events, but MSOF then intervened as the subsequent pattern of death.

The physiologic correlations with the human septic state were carefully detailed and characterized in the studies of Siegel et al. [8]. Large numbers of critically ill patients were longitudinally followed in an effort to define the stages of the stress and septic responses. These authors identified four states of the human stress/septic response.

State A was the obligatory stress response that is identified among all patients who experience major injury or operations. The patients develop a modest (20%-30%) elevation of cardiac output and a modest reduction in systemic vascular resistance. The net effect of these changes is to increase systemic oxygen delivery. Arteriovenous oxygen content differences remained essentially unchanged, such that increased systemic cardiac output resulted in increased oxygen consumption. Lactic acidemia was not a feature of State A patient.

State B represented the compensated physiologic state of human sepsis. It was compensated by virtue of the fact that the patients had a normal arterial blood pressure. The cardiac output was quite elevated in response to the profound reduction in systemic vascular resistance. The arteriovenous oxygen content was narrowed. Lactic acidemia was documented at this stage in the process but compensatory mechanisms prevented the development of a metabolic acidosis. The sustained state B becomes the physiologic environment that is associated with the development of the adult respiratory distress syndrome and other elements of MSOF.

During state B, the metabolic features of the true septic response can be identified. Hypermetabolism and accelerated gluconeogenesis develop which are refractory to manipulation by exogenous nutritional support [9]. The accelerated gluconeogenesis appears to be driven by dramatically elevated circulating concentrations of glucagon. Proteolysis of skeletal muscle provides the amino acids which are deaminated and incorporated into new glucose production. Hepatic ureagenesis is increased because of the gluconeogenic process. Accelerated urinary nitrogen losses are an obligatory result of the entire process. Despite the state B patient having an increased blood sugar and an increased insulin concentration, a relative insulin resistance exists in these patients.

State C represents the decompensation of systemic hemodynamics in the septic response patient. Cardiac output, while normal or slightly elevated by normal standards, is adequate to meed the demands of a profoundly reduced peripheral vascular resistance. The disparate relationship between cardiac output and systemic vascular resistance results in clinical shock. Because actual cardiac output is normal-to-elevated, these patients are commonly viewed as being in "hot" shock. Lactic acidemia now becomes evident as metabolic acidosis. Inotropic support is necessary to elevate cardiac output to a level necessary to support arterial pressure.

State D represents the superimposition of cardiac failure upon the fundamental septic response picture. Cardiac output in this state is depressed and apparent autonomic control overrides peripheral vasodilatory mechanisms and the patients become vasoconstricted. These "cold" shock patients have severe lactic acidosis and generally are in the immediate preterminal phases of the disease process.

Defective Oxygen Metabolism and Multiple System Organ Failure

From the foregoing discussion, it is apparent that a peripheral defect in oxidative metabolism is operational in the septic patient. This is most clearly seen in the state B septic response patient. The hyperdynamic circulation can be viewed teleological as an attempt to increase the peripheral delivery of oxygen. The narrowed arteriovenous oxygen content illustrates that a defect in peripheral extraction is present. Lactic acidemia is further testimony to peripheral anaerobic glycolysis. The shift in the body substrate economy to the production of glucose would appear to be an adaptive response to fuel glycolysis during this period of glycolytic dependence for energy production.

During the early 1970s, several authors examined models of experimental endotoxemia to identify potential cellular mechanisms which may account for the altered oxygen metabolism of the septic state [10, 11]. These experiments with endotoxin showed that isolated hepatic mitochondria demonstrated severe uncoupling and inhibition of oxidative phosphorylation. These data indicated that, like cyanide poisoning, endotoxemia may inhibit electron transport and impair oxygen utilization.

Our laboratory explored similar experiments except that a clinically relevant model of peritonitis was used [12]. Rats underwent ligation and perforation of the cecum. A fulminant peritonitis ensued and all animals became bacteremic with a polymicrobial microflora by 6 h after the onset of peritonitis. As opposed to the endotoxic experiments, bacterial peritonitis resulted in *increased* efficiency of oxygen utilization by the isolated hepatic mitochondria. The mitochondrial response in rats with peritonitis was analogous to that observed when rats had been subjected to systemic hypoxemia [13]. However, the peritonitis animals in our experiments had normal arterial pressures and a normal arterial pO_2. Interestingly, the peritonitis rats did develop a metabolic acidosis. Studies were then undertaken to directly examine the oxygenation of the liver during both peritonitis and in experimental bacteriemia [12, 14]. Using a surface poly-tipped oxygen electrode, reduced oxygenation of the liver was identified during the course of both peritonitis and gram-negative bacteremia. As in our previous experiments, arterial pO_2 and mean arterial pressure were unchanged from the control animals. It appeared that oxygen delivery to the liver was inadequate even though systemic measurements did not indicate either hypoxemia or shock. Initial experiments with indocyanine green clearance as an indirect method to measure liver blood flow in experimental models of systemic infection demonstrated a reduction in effective hepatic flow in rats with normal mean arterial pressures and normal arterial pO_2 [15-17].

A question remained whether cardiac output was truly adequate in these animals. Furthermore, technical problems that many authors have had using the indocyanine green clearance methodology for the measurement of liver blood flow left an uncertainty about the presumed defect in oxygen delivery to the liver. We then developed a thermodilution technique to measure cardiac output in rats and validated galactose elimination kinetics as a method to measure effective hepatic blood flow. These studies of peritonitis demonstrated normal-to-elevated cardiac output in the rats with peritonitis at points in time when effective hepatic blood flow was diminished [18]. These data led to the conclusion that hepatic blood flow was dissociated from systemic hemodynamics and that a microcirculatory injury may be responsible for the defective oxygen utilization of the septic response. Persistence in defective oxygen utilization may be of mechanistic significance to the development of MSOF.

The Genesis of Multiple System Organ Failure: Microcirculatory Arrest

The histologic evaluation of liver from septic patients and from experimental animals with bacteremic infection have demonstrated focal inflammatory lesions and focal cellular necrosis [16, 19]. As the process continues, the number and size of these necrotic inflammatory lesions increase. Histologic examination during the course of septic models of the hepatic microcirculation identifies sequestered neutrophils in a fibrin cast. These observations led us to explore whether sequestered neutrophils within the hepatic circulation could have relevance to our observed defect in effective hepatic blood flow.

Biological mediators that might activate human neutrophils then became the focus of attention. Complement cleavage products are chemotactic agents which bind to specific membrane receptors on neutrophils and also up-regulate certain neutrophil functions such as the production of superoxide anion and production of lysosomal enzymes. Systemic activation of complement proteins via the alternative pathway had previously been observed in bacteremic humans and gave credibility to this component of the human inflammatory response as a potential "trigger" to the septic response [20].

Rats with peritonitis were then studied with respect to activation of total hemolytic complement [21]. Nearly 70% of total hemolytic complement was activated by peritonitis. Regression analysis demonstrated a statistically significant relationship between the magnitude of complement activation and the reduction of both effective hepatic blood flow and effective renal plasma flow.

If complement activation was an important trigger in the septic response, then could systemic complement activation provoke the septic response in the absence of bacteria or endotoxin? We infused intravenously varying concentrations of zymosan into rats to activate the complement cascade by the alternative pathway [22]. Rats at lower concentrations developed an increased cardiac output and likewise developed a reduction of effective hepatic blood flow. All physiologic and metabolic responses were identical to rats with bacteremia except that no culturable bacteria in blood were present in these animals. Large dose zymosan infusion resulted in hemodynamic responses similar to rats which receive bolus endotoxin in that they developed depressed cardiac output and rapidly progressed to death. These experiments led us to the conclusion that complement activation appeared to be a potent activator of the septic response.

The zymosan experiments raised the interesting question whether infection was necessary at all to activate the inflammatory response and potential organ failure. Previous studies have noted organ failure complexes in patients with femoral fractures and fulminant acute pancreatitis [23, 24]. This raised the experimental question whether biological insults of sufficient severity to systematically activate the complement cascade could provoke a septic response without actual infection. Closed femoral fractures in rats were associated with a 70% activation of systemic hemolytic complement and with a reduction in effective hepatic blood flow [25]. Open fractures without massive soft tissue injury did not activate the complement cascade and were not associated with any reduction in liver blood flow. These data support the hypothesis that sterile, noninfectious inflammatory insults can provoke the physiologic and metabolic consequences of "sepsis" but without infection. These experiments would imply that mediator substances from the site of sterile inflammatory injury must orchestrate the systemic response.

Tumor necrosis factor (TNF) is one such putative substance. TNF is known to up-regulate neutrophils as part of its proinflammatory effects [26]. Complement cleavage products stimulate TNF production from macrophages. TNF may be an effector mechanism of the complement-mediated septic response.

The administration of human recombinant TNF to rats gave most interesting results despite the cross-species nature of these experiments [27], TNF produced and increased cardiac output, reduced peripheral vascular resistance, and reduction in effective hepatic blood flow. Of interest, TNF infusion did not activate the complement cascade.

A hypothesis was thus formulated which proposed that systemic activation of neutrophils results in neutrophil-endothelial cell adhesion. Activated neutrophils within the microcirculation produce reactive oxygen intermediates and hydrolytic enzymes which mediate a microcirculatory injury which may lead to tissue ischemia and organ failure. Treatment with superoxide dismutase and catalase reduced the microcirculatory injury [28]. Specific inhibition of xanthine oxidase did not provide microcirculatory protection, which led to the conclusion that neutrophils are the source of the reactive oxygen intermediates that are responsible for the impaired liver blood flow [29].

Clinicians have all been confronted with relentless down-hill progression of MSOF once the process has been activated. It seems that even arrest and correction of the primary infectious event which triggered the process does not reverse the clinical course. It is hypothesized that the tissue level, necrotic inflammatory lesion that is the product of the microcirculatory injury may actually be the bases for sustained activation of all the proinflammatory mediators which are responsible for continuation of the process (Fig. 2). Simply stated, the end products of systemic inflammation produces tissue level necrosis which reactivates and sustains the entire process.

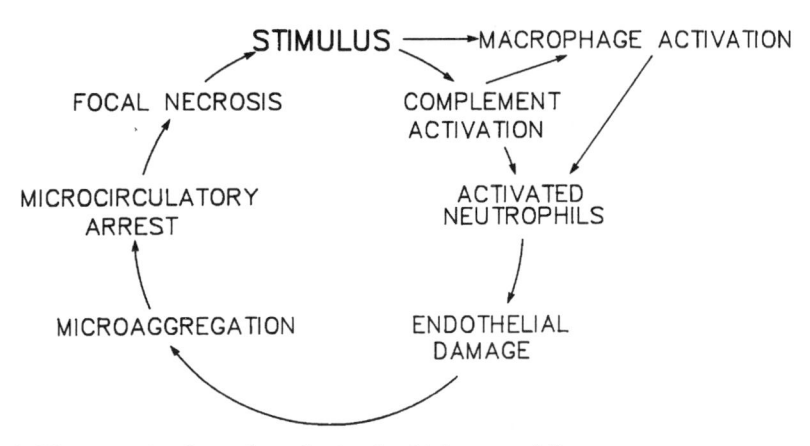

Fig. 2: The microcirculatory hypothesis of multiple organ failure

Perspectives in Future Management of Multiple System Organ Failure

The proposed microcirculatory hypothesis of MSOF represents the systemic activation of the normal local inflammatory response. Complement activation and TNF are normal mediators and effector signals as part of the salutory benefits of inflammation following tissue injury and wound contamination. The systemic amplification of salutory local inflammatory mechanisms poses a most interesting problem in proposing newer treatment modalities.

Some have advocated attempts to blunt activation of the inflammatory cascade. The monoclonal antibody for gram-negative endotoxin had been one such attempt [30, 31]. Unfortunately, the septic response is activated by many putative stimuli other than endotoxin. Our current lack of specificity in the identification of the activator substance or process means that many more patients would have to be treated to benefit a few. Establishing the cohort of patients to receive this therapy will be difficult but potentially productive.

Mediator blockade has also been demonstrated in experimental models to be potentially effective therapy. Anti-TNF monoclonal antibodies [32, 33], TNF receptor antagonists [34, 35], and interleukin-1 receptor antagonists [36-38] have been advocated. While some benefit can be seen in short-term experimental models, the complete ablation of these biological messenger systems may not be desirable. Likewise, neutralization of reactive oxygen intermediates and blockade of prostaglandin metabolites is to ignore the salutary benefits of these mediators.

The focus of attention in recent years has been in studying the proinflammatory cascade of the septic response. Perhaps a preferable strategy for the development of patient treatment will be a better understanding of intrinsic down-regulating mechanisms. These are clearly down-regulatory messages which blunt the progression of local inflammation without impairing host defense. Emulation of these down-regulatory signals into a future treatment strategy would appear to have the greatest prospect for meaningful new therapy of MSOF.

References

1. Fry DE, Pearlstein L, Fulton RL, Polk HC Jr (1980) Multiple system organ failure: the role of uncontrolled infection. Arch Surg 115: 136-140
2. Fry DE, Garrison RN, Heitch RC. et al. (1980) Determinants of death in patients with intraabdominal abscess. Surgery 89: 517-523
3. Fry DE, Garrison RN, Polk HC Jr (1979) Clinical implications in bacteroides bacteremia. Surg Gynecol Obstet 149: 189-192
4. Fry DE, Garrison RN, Williams HC (1980) Patterns of morbidity and mortality in splenectomy for trauma. Am Surg 46: 28-32
5. Eiseman B, Beart R, Norton L (1977) Multiple organ failure. Surg Gynecol Obstet 144: 323-326
6. Baue AE (1975) Multiple, progressive, or sequential systems failure. Arch Surg 110: 779-781
7. Tilney NL, Bailey GL, Morgan AP (1973) Sequential system failure after rupture of abdominal aortic aneurysms: an unresolved problem in postoperative care. Ann Surg 178: 117-122
8. Siegel JH, Cerra FB, Coleman B, et al. (1979) Physiologic and metabolic correlations in human sepsis. Surgery 86: 163-193
9. Cerra FB, Siegel JH, Coleman B, et al. (1980) Septic autocannibalism: a failure of exogenous nutritional support. Ann Surg 192: 570-580
10. Mela L, Bacalzo LV, Miller LD (1971) Defective oxidative metabolism of rat liver mitochondria in hemorrhage and endotoxin shock. Am J Physiol 220: 571-576
11. Schumer W, Das Gupta TK, Moss GS, et al. (1970) Effect of endotoxemia on liver cell mitochondria in man. Ann Surg 171: 875-879
12. Fry DE, Silver BB, Rink RD, et al. (1979) Hepatic cellular hypoxia in murine peritonitis. Surgery 85: 652-661
13. Mela L, Olofsson K, Miller LD, et al. (1971) Effect of lysosomes and hypoxia on mitochondria in shock. Surg Forum 22: 19-21
14. Fry DE, Kaelin CR, Giammara BL, Rink RD (1981) Alterations of oxygen metabolism in experimental bacteremia. Adv Shock Res 6: 45-54
15. Asher EF, Garrison RN, Ratcliffe DJ, Fry DE (1983) Endotoxin, cellular function and nutrient blood flow. Arch Surg 118: 441-445
16. Asher EF, Rowe RL, Garrison RN, Fry DE (1986) Experimental bacteremia and nutrient hepatic blood flow. Circ Shock 20: 43-49
17. Garrison RN, Ratcliffe DJ, Fry DE (1982) Hepatocellular function and nutrient blood flow in experimental peritonitis. Surgery 92: 713-719
18. Townsend MC, Hampton WW, Haybron DM, et al. (1986) Effective organ blood flow and bioenergy status in murine peritonitis. Surgery 100: 205-213

19. Fry DE (1992) Multiple system organ failure. In: Fry DE (ed.) Multiple system organ failure. Mosby Year Book, Chicago, pp. 3-14
20. Fearon DT, Ruddy S, Schur PH, et al. (1975) Activation of the properdin pathway of complement in patients with gram-negative bacteremia. N Engl J Med 292: 937-940
21. Schirmer WJ, Schirmer JM, Naff GB, Fry DE (1987) Complement activation in peritonitis: association with hepatic and renal perfusion abnormalities. Am Surg 53: 683-687
22. Schirmer WJ, Schirmer JM, Naff GB, Fry DE (1988) Systematic complement activation produces hemodynamic changes characteristic of sepsis. Arch Surg 123: 316-321
23. Seibel R, LaDuca J, Hassett JM, et al. (1985) Blunt multiple trauma (ISS 36), femur fracture, and the pulmonary failure-septic state. Ann Surg 202: 283-295
24. Ranson JHC, Rifkind KMK, Roses DF, et al. (1974) Prognostic signs and the role of operative management in acute pancreatitis. Ann Surg 139: 69-74
25. Schirmer WJ, Schirmer JM, Townsend MC, Fry DE (1988) Femur fracture with associated soft-tissue injury produces hepatic ischemia: possible cause of hepatic dysfunction. Arch Surg 123: 412-415
26. Klebanoff SJ, Vedes MA, Harlan JM, et al. (1986) Stimulation of neutrophils by tumor necrosis factor. J Immunol 136: 4220-4225
27. Schirmer WJ, Schirmer JM, Fry DE (1989) Recombinant human tumor necrosis factor produces hemodynamic changes characteristic of sepsis and endotoxemia. Arch Surg 124: 445-448
28. Schirmer WJ, Schirmer JM, Naff GB, Fry DE (1988) Contribution of toxic oxygen intermediates to complement-induced reduction in effective hepatic blood flow. J Trauma 28: 1295-1300
29. Schirmer WJ, Schirmer JM, Naff GB, Fry DE (1988) Effects of allopurinol and Iodoxamide on complement induced hepatic ischemia. J Surg Res 45: 28-36
30. Ziegler EJ, Fisher CJ, Sprung CL, et al. (1991) Treatment of gram negative bacteremia and septic shock with HA-1A human monoclonal antibody against endotoxin. N Engl J Med 324: 429-436
31. Greenman RL, Schein RM, Martin MA, et al. (1991) A controlled clinical trial of E5 murine monoclonal IgM antibody to endotoxin in the treatment of gram-negative sepsis. The XOMA sepsis study group. JAMA 266: 1097-1102
32. Beutler B, Milsark JA, Cerami AC (1985) Passive immunization against cachectin/tumor necrosis factor protects mice from the lethal effect of endotoxin. Science 229: 869-871
33. Tracey KJ, Fong Y, Hesse DG, et al. (1987) Anticachectin/TNF monoclonal antibodies prevent septic shock during lethal bacteremia. Nature 330: 662-664
34. Gatanga T, Hwang CD, Kohr W, et al. (1990) Purification and characterization of an inhibitor (soluble tumor necrosis factor inhibitor) for tumor necrosis factor and lymphotoxin obtained from the serum ultrafiltrates of human cancer patients. Proc Natl Acad Sci USA 87: 8781-8784
35. Mohler KM, Torrance DS, Smith CA, et al. (1993) Soluble tumor necrosis factor (TNF) receptors are effective therapeutic agents in lethal endotoxemia and function simultaneously as both TNF carriers and TNF antagonists. J Immunol 151: 1548-1561
36. Ohlsson K, Bjork P, Bergenfeldt M, et al. (1990) Interleukin-1 receptor antagonist reduces mortality from endotoxin shock. Nature 348: 550-551
37. Okusawa S, Gelfand JA, Ikejima T, et al. (1988) Interleukin 1 induces a shock-like state in rabbits: synergism with tumor necrosis factor and the effect of cyclooxygenase inhibition. J Clin Invest 81: 1162-1172
38. Wakabayashi G, Gelfand JA, Burke JF, et al. (1991) A specific receptor antagonist for interleukin 1 prevents Escherichia coli - induced shock in rabbits. FASEB J 5: 338-343

SEPSIS, SIRS, and MODS:
Consensus, Controversy, and Challenge

J. C. Marshall

Introduction

The definition of a clinical syndrome serves two purposes: it identifies a group of clinical and laboratory abnormalities as manifestations of a single pathologic process, and it suggests a unifying approach to therapy. Because terminology reflects prevailing views of biology, significant advances in the understanding of biology can render existing definitions confusing or even obsolete.

During the nineteenth century, the terms "consumption" and "phthisis" were applied to describe a group of patients with a chronic wasting disease associated with cough, dyspnea, intermittent fever, and purulent sputum [1]. Today this description could include not only patients with pulmonary tuberculosis, but also those with lung cancer, chronic congestive heart failure, and contemporary diseases such as AIDS. However, it was only with the identification of the tubercle bacillus and the introduction of effective antituberculous therapy that there arose a need to define tuberculosis on the basis of a common pathologic process rather than on the basis of common clinical manifestations. Similarly the classic features of hypoperfusion - tachycardia, tachypnea, hypotension, and characteristic sense of anxiety in the facial expression - suggested that the fundamental biologic process was one of fear and pain and the word "shock" has persisted in common usage as a reflection of this early hypothesis. Much later, Blalock [2] demonstrated the critical role of reduced intravascular volume in the pathogenesis of shock and it became clear that the fundamental problem was one of circulatory inadequacy, rather than sympathetic overactivity.

The leading cause of death for patients admitted to a contemporary intensive care unit following multiple trauma, overwhelming infection, or a heterogeneous group of disorders characterized by an acute disruption of normal homeostasis is a complex process that has been termed the "multiple organ dysfunction syndrome (MODS)" [3]. MODS, like phthisis or consumption, is a purely descriptive term. It is unknown whether patients manifesting the syndrome share a common pathologic disorder; moreover, there is only the most general form of consensus on what clinical or laboratory abnormalities comprise the syndrome [4]. It is widely believed that the evolution of MODS is a consequence of the activation of the host septic response [3,5-7], yet the word "sepsis", like the word "shock", has its origins in an outdated model of biology.

MODS can be prevented, or its severity minimized, by careful adherence to time-honored principles of good surgical care [8]. Treatment of the syndrome once established, however, is entirely supportive and expectant. Advances in specific therapy are dependent as much on an improved conceptual and linguistic understanding of the process as they are on studies of its cellular biology.

Sepsis and Infection: Evolving Concepts

The word "sepsis" was first used by Hippocrates to denote a process of tissue breakdown accompanied by putrefaction and a bad smell, and differentiated from a companion process of "pepsis" - breakdown of tissue through a process of fermentation [9]. These contrasting Greek concepts represented a fusion of opposites in much the same way that the Oriental concepts of *yin* and *yang* define two opposite, but necessarily interdependent processes. Pepsis occurred in the fermentation of wine, and gave rise to life, health, and happiness. Sepsis occurred in swamps: it produced death, disease, and misery. The concept of pepsis encompassed the processes involved in the digestion of food and persists in our vocabulary in terms such as peptic ulcer disease. Sepsis on the other hand described the processes involved in the formation of abscesses following trauma and in death from infectious disease. When it was learned in the nineteenth century that infection was caused by transmissable microorganisms, it was a natural conceptual leap that the word sepsis came to be applied to denote the clinical syndrome of overwhelming infection. Until very recently, the terms sepsis and infection have been used interchangeably; indeed a recent edition of a standard medical dictionary defines sepsis as "the presence of various pus-forming and other pathogenic organisms, or their toxins in the blood or tissues" [10].
Within such a paradigm, the clinical manifestations of sepsis reflected the direct action of microbes or their toxins, and the clinical syndrome of sepsis was held to be the expression of disseminated and uncontrolled infection. In the absence of effective therapy to eradicate microorganisms in the host, this model persisted unchallenged for more than a century. But with the increasing availability of antibiotics, flaws in the paradigm came to be recognized. First it became evident that the major impact of antimicrobial therapy was not a reduction in the prevalence or lethality of infection, but rather a change in its epidemiology and bacteriology [11]. In the period following the widespread availability of penicillin and the sulfonamides, gram-negative bacteria, previously believed to be of low intrinsic virulence, emerged as the most prominent infecting organisms in hospitalized critically ill patients [12,13]. The clinical syndrome of sepsis was seen most commonly in patients with overwhelming gram-negative infection [14], and the focus of studies of the pathogenesis of sepsis shifted from gram-positive exotoxins to the role of lipopolysaccharide from the gram-negative bacterial cell wall [15].
Two separate lines of investigation, however, challenged the concept that clinical sepsis was a direct consequence of the action of bacterial endotoxin. A series of clinical studies of the septic response showed that it was not specific for gram-negative infection, but that the identical clinical syndrome occurred during gram-positive infection [16], viral infection [17], and even in the absence of infection following the systemic infusion of stress hormones [18]. At the same time, experimental studies demonstrated that the response to endotoxin arose indirectly through the release of endogenous mediator molecules from host myeloid cells [19-21]. These advances in the understanding of the biology of infection have opened the door to an entirely novel therapeutic approach based on modulation of the host response,

but have created clinical and diagnostic confusion, for it is now apparent that the host septic response is not specific for infection, and may be either beneficial or detrimental, depending on the clinical situation [22]. The septic response can be triggered by a wide spectrum of infections, but also by noninfectious insults such as sterile inflammation, tissue injury, autoimmune disease, ischemia, and various nonmicrobial toxins.

Controversy regarding the clinical meaning of the word "sepsis" led a group of North American intensivists in 1991 to propose a new term - the "systemic inflammatory response syndrome or SIRS" - to describe the clinical response independent of its etiology [3]. This same consensus conference advocated that the word "sepsis" be used to denote SIRS when it arises as a result of infection.

Infection and the Septic Response: Contemporary Perspectives

Infection denotes a microbial phenomenon - the invasion of host tissues by microorganisms or their toxins; tissue invasion differentiates infection from colonization. Implicit in the concept is the persistence of the process over time, so that a transient bacteremia associated with colonoscopy or endotoxemia caused by experimental bolus injection does not truly represent infection. Rather infection implies both tissue invasion and subsequent microbial proliferation. Such a definition suggests a logical therapeutic approach - the drainage of abscesses, the debridement of injured tissues where bacteria proliferate, and the administration of systemic antibiotics.

Infection is a dichotomous state that is either present or absent, although it may be local or disseminated and the actual microbial load may vary. Its diagnosis hinges on the demonstration of an infecting organism. Infection in the critically ill may be difficult to diagnose. It may prove impossible, for example, to determine whether a chest X-ray infiltrate results from pneumonia or noninfectious acute lung injury [23], or to differentiate drain or wound colonization from invasive infection in the patient with persistent peritonitis [24]. Detection of microbial toxins such as endotoxin in body fluids is technically difficult and not presently feasible in clinical practise. Once the diagnosis of infection is made, however, therapy is generally both straightforward and effective in eliminating the infecting organism; reversing the systemic sequelae of the infectious process remains an unsolved problem [25]. The challenge of infection is primarily diagnosis, the challenge of the host septic response is therapy.

The host septic response or SIRS is an adaptive process, rather than a pathologic state. It is not simply present or absent, but present in varying degrees of intensity and probably in varying biologic patterns. Moreover the septic response is an appropriate homeostatic response that serves to optimize the internal milieu of the host for the clearance and killing of bacteria, the removal of injured tissue, and the initiation of the process of tissue repair. The still unsolved clinical paradox is that this protective response can itself produce disease and death.

SIRS criteria as enunciated by the ACCP/SCCM Consensus Conference [3] successfully differentiate the host response from the process that initiates it, however they fail in two important respects. The specific SIRS criteria proposed do not embody the clinical variability of the response, but rather limit it to a specific combination of manifestations - alterations in temperature and white blood cell count, tachycardia, and tachypnea. More importantly they define the response as a state that is present or absent, rather than as a process that is dynamic and that evolves with graded degrees of severity.

Current criteria for SIRS are derived from those previously used to define sepsis syndrome [26]. These, in turn, were established not empirically through study of the epidemiology of the process, but arbitrarily through an imperfect process of consensus in the context of the design of entry criteria for a clinical trial [27]. There have been few studies of the epidemiology of the septic response as a process distinct from infection, and none to evaluate whether distinct clinical patterns can be discriminated, nor whether, for example, the presence of a high temperature and insulin resistance with a normal white blood cell count has the same diagnostic or prognostic implications as a normal temperature in association with marked leukocytosis and a hyperdynamic circulatory response. Studies of the epidemiology of SIRS and the associations of its manifestations with its causes, with its outcome, or with its mediator profile are needed before definitive conclusions regarding its optimal management can be made.

Infection, SIRS, and the Roots of MODS

Intensive care units evolved in the late 1950s to provide organ system specific support to critically ill patients who had survived the immediate sequelae of previously lethal injuries or diseases [28]. In a relatively short period of time, techniques were developed to provide respiratory support in the form of tracheal intubation and positive pressure ventilation, renal support in the form of dialysis, hemodynamic support in the form of invasive monitoring and vasoactive therapy, and metabolic and gut support in the form of total parenteral nutrition. It was natural therefore, that the need for such support would come to define the nature of critical illness, and that the failure of such support, the limitations of intensive therapy [29]. The concept of multiple organ failure emerged as a central paradigm of critical care practise.
It quickly became evident that multiple organ failure was more than the terminal event for a disparate group of diseases requiring ICU supportive care. The demonstration that organ failure was often the presenting manifestation of occult infection in the critically ill suggested a causal association with infection [5, 30]. The nature of that association was unclear, for although organ failure frequently occurred in association with infection, it could arise in the absence of infection and the control of infection did not necessarily lead to the reversal of organ failure [25, 31].
The conceptual evolution of the pathophysiology of multiple organ failure faithfully mirrors that of the septic response. Organ failure is not specific for infection, but develops in association with the same group of stimuli that lead to the expression of a host septic response (Table 1). Like the septic response, organ failure is not a discrete event, but a continuous process of graded severity and variable clinical expression. This recognition prompted the ACCP/SCCM consensus conference to propose the term "the multiple organ dysfunction syndrome" to describe the clinical syndrome [3]. Finally, animal models of organ dysfunction show that it develops following the same stimuli as produce a septic response [32], and involves the same host derived mediators [20, 33].
MODS can be defined as a clinical syndrome of altered physiologic organ system function that arises in the wake of an acute severe insult to normal homeostasis. There is as yet no clear consensus on what systems comprise MODS, nor what variables best define altered function in each of these. A review of the published literature shows that seven organ systems - respiratory, renal, hepatic, cardiovascular, gastrointestinal, neurologic, and hematologic - are most widely held to be the systems whose dysfunction defines MODS [4]. As is the case for

Table 1: The clinical setting of the multiple organ dysfunction syndrome (MODS)

Stimulus	Examples	References
Infection	Peritonitis	[5, 30, 34]
	Pneumonia	[35]
	Emergency surgery	[5]
Injury	Multiple trauma	[36, 37]
	Burns	[38]
Inflammation	Pancreatitis	[39]
Ischemia	Hypotension	[5, 37]
	Ruptured aneurysm	[40]
	Aortic occlusion	[41]
	Pheochromocytoma	[42]
Intoxication	Salicylates	[43]
	Arsenic	[44]
	Cresol	[45]
	Heat stroke	[46]
Immunologic Activation	IL-2 therapy	[47]
Iatrogenic	Missed or delayed diagnosis of above	[37]
Idiopathic		

SIRS (and likely because diagnostic criteria have not been established) there are no sophisticated studies of the epidemiology of MODS.

MODS therefore mirrors the septic response in its clinical setting, its biology, and its conceptual confusion. Indeed MODS and the septic response are, in reality, differing manifestations of the same process: if the septic response is an adaptive process that serves to modify the internal milieu to confront an acute insult to normal homeostasis, then the multiple organ dysfunction syndrome is the maladaptive outcome of that response.

Conclusion: Consensus, Controversy, and Challenges

It is now generally accepted that the host septic response itself plays a significant role in the pathogenesis of the complex physiologic changes in the patient with evolving multiple organ dysfunction, and that the clinical syndrome reflects more than the sequelae of inadequate antimicrobial therapy or the presence of an occult or untreated focus of infection [3, 6, 7]. The introduction of such new terminology as the "systemic inflammatory response syndrome" has served to crystallize the paradigm shift that has occurred as the biology of the host response to infection becomes better understood. However, while SIRS is appealing as a concept, it leaves much to be desired as a clinical definition, for its published criteria are sufficiently broad as to include the majority of patients admitted to an ICU [48].

One of the unsolved challenges confronting those who attempt to better characterize the clinical phenomenon of sepsis is that the clinical manifestations of systemic inflammation can occur in response to overwhelming and life-threatening infection, noninfectious but life-threatening inflammatory processes such as pancreatitis, clinically minor viral infections, and such non-pathogenic processes as active exercise [49]. We do not currently have a satisfactory clinical or laboratory method of differentiating infectious and noninfectious causes of SIRS, nor of grading the severity of the response so that valid decisions can be made regarding therapeutic manipulation of the host response.

On the basis of a retrospective subgroup analysis of patients enrolled in a clinical trial of mediator manipulation using the interleukin-1 receptor antagonist [50], it has been proposed that the use of clinical criteria for SIRS in conjunction with a validated severity of illness measure can reliably identify patients who might benefit from such novel therapies [51]. While such an approach can identify a sicker group of patients at a higher risk of death, it remains to be proven that this is an homogeneous group whose mechanism of mortality is similar.

The need to stratify patients on the basis of a common pathologic process is particularly compelling in the context of clinical trials of agents that can modify the endogenous host response. Animal studies demonstrate that the effects of mediator antagonism are highly model-dependent. For example, neutralization of tumour necrosis factor (TNF) by pretreatment with a blocking antibody improves survival in experimental endotoxemia [52], whereas pretreatment with recombinant TNF improves survival in cecal ligation and puncture [53]. Similarly administration of the anti-inflammatory cytokine interleukin-10 (IL-10) improves survival in experimental endotoxemia [54], while blockade of IL-10 is associated with enhanced survival in experimental candidiasis [55]. The explanation for these divergent results is speculative: a reasonable explanation would be that the beneficial consequences of the proinflammatory cytokine response are evident when uncontrolled infection is the problem, but that once infection has been controlled, the adverse effects of the response dominate. Nonetheless it is clear that results from animal models must be interpreted cautiously, and that we do not have a truly satisfactory model for clinical sepsis.

With the advent of multimodal therapy for life-threatening inflammatory disorders - surgical, antimicrobial, immunomodulatory, and supportive - it may well be necessary to adopt a more sophisticated approach to patient stratification analogous to staging systems now widely in use to plan and evaluate multimodal therapy for patients with malignancy [56].

Although MODS is the leading cause of contemporary ICU mortality, it remains in many ways an elusive and enigmatic process. It is unclear, for example, whether MODS is a single pathologic process wth variable clinical expression, or many separate processes with common clinical manifestations dictated by a common mode of ICU support. Is MODS a disease process itself, or the consequence of a disease, and if the latter, what is the disease process? Are there discrete patterns of MODS that can be differentiated on the basis of preceding cause or differential response to therapy? Can MODS be defined by distinct biochemical markers? How is it best defined using clinical parameters? Does MODS arise because of a failure of host defense mechanisms, or as a consequence of the activation of those mechanisms? Should our therapeutic goal be to augment or suppress the host response, or if the goal depends on the clinical context, how can we decide when to fan the flames and when to put them out?

There is at present no consensus on the answers to these questions, and the challenges of their resolution are both conceptual and biologic. Within the framework of the model presented here, the conceptual challenge can be expressed as the manipulation of the endogenous host reponse to maximize its adaptive benefits in restoring normal homeostasis while minimizing the maladaptive consequences of its activation. By this model, MODS is not a disease to be treated, but an adverse outcome to be prevented. Because the very interventions we use to support the patient with clinical sepsis may inadvertently result in worsening of organ dysfunction [56-59], it is vital that approaches be developed to permit the optimal evaluation, not only of expensive mediator-directed therapy, but of many of the standard practises routinely used in the care of the multiply traumatized and critically ill.

References

1. Bayle G-L (1945) Essential character of pulmonary phthisis. In: Major RH (ed.) Classic descriptions of disease. Thomas, Springfield, pp. 64-66
2. Blalock A (1930) Experimental shock: the cause of the low blood pressure produced by muscle injury. Arch Surg 20: 959-996
3. ACCP-SCCM Consensus Conference (1992) Definitions of sepsis and multiple organ failure. Crit Care Med 20: 864-874
4. Marshall JC (1994) Descriptors of organ system dysfunction for the multiple organ dysfunction syndrome (MODS). In: Sibbald WJ, Vincent J-L, Cook DJ (eds.) Design of clinical trials for sepsis. Springer, Berlin, Heidelberg, New York (in press)
5. Fry DE, Pearlstein L, Fulton RL, Polk HC (1980) Multiple system organ failure. The role of uncontrolled infection. Arch Surg 115: 136-140
6. Carrico CJ, Meakins JL, Marshall JC, Fry D, Maier RV (1986) Multiple-organ-failure-syndrome. Arch Surg 121: 196-208
7. Deitch EA (1992) Multiple organ failure: pathophysiology and potential future therapy. Ann Surg 216: 117-134
8. Baue AE, Chaudry IH (1980) Prevention of multiple systems failure. Surg Clin North Am 60: 1167-1178
9. Majno G (1991) The ancient riddle of sepsis. J Infect Dis 163: 937-945
10. Stedman's Medical Dictionary, 24th edn. (1982) Williams and Wilkins, Baltimore/MD
11. Rogers DE (1959) The changing pattern of life-threatening microbial disease. N Engl J Med 261: 677-683
12. McGowan JE, Barnes MW, Finland M (1975) Bacteremia at Boston City Hospital: occurrence and mortality during 12 selected years (1935-1972), with special reference to hospital-acquired cases. J Infect Dis 132: 316-335
13. Altemeier WA, Todd JC, Inge WW (1967) Gram-negative septicemia: a growing threat. Ann Surg 166: 530-542
14. MacLean LD, Mulligan WG, McLean APH, Duff JH (1967) Patterns of septic shock in man - a detailed study of 56 patients. Ann Surg 166: 543-562
15. Morrison DC, Ulevitch RJ (1978) The effects of bacterial endotoxins on host mediation systems. Am J Pathol 93: 527-617
16. Wiles JB, Cerra FB, Siegel JH, Border JR (1980) The systemic septic response: does the organism matter? Crit Care Med 8: 55-60
17. Deutschmann CS, Konstantinides FN, Tsai M, Simmons RL, Cerra FB (1987) Physiology and metabolism in isolated viral septicemia. Further evidence of an organism-independent, host-dependent response. Arch Surg 122: 21-25

18. Watters JM, Bessey PQ, Dinarello CA, Wolff SM, Wilmore DW (1986) Both inflammatory and endocrine mediators stimulate host responses to sepsis. Arch Surg 121: 179-190
19. Michalek SM, Moore RN, McGhee JR, Rosenstreich DL, Mergenhagen SE (1980) The primary role of lymphoreticular cells in the mediation of host responses to bacterial endotoxin. J Infect Dis 141: 55-63
20. Tracey KJ, Beutler JB, Lowry SF, Merryweather J, Wolpe S, Milsark IW, Hariri RJ, Fahey TJ, Zentella A, Albert JD, et al. (1986) Shock and tissue injury induced by recombinant human cachectin. Science 234: 470-474
21. Ohlsson K, Bjork P, Bergenfeldt M, Hageman R, Thompson RC (1990) Interleukin-1 receptor antagonist reduces mortality from endotoxin shock. Nature 348: 550-552
22. Natanson C, Hoffman WD, Suffredini AF, Eichaker PQ, Danner RL (1994) Selected treatment strategies for septic shock based on proposed mechanisms of pathogenesis. Ann Intern Med 120: 771-783
23. Fagon J-Y, Chastre J, Domart Y, Trouillet J-L, Pierre J, Darne C, Gibert C (1989) Nosocomial pneumonia in patients receiving continuous mechanical ventilation. Am Rev Respir Dis 139: 877-884
24. Nathens A, Rotstein OD, Marshall JC (1993) Tertiary peritonitis: clinical features of a complex nosocomial infection (Abstr). Crit Care Med 21 Suppl:S129
25. Norton LW (1985) Does drainage of intra-abdominal pus reverse multiple organ failure? Am J Surg 149: 347-350
26. Bone RC, Fisher CJ, Clemmer TP, Slotman GJ, Metz CA, Balk RA, the Methylprenisolone Severe Sepsis Study Group (1989) Sepsis syndrome: a valid clinical entity. Crit Care Med 17: 389-393
27. Bone RC, Fisher CJ, Clemmer TP, Slotman GJ, Metz CA, Balk RA, the Methylprednisolone Severe Sepsis Study Group (1987) A controlled clinical trial of high-dose methylprednisolone in the treatment of severe sepsis and septic shock. N Engl J Med 317: 653-658
28. Safar P, DeKornfeld TJ, Pearson JW, Redding JS (1961) The intensive care unit. A three year experience at Baltimore city hospitals. Anesthesia 16: 275-284
29. Baue AE (1975) Multiple, progressive, or sequential systems failure. A syndrome of the 1970's. Arch Surg 110: 779-781
30. Polk HC, Shields CL (1977) Remote organ failure: a valid sign of occult intra-abdominal infection. Surgery 81: 310-313
31. Marshall JC, Christou NV, Horn R, Meakins JL (1988) The microbiology of multiple organ failure. The proximal GI tract as an occult reservoir of pathogens. Arch Surg 123: 309-315
32. Steinberg S, Flynn W, Kelley K, Bitzer L, Sharma P, Gutierrez C, Baxter J, Lalka D, van Liew J, Hassett J, Price R, Beam T, Flint L (1989) Development of a bacteria-independent model of the multiple organ failure syndrome. Arch Surg 124: 1390-1395
33. Okusawa S, Gelfand JA, Ikejima T, Connolly RJ, Dinarello CA (1988) Interleukin 1 induces a shock-like state in rabits. Synergism with tumor necrosis factor and the effect of cyclooxygenase inhibition. J Clin Invest 81: 1162-1172
34. Pine RW, Wertz MJ, Lennard ES, Dellinger EP, Carrico CJ, Minshew BH (1983) Determinants of organ malfunction or death in patients with intra-abdominal sepsis. Arch Surg 118: 242-249
35. Bell RC, Coalson JJ, Smith JD, Johanson WG (1983) Multiple organ system failure and infection in adult respiratory distress syndrome. Ann Intern Med 99: 293-298
36. Faist E, Baue AE, Dittmer H, Heberer G (1983) Multiple organ failure in polytrauma patients. J Trauma 23: 775-786

37. Henao FJ, Daes JE, Dennis RJ (1991) Risk factors for multiorgan failure: a case-control study. J Trauma 31: 74-80
38. Marshall WG, Dimick AR (1983) The natural history of major burns with multiple subsystem failure. J Trauma 23: 102-105
39. McFadden DW (1991) Organ failure and multiple systems organ failure in pancreatitis. Pancreas 6 Suppl 1: S37-S43
40. Tilney NL, Bailey GL, Morgan AP (1973) Sequential system failure after rupture of abdominal aortic aneurysms: An unsolved problem in postoperative care. Ann Surg 178: 117-122
41. Porembka DT, Johnson DJ, Fowl RJ, Reising J, Dick BL (1992) Descending thoracic aortic aneurysm as a cause of MOF. Crit Care Med 20: 1184-1187
42. Lorz W, Cottier C, Imhof E, Gyr N (1993) Multiple organ failure and coma as initial presentation of pheochromocytoma in a patient with multiple endocrine neoplasia (MEN) type II A. Intensive Care Med 19: 235-238
43. Leatherman JW, Schmitz PG (1991) Fever, hyperdynamic shock, and multiple-system organ failure. A pseudo-sepsis syndrome associated with chronic salicylate intoxication. Chest 100: 1391-1396
44. Bolliger CT, van Zijl P, Louw JA (1992) Multiple organ failure with ARDS in homicidal arsenic poisoning. Respiration 59:57-61
45. Lin CH, Yang JY (1992) Chemical burn with cresol intoxication and multiple organ failure. Burns 18:162-166
46. Lumlertgul D, Chuaychoo B, Thitiarchakul S, Srimahachota S, Sangchun K, Keoplung M (1992) Heat-stroke induced multiple organ failure. Ren Fail 14: 77-80
47. Sculier JP, Bron D, Verboven N, Klastersky J (1988) Multiple organ failure during interleukin-2 and LAK cells infusion. Intensive Care Med 14: 666-667
48. Vincent J-L (1994) Sepsis and septic shock: update on definitions. In: Reinhart K, Eyrich K, Sprung C (eds.) Sepsis. Current perspectives in pathophysiology and therapy. Springer, Berlin, Heidelberg, New York, pp. 3-15
49. Camus G, Pincemail J, Lamy M (1992) Sepsis and strenuous exercise: common inflammatory factors. In: Lamy M, Thijs LJ (eds.) Mediators of sepsis. Update in intensive care and emergency medicine. Springer, Berlin, Heidelberg, New York, pp. 206-219
50. Fisher CJ, Dhainaut J-FA, Opal SM et al., the Phase III IL-1ra Sepsis Syndrome Study Group (1994) Recombinant human interleukin 1 receptor antagonist in the treatment of patients with sepsis syndrome. Results from a randomized, double-blind, placebo-controlled trial. JAMA 271: 1836-1842
51. Knaus WA, Harrell FE, Fisher CJ, Wagner DP, Opal SM, Sadoff JC, Draper EA, Walawander CA, Conboy K, Grasela TH (1993) The clinical evaluation of new drugs for sepsis. A prospective study design based on survival analysis. JAMA 270: 1233-1241
52. Beutler B, Milsark IW, Cerami AC (1985) Passive immunization against cachectin/tumor necrosis factor protects mice from lethal effect of endotoxin. Science 228: 869-871
53. Alexander HR, Sheppard BC, Jensen JC, Langstein HN, Buresh CM, Venzon D, Walker EC, Fraker DL, Stovroff MC, Norton JA (1991) Treatment with recombinant human tumor necrosis factor-alpha protects rats against the lethality, hypotension and hypothermia of gram negative sepsis. J Clin Invest 88: 34-39
54. Gerard C, Bruyns C, Marchant A, et al (1993) Interleukin 10 reduces the release of tumor necrosis factor and prevents lethality in experimental endotoxemia. J Exp Med 177: 547-550
55. Romani L, Puccetti P, Mencacci A, Cenci E, Spaccapelo R, Tonnetti L, Grohmann U, Bistoni F (1994) Neutralization of IL-10 up-regulates nitric oxide production and protects susceptible mice from challenge with Candida albicans. J Immunol 152: 3514-3521

56. Marshall JC, Shields J (1994) Infection, host response, and organ dysfunction contribute independently to outcome in sepsis syndrome: towards a staging system for clinical sepsis. 14th annual meeting of the Surgical Infection Society, Toronto, Canada
57. Maetani S, Nishikawa T, Hirakawa A, Tobe T (1986) Role of blood transfusion in organ system failure following major abdominal surgery. Ann Surg 203: 275-281
58. Rello J, Ausina V, Ricart M, Castella J, Prats G (1993) Impact of previous antimicrobial therapy on the etiology and outcome of ventilator-associated pneumonia. Chest 104: 1230-1235
59. Hayes MA, Timmins AC, Yau EHS, Palazzo M, Hinds CJ, Watson D (1994) Evaluation of systemic oxygen delivery in the treatment of critically ill patients. N Engl J Med 330: 1717-1722

Development, Validation and Use of the SAPS II Model for Early Severe Sepsis

J. R. Le Gall

Introduction

The new drugs proposed for the treatment of sepsis are very expensive. Despite the well-designed phase III studies, the results are often controversial. A precise methodology must be used to develop and validate probability models giving the risk of hospital death for intensive care unit (ICU) patients. This methodology has been used to establish the new Simplified Acute Physiology Score (SAPS II) system. The same principles are applied to specific models for sepsis.

General Principles

Development of a Probability Model

The development of a multipurpose probability model needs a large database, collecting data from many ICUs. The collected variables can be classified into four groups: age, comorbidity, physiologic abnormality and acute diagnosis. Some systems have introduced variables to decrease the lead time bias. The collected outcome is usually the hospital outcome but may be different, such as the 28-day death rate. Using the logistic regression technique, the Lowess curves, and clinical judgement, the variables are selected, the ranges determined, and the weights calculated. The result is a score, such as the SAPS II, which is introduced into a logistic regression equation to give the risk of death.

Validation of a Probability Model

In order to answer the questions about the ability of models to provide accurate estimates of hospital mortality, two important statistical criteria must be defined: discrimination and calibration. Discrimination uses the area under the receiver-operating characteristic (ROC) curve to evaluate the ability of a model to distinguish patients who die from patients who live, based on the estimated probabilities of mortality. Calibration evaluates the degree of correspondence between a model's estimated probabilities of mortality and the actual mortality experience of patients within severity strata using formal goodness-of-fit tests.

Discrimination

To construct the ROC curve, a sequence of cutoff points is specified and, for each, a 2x2 classification table is constructed. For example, if the cutoff point chosen is 0.35, then any patient whose probability of mortality is 0.35 or higher is "predicted" to die, whereas any patient whose probability is less than 0.35 is "predicted" to live. Observed mortality is noted for each positive rate and determined. These points are then plotted for the sequence of cutoff points. The higher the true-positive rate relative to the false-positive rate, the greater the area under the ROC curve.

The interpretation of the area under the ROC curve is quite simple. If the entire sample were divided into patients who lived and patients who died and each patient who lived was paired with each patient who died, there would be $n_L \times n_D$ such pairs, where n_L is the number of patients who live and n_D is the number of patients who died. The area under the ROC curve is the proportion of the total number of pairings in which the patient who died had the higher of the two probabilities. Clearly, if this area is in the neighborhood of 0.50, the model is performing no better than a coin toss, and developers of models are typically not satisfied unless the ROC area of a model exceeds 0.70 [1].

Calibration

Calibration can be statistically evaluated using goodness-of-fit tests. What information does the assessment of calibration provide? If a model estimates that a patient has a probability of hospital mortality of 0.38, it means that among 100 patients with that probability of dying, 38 would be expected to die and 62 would be expected to live. When the observed number of deaths is close to the number expected from the model across the strata of probabilities, the model is considered to be well calibrated.

To formally test calibration, patients are rank-ordered according to their probabilities and mortality and are stratified into groups. Typically, ten such groups are formed, each containing approximately the same number of patients (these are called "deciles of risk"). Alternatively, patients could be divided into ten equal possibility groups, whereby patients with probabilities of mortality between 0.0001 and 0.0999 would constitute the first group, those with probabilities of mortality between 0.1000 and 0.1999 would constitute the second group, and so on to the last group comprising patients with probabilities between 0.9000 and 0.9999. To obtain the expected number of deaths in a stratum, the probability of mortality for every patient in the stratum is summed. The observed deaths are known. A formal goodness-of-fit test to compare the observed to expected number of deaths in each cell of the table is computed and it can be statistically determined whether the discrepancy between observed and expected numbers of deaths over all 20 cells in the table is unacceptably large [2].

In Summary

Both discrimination and calibration should be used to evaluate and compare the predictive efficacy of competing models. The area under an ROC curve provides an assessment of a model's ability to discriminate between patients who live and patients who die. Goodness-of-fit testing indicates whether the model is well calibrated. Calibration and discrimination provide different and useful information about a model's performance. Both techniques should be used routinely to evaluate models prior to their dissemination for general use. Whether a model fits well or not tells us nothing about the discrimination ability of the model, and the reverse is also true. Once it has been determined that a model does fit well, ROC analysis should be used to assess a model's performance with regard to discrimination, so that both parameters of model performance are applied to models in development.

The SAPS II System

The SAPS II was developed and validated among 12 997 patients from the ENAS database [3]. Like the original SAPS and APACHE systems, the SAPS II comprises primarily physiologic variables, with increasing derangement from normal limits being assigned progressively higher values to be included in the calculation of the score. In the original SAPS, no algorithm existed for producing a probability of hospital mortality, a measure that was available with both the APACHE II and MPM systems. The SAPS II now has the feature of providing, in addition to the score, a simple method to convert the score to a probability of hospital mortality using a chart. Table 1 presents the variable ranges and points that constitute the SAPS II score, which may range from 0 to 182 points, this being made up of from 0 to 120 points for the physiology variables, 0 to 36 points for the chronic health variables, 0 to 18 points for age, and 0 to 8 points for type of admission (emergency surgical, scheduled surgical, nonsurgical). The $\hat{\beta}$'s for conversion of the SAPS II score to a probability of hospital mortality are available, and the following formula is used:

$$\text{Probability of mortality} = \frac{e^{-7.7631 - 0.0737(\text{SAPS II Score}) + 0.9971\{\ln(\text{SAPS II Score} + 1)\}}}{1 - e^{-7.7631 - 0.0737(\text{SAPS II Score}) + 0.9971\{\ln(\text{SAPS II Score} + 1)\}}}$$

where Pr indicates probability, and e indicates a mathematical constant 2.71812818, which represents the base of the natural logarithm.

Evaluation of SAPS II

The SAPS II model developed from a sample of 65% of the patients, was validated on another sample of 35% of the patients of the European-North American study. This system gives excellent calibration and discrimination.

In a recent editorial, Selker [4] stated that the specific characteristics of the risk-adjusted mortality predictors are: time-intensive predictive instruments, they must be based on the first minutes of hospital presentation, not affected by whether a patient is hospitalized, use data collected in the usual care of the patients, must have excellent calibration, be computer system integrated, and be open for inspection and testing. These criteria are probably utopian. How could a scoring system at the same time be perfectly calibrated, based on the first minutes of hospital presentation, and not be affected by whether the patient is hospitalized? Other factors are included in the SAPS II system: use of data collected during the usual care of patients, open publication for inspection and testing, and time-insensitive predictive instruments.

Table 1: SAPS II scoring sheet

VARIABLE/POINTS	26	13	12	11	9	7	6	5	4	3	2	0	1	2	3	4	6	7	8	9	10	12	15	16	17	18
Age (years)												<40						40-59				60-69	70-74	75-79		≥80
Heart rate (beats/min)				<40							40-69	70-199				120-159		≥160								
Systolic BP (mmHg)		<70						70-99			≥200	100-199														
Body temperature (°C)(°F)												<39°/<102.2°			≥39°/≥102.2°											
Only if VENT or CPAP: PaO_2 (mmHg)/FiO_2 (0.XX) / PaO_2 (kPa)/FiO_2 (0.XX)				<100 / <13.3	100-199 / 13.3-26.5		≥200 / ≥26.6																			
Urinary output (l/day)				<0.500					0.500-0.999			≥1.000														
Blood urea (mmol/l)(g/l)												<10.0 / <0.60					10.0-29.9 / 0.60-1.79				≥30.0 / ≥1.80					
WBC count (10^3/cu.mm)			<1.0									1.0-19.9			≥20.0											
Serum K (mEq/l)										<3.0		3.0-4.9			≥5.0											
Serum Na (mEq/l)								<125				125-144	≥145													
Serum HCO3 (mEq/l)							<15			15-19		≥20														
Bilirubin (μmol/l)(mg/l)												<68.4 / <40.0				68.4-102.5 / 40.0-59.9				≥102.6 / ≥60.0						
Glasgow Coma Score	<6	6-8				9-10		11-13				14-15														
Chronic diseases:																				Met. Can.	Hem. Mal.				AIDS	
Type of admission												Scheduled Surgical					Medical		Unscheduled Surgical							
sum of points																										

Total SAPS II = ☐ pts.

Risk of hospital death = ☐ %

SAPS II Model for Early Severe Sepsis

The "sepsis syndrome" means the clinical and biological manifestations of infection, no matter what the intensity of the symptoms or the type and timing of infection.

What Are the Problems?

Two main problems exist regarding the definition and grading of sepsis. First the sepsis syndrome is not a diagnosis. It includes urinary infection, pneumonia, septicemia of all origins, and bacteriologic, fungal and viral infections. Is it possible to use a unique model for all these pathologies? Besides, the definitions used in the database can be different from those from the target population. Since the appearance of the anti-endotoxins or anti-cytokine antibodies, therapeutic trials on patients with sepsis have been more frequently conducted. The results, however, are often controversial, which may be due at least in part to the inclusion of all patients with sepsis in the studies, without taking into account the many different types of sepsis. Is it reasonable to include in the same study patients who are septic from urinary sources and patients who have pneumonia, peritonitis, or catheter-related infection? An obviously limiting factor has been the necessity to obtain information on a sufficiently large number of patients to perform the desired statistical comparisons.

Secondly, until recently, there has been no proposed grading of sepsis, which is why the reported mortality rates from sepsis have differed widely: 30% in steroid trials [5], 20% in the Veterans Administration Cooperative Study [6], 35% in the HAIA [7].

Subjective Grading of Sepsis

In 1991, the American College of Chest Physicians (ACCP) [8] proposed a grading of severity of sepsis based on clinical and biologic symptoms assessed at the bedside. Four stages of increasing severity were defined: sepsis, severe sepsis, septic shock, and multiple organ dysfunction syndrome. One of the primary criticisms of the proposed grading system is that, in order to be useful for the selection of patients, the severity of illness as reflected in a probability of mortality should be accurately assessed.

Model Development Strategy

The European North American Study was not specifically designed to build models for patients with sepsis. We collected data for the first ICU day, so the proposed model is only for early ICU sepsis. The definition of confirmed infection at the 24th h was as follows: "Enter "yes" only if cultures, gram stains, or X-rays confirm a suspected infection on admission or new infection that developed in the 1st 24 h, or there is evidence of gross purulence. Laboratory confirmation (including verbal or "fax"-type confirmation) must be obtained by the 24-h stage for "confirmed" to be entered. A confirmed diagnosis from another source is acceptable if cultures are negative because the patient has been on antibiotics.

Patients were classified as having severe sepsis if they manifested systemic inflammatory response syndrome (SIRS) and infection, along with evidence of hypotension, hypoperfusion, or multiple organ dysfunction.

The lack of fit of the original SAPS II model among the patients with sepsis indicates the desirability, especially for clinical trials, of being able to adjust models to correctly reflect the mortality of a specific subgroup of ICU patients. This is important both to verify the success of randomization as evaluated by the comparable severity of illness of control and experimental groups, and to derive a model that can be used to evaluate the success of the trial by comparing the observed and expected outcomes among the control and experimental groups across all strata of probabilities of hospital mortality. Models designed for a precise category of patients can be developed in several ways. One way is to generate entirely independent models with a new set of variables, but this requires a very large developmental effort and enrollment of a large patient database [9]. Another way is to use a variety of factors such as physiology, previous hospitalization, underlying disease, and precipitating factors to generate models with different model coefficients for different subgroups of patients.

Our model development strategy focused on keeping the new models as similar as possible to the existing models, ideally eliminating the need for additional data collection. In a preliminary analysis, we developed models for patients with sepsis by incorporating additional variables into the existing model. This was successful, resulting in a good-fitting model. The ease of customizing the logit rather than adding the variables, however, and the reduced sample size necessary for customizing the logit, made it a more appealing alternative for developing models that can be useful for patients with severe sepsis.

Our purpose was not necessarily to develop the definitive model for this group, especially given the limitations on our ability to define them precisely with the available data. Our goal was to demonstrated the success of the customization technique using information already easily collected for SAPS II.

The customized SAPS II model for patients with early severe sepsis (number of patients 1128) (from [11])

Constant $\beta = -3.5524$

SAPS II score $\beta = 0.0694$

$$\text{Probability of mortality} = \frac{e^{\beta_0 + \beta_1 \times \text{SAPS II score}}}{1 + e^{\beta_0 + \beta_1 (\text{SAPS II score})}}$$

At this point, this model is appropriate only for patients with severe sepsis who are defined in the same manner as in our study, and it needs to first be validated in another independent group of patients, using the same definitions. For a therapeutic trial with different definitions, it would be necessary to evaluate the fit of this model in that group to determine whether customized models needed to be generated.

It would be possible, for example, to develop customized models for pneumonia, urinary sepsis, abdominal sepsis, or sepsis with gram-positive microorganisms. In these cases it would be much easier to use the published scores and to customize them if necessary, rather than to add more variables and generate new models.

The customized models we present were developed among patients hospitalized for at least 1 day in the ICU. They use the worst physiologic measurements in the 1st 24 h (SAPS II). Models that are applicable at later time periods in the ICU for assessing the severity of patients with sepsis and evaluating the outcome of clinical trials for patients becoming septic after 24 h still need to be developed.

All the proposed models are derived from a large database, in which diseases are recorded with definitions - or more often without precise definitions - spectrum and inclusion criteria which may not be the same as those used in a trial. Inclusion or exclusion criteria in a trial may concern characteristics which could hardly be prospectively recorded in the original data base. It is not conceivable that a large database could contain all the information which could fulfill all the requirements of actual and future trials. This must lead to the rejection of comparisons between an expected mortality rate, given by a model derived from a large database, and an observed mortality rate in a treatment group. In a recent critique of scoring systems, Loirat [10] favors the opposite method by using a simpler tool without any weight for acute disease. For a trial, a specific model could be derived from the score and patients or disease characteristics in one-half of the control group. This model could be used to assess comparability between the second control half and the treatment group, which would be less expensive than repetition of trials without significant result.

Conclusions

The customization technique using SAPS II gives a model for early severe ICU sepsis, evaluated not only by the are under the ROC curves but with the goodness-of-fit test. In the future, therapeutic trials must be conducted on more narrowly defined groups of patients with sepsis. It would be more scientifically desirable to conduct trials on sepsis from a single cause, although the number of patients may be small. In these trials, the use of a customized model may be the simplest and best method for assessing the success of the study therapy.

References

1. Haneley JA, McNeil BJ (1982) The meaning and use of the area under a receiver operating characteristic (ROC) curve. Radiology 143: 29-36
2. Hosmer DW, Lemeshow S (1989) Applied Logistic Regression. Wiley, New York
3. Le Gall Jr, Lemeshow S, Saulnier F (1993) A new simplified acute physiology score (SAPS II) based on a European North American Multicenter Study. JAMA 270: 2957-2963
4. Selker HP (1993) Systems for comparing actual and predicted mortality rates: characteristics to promote cooperation in improving hospital care. Ann Intern Med 118: 820-822
5. Bone RC, Fisher CJ Jr, Clemmer TP, Slotman GJ, Metz CA, Balk RA (1987) A controlled clinical trial of high dose methylprednisolone in the treatment of severe sepsis and septic shock. N Engl J Med 317: 653-658
6. Veterans Administration Systemic Sepsis Comparative Study Groups (1987) Effects of high dose glucocorticoid therapy on mortality in patients with clinical signs of sepsis. N Engl J Med 317: 659-665
7. Ziegler EJ, Fisher CJ Jr, Sprung CL, et al. (1991) Treatment of gram negative bacteremia and septic shock with HA 1 A human monoclonal antibody against endotoxin. N Engl J Med 324: 429-436
8. American College of Chest Physicians/Society of Critical Care Medicine Consensus Conference (1992) Definitions for sepsis and organ failure and guidelines for the use of innovative therapies in sepsis. Crit Care Med 20: 864-874
9. Knaus WA, Harrel FE, Fisher CJ, Wagner DP, Obal SM, Sadoff JC, Draper EA, Walawander LA, Conboy KGR, Grasela TH (1993) The clinical evaluation of new drugs for sepsis. A prospective study design based on survival analysis. JAMA 270: 1233-1241
10. Loirat P (1994) Critique of existing scoring systems: admission scores. Rean Urg: 173-175
11. Le Gall JR, LeMesnow S, LeLeu G, Klar J, Huillard J, Rué M, Teres D, Artigas A (1995) JAMA 273: 644-650

Physiologic State Classification and Bayesian Probability Analysis as a Technique for Stratification of Severity and Prediction of Outcome in Human Post-Traumatic Sepsis and ARDS

J.H. Siegel, D. Rixen, A. Abu-Salih, M. Bertolini, F. Panagakos, N. Espina

A technique of Physiologic State classification has been developed based in the multivariable analysis of patient-derived data sets of 17 physiologic variables: mean arterial pressure (MAP), right arterial pressure (RAP), heart rate (HR), systolic ejection time (ET), mixed venous oxygen tension (PvO_2), mixed venous carbon dioxide tension ($PvCO_2$), mixed venous pH (pHv), arteriovenous oxygen content difference (Ca-vO_2D), and three variables obtained from the indocyanine green dye dilution curve, the cardiac index (CI), the cardiac mixing time (Tm) obtained from the exponential dye washout, which is related to the cardiac ejection fraction (EFx), and the dispersive mean transit time (Td), which is related to the pulmonary blood flow mean transit time through the lung. In addition, derived variables are included which are related to oxygen consumption per square mater body surface area (VO_2/m^2), the arterial base excess (BEA), the total peripheral resistance (TPR), the respiratory index (RI) which is the alveolar-arterial oxygen gradient normalized by the arterial oxygen tension, the percent shunt (Qs/Qt) and the carbon dioxide tension ($PaCO_2$).

To develop this physiologic classification system, 1120 multivariable data sets obtained from 338 critically ill patients requiring intensive care were normalized by the mean and the standard deviation of this same data set in a group of recovering trauma patients who were not critically ill. The resulting normalized 17 variable sets were then clustered so as to allow the data-derived physiologic patterns to become evident [1-3]. Seven independent data groupings were developed. These were: a pattern characteristic of the normal stress response hyperdynamic state seen post-trauma and in compensated sepsis (A State); a pattern characteristic of the metabolic insufficiency seen in septic decompensation and in patients with end-state cirrhotic liver disease (B State); two State patterns characteristic of early (C_1) and late (C_2) respiratory insufficiency associated with the development of the adult respiratory distress syndrome (ARDS); a pattern characteristic of cardiogenic decompensation seen in myocardial infarction, or with septic or ischemic myocardial decompensation (D State); and a State seen in post-trauma patients who have hypovolemia without shock (H state).

Figure 1 shows the prototype patterns for the A, B, C_2 and D States normalized by the mean and standard deviations of the reference recovering trauma patients (perfect circle at 0 standard deviations).

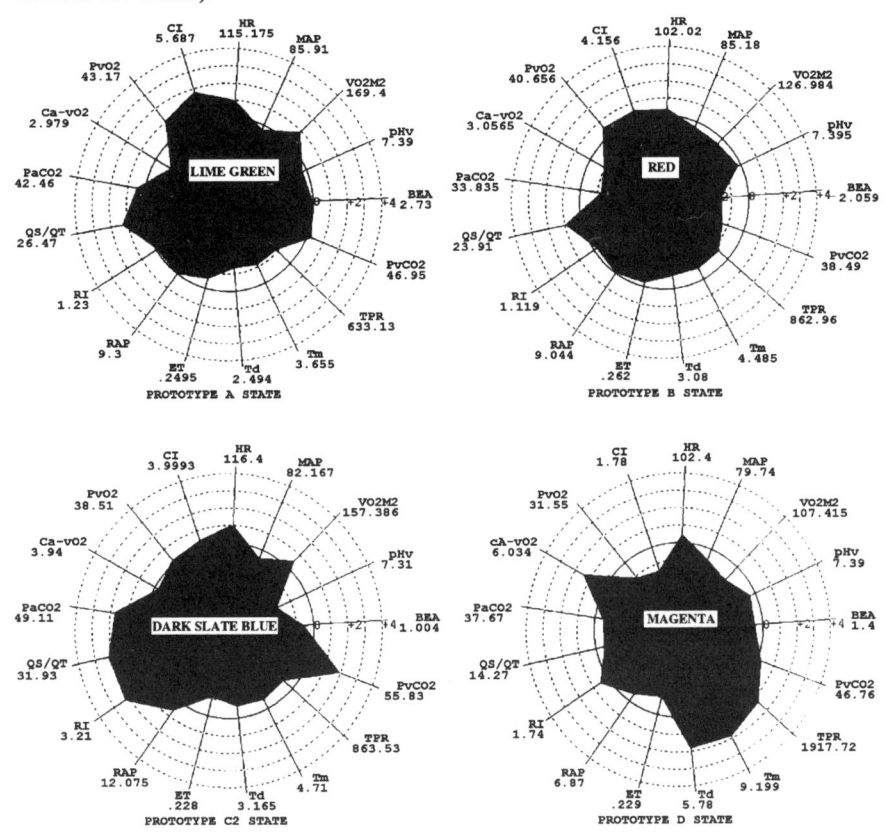

Fig. 1: Prototype of Physiologic States referenced to R State of control nonseptic recovering of trauma patients at zero standard deviations. All values are shown scaled by mean and standard deviation of R State controls: A State, normal stress response; B State, metabolic insufficiency; C_2 State, late combined metabolic and respiratory insufficiency; D State, cardiogenic decompensation. Each pattern is colored to assist recognition

Each of these State cluster centers forms a nodal point in a physiologic hyperspace to which new patients can be referenced, on the basis of their individual physiologic pattern. This allows a pseudo-distance within the hyperspace to be developed for each patient at a given time from each of the State centers (A, B, C_1, C_2, D, etc.) (Fig. 2). The center closest to the patient values allows patient classification with regard to the physiologic State. Since every real patient has some similarity to all of the States, given the limited dimensions of the physiologic universe, a "distance" from each prototypic State also can be developed. More important, our experience in classifying observations from patients who lived or died with various clinical conditions, who fell into these Physiologic States at various times in their clinical course, has enabled us to gather a body of data by which the likelihood of death in each Physiologic State can be determined. This concept is shown in figure 2.

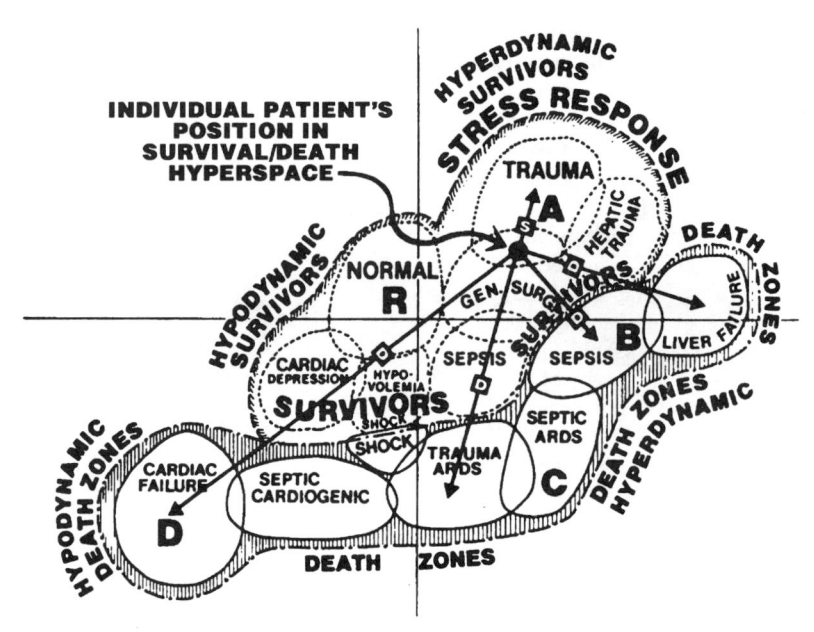

Fig. 2: Conceptual diagram of physiologic hyperspace with State centers noted and "distance" between a given new patient and various State prototypes, in terms of probabilities of being more like the survivors or the deaths in any given State. (From Siegel et al. [1] with permission)

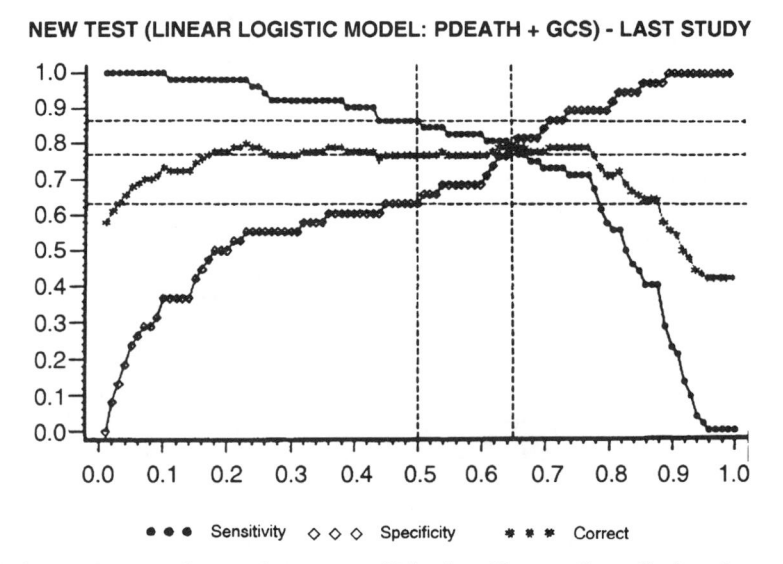

Fig. 3: Sensitivity, specificity and accuracy of Pdeath + Glasgow Coma Scale estimate. Note consistent accuracy over wide range of prior probabilities. For 205 trauma patients not in original development group for Pdeath. (From Siegel et al. [1] with permission)

Since patients move through this physiologic hyperspace with regard to recovery or death, there is the potential for the patient's outcome to be related to some degree to every one of the States. Therefore a set of probabilities of survival or death can be developed for each patient in terms of his or her own pattern's closeness to the pattern of each State. Since the sum of all probabilities must equal one, a probability of death (P death) can be directly obtained by summing the probabilities of survival or death with regard to each of the physiologic prototypic States in the hyperspace. This Bayesian statistical methodology was tested on 205 trauma patients not in the original reference group and shown to be highly accurate [1]. It can be combined with the Glasgow Coma Scale (GCS) in a statistical model which enables the metabolic physiologic probability of death to be estimated in conjunction with the neurologic probability of death. This combined model was tested on the 205 trauma patients at the 0.5 threshold (in order words a 50%/50% prior probability of survival or death), and gave a sensitivity of 87%, a specificity of 63% and a correctness or accuracy of 77%. However, the level of accuracy was highly consistent over a range of thresholds (prior probabilities) from 0.3 to 0.75 [1] (Fig. 3). These data suggest that this probability model can be used in a wide range of cases, even where the real outcome on first seeing the case is actually better or worse than a 50%/50% chance of survival or death. This is often true in Intensive Care Unit patients. The correctness of prediction is shown in Fig. 4, where the observed versus the predicted death rates for the combined Bayesian Pdeath and GCS model are compared for the 205 trauma patients used as a test group for the model [1]. It is important to stress that the predicted Pdeath was made from the first observation data set, but the actual deaths occurred up to 40 days later. The importance of using a physiologically based predictor of outcome rather than an anatomic index only is shown in Fig. 5, which compares the Injury Severity Score (ISS) to the Bayesian Pdeath for the 205 trauma patients with severe injuries requiring ICU care. Note that virtually all of the discrimination between survivors (S) versus deaths (D) occurs in the Bayesian Pdeath axis.

OBSERVED DEATH VERSUS PREDICTED DEATH
NEW TEST (LINEAR LOG. MODEL – PDEATH + GCS) – FIRST STUDY

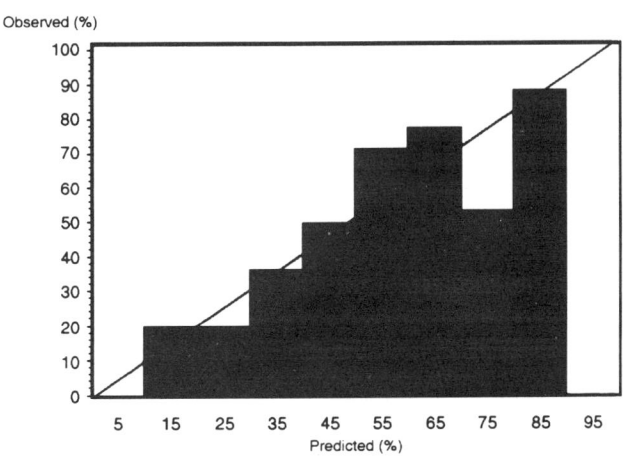

Fig. 4: Correctness of Pdeath + GCS estimate compared to actual patient outcomes based on first observation period. Deaths may have occurred up to 40 days after first estimate of Pdeath. For 205 trauma patients not in original development group for Pdeath (From Siegel et al. [1], with permission)

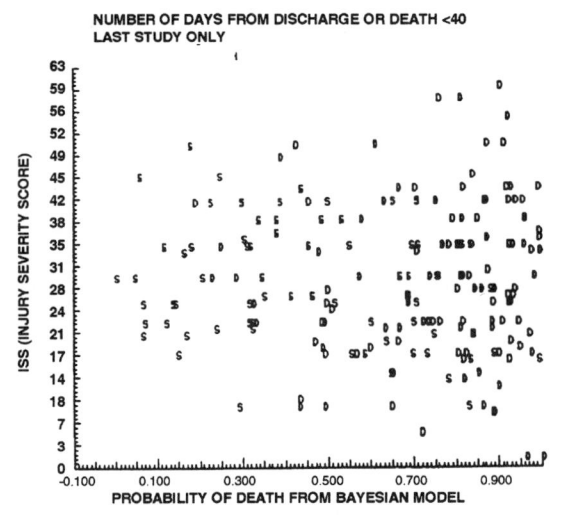

Fig. 5: Comparing Injury Severity Score (ISS) with Pdeath + GCS estimate of severity with regard to patient outcome. Note that nearly all of the discriminant ability is on the Pdeath axis. (From Siegel et al. [1], with permission). Labeled by survival (S) and death (D)

To prospectively evaluate the predictive ability of the Physiologic State classification system to quantify the severity of a given patient's response to traumatic injury and sepsis, a new group of 44 multiple trauma patients were studied from the time of admission to the Surgical Trauma Intensive Care Unit until their successful recovery with discharge from the Critical Care Unit, or until patient demise. In these 44 multiple trauma patients, 273 observation periods were obtained. In addition to the 17 variable staging criteria used for classification of physiologic state, the plasma levels of the cytokines, tumor necrosis factor (TNF), interleukin 1 (IL-1) and interleukin 6 (IL-6) were also determined. The plasma levels of the circulating amino acids, urea, lactate, glucose and the hepatic acute phase proteins: C-reactive protein (CRP), $_1$-antitrypsin (A1TRIP), fibrinogen (FIBRIN), $_2$-macroglobulin (AMACRO), ceruloplasmin (CERUL), transferrin (TRANSF) and albumin (ALBU) were obtained. The urinary levels of the circulating amino acids, urinary urea nitrogen, creatinine and 3-methylhistidine (3MH) were also obtained, as was urinary volume on a 12-h basis. The patients were maintained on nutritional support using either TPN, or a combination of TPN and enteral nutrition. As has been shown previously, the administration of a constant full level of TPN for nutritional support allows the plasma levels of each amino acid to reflect the relative cellular clearance of that amino acid from the circulation.

These 44 multiple trauma patients had a mean age of 42 years (range, 16-79 years) and 77% were males. The mean Injury Severity Score was 28.4 with a range of 16-45, but 21% of these patients had a head injury with a Glasgow Coma Scale (GCS) less than or equal to 12. The causative mechanisms of injury were motor vehicle crash 42.2%, a gunshot wound 24.4%, pedestrian injury 17.8%, a motor cycle crash 6.7%, fall 6.7% and assault 2.2%. Forty-seven percent of these patients had shock on admission to the Trauma Admitting Area and following resuscitation emergency surgery was necessary in 72%. Of these 44 patients, 72% developed sepsis, 36% septic ARDS and exactly 50%, 22 patients, survived to leave the hospital and the other 50% died in the Intensive Care Unit. It is important to emphasize that all but one of these patients (a 64-year-old male who had a previous history of chronic

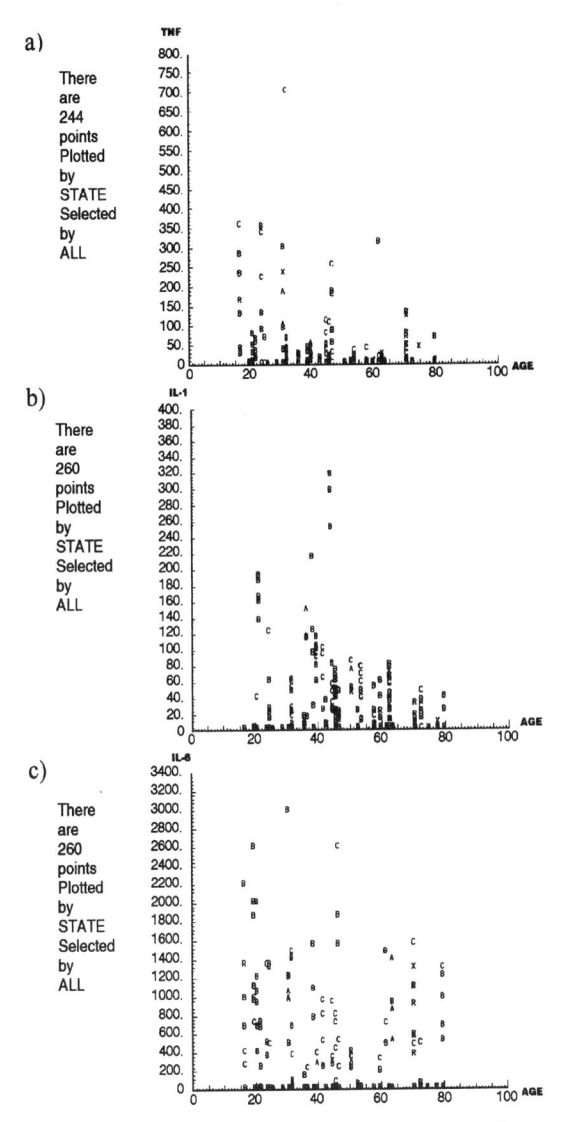

Fig. 6: a) Distribution of plasma TNF (by ELISA) as function of patient age labeled by Physiologic State. Note that nearly all the patient samples with elevated TNF levels were from patients in the B State of metabolic insufficiency or the C_2 State of combined metabolic and respiratory insufficiency. b) Distribution of plasma IL-1 (by ELISA) as a function of patient age labeled by Physiologic State. Note that nearly all these patient samples with elevated IL-1 levels were from patients in the B State of metabolic insufficiency or the C_2 State of combined metabolic and respiratory insufficiency. c) Distribution of plasma IL-6 (by ELISA) as a function of patient age labeled by Physiologic State. Note that nearly all these patient samples with elevated IL-6 levels were from patients in the B State of metabolic insufficiency or the C_2 State of combined metabolic and respiratory insufficiency

obstructive lung disease with prior heart failure) developed a hyperdynamic state following resuscitation and/or surgery, all demonstrated some elevation of fever and all had leukocytosis. Thus, all would have met the criteria for the sepsis syndrome or SIRS [4]. Taken in the aggregate, neither the SIRS nor the sepsis syndrome criteria provided any useful discrimination with regard to true severity or outcome.

However, when the Physiologic State classification was used as a basis for stratification of the cytokine mediator response (Table 1), it can be seen that compared to the control group of nonseptic recovering trauma patients, or to the patients with the A State normal stress response seen in sepsis, the patients with the metabolic insufficiency B State or those with the combined metabolic and respiratory insufficiency C_2 State seen in septic ARDS showed an increased incidence (%) of detectable plasma levels of TNF and IL-1. Since there is a wide range of plasma cytokine levels in critically ill patients it is important to examine the actual spread with respect to the Physiologic State classifications. These are shown in Fig. 6a-c; Fig 6a demonstrates the range of TNF plasma values as a function of age and Physiologic State, Fig. 6b represents the distribution of age and State versus plasma levels of IL-1 and Fig. 6c demonstrates the range of age and State versus plasma levels of IL-6. What is evident in all of these three figures is that, while there are many patients with no circulating levels of cytokines, the overwhelming number of samples with elevated cytokines levels come from patients in the B or C_2 States of metabolic, or combined metabolic and respiratory insufficiency. While there are small number of patient samples taken in the A State and a few in the C_1 State (X), these are mostly from patients in transition between the A and B States or the C_1 and C_2 States. This transition can be quantified by the Physiologic State distances, which enable precise quantification of a patient's movement in the physiologic hyperspace, as shown in Fig. 2.

Utilizing the Physiologic State criteria for the staging of severity in these 44 recent trauma patients not in either of the previously studied patient groups, it was shown that not only did the Physiologic States accurately and significantly predict the likelihood that the patient has a detectable circulating level of the cytokines TNF and IL-1 [5] but, more important, the probability of death (P death) as well as the cytokine levels appeared to be a function of the specific Physiologic State, with the highest levels being seen in the B State of metabolic insufficiency and the C_2 State of combined respiratory and metabolic insufficiency characteristic of septic ARDS. As shown in Table 2, the increase in the magnitude of metabolic abnormalities associated with the transition from nonsepsis to septic A, septic B or septic C_2 States was associated with an increasing probability of death (P death) statistic (mean A State = 0.28, mean B State = 0.57, mean C_2 State = 0.61).

Table 1: Physiologic State classification indicates cytokine response

	Control	A Sepsis	B Sepsis	C_2 Sepsis
Number of observations	17	26	127	80
%Detectable TNF	21	35	53*	55*
(mean plasma level in pg/ml)	(19.2)	(48.5)	(53.5)	(74.4)
% Detectable IL-1	35	35	58**	61*,**
(mean plasma level in pg/ml)	(76.3)	(53.3)	(58.9)	(44.2)
% Detectable IL-6	24	31	39	49
(mean plasma level in pg/ml)	(661)	(785)	(919)	(703)

* p <0.05 vs. control (nonseptic trauma recovery); ** p<0.05 vs. A state

While the Physiologic States are developed on the basis of cardiovascular and blood gas variables, these Physiologic States reflect underlying patterns of metabolic abnormalities [3]. This is also true of the post-trauma septic and ARDS patients whose Physiologic State classification was quantified using the 17-variable Physiologic pattern. As also can be seen in Table 2, progression from the A to B to C_2 State was associated with a significant rise in the mean circulating plasma levels of the gluconeogenic amino acid alanine and in lactate, and these increases in gluconeogenic precursors were associated with a rise in the mean plasma glucose level. The mean plasma levels of other amino acids that were seen to rise, most significantly elevated with these State transitions, were phenylalanine, which to a large extent reflects phenylalanine liberated by muscle proteolysis, and leucine. An effective reprioritization of hepatic acute phase proteins [6] also occurred. There was a progressive rise in C-reactive protein (CRP) as the Physiologic State became more severe. This was associated with a rise in $_2$-macroglobulin (AMACRO) and a fall in transferrin (TRANSF) from control levels. While the mean transferrin level did not decrease further as the patient condition worsened from the A to B to C_2 State, its relative decrease compared to the corresponding circulating levels of CRP, $_2$-macroglobulin and the other acute phase proteins measured was worse in the C_2 State. As also noted, the magnitude of the combined acidosis was also a function of the transition from the A to the B State of metabolic insufficiency, or the C_2 State of combined metabolic and respiratory insufficiency. The increasing base deficit of the B and C_2 States reflects the rise in the total of all metabolic acids released into the extracellular fluid, including lactate, amino acids, and other acid products released by an inadequate oxidative metabolism. In Table 2, it can also be seen that the mean Pdeath (computed from metabolic parameters only, for all samples in each of the Physiologic States) shows a progressive rise in Pdeath compared to either control or the A State as the patient's Physiologic State classifications worsened to the B and C_2 States. The increase in Pdeath in these two States was shown to be statistically significant ($p < 0.05$) compared to that found in either the A State or in the control nonseptic trauma recovering patients.

Table 2: Associated mean plasma levels of amino acids, acute phase proteins, lactate, glucose and base excess

	Control	A Sepsis	B Sepsis	C_2 Sepsis
Alanine (mM/l)	103.7	96.73	118.8[a]	145.7[c]
Phenylalanine (mM/l)	38.51	44.76	49.88	64.21[d,e]
Leucine (mM/l)	42.36	68.95	78.02	85.15[d]
C-Reactive protein (µg/ml)	185.3	208.6	249.7	257.5
α_2-Macroglobulin (mg/ml)	1.23	1.16	1.24	1.47
Transferrin (mg/ml)	1.37	1.29	1.26	1.28
Lactate (mM/l)	1.22	1.25	1.61	1.89
Glucose (mg/ml)	141	139	154	158
Base excess (mM/l)*	0.99	2.20	-1.07[a,b]	-2.0[c]
Pdeath for State	0.27	0.28	0.57[a,b]	0.61[c,d]

[a]$p < 0.05$, B vs. A, [b]$p < 0.05$, B vs. control, [c]$p < 0.05$ C_2 vs. A, [d]$p < 0.05$, C_2 vs. control
[e]$p < 0.05$, C_2 vs. B
* Negative base excess = Base deficit

Finally, each patient was considered as a single entity with regard to the prediction of outcome as a function of the predominant Physiologic State classification manifested by that patient during his or her entire ICU clinical course. When this was done (Table 3) examination of the mean Pdeath for each patient as a function of his or her predominant State showed that there were no deaths of patients whose predominant State was that of a normal stress response A State. The average of the mean Pdeath for all these patients, both survivors and deaths, was only 0.26. However, as the predominant State classification became more severe, the overall average of the mean Pdeath increased to 0.53 for those in a B State and 0.64 for C_2 State patients. Considering survivors versus deaths it can be seen that the overall Pdeath for all survivors in any State was 0.39, compared to the overall Pdeath of 0.63 for all of the deaths regardless of State. Interestingly, the average of the estimates mean Pdeath for all 44 patients was 0.50 and the actual death rate was also 50%. Most important, however, was the fact that within a given State the deaths had a higher Pdeath than the survivors. In patients with the B State the survivors had a mean Pdeath of 0.47, whereas the deaths had a mean of Pdeath of 0.59. In the C_2 State, only one patient who had predominant C_2 State was found in the survivors; he had a Pdeath of 0.09 and was probably inadequately ventilated, producing a false C_2 State due to a rise in transient $PaCO_2$. However, the mean Pdeath in the C_2 State deaths was 0.72.

A summary of the pattern of changes in metabolic parameters and cytokine mediators as a function of the States is shown in Fig. 7, where the variables of interest are demonstrated, not in terms of their actual values but in terms of their standard deviations, increased or decreased, from the reference group of recovering nonseptic Trauma patients at zero standard deviations. Examining septic patient observation periods in A, B or C_2 States, it can be seen that there was a progressive increase in TNF and in the plasma levels of alanine, leucine, tyrosine, phenylalanine and lactate as well as glucose as the State classification increased in severity. A reprioritization of the acute phase proteins was seen in the more severe states and there was a progressive increase in base deficit (negative base excess) with patient transitions from the A to B to C_2 States. Of great interest, as noted previously [3], is the fact that B State patients with severe metabolic insufficiency have a markedly reduced $VO2/m^2$ compared to the other States. The progressive rise in calculated Pdeath as a function of the severity of State classification is also shown.

Table 3: Pdeath as a function of the predominant physiologic state manifested by patients during the entire ICU clinical course

	Mean Pdeath for patients with predominant			
	A	B	C_2	All states
Survivors				
Mean Pdeath	0.26	0.47	0.09	0.39
(n)	(7)	(14)	(1)	(22)
Death				
Mean Pdeath	0a	0.59a,b	0.72a,b	0.63a
(n)	(0)	(14)	(7)	(22)
All survivors and deaths				
Mean Pdeath	0.26	0.53b	0.64b	0.50
(n)	(7)	(28)	(8)	(44)

[a]p <0.05 death vs. survivors, [b]p <0.05 vs. A state

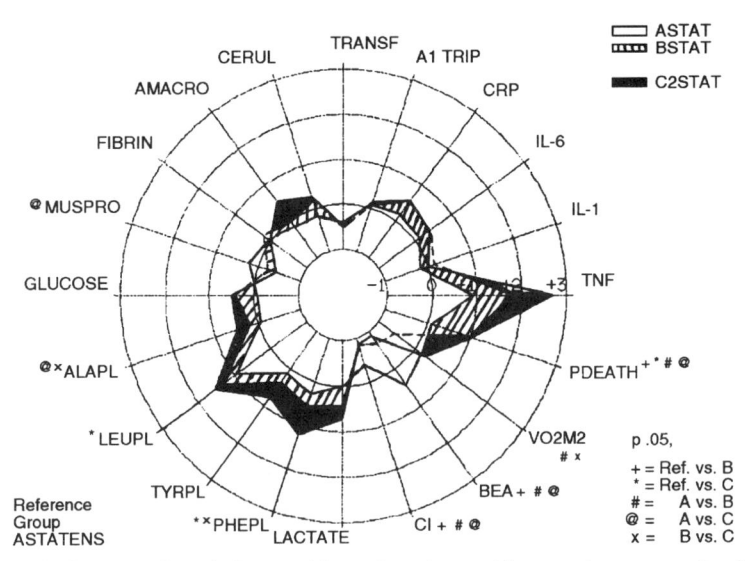

Fig. 7: Circle diagram of metabolic variables and cytokines with mean changes noted as functions of the patient's Physiologic State classification at time of plasma or urine samples. Scale in standard deviation from nonseptic A State control patients recovering from trauma. Significance levels noted at p<0.05. TNF, tumor necrosis factor; IL-1, interleukin 1; IL-6, interleukin 6; CRP, C-reactive protein; A1TRIP, α_1-antitrypsin; TRANSF, transferrin; CERUL, ceruloplasmin; AMACRO, α_2-macroglobulin; FIBRIN, fibrinogen; MUSPRO, muscleproteolysis/12h; GLUCOSE, glucose plasma level; ALAPL, alanine plasma level; LEUPL, leucine plasma level; TYRPL, tyrosine plasma level; PHEPL, phenylalanine plasma level; LACTATE, lactate plasma level; CI, cardiac index; BEA, base excess; VO_2m^2, oxygen consumption per square meter body surface area; PDEATH, probability of death

Finally the time course of a specific patient with respect to the change in cytokine levels, cardiac index, and shunt is shown in Fig. 8. Figures 9-13 show the Physiologic State profile classifications at various time periods during the patient's physiologic course. This patient was a 31-year-old man involved in a serious motor vehicle crash who sustained a major grade IV laceration of the right lobe of the liver, a left femur fracture and a left open fracture of the left tibia and fibula. On admission he had an ISS of 34, was profoundly hypotensive and was taken immediately to the operating room where the abdomen was opened, the laceration partially repaired by suture and the liver then packed because of the patient's hypothermia and coagulopathy. The fractures of the left lower extremity were stabilized and the open tibial fracture lavaged, but no attempt was made to perform internal fixation because of the severe post-injury and emergency surgery physiologic instability. On admission to the Intensive Care Unit the patient manifested a persistent base deficit, but was able to maintain a hyperdynamic cardiovascular response which was progressively increased by volume and inotropic support. After the 1st postoperative day, the patient became mildly febrile and had leukocytosis and would therefore have qualified for the SIRS syndrome. He developed an immediate post-trauma fulminant ARDS syndrome [7] with a 39% shunt (Qs/Qt) manifested by a C_2 State (Fig. 9), which was managed by ventilatory support and diuresis. As shown in Fig. 8, during this immediate postinjury ARDS phase the patient maintained a plasma level of IL-1. By the 4th postinjury day (Fig. 10) the postinjury ARDS had resolved but the patient began to show signs of sepsis syndrome but was in A State physiologic response. Sepsis progressed and he developed evidence of septic ARDS and oscillated between the C_2 and B State from the 5th to the 9th postinjury day. As the septic ARDS developed, he had plasma levels first of IL-1 and then a progressive and sustained, though failing, level of TNF with large pulses of IL-6, all the while maintaining a hyperdynamic state with cardiac index ranging between 7 and 8 liters per minute per square meter BSA and a shunt (Qs/Qt) which reached 30%. As control of the sepsis was achieved with antibiotics and by CT-guided drainage of a perihepatic collection the patient returned to an A State physiologic response (though with acidosis which later resolved) with a decrease in all cytokine levels to nondetectable values by ELISA. The physiologic profiles of this patient are shown during the peak septic ARDS response (C_2 State) on day 7 (Fig. 11) at which time he had high levels of both TNF and IL-6 (Fig. 8); on day 9 (B State) (Fig. 12) when the TNF level was declining, although there was a pulse level of IL-6; and on day 10 (Fig. 13) when he returned to the A State with nondetectable cytokine levels. It is clear that the physiologic classification staging was of value in understanding the physiologic host defense response of the patient and was also useful in determining whether the therapeutic modalities utilized were resulting in a reduction of severity earlier than might have been detected by conventional means.

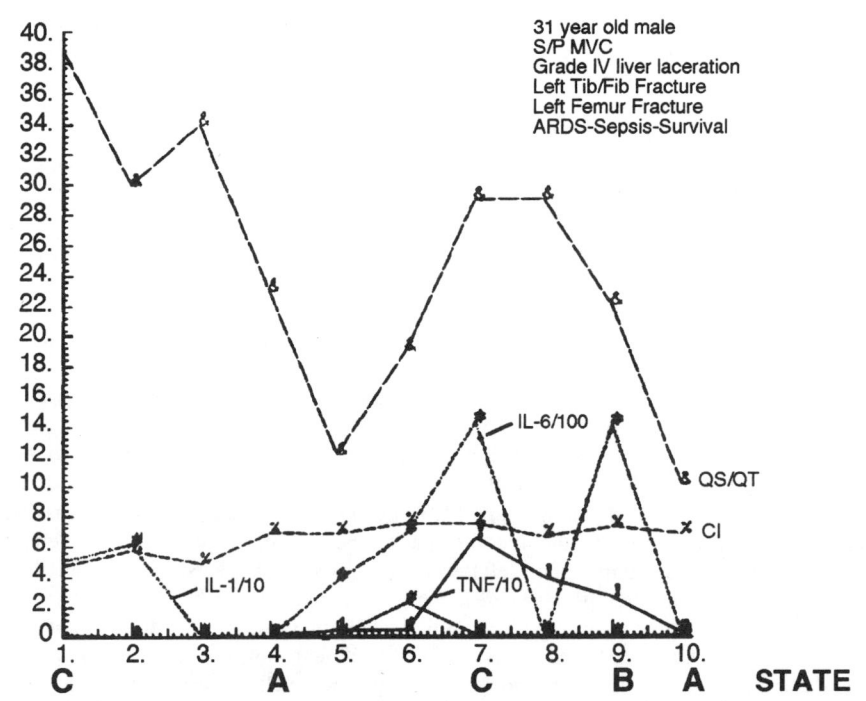

Fig. 8: Patient #0729, a 31-year-old motor vehicle crash patient. Time course of cardiac index (CI), percent shunt (QS/QT) and plasma cytokine levels (ELISA) of TNF (pg/ml), IL-1 (pg/ml divided by 10) and IL-6 (pg/ml divided by 100). Below are noted Physiologic State classifications of patient at time of samples (see Figs. 9-13 for actual patient circle diagrams of States at time noted. This patient was previously shown in ref. [5])

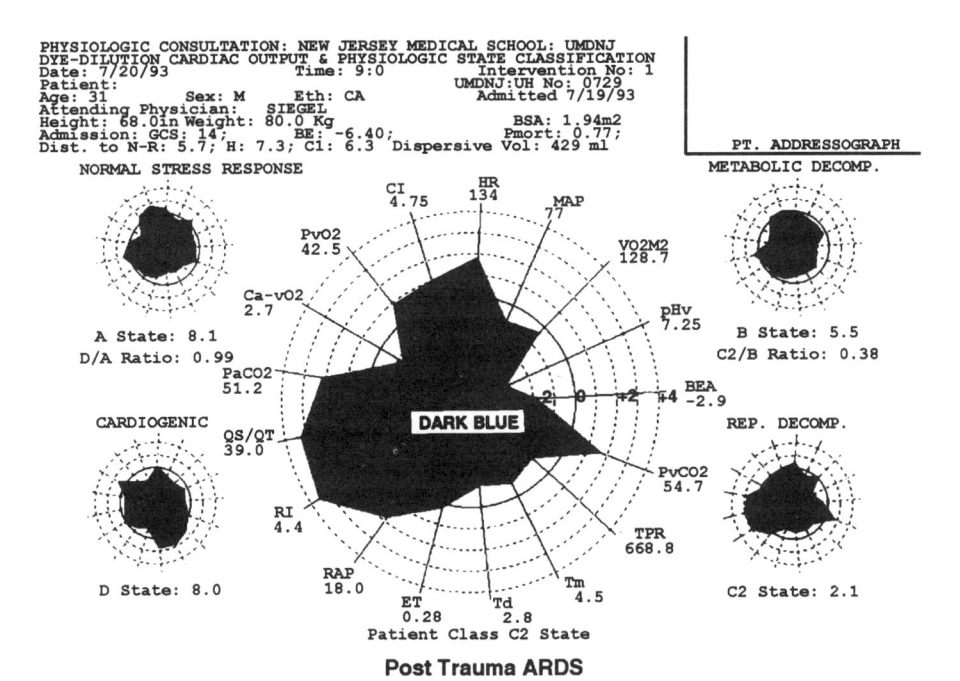

Fig. 9: Patient #0729; initial study, C2 State, post-trauma ARDS

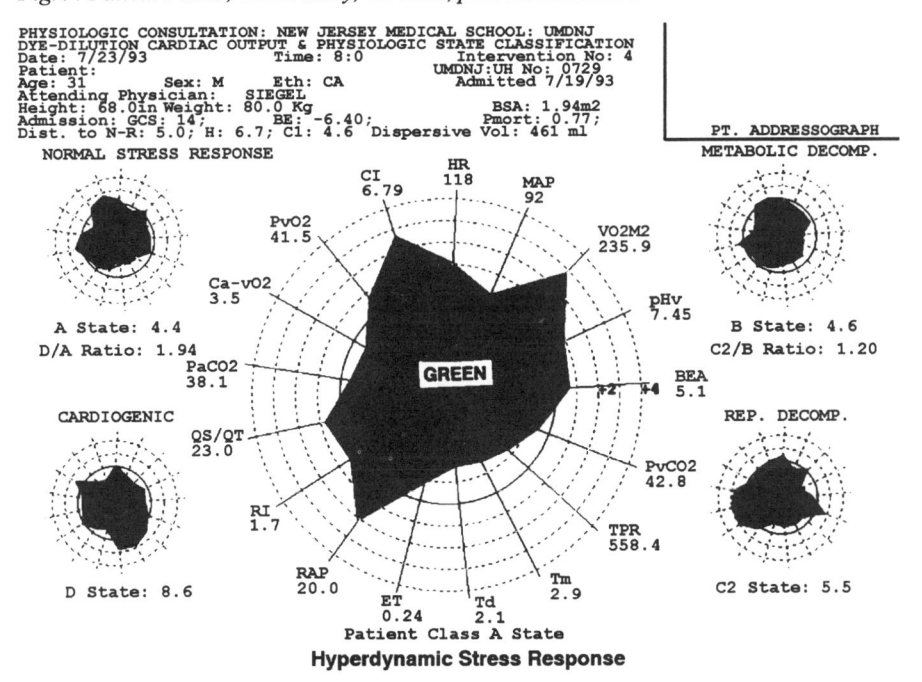

Fig. 10: Patient #0729; 4th postinjury day, A State, hyperdynamic stress response

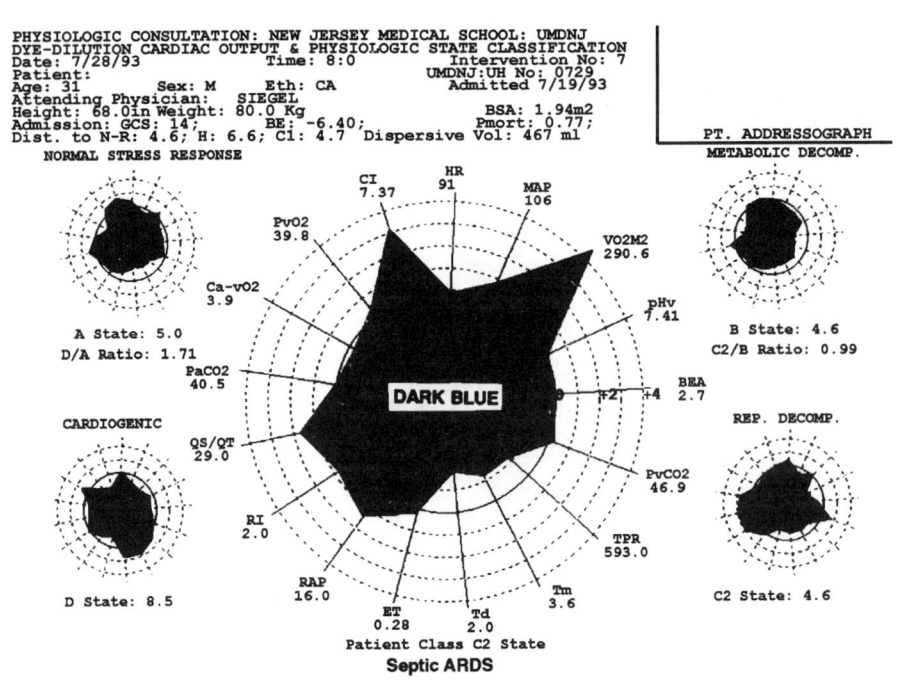

Fig. 11: Patient #0729; 7th postinjury day, C2 State, septic ARDS

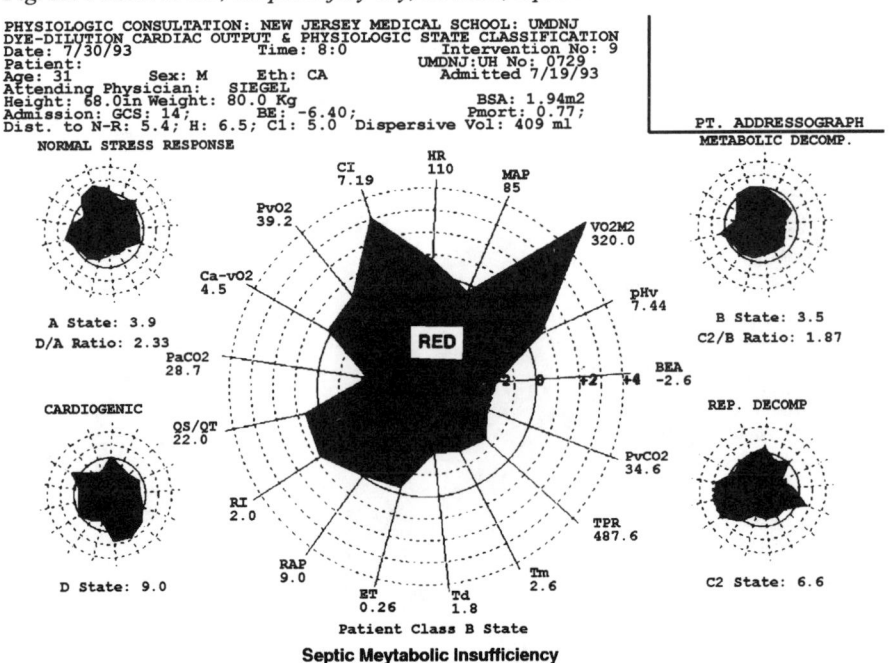

Fig. 12. Patient #0729; 9th postinjury day, B State, septic metabolic insufficiency

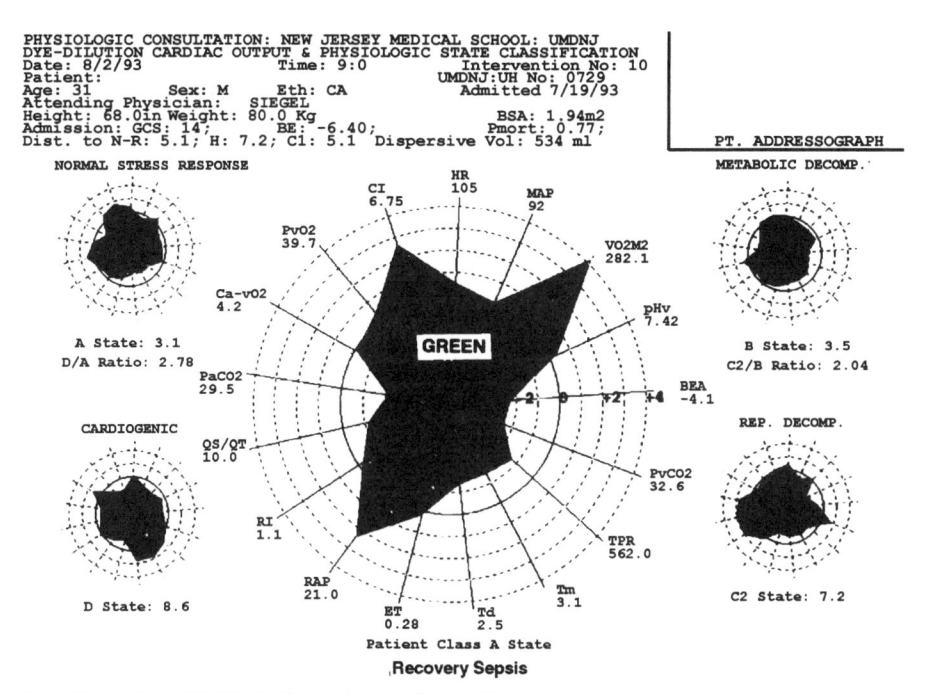

Fig. 13: Patient #0729; 10th postinjury day, A State, recovering sepsis

Conclusion

These data suggest that the severity of post-traumatic septic critical illness can be quantified by a precise statistical procedure using multivariable pattern recognition and Bayesian probability analysis. An immediately obtainable computer-generated probability of survival and Physiologic State classification enables the stratification of patients into classes which reflect underlying cytokine mediator and metabolic response abnormalities not present in the original classification data. Moreover, this technique accurately stratifies the patient with regard to the physiologic type of disease process, and ranks their present degree of severity based on the instantaneous Bayesian probability of death related to the patient's physiologic pattern and the moment of observation. Thus, not only can appropriate stratification for clinical trials be determined, but patients of comparable severity can be then randomized in a prospective fashion with regard to a new therapeutic program and this program validly compared to best standard therapy.

These data also suggest that post-trauma patients with sepsis and/or septic ARDS can be stratified by the Physiologic State classification [1] with a greater degree of precision than can be carried out by the more heuristic criteria such as those used for determining sepsis syndrome - SIRS [4]. Septic patients who manifest either a B State of metabolic insufficiency or a C_2 State of combined metabolic and respiratory insufficiency have a higher frequency of elevated cytokine levels, with detectable TNF and IL-1 being statistically significant in the B and C_2 States compared to A State septic patients or to control nonseptic recovering trauma patients. In addition, patients with B and C_2 States demonstrated increased levels of circulating leucine, phenylalanine and lactate with the gluconeogenic amino acid and lactate increases being associated with hyperglycemia. They also manifested evidence of reprioritization of hepatic acute phase proteins and metabolic acidosis. These patterns of physiologic mediator and metabolic abnormalities were associated with a higher probability of death (Pdeath). It is suggested that the use of Physiologic State classification provides a quantifiable means of stratification (the States) and an index of severity (Pdeath) which can be utilized in prospective randomized trials of new therapeutic modalities.

Acknowledgement. This study met requirements for human investigations by the IRB of New Jersey Medical School: UMDNJ. The metabolic studies were supported in part by the Wesley J. Howe endowed Professorial Chair in Trauma Surgery, held by Dr. John H. Siegel, M.D.

References

1. *Siegel JH, Goodzari S, Coleman WP, Malcolm D, et al. (1993) Quantifying the severity of the human response to injury and sepsis as a guide to the interpretation of pathophysiologic cytokine effects. In: Schlag G, Redl H, Traver D (eds.) 3rd Wiggers Bernard conference on shock, sepsis and organ failure. Springer, Berlin, Heidelberg, New York, pp. 163-204*
2. *Friedman HP, Goldwyn RM, Siegel JH (1975) The use and interpretation of multivariable methods in the classification stages of serious infectious disease processes in the critically ill. In: Elashoff R (ed.) Perspectives in biometrics. Academic, New York, pp. 81-122*
3. *Siegel JH, Cerra FB, Coleman B, et al. Physiologic and metabolic patterns in human sepsis. Surgery 85: 163-193*
4. *Bone RC and members of the American College of Chest Physicians/Societies of Critical Care Medicine Consensus Conference Committee (1992) Definitions for sepsis and organ failure and guidelines for the use of innovative therapies in sepsis. Crit Care Med 20: 8664-8874*
5. *Rixen D, Siegel JH, Abu-Salih A, Bertolini M, Panagakos F, Espina N (1995) Physiology state severity classification as an indicator of posttrauma cytokine response. Shock 4: 27-38*
6. *Sganga G, Siegel JH, Brown G, et al. (1985) Reprioritization of hepatic plasma protein release in trauma and sepsis. Arch Surg 120: 187-199*
7. *Rivkind AI, Siegel JH, Guadalupi P, Littleton M (1989) Sequential patterns of eicosanoid, platelet and neutrophil interactions in the evolution of the fulminant post traumatic adult respiratory distress syndrome. Ann Surg 210: 355-373*

Epilogue - Toward a Consensus

A.E. Baue

Introduction

An important characteristic of a physician is his or her curiosity about human disease. Patients expect diagnosis, treatment, and sympathetic care, but advances result from observation of changing disease patterns, new syndromes, research contributions, and better methods of support and therapy. Significant recent advances in technology and in molecular biology have contributed to the development and understanding of new disease processes and syndromes in which patients may initially survive an illness or an injury that would previously have been fatal in an early period, only to develop complications later. So it is with multiple organ failure (MOF), which was clearly defined in 1975 as a "syndrome" of surgical progress [1].
Physicians also have a great interest in naming things, particularly disease entities. We may aspire to be an Osler, Halsted, Blalock, Graham, or Churchill. Some may also hope to describe a disease, syndrome, or an operation and then be a follower of Zollinger, Ellison, Mallory, Weiss, Fallot, or Taussig. Eponyms, when used appropriately, give credit to our heros and those who labor in the vineyards of surgery and medicine. Original terms, eponyms, phrases, or acronyms are fun. They acknowledge those who have made contributions and remind us of our medical history. Our heritage is important to all of us. There also seems to be some interest or desire to modify, rename, redesignate, or develop a totally new description of a disease, a clinical entity, or a syndrome. Reasons, of course, can be very appropriate to change from an eponym to a descriptive phase so as to better describe a disease entity. For this reason, the Pancoast tumor or syndrome has now become known as the superior sulcus syndrome, but both descriptions are still used. One did not supplant the other. The Mallory-Weiss syndrome is a much more interesting term than post-emetic esophageal mucosal tears with bleeding. The Boerhaave syndrome is as descriptive a term as post-emetic esophageal rupture. This also includes acronyms such as the WPW syndrome (Wolf-Parkinson-White). A number of acronyms catch on such as ARDS, the adult respiratory distress syndrome. This is written as such but spelled out when spoken. The earlier term developed by surgeons for what was happening during the time of the Vietnam conflict was post-traumatic pulmonary insufficiency, but this expression never caught on. The acquired immunodeficiency syndrome (AIDS) is brief, descriptive and certainly irreplaceable.
It is appropriate and worthwhile to participate in evolving terminology as patient care and syndromes evolve and as we attempt to better clarify or describe what is happening. Some

individuals may have the need to name an entity themselves. So it has been with MOF, which has been written MOF but also spelled out when spoken. It has caught on. It is well established in medical terminology and recognized internationally. Despite this situation, changes continue to be recommended. Could some of these recommendations strive to fulfill the couplet of James Russell Lowell? "Though old the thought and oft expressed, tis his at last who says it best" (from *An Autograph*).

The MODS Proposal

You have now read about the proposals to use the expressions SIRS, the systemic inflammatory response syndrome, and the multiple organ dysfunction syndrome (MODS). The origin of these expressions and proposals may be of interest to the reader as we evaluate how they came about.

Dr. Roger Bone and the Methylprednisone Sepsis Study Group reported in 1987 on the negative results of a clinical trial of this drug in sepsis [2]. As an addendum to that study, they described the sepsis syndrome in 1989 as the systemic response to infection, which was expressed as tachycardia, either fever or hypothermia, and evidence of inadequate organ perfusion or dysfunction [3]. This they stated was a valid clinical entity. In February 1991, Bone [4] appropriately made a plea for comparable definitions and defined the terms bacteremia, septicemia (which he recommended no longer be used), sepsis, the sepsis syndrome, septic shock, and refractory shock. Other terms were proposed such as the septic response without infection or the non-bacteremic septic inflammatory state and a slang expression-septoid (Table 1). In July 1991 Bone [5] again proposed the creation of a standard specific nomenclature for sepsis and related terms in order to eliminate confusion and promote comparative clinical investigation. The sepsis syndrome was further defined as a clinical state of pyrexia, leukocytosis, altered mentation with hypermetabolism, and a hyperdynamic circulation. Certainly, Bone's recommendations were important, well thought out and also well-intentioned. In that same month, Sprung [6] wrote that septicemia is an essential term that should be preserved. Sprung disagreed with the other definitions of Bone but saluted his efforts for trying to reach a consensus on terminology. In August, 1991 the Canadian Multiple Organ Failure Study Group published an article titled "Sepsis - Clarity of existing terminology - or more confusion" [7]. They stressed the importance of separating infection as a microbial phenomenon from the septic or inflammatory response of the host from a number of other causes. They also reemphasized the need to reach agreement on the definitions of MOF. This was in spite of the fact that comparable definitions had been provided by Faist et al. [8], Knaus et al. [9], and many others. These definitions are similar and have been generally accepted by many investigators. It would be easy to agree on definitions of organ failures, if anyone wished to agree. The authors of various descriptions and scores for MOF are shown in Table 2 of my previous chapter - Prologue. I am reminded that, many years ago, Hinshaw [10] proposed the use of a common shock model, so that results from various laboratories could be compared. Of course, no one used it. In fact, Hinshaw invited a number of shock investigators to come to Oklahoma City and demonstrate their sepsis models, which were all different. This was done but, in spite of this, there was never general agreement on a sepsis model to be used by many other laboratories. In May of 1992, Benjamin et al. [11] proposed a new expression "the systemic hypoxic and inflammatory syndrome" which they wished to substitute for Bone's sepsis syndrome. This neologism of Benjamin et al. sought to emphasize cellular hypoxia and unregulated inflammation.

Table 1: Terms proposed for infection and inflammation

Infection - bacteria
Bacteremia - bacteria
Sepsis - originally bacteria
Sepsis syndrome, infection, or inflammation or necrotic or ischemic tissue
Septic response without infection
Non-bacteremic septic inflammatory state
Septoid

Certainly, this was a good principal. Unbeknownst to some of these authors, a consensus conference of the Society of Critical Care Medicine and the American College of Chest Physicians was held in August 1991 and reported, along with accompanying editorials, but with different titles, in the journals of these societies in 1992 [12-15]. The conference group hoped to standardize the terminology in this area. They made two recommendations. The first was to use the phrase "systemic inflammatory response syndrome" (SIRS) for an inflammatory response. They recommended that if SIRS was due to infection, that it then be termed sepsis. Infection, bacteremia, and sepsis were defined, and the term bacteremia was eliminated. Sprung attended the conference but must not have prevailed on that point. The term sepsis syndrome described by Bone et al. was also discarded. The consensus group defined severe sepsis and sepsis-induced hypotension with septic shock being a subset of severe sepsis. The group then indicated that conventional terminology for MOF was "inadequate to accurately characterize this syndrome." They then proposed the expression "multiple organ dysfunction syndrome" (MODS) to correct this "inadequacy." They stated "the detection of altered organ function in the acutely ill patient constitutes a syndrome." MODS was defined as the "presence of altered function in an acutely ill patient such that homeostasis cannot be maintained without intervention." Individual organ dysfunctions were not defined, and a classification of MODS was not developed at this conference. The consensus makers, however, did indicate that MODS may be either primary, such as early dysfunction after an insult, or secondary, developing as a result of a host response such as with infection. This sounds identical to the early or first stage and late or second stage, or double-hit development of MOF, which had been described by Faist et al. [8] previously. The consensus group seemed to be starting all over again to develop a new set of definitions. Many who attended the conference could probably modify their previous descriptions of various organ failures and quickly come up with a new set of organ dysfunctions rather than failures.

Will These Proposals Succeed?

"And the whole world was of one language and of one speech." "Therefore is the name of it called Babel because the Lord did there confound the language of all of the Earth: and from thence did the Lord scatter them abroad upon the face of the Earth." Genesis 11:1-9.
The proposal to supplant MOF with MODS and SIRS has some advantages and has certainly stirred up the world of intensivists, surgeons, and physicians. In that sense, the proposal has already made a contribution, because it has made all of us think more clearly and carefully about what we are doing. The matter of a common terminology accepted by everyone with

definitions of the various categories may be difficult to achieve. The reason why I say this is it has never happened before in medical history that a large group has ever been totally in agreement on terminology or methodology. This is illustrated in Fig. 1. Although MOF has served us well, there will always be new classifications proposed, with good reasons for them. Thus MODS and SIRS are not the final expressions in the lexicographic sweepstakes. Attempts to develop standard animal shock and sepsis models (hemorrhage, endotoxin, fecal pellets, cecal ligation and puncture, *E. coli* infusion, and others) to evaluate therapy have not been successful. Clinical symptoms of MOF, sepsis, sepsis syndrome, and others have not been accepted by all.

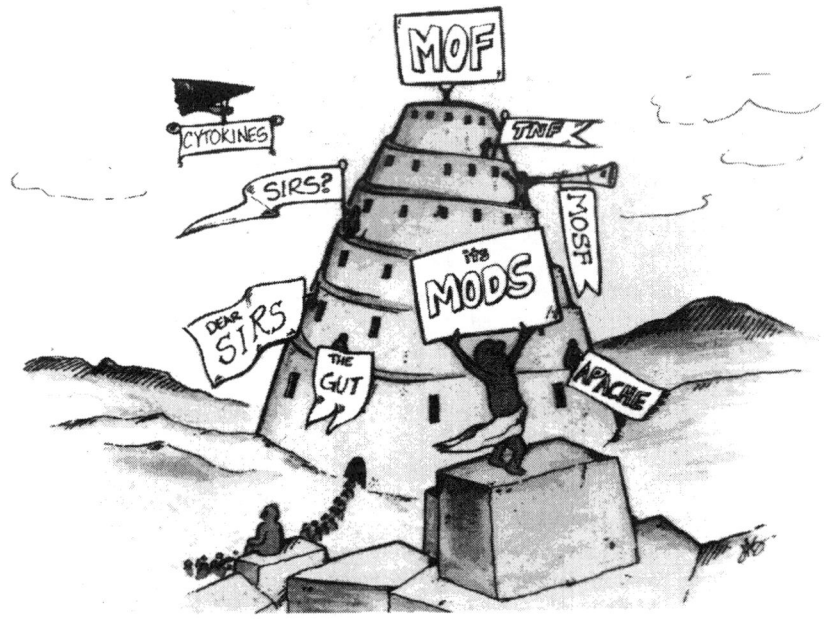

Fig. 1: The Tower of Babel adapted from Genesis 11: 1-9 with the MODS, MOF, and SIRS terminology

MOF, MODS, and SIRS are Nonentities

Part of our problem is that we are trying to define a nonentity. MOF or MODS or SIRS is not a disease or even a syndrome. Perhaps we have done the world of intensive care a disservice by referring to MOF as a syndrome. It is a series of complications of injury, disease, and intensive care which lead to death for many patients in ICUs. It is not a fixed entity but an evolving picture. We have lumped together for therapy and definition a number of diseases and problems according to clinical manifestations rather than the cause of the problem. The search for unified mechanisms has not been successful. Beale and Bihari [16] commented in 1993 on MOF, and said "the search for a unified mechanism and hence, perhaps an effective therapy has been intense." Beal and Cerra [17] stated that "the cause of SIRS/MODS is complex and not fully understood, but multiple mediators and stimulated macrophages likely are important components." Cerra [18] asked the question "What is MOF? I wish I knew. A lot of people in this room have done a lot of work, and I think we know a lot about what it is not, but what it is remains elusive and needs a lot more research." The question I raise then is, will we benefit from a more precise classification and definition of a nonentity, a hodgepodge of human disorders which have characteristics and manifestations of tissue injury, inflammation, and infection. Certainly, there is much to be learned about sick patients, the response to injury, the inflammatory response, the immune response, and many other factors. Powerful molecular biology will make great contributions to this, and out of this can come positive therapeutic efforts. However, recent clinical trials of potential "magic bullets" suggest that we should go in a different direction - instead of lumpers, we should be splitters. To seek effective therapy we must focus on specific disorders such as trauma, specific infections, inflammatory disease, and chronic or acute organ damage (chronic obstructive pulmonary disease - renal failure, etc.). I will write more about this in a later discussion titled "The Causality of Disease."

What's in a Name? An Acronym or a Response?

"What's in a name? That which we call a rose by any other name would smell as sweet:" William Shakespeare, *Romeo and Juliet* II-2, 43.

Many terms have been proposed to better describe what we are dealing with. Some of these are shown in Table 2. The multiplicity of terms is shown in Table 1 in my previous chapter - "Prologue." Other expressions have included cooperative, concentrated destruction, polytrauma schlussel (the key to injured patients), angry macrophages and leaky gut. Sepsis has been described as peripheral vascular failure, the gastrointestinal tract as the undrained abscess of MOF, and Goris has described a severe, generalized, autoinflammatory response. Thus one could have the M&M classification of MODS, minimal MODS which is pre-MOF or moderate MODS which is early MOF or maximal MODS which certainly is MOF. Another proposal would include asking the question, which patients will develop early SIRS which could be called incipient SIRS, SIRS which is basic SIRS, severe SIRS which is bad SIRS or dying-of-SIRS which would be fatal SIRS. The new terminology is a lot more fun

Table 2: New terms

Organ in shock	ASCOT - severity characterization of trauma - Champion et al. [22]
Early organ failure	MTOS - major trauma outcome study
Sepsis-related mortality score	Shock and ischemia
Prognostic nutritional index - PNI	Immunologic dyshomeostasis
Hospital prognostic index - HPI	Post-traumatic host defense failure syndrome
Anatomic profile - AP	Host defense failure
Probability of death score - PODS	Malignant systemic inflammation
Acute inflammatory phase	Multiple organ failure syndrome (MOFS)
Intermittent inflammatory phase	Whole body inflammation
Macro-endocrine stress (mediator) hormones	

than the old MOF because we can use the old song "yes SIRS that's my baby, no SIRS I don't mean maybe" (popularized by Eddie Cantor).

The inflammatory response syndromes (IRS) could be separated into local which would be LIRS, progressive which would be PIRS, regional which would be RIRS, systemic which would be SIRS, and fatal which would be FIRS. Also, predictors of MODS would be the risk factors for MOF. There could be initiators of MODS, pre-MODS, early MODS which is pre-MOF, established MODS which is early MOF, and late MODS which is the equivalent of MOF. I am reminded of an expression in India about the religious group in the Punjab called Sikhs. The expression is "all Sikhs are Singhs but not all Singhs are Sikhs." Thus we could say that all patients with sepsis have SIRS but not all SIRS have sepsis. Is this recent proposal then a scientific advance or an example of acronymia [19] or acronymitis [20]? Will this help us clarify the matter of acutely ill patients with organ failure, or will it further confuse things? Certainly, the standardization of definitions is worthwhile and should be applauded. Invention of a whole new language in this scientific Sarajevo of words reminds me of the previous cited couplet by James Russell Lowell.

SIRS is a manifestation of many diseases, and treatment may ameliorate some of these manifestations. MODS is really pre-MOF from a number of diseases, and treatment could lead to prevention of MOF, whereas MOF is a final complication before death in the ICU patients and if not prevented is lethal.

There is one excellent part of the MODS proposal. If, in the early care of very sick or injured patients we can shift to measurement of early organ dysfunctions, we may well develop better support mechanisms, better treatment opportunities and prevent the development of organ failure. Once organ failure develops with our present state of knowledge, the mortality remains high. Better support mechanisms in an ICU certainly can lead to better care and improvement of outcome. However, I remain convinced that prevention is the only final answer.

Toward a Consensus

This entire conference from now until Saturday is dedicated to seeking a consensus. Certainly, agreement on certain principals would be important. Terminology and classifications are important. However, since 1975 there has been no agreement on the definitions of organ failure. The different definitions proposed are very similar. It should be possible to develop a common set of descriptions of what is meant by respiratory, renal, hepatic, and cardiovascular failure. Will everyone agree? Will all accept and use them if it is done? It has not happened before. Other examples of the redundancy, overlap, and continuing development of new terminology are the many injury severity scores (Table 3), severity of illness scoring (Table 4) and sepsis scoring (Table 5).

What I propose then for a consensus is not more terminology or even trying to get the agreement of everyone on a common terminology but to agree on the importance of the prevention of organ failure, single and multiple, to focus on organ dysfunction and organ support and on specific disease entities. Certainly, we can use our discussions of MODS, MOF, and SIRS for fun and discussion and review but not for therapeutic considerations, mechanistic resolutions, or randomized trials. I believe that the agents studied in many of the recent clinical trials which have been less than successful could be helpful in specific circumstances if the patient population can be identified and specific abnormalities are described. Our ability to develop terminology and descriptions exceeds our ability to prevent organ failures - MOF, MODS, SIRS or whatever you prefer to call it. Perhaps we can all agree on prevention.

Table 3: Injury severity scoring

ISS	-	injury severity score
AI	-	anatomic index - HICDA-8 code
PEBL	-	penetrating and blunt injury code
ASCOT		
OIS	-	organ injury scales
AIS	-	abbreviated injury score
GCS	-	Glasgow coma scale
TS	-	trauma score
TI	-	trauma index
MTOS	-	major trauma outcome study
HTI	-	hospital trauma index
CRAMS	-	circulation, respiration, abdomen, motor, speech
MESS	-	mangled extremity score

Table 4: Severity of illness scoring (predictors of mortality)

APACHE I, II, III - acute physiology and chronic health evaluation system
Simplified acute physiology score (SAPS I and II)
Mortality probability mode (MPM 11, 0, 24)
CARE - Clinical assessment, research scoring system
Probability of death score (PODS)
MOF scoring
MSOF score
MODS score
Hospital prognostic index
TISS - therapeutic intervention scoring system
Prognostic nutritional index
PRISM - pediatric risk of mortality

Table 5: Sepsis scoring

Sepsis score - sepsis severity score (Elebute-Stoner)
Complete septic shock score
Simplified septic shock score
Sepsis related mortality score
Risk of operative site infection formula
Surgical stratification system for intraabdominal infections
DTH skin test score
LPS - cytokine score - LPS - IL-1 - IL-6

Conclusions

MOF, MODS, and SIRS are the final series of events leading to death in many patients in an ICU. This problem only became recognized when modern intensive care provided circulatory, ventilatory, gastrointestinal, renal, and metabolic support. The central nervous system remains a problem. Coagulation failure may be treatable, and extracorporeal therapy for hepatic failure is on the horizon.

Thus a number of diseases have been lumped together for therapy according to clinical manifestations rather than the cause of the problem. I suspect that this is the major reason why previous clinical trials of potential magic bullets have not been positive. In fact, some involved in the trials broke down their study into subgroups after the studies were completed. Positive results were suggested in various retrospective subgroups. New trials have been proposed for more specific groups or patients. Thus the original lumpers are becoming splitters. There is no magic bullet now for the manifestations of infection, sepsis, the sepsis syndrome, MOF, MODS, SIRS, or whatever. I predict that there will be no magic bullet. We must go back to the causes of diseases [21].

References

1. Baue AE (1975) Multiple, progressive or sequential systems failure. Arch Surg 110: 779-181
2. Bone RC, Fisher CJ Jr, Clemmer TP et al. (1987) A controlled clinical trial of high dose methylprednisolone in the treatment of severe sepsis and septic shock. N Engl J Med 317: 653-658
3. Bone RC, Fisher CJ Jr, Clemmer TP et al. (1989) Sepsis syndrome: a valid clinical entity. Crit Care Med 17: 389-393
4. Bone RC (1991) The sepsis syndrome, multi-organ failure: a plea for comparable definitions. Ann Intern Med 114: 332-333
5. Bone RC (1991) Let's agree on terminology: definitions of sepsis. Crit Care Med 19: 973-976
6. Sprung CL (1991) Definitions of sepsis - have we reached a consensus? Crit Care Med 19: 849-851
7. Sibbald WJ, Marshall J, Christou N et al. (1991) "Sepsis" clarity of existing terminology or more confusion. Crit Care Med 19: 996-998
8. Faist E, Baue AE, Dittmer A, Heberer G (1983) Multiple organ failure in polytrauma patients. J Trauma 23: 775-787
9. Knaus WA, Draper EA, Wagner DP, Zimmerman JE (1985) Prognosis in acute organ-system failure. Ann Surg 202: 685-693
10. Hinshaw L (1966) Therapy of endotoxin shock. Oklahoma State Med Assoc 59: 407-484
11. Benjamin E, Leibowitz AB, Oropello J, Iberti TJ (1992) Systemic hypoxic and inflammatory syndrome: an alternative designation for "sepsis syndrome". Crit Care Med 20: 680-682
12. Bone RC, Balk RA, Cerra FB et al. (1992) Definitions for sepsis and organ failure and guidelines for the use of innovative therapies in sepsis. Chest 101: 1644-1655
13. American College of Chest Physicians/Society of Critical Care Medicine Consensus Conference Committee (1992) Definitions for sepsis and organ failure and guidelines for the use of innovative therapies in sepsis. Crit Care Med 20: 864-874
14. Bone RC, Sibbald WJ, Sprung CL (1992) The ACCP-SCCM Consensus Conference on sepsis and organ failure. Chest 101: 1481-1483

15. Bone RC, Sprung CL, Sibbald WJ (1992) Definitions for sepsis and organ failure. Crit Care Med 20: 724-726
16. Beale R, Bihari DJ (1993) Multiple organ failure: the pilgrim's progress. Crit Care Med 21: 51-53
17. Beal AL, Cerra FB (1994) Multiple organ failure syndrome in the 1990's. JAMA 271: 226-233
18. Cerra FB (1992) Closing discussion. Arch Surg 129: 169
19. Beck WC (1990) Acronymia. Surg Gynecol Obstet 76: 509
20. Jaffe BM (1990) Acronymitis. Surg Rounds 10: 11-12
21. Stehbens WE (1992) Causality in medical science with particular reference to heart disease and atherosclerosis. Perspect Biol Med 36: 97-117
22. Champion HR, Copes WS, Sacco WJ, Lawnick MM, Bain LW, Gann DS, Gennarelli T, MacKenzie E, Schwaitzberg S (1990) A new characterization of injury severity. J Trauma 30: 539-546

Section 2:

Mechanistic and Biochemical Profiles of Specific Organ Dysfunction/Failure

Pathogenic Mechanisms of Brain Failure

J. Cervós-Navarro

The causative factors of brain dysfunction are firstly breakdown of the blood-brain barrier and increased intracranial pressure (ICP) and secondly decreased systemic blood pressure and disorders of metabolism, blood coagulation and respiratory function.

Blood-Brain Barrier and Edema

Compared with other organs of the body, the central nervous system (CNS) behaves uniquely with regard to exchange of metabolites that are not freely transferred to and from the blood. This phenomenon has led to the concept of the "blood-brain barrier" (BBB). In spite of the fact that the first concept of the BBB itself was a physiological phenomenon, morphologists have been repeatedly called upon to identify the localization of this barrier system. The BBB comprises tightly apposed endothelial cells (Fig. 1) that lack fenestra and typically possess few pinocytic vesicles [5]. Breakdown of the BBB is a general response of the brain to global ischemia, stroke, cerebral trauma, surgical procedures, inflammation, convulsions, acute hypertension, changes in blood osmolarity, brain tumors, abscess and intoxication. Transport of protein tracers through endothelium of cerebral capillaries after experimental damage to the BBB has been reported to occur by various pathways. These include passage between adjacent endothelial cells by the opening of tight junctions, and vesicular transport, through endothelial channels and diffusely through the endothelial cytoplasm.

The breakdown of the BBB results in brain edema formation with accumulation of water and proteins in the extracellular spaces (Fig. 2). The effect of edema in the brain is an increase in volume and since the brain is encased within a rigid structure allowing little room for expansion ICP is also increased. The problem of brain edema is unique and differs from edema in other parts of the body, chiefly on the basis of its more serious implications within the CNS. In clinical practice it can be a devastating process. Acute syndromes with a fulminant course are seen after intracranial hemorrhages, rupture of aneurysms, malignant cerebral tumors, inflammatory diseases, circulatory disorders, poisoning and severe craniocerebral injuries. Such events are soon followed by loss of consciousness and acute signs of cerebral and brain stem compression. It has yet to be proved clinically that edema as such - especially protein-free edema - has a damaging effect on nervous tissue. Rather it appears that many of the problems encountered in the patient with brain edema result from the elevation of ICP (Fig. 3).

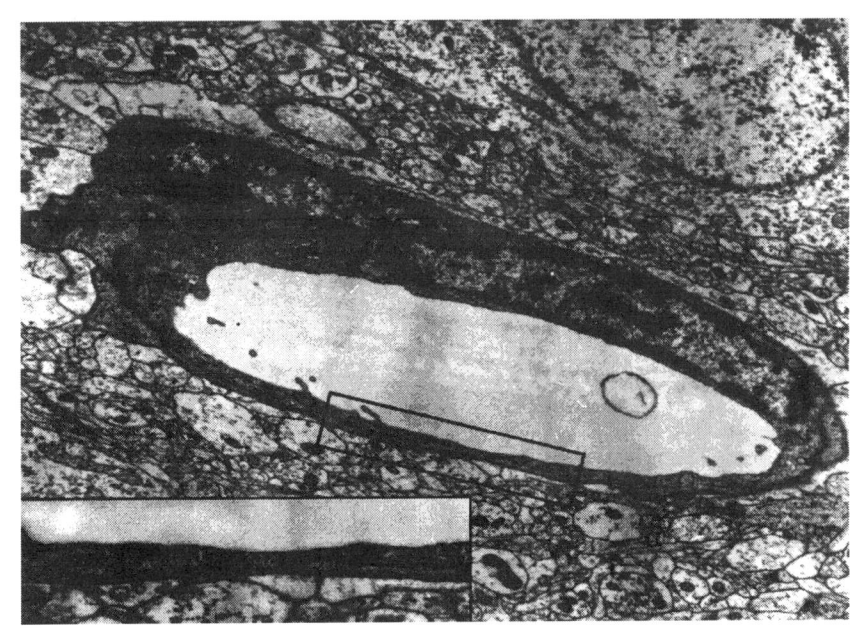

Fig. 1: Normal capillary in the cortex. No fenestration or pinocytosis is found in the endothelium, x9000

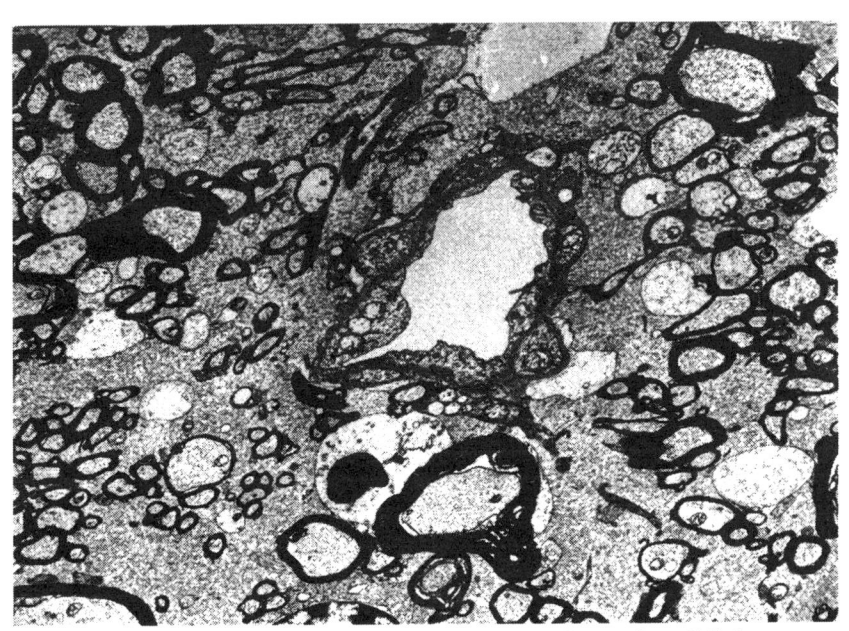

Fig. 2: White matter of postirradiation brain edema in the monkey. Cellular structures surrounding venules are distended by marked protein-rich edema, x6000

Brain Failure

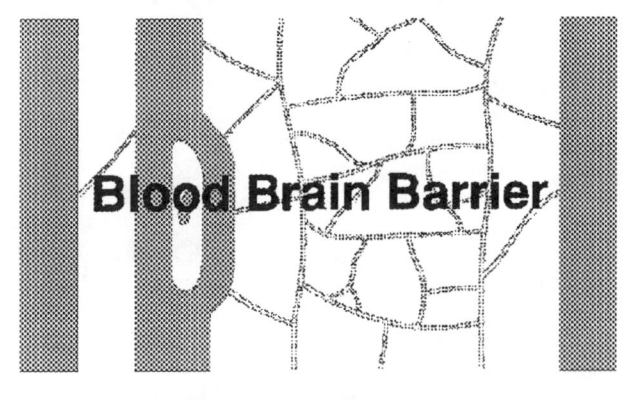

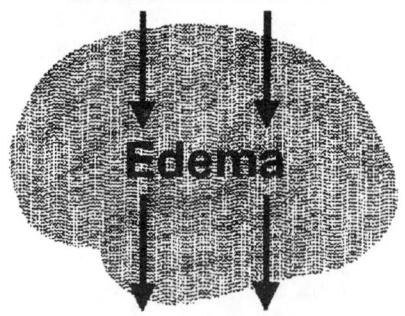

Blood Brain Barrier

Breakdown

Edema

Increase of Intracranial Pressure (ICP)

Fig. 3: Elevation of ICP

The accumulation of water in a tissue is common during ischemia and subsequent reflow. The pathogenic mechanisms involved in the development of ischemic brain edema are complex. It seems that brain edema after ischemia is related to the degree of cerebral blood flow (CBF) reduction and the duration of interruption of the blood supply. Mrsulja et al. [22] showed that edematous changes associated with bilateral occlusion of the carotid arteries were insignificant (0.4%) when CBF remained above 10 ml/min/100 g tissue (5 min of ischemia). Below 10 ml/min/100 g tissue the brain swelling was marked (1.9%). It might be expected that an increase in tissue water content would occur when the ionic pump breaks down as a consequence of energy failure caused by the cessation of blood supply. However, depletion of tissue energy reserves seems not to be a major mechanism of edema formation, because time courses of the decrease in high-energy phosphates (ATP+P-creatine) and the development of ischemic brain edema do not appear to be related. The rates of cerebral consumption of energy during hypoxia and ischemia anoxia were inversely related to hypoxic tolerance. Energy requirements rather than mere levels of energy reserves or the anaerobic generation of ATP are critical determinants of hypoxic tolerance of the brain.

In cerebral trauma the course of brain edema syndrome may be obscured by the impaired consciousness due to cerebral concussion. When the head is struck, the brain, it its semirigid, uneven housing, is subjected to varying degrees of acceleration, rotation, compression, expansion and swirling movements about its points of attachment. As a result there may be diffuse neuronal injury, contusion, laceration or all the three. Following the impact, and depending roughly on the site and extent of the injury, secondary physical and biochemical changes, local or general, extend the brain damage. The more apparent changes include brain anoxia, edema, stasis and lactic acidosis. Post-traumatic brain edema is a cherished concept long held by neurosurgeons to explain delayed deterioration in patients with severe head injury. Lundberg et al. [19] showed that elevation of ICP is common in patient with severe head injury, and the occurrence of elevated ICP often corresponds to neurological deterioration [20, 21]. Langfitt and his school have argued very strongly from a wealth of experimental and clinical evidence that in patients with severe head injury the most common cause of acute raised ICP and neurological deterioration is vascular engorgement, not brain edema as strictly defined [8, 18].

Intracranial Pressure

Increased ICP results (Fig. 4) in an impairment of CBF with subsequent cerebral ischemia and cell death which, when coupled with the lack of regenerative powers of the CNS, lead to serious after effects. In brain trauma greater mortality and poorer neurological status have been reported after ICP elevations and diffuse CT lesions. However, ICP levels, rather than CT lesions, have been found to contribute to prognosis after severe head injury [35].

Brain Failure

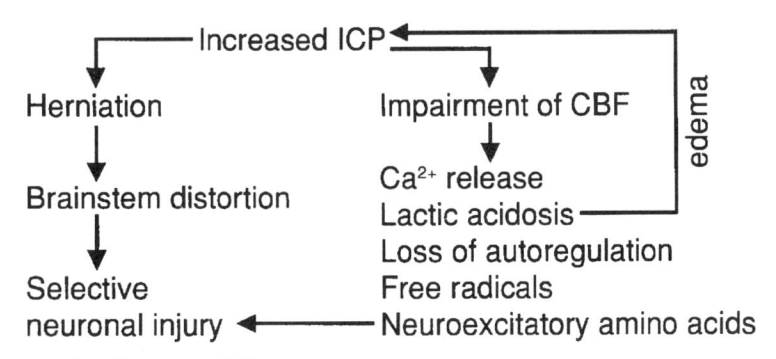

```
                ┌────── Increased ICP ◄──────┐
                ▼                ▼            │
          Herniation      Impairment of CBF   │ edema
              ▼                ▼              │
      Brainstem distortion  Ca²⁺ release      │
              ▼             Lactic acidosis ──┘
          Selective         Loss of autoregulation
       neuronal injury ◄── Free radicals
                            Neuroexcitatory amino acids
```

Fig. 4: Results of increased ICP

The breakdown of the intracranial circulation in any type of severe brain edema is a process which occurs in several stages. The first impairment is caused by a compression of the superficial cerebral veins [10]. This results in an increased venous pressure, which leads to a reduction of cerebral perfusion pressure, and thus - beyond certain limit - to a reduction or even breakdown of the CBF. The intracranial hypertension venous blood pressure is at least as high as the intracranial and tissue pressures [23a, 28]. If, therefore, the ICP rises to the level of the systemic blood pressure, any circulation would have to cease. These have often occurred since it became possible to maintain vegetative functions by artificial means in a hopelessly injured person without viable centers of the CNS.

Brain death may be defined as the survival of the organism after the complete and permanent breakdown of the cerebral circulation. Morphologically it can be regarded as an infarction of all the structures enclosed by the skull (Fig. 5a). The most reliable sign of brain death thus far seems to be the arrest of the cerebral circulation as established by angiography. Axial distortion of the brain stem occurs and caudal parts of the cerebellum are pressed into the foramen occipitale magnum (Fig. 5b). The resulting cerebellar pressure cone may be cut off and displaced into the spinal subarachnoid space (Fig. 5c), lying as a cuff around the spinal cord.

Pressure Gradients in the Brain

Focal brain edema may cause shifts of brain substance with cerebral herniation (Fig. 6a), and compression of adjacent cerebral tissue, producing distortion and interference with the function of the respiratory and circulatory centers in the brain stem. In stroke and in brain trauma when the edematogenous condition is initially localized the tissue pressure variance within and between the hemispheres leads to tentorial and falciform herniations, which are the common cause of death even before the critical threshold of ICP is reached. The midbrain and brain stem hemorrhages are of special interest (Fig. 6b). They arise as a result of the biphasic development of extreme brain edema.

If the tissue pressure, acting on the outer surface of the veins, remains low, a high positive pressure gradient between the lumen of the veins and the environment results. This gradient certainly facilitates venous hemorrhages, since the veins are not built for such high pressures. The occurrence of midbrain hemorrhages indicates the end of the first stage of breakdown of the intracranial circulation. If no treatment stops the process, this stage is inevitably followed by progressing hypertension in the infratentorial space. In stroke, a common cause of death, the tentorial herniation is induced by brain swelling following acute infarction, whereas in surgery of subarachnoid hemorrhage a lethal outcome is frequently associated with extensive brain swelling secondary to focal cerebral edema.

Metabolic Failure

The biochemical sequelae following impairment of CBF are a host of metabolic events, namely lactic acidosis, ionic fluxes especially of calcium, breakdown of phospholipids with release of free fatty acids, prostanoid synthesis, transmitter release and free radical formation (Fig. 7). These events follow one another in a deleterious cascade which results in structural defects and, finally, in the death of the neuron. Release of edema factors simultaneously or in cascades in the form of a positive feedback cycle may constitute the basic mechanism, which may explain the often rapid development of tissue damage and edema secondary to a relatively small initial insult.

Lactic acidosis is a more general reaction to various noxious stimuli and is by no means specific. It may occur in ischemia as well as in head trauma, meningitis, status epilepticus and intoxications. Fatal brain edema is strongly associated with hyperglycemia, which causes

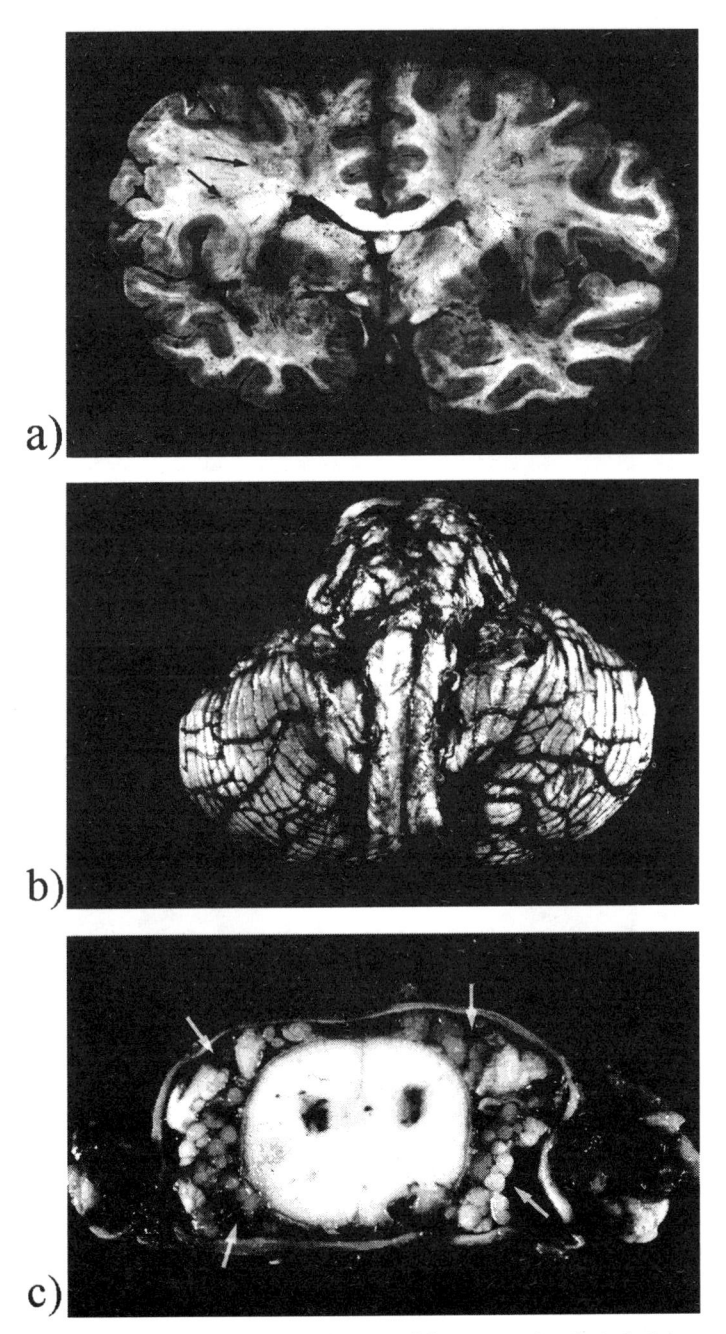

Fig. 5: Brain death for 72 h. a) *Diffuse softening of the cortex. Autolysis lesions are seen on the white matter (arrows).* b) *Caudal parts of the cerebellum are pressed into the foramen magnum.* c) *In the subarachnoid space there is amorphous necrotic material*

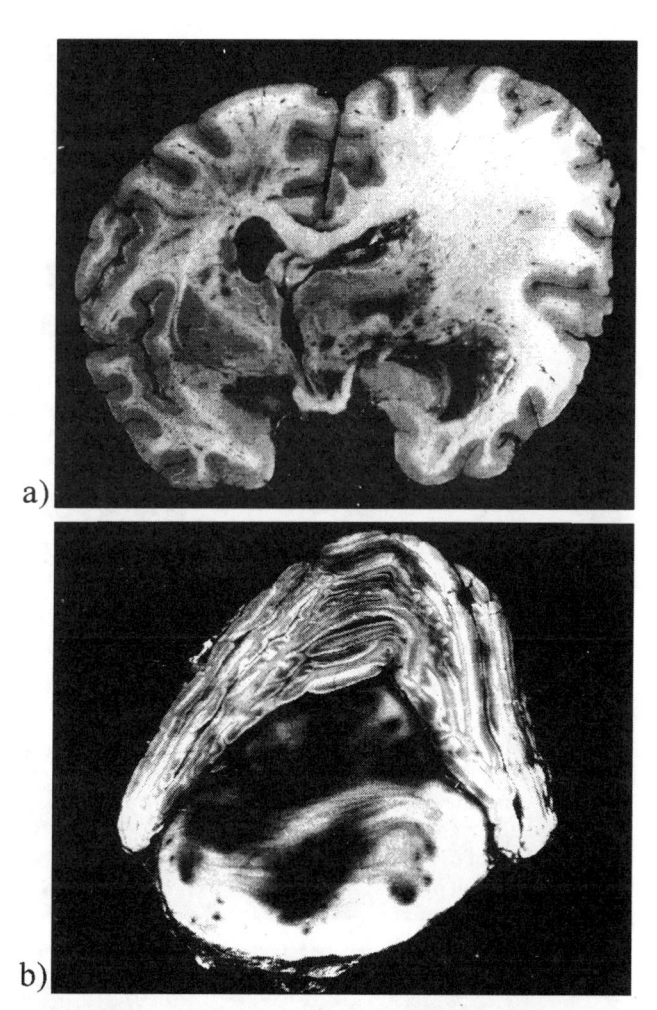

Fig. 6: Focal brain edema of the right cerebral hemisphere after contusion trauma on the same side. a) *Tentorial hernia of brain tissue. Multiple hemorrhages in the capsula interna, basal ganglia and midbrain.* b) *Large hemorrhagic lesions in the brain stem.*

more marked ischemic brain tissue lactic acidosis, apparently damaging blood vessels and synergistically causing augmentation of edema. Hyperglycemia with the consequent increase in lactic acidosis may also be harmful to calcium recovery during the early recirculation period following focal cerebral ischemia [1]. Mean CSF lactate and pyruvate values as well as lactate-pyruvate ratio are significantly higher in those neurological patients who have lost consciousness than in those who have not. However, a simple correlation between CSF lactic acidosis and survival does not seem justified, since lactate can penetrate the BBB by a carrier-mediated transport mechanism. Thus, high lactate concentrations in the blood can be transmitted into the CSF. Such exogenous lactic acidosis is caused by brain hypoxia.

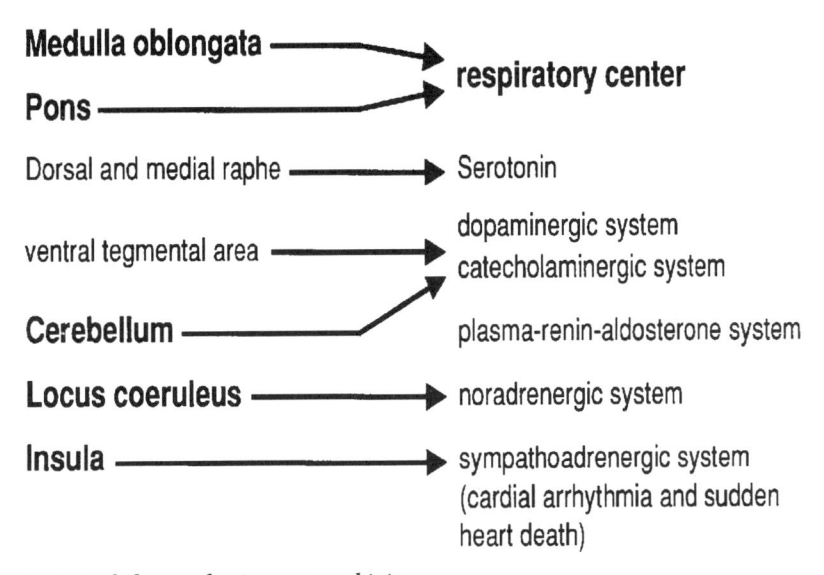

Medulla oblongata →	**respiratory center**
Pons →	
Dorsal and medial raphe →	Serotonin
ventral tegmental area →	dopaminergic system
	catecholaminergic system
Cerebellum →	plasma-renin-aldosterone system
Locus coeruleus →	noradrenergic system
Insula →	sympathoadrenergic system (cardial arrhythmia and sudden heart death)

Fig. 7: Brain failure: selective neuronal injury

Neuronal response to ischemia initially consists of a breakdown of ATP-dependent membrane carrier mechanisms, culminating in the depolarization of the cell. As a consequence, a sharp increase within the cellular membrane permeability appears, leading to abnormal transmembranal ionic shift. Similarly, compression contusion trauma produces a transient membrane depolarization associated with a pronounced cellular release of K^+ and a massive Ca^{2+} entry into the intracellular compartment. The intraneuronal presence of serum proteins on the one hand and the loss of cytoplasmic enzymes on the other hand reflect disturbances of membrane function as a result of preceding ischemia [13].

The role of calcium is irreversible cell damage during cerebral ischemia and reperfusion has been a focus of special attention over the past decade [30, 31]. The acute functional impairment and the subsequent neuronal injury in the affected areas of the brain are caused by the prolonged disturbance of cellular calcium homeostasis mediated by leaky membranes exposed to shear stress [23]. Calcium activates enzyme-degrading structures, particularly lipases, proteases and endonucleases [25, 32]. Influx of calcium, or its release from intracellular stores, could be responsible for the extreme vulnerability of some neuronal populations to ischemia/anoxia.

The correlation between the profile of PGE_2 and Evans-Blue extravasation suggests that ischemia damages the vascular endothelium, which produces PGE_2 when the circulation is restored and in turn increases vascular permeability allowing the egress of proteins.

Immediately after interrupting the blood supply to the brain, a strikingly rapid production of free fatty acids (FFAs) takes place. The rate of production is of the same order of magnitude as observed in adipose tissue under maximal lipolytic hormonal situation. FFAs, e.g., palmitic acid, were markedly increased in edema fluid as compared with normal CSF. Arachidonic acid concentration was almost twice as high in edema fluid as in plasma, indicative of the cerebral origin of its accumulation in interstitial fluid. However, the concentrations of FFAs in edema fluid are not affected by additional cerebral ischemia.

There is experimental literature that supports a role for free radicals in the genesis of the permeability changes that underlie brain edema [6]. Free radicals are ions possessing unusual chemical reactivity, including an ability to alter and to fragment membrane lipids.

A proposed mechanism to account for vulnerability in neuronal ischemia involves pathological neuronal excitation via glutamate or other excitatory amino acids (EAAs) [16]. In experimental edema after frozen lesion Baethmann [2] found accumulation of the glutamate in interstitial edema fluid, which he attributed to a release from damaged brain tissue areas rather than to transport from the intravascular space. Faden et al. [7] demonstrated that levels of EAAs increase in the extracellular space after brain trauma. Ischemia does in fact result in a significant increase in the extracellular concentration of L-glutamate and L-aspartate [9], probably due to decreased reuptake of released EAAs.

Under physiological conditions, glutamate is compartmentalized in the brain, and the BBB prevents an uncontrolled influx of glutamate from the intravascular compartment. Under conditions of brain trauma when the BBB is damaged, increased glutamate levels in the edema fluid could additionally contribute to neuronal injury. The disturbances of EAAs during hypoxia/ischemia are also accompanied by changes in calcium homeostasis [30]

The biological actions of the EAAs are exclusively mediated via receptor-linked second-messenger systems. Regional derangement of the second-messenger system may thus be tightly linked with the mechanisms of selective vulnerability. Adenylate cyclase catalyzes the receptor-mediated generation of cyclic adenosine monophosphate. Similarly, protein kinase C in the phosphoionositide system regulates the amount of neurotransmitters released by nerve cells as well as the intracellular ion concentrations.

As a consequence of both metabolic failure and mechanical damage, strategically located neuronal cells can be selectively injured. The hippocampus is selectively vulnerable to a variety of insults, including cardiac arrest, status epilepticus and hypoglycemia [3]. Additionally, the hippocampus is known to be frequently damaged in fatal nonmissile head injury [17]. Hypoxia and high ICP are likely to contribute to the occurrence of hippocampal damage but other mechanisms such as excitotoxcity are likely to be operative. Different factors support a pathogenic role of glutamate in this selective vulnerability. EAAs are presumed to cause neuronal injury as a result of persistent depolarization, causing normal cationic channels to be held in the "open" position, with a resultant intracellular accumulation of cations.

By employing fluid percussion injury in rabbit, significant fluorescence has been demonstrated within the brain stem vasculature of the traumatized animals. The localization of vasculature permeability changes within both the raphe and reticular regions corresponds to neuronal alterations occurring with brain injuries [25].

Disorders of Other Organs and Systems (Fig. 8)

Cessation of the circulation to the brain due to systemic disorders occurs only in the event of systemic circulatory arrest. The prognosis is good in patients who, after resuscitation, regain consciousness quickly with complete neurological recovery. However, many remain unconscious and die within 24 h of the cardiac arrest. With longer survival there may be an appreciable reduction in the weight of the brain [3].

Global oligemia implies some reduction in the overall flow of blood through the brain. However, a reduction of blood flow in all or part of an arterial territory is unusually due to a combination of systemic hypotension and stenosis. Provided that thrombosis and embolism

Heart dysfunction Shock	Systemic hypotension

Kidney dysfunction	Edema

Hypercoagulation (platelet activating factor)	Sinus and venous thrombosis Microthrombosis

Acute viral infections Gram-negative septicemia Drug hypersensitivity	Hemorrhagic leukoencephalopathy Brain purpura

Fig. 8: Brain failure

can be excluded, such local oligemia is a not uncommon cause of ischemic brain damage, and if blood flow is sufficiently impaired the outcome will be an infarct involving gray and white matter.

Factors that may result in brain damage after a period of relatively moderate hypotension are some degree of hypoxemia, some preexisting vascular disease (particularly atheroma of the extra- and intracranial arteries and hypertensive arteriosclerosis) and also variations in the configuration of the circle of Willis. The frequency of these complications of reduced CBF due to systemic hypotension is largely responsible for hypoxic brain damage along the arterial boundary zones. The boundary zone pattern of ischemic brain damage is usually seen after a conscious subject has collapsed as a result of a sudden reduction in cardiac output or an episode of anoxemia or hypoxemia has led to impaired myocardial activity.

A clinical episode of shock, which is accompanied by circulatory deficiency and systemic hypotension, is a common critical care emergency [34]. It is well accepted that ischemia caused by reduction in blood flow plays a key role in the pathogenesis of cell injury during shock. Systemic hypotension below the autoregulatory range of cerebral circulation, therefore, can induce cerebral ischemia and cause brain damage.

Central and peripheral neurological disturbances are often the leading symptoms in chronic renal insufficiency. Without successful treatment, loss of mental activity and finally precomatose and comatose states are the fate of these patients. Cerebral edema is associated with acute hypo-osmolarity due to inappropriate secretion of antidiuretic hormone, sodium depletion or the dialysis disequilibrium syndrome. Acute hypo-osmolarity causes an increase in brain water followed by a loss of intracellular potassium.

Following cerebral ischemia and after severe head injury a tendency to develop hypercoagulation can be detected. Vascular occlusion may develop either as a result of local thrombus formation or from emboli caused by circulating platelet aggregates.

In ischemic brain tissue the main mechanisms of coagulation and vessel occlusion are platelet-endothelium and platelet-collagen interactions as well as reduction of local CBF [24]. Platelet hyperaggregability, circulating platelet aggregates, increased levels of -thromboglobulin and reduced megakaryocyte-platelet regeneration time are common findings associated with increased platelet activity in stroke. The formation of microthrombi is triggered by the platelet-activating factor, a mediator in a central injury also responsible for aggravation of post-traumatic brain edema.

At the early postischemic stage there is an initial contact between endothelial cells and platelets, with thrombi formation in the ischemic tissue. At a later necrotic stage increased numbers of circulating microthrombi are then deposited in the penumbra and the contralateral, healthy brain. At the stage of disintegration, the locally released and circulating aggregation substances play a minor role. Aggregation is then triggered mainly by contact with exposed vascular collagen and macrophage-dependent factors in the necrotic area. Fresh brain infarcts showed a large number of microthrombi limited to the ischemic region. In more advanced infarcts they were found mainly at the border of the necrosis and diffusely distributed over both hemispheres. Older, subsiding infarcts showed only isolated microthrombi limited to the area of the necrosis. This indicates that great importance must be attached to microthrombi in infarct progression [12, 27].

The development of postischemic microthrombi has been described in experimental and clinical studies by Cervós-Navarro et al. [4], Sampaolo et al. [27] and Heye et al. [11]. In 1987 Hekmatpanah [10] demonstrated the occurrence of collapsed vessels and intravascular clots after brain trauma in rats. In human brains with head trauma, Huber et al. [14] demonstrated fibrinous microthrombi in the contusional areas as well as in lower numbers in the contralateral hemisphere (Fig. 9).

Acute hemorrhagic leukoencephalitis and brain purpura (Fig. 10) are known to arise as complications of acute viral infections and following gram-negative septicemia. Endotoxin shock has a crucial role in initiating the events leading to brain damage. Derangement of the BBB functions has been demonstrated in sepsis [15]; increased permeability establishes the conditions for an antigen-antibody reaction in the wall of cerebral vessels. Schwenk and Gosztonyi [29] postulated that septic shock due to gram-negative bacteria leads to endothelial damage in the cerebral vessels by complement activation.

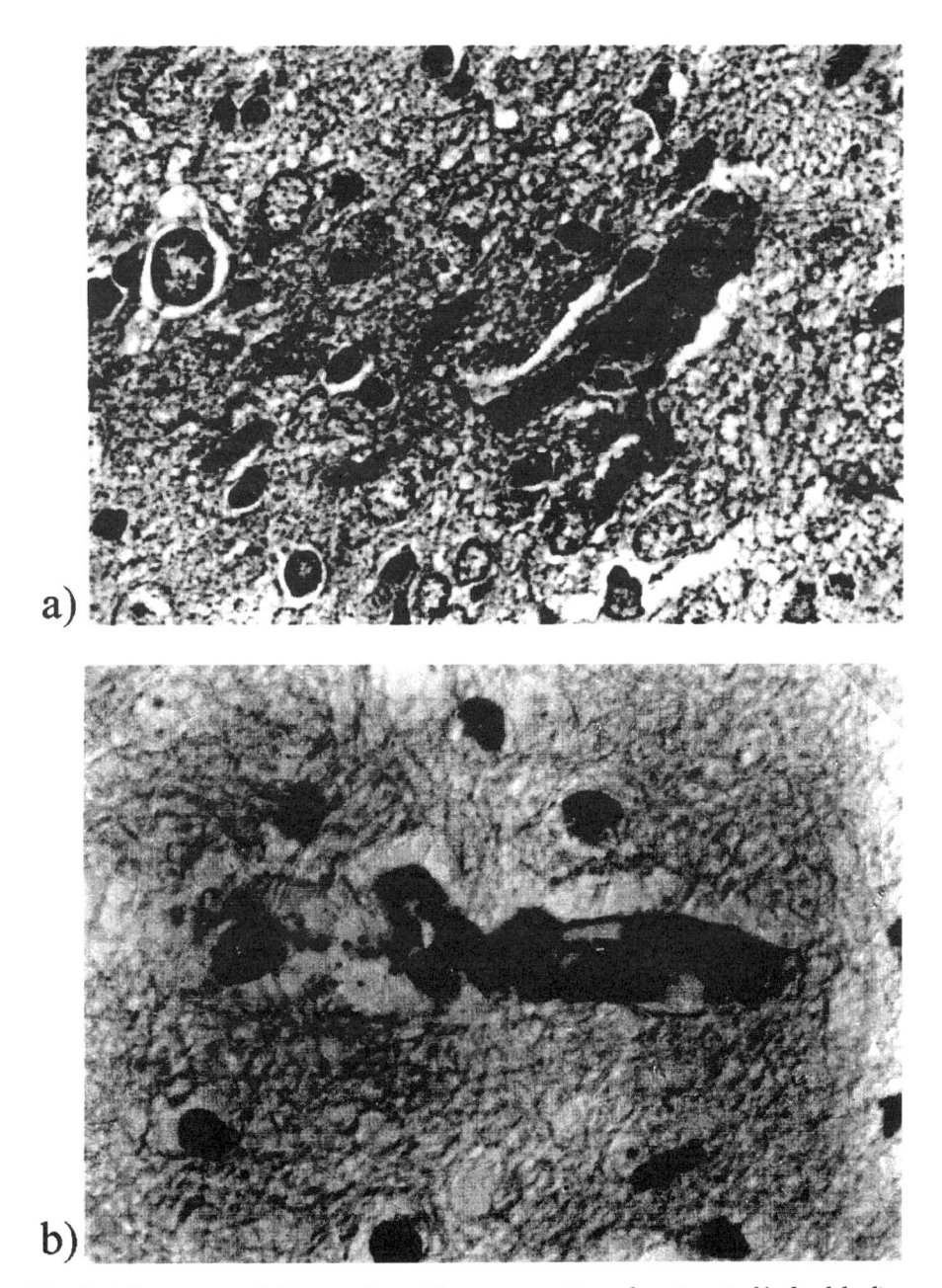

Fig. 9: a) *Purpura cerebri in a patient with acute enteritis and septicemia.* b) *shock bodies in bronchopneumonia complicated with right heart insufficiency. Capillary of the white matter. Kranland stain, x600*

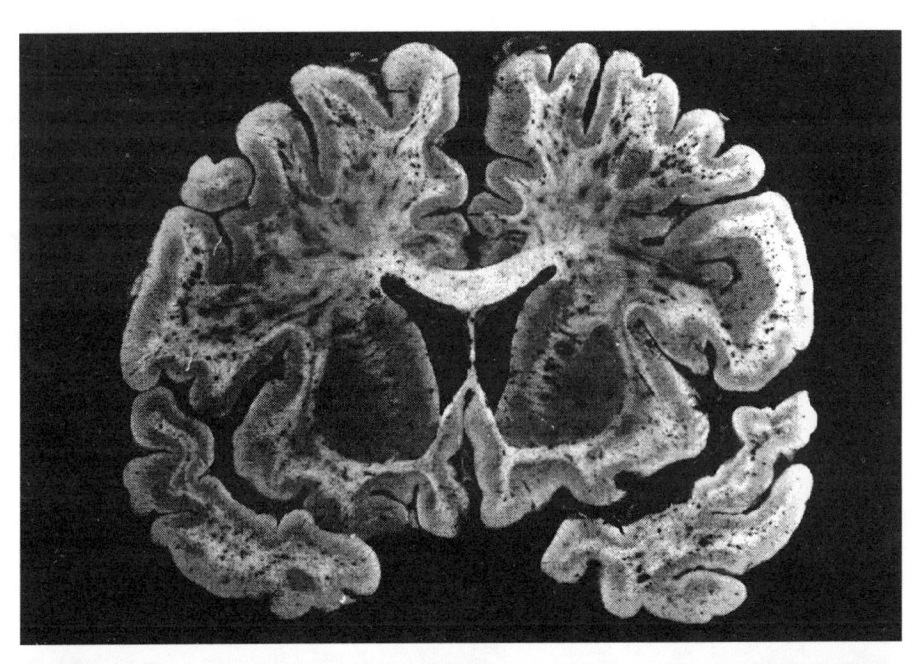

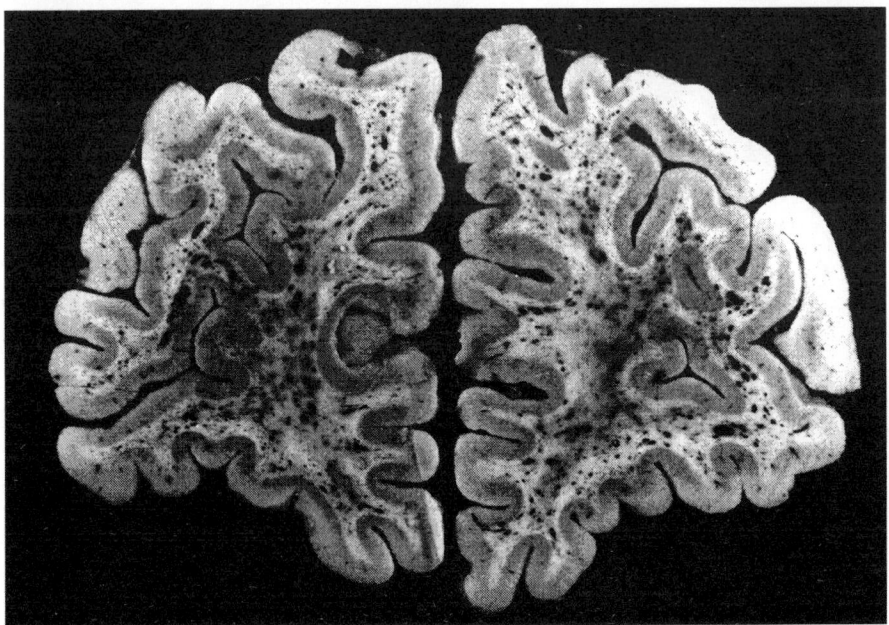

Fig. 10: Brain infarct 1 day old. Occlusion of a capillary by fibrin microthrombus in the contralateral hemisphere to the infarct. PTAH, x20

References

1. Araki N, Greenberg JH, Sladky JT, Uematsu D, Karp A, Reivich M (1992) The effect of hyperglycemia on intracellular calcium in stroke. J Cereb Blood Flow Metab 12: 43-52
2. Baethman A (1986) Secondary events accompanying brain trauma. In: Mchedlishivili G, Cervós-Navarro J, Hossmann K-A, Klatzo I (eds.) Brain edema, a pathogenic analysis. Akademiai Kiado, Budapest, pp. 287-289
3. Brierly JB, Graham DI (1984) Hypoxia and vascular disorders of the central nervous system. In: Adams JH, Corsellis JAN, Duchen LW (eds.) Greenfield neuropathology. Arnold, London, pp. 125-207
4. Cervós-Navarro J, Figols J, Ebhardt G (1984) Microthrombosis: a contributing factor to the progression of cerebral ischemia. In: Baethmann A, Go KG, Unterberg A (eds.) Mechanisms of secondary brain damage. Plenum, New York, pp. 109-119
5. Cervós-Navarro J, Kannuki S, Nakagawa Y (1988) Blood-brain barrier. Review from morphological aspect. Histol Histopathol 3: 203
6. Demopoulos HB, Flamm ES, Seligmann ML (1977) Antioxidant effects of barbiturates in model membranes undergoing free radical damage. Acta Neurol Scand 56 (Suppl 64): 152-153
7. Faden IF, Demediuk P, Panter SS, Vink R (1989) The role of excitatory amino acids and NMDA receptors in traumatic brain injury. Science 244: 798-800
8. Gennarelli TA, Obrist WD, Langfitt TW, Segawa H (1979) Vascular and metabolic reactivity to changes in PCO_2 in head injured patients. In: Popp AJ, Bourke RS, Nelson LR, Kimelberg HK (eds.) Neural trauma. Raven, New York, pp. 1-8
9. Hagberg A, Lehmann A, Sandberg M, Nystrom B, Jacobson I, Hamberger A (1985) Ischemia-induced shift of inhibitory and excitatory amino acids from intra- to extracellular compartments. J Cereb Blood Flow Metab 5: 413
10. Hekmatpanah J (1970) Cerebral circulation and perfusion in experimental increased intracranial pressure. J Neurosurg 31: 21-29
11. Heye N, Campos A, Kannuki S, Cervós-Navarro J (1991) Effects of triflusal and acetylsalicylic acid on microthrombi formation in experimental brain ischemia. Exp Pathol 41: 31-36
12. Heye N, Paetzold C, Steinberg R, Cervós-Navarro J (1992) The topography of microthrombi in ischemic brain infarct. Acta Neurol Scand 86: 450-454
13. Horn M, Schlote W (1993) Cytoplasmic protein loss and serum protein uptake in hippocampal neurons indicate early post-ischemic bi-directional membrane dysfunction. Clin Neuropathol 12: 284
14. Huber A, Dorn A, Witzmann A, Cervós-Navarro J (1993) Microthrombi formation after severe head trauma. Int J Legal Med 106: 152-155
15. Jeppsson B, Freund HR, Gimmon A, James JH (1981) Blood-brain barrier derangement in sepsis: cause of septic encephalopathy? Am J Surg 141: 136-142
16. Kotapka MJ, Gennarelli TA, Graham DI, Adams JH, Thibault LA, Ross DT, Ford I (1991) Selective vulnerability of hippocampal neurons in acceleration-induced experimental head injury. J Neurotrauma 8: 247-258
17. Kotapka MJ, Graham DI, Adams JH, Gennarelli TA (1992) Hippocampal pathology in fatal non-missile human head injury. Acta Neuropathol (Bol) 83: 530-534
18. Langfitt TW, Marschall WJS, Kassel NF, Schutta AS (1968) The pathophysiology of brain swelling produced by mechanical trauma and hypertension. Scand J Clin Lab Invest Suppl 102: 545-553

19. Lundberg NN, Conquist S, Kjallquist A (1968) Clinical investigations on interrelations between intracranial pressure and intracranial hemodynamics. Brain Res 30: 69-75
20. Marshall LF, Smith RW, Shapiro HM (1979) The outcome with aggressive treatment in severe head injuries. Part I: the significance of intracranial pressure monitoring. J Neurosurg 50: 20-25
21. Miller JD, Sweet RC, Narayan R, Becker DP (1978) Early insults to the injured brain. JAMA 240: 439-442
22. Mrsulja BB, Djuricic BM, Ueki Y, Cahn R, Cvejic V, Martinez H, Micic DV, Stojanovic T, Spatz M (1985) Cerebral blood flow, energy utilization, serotonin metabolism, (Na, K)ATPase activity, and postischemic brain swelling. In: Inaba Y, Klatzo I, Spatz M (eds.) Brain edema. Springer, Berlin, Heidelberg, New York, pp. 170-177
23. Nilsson P, Hillered L, Olsson Y, Sheardown MJ, Hansen AJ (1993) Regional changes in interstitial K^+ and Ca^{2+} levels following cortical compression contusion trauma in rats. J Cereb Blood Flow Metab 13: 183-192
24. Oates JA, Fitzgerald GA, Branch RA, Jackson EK, Knapp HR, Roberts LJ (1988) Clinical implications of prostaglandins and thromboxane A_2-formation. N Engl J Med 319: 689-698, 761-767
25. Orrenius S, McConkey DJ, Jones DP, Nicotera P (1988) Ca^{2+}-activated mechanisms in toxicity and programmed cell death. ISI Atlas Sci Pharmacol 2: 319
26. Povlishock JT, Becker DP, Sullivan HG, Miller JD (1978) Vascular permeability alterations to horseradish peroxidase in experimental brain injury. Brain Res 153: 223-239
27. Sampaolo S, Cervós-Navarro J, Djouchadar D, Figols J (1987) Clinical and experimental evidence of microthrombosis in cerebral ischemia. In: Hartmann A, Kuschinsky W (eds.) Cerebral ischemia and hemorrheology. Springer, Berlin, Heidelberg, New York, pp. 386-393
28. Schneider H, Matakas F (1971) Pathological changes of the spinal cord after brain death. Acta Neuropathol (Bol) 18: 234-247
29. Schwenk J, Gosztonyi G (1987) Purpura cerebri in gram-negative septicaemia. A histological and histochemical study. Histol Histopathol 2: 57-66
30. Siesjö BK (1981) Cell damage in the brain: a speculative synthesis. J Cereb Blood Flow Metab 1: 155-185
31. Siesjö BK, Bengtsson F (1989) Calcium fluxes, calcium antagonists, and calcium-related pathology in brain ischemia, hypoglycemia and spreading depression: a unifying hypothesis. J Cereb Blood Flow Metab 9: 127-140
32. Siesjö BK, Wieloch T (1985) Calcium homeostasis, calcium entry blockers, and brain ischemia. In: Auer LM (ed.) Timing of aneurism surgery. de Gruyter, Berlin
33. Uzzell BP, Dolinskas CA, Wiser RF (1990) Relation between intracranial pressure, computed tomographic lesion, and neuropsychological outcome. Adv Neurol 52: 269-274
34. Yamauchi Y, Kato H, Kogure K (1990) Brain damage in a new hemorrhagic shock model in the rat using long-term recovery. J Cereb Blood Flow Metab 10: 207-212

Definition of Cardiovascular Dysfunction/Failure

J.-L. Vincent, G. Friedman

Introduction

To quantify as objectively as possible the degree of dysfunction of the various organs is very important not only to evaluate the critically ill patient at the bedside but also to assess the effects of new therapeutic interventions in clinical trials. Study of the time course of organ failure is also important to better understand its pathophysiology, from which new therapeutic options can be proposed. Definitions of organ failure can be provided for several organs, and especially for the lungs, kidneys, liver and coagulation system. However, each of these organs may individually fail while the other organs sill function relatively well. Even severe lung failure can be supported for many days by the use of oxygen mixtures and elevated end-expiratory pressure without major consequences for the other organs. The cardiovascular system has a specific role in that cardiovascular failure is rapidly and inevitably followed by the failure of the other organs. Even though arterial hypotension may be controlled by the use of adrenergic agents, the alterations in microvascular blood flow will rapidly lead to multiple organ dysfunction and failure. Hence the development of acute circulatory failure (shock) is usually a cause rather than a part of organ failure.

The present chapter will review the criteria used by various authors to define cardiovascular dysfunction/failure in the context of multiple organ dysfunction/failure and discuss these observations.

We reviewed the articles dealing with organ failure in the past 10 years (1983-1994) and completed this series by a Medline search [1-20]. Only articles (original or review articles) published in peer-reviewed journals were included, and book chapters were not considered. We found 20 articles which introduced a definition of cardiovascular dysfunction/failure. Table 1 summarizes the definitions used in these articles.

The criteria used can be grouped into four broad categories:

Circulatory Shock. In a number of articles, cardiovascular failure was assimilated with circulatory shock, and primarily defined as arterial hypotension [4, 6, 8, 13, 18]. For some authors, arterial hypotension requires the use of vasopressor agents [10, 15, 19], whereas for others the administration of vasoactive agents suffices to diagnose shock [9, 14, 16]. For some authors, fluid requirements may be high [8, 9], whereas for others hypotension should be resistant to fluid administration [17]. In only a few articles was it stated that hypotension should be associated with signs of tissue hypoperfusion [18].

Table 1: Definitions of organ dysfunction/failure

Author	Year	Definition
Borzotta and Polk [1]	1983	Hypotension, CI <1.5 l/min.m^2, no myocardial infarction
Bell et al. [5]	1983	Tamponade, endocarditis, or myocardial infarction
Faist et al. [2]	1983	High filling pressure with inadequate circulation, arrhythmia
Pine et al. [3]	1983	Heart failure needing inotropic agents or diuretics; pulmonary edema with PAOP ≥19 mmHg, myocardial infarction, cardiogenic shock
Bohnen et al. [4]	1983	Systolic AP <100 mmHg
Knaus WA et al. [6]	1985	HR ≤54 bpm, MAP ≤49 mmHg, ventricular tachycardia/fibrillation, metabolic acidosis
Goris and Boekhorst [7]	1985	Hypotensive requiring fluid and/or vasoactive drugs (dopamine or nitroglycerin)
Knaus et al. [6]	1985	APACHE II (HR >109 or <70 bpm, MAP >109 or <69 mmHg)
Carrico et al. [9]	1986	Increased volume requirements, volume-dependent hyperdynamic state or low CO, shock, inotropic support or volume overload/edema
Bihari et al. [10]	1987	Dopamine therapy for MAP >45 mmHg in the absence of hypovolemia (PAOP >6 mmHg)
Marshall et al. [11]	1988	CO >7 l.min, or PAOP ≥20 mmHg, inotropic support
DeCamp and Demling [12]	1988	Decreased ejection fraction
Tran et al. [13]	1990	MAP ≤50 mmHg, need for volume loading and/or vasoactive drugs to maintain systolic BP >100 mmHg, HR ≤50 bpm, ventricular arrhythmia, cardiac arrest, myocardial infarction
Moore et al. [14]	1991	Inotropic support or treated arrhythmia or cardiac arrest
Ruokonen et al. [15]	1991	Vasoactive drug infusion required to treat hypotension or decreased CO (excluding low-dose dopamine for renal perfusion)
Pinsky et al. [16]	1993	54 >HR 140 bpm, MAP <50 mmHg, PAOP >18 mmHg, or requirement of inotropic agents for >12 h
Marik [19]	1993	PAOP >16 mmHg and requirement for dopamine, dobutamine, epinephrine, and/or norepinephrine to maintain MAP >80 mmHg
Hebert et al. [17]	1993	Adrenergic agents to maintain MAP ≥55 mmHg in the absence of hypovolemia (PAOP ≥6 mmHg)
Fagon et al. [18]	1993	Systolic BP <90 mmHg with signs of hypoperfusion and/or requirement for inotropic support to maintain systolic BP >90 mmHg in the absence of hypovolemia
Sauaia et al. [20]	1994	CI <3.0 l/min.m^2 requiring inotropic support (dopamine or dobutamine)

PAOP, pulmonary artery balloon-occluded pressure; MAP, mean arterial pressure; CO, cardiac output; CI, cardiac index; HR, heart rate; BP, blood pressure

Heart Failure. Some articles used a categorical definition of heart failure [3], low cardiac output [15, 10] or low ventricular ejection fraction [12]. In some articles it was stated that cardiovascular dysfunction must be associated with elevated cardiac filling pressures [2, 3, 11, 16, 19] or requires the administration of inotropic agents [3, 20].

Increased Cardiac Output or Decreased Systemic Vascular Resistance. Here, e.g., Marshall et al. [11] considered a cardiac output above 7 l/min as a sign of cardiovascular dysfunction. The criteria used by Bone et al. [21] to define sepsis syndrome included elevated cardiac index and/or decreased systemic vascular resistance.

Specific Diagnoses. Diagnoses such as tamponade or endocarditis were sometimes included [5, 13]. Some authors also included myocardial infarction [3, 5, 13] while others specifically excluded this diagnosis [1]. Arrhythmias were also sometimes considered as a sign of cardiovascular dysfunction [2, 6, 14].

Discussion

We will successively review the problems associated with these four categories of signs of cardiovascular dysfunction/failure.

Circulatory Shock

Circulatory shock is clearly a very important entity, but also a complex one. Although arterial hypotension is an important sign of shock, acute perfusion failure involves more complex mechanisms than a reduction in perfusion pressure. Yet many authors use only hypotension in their definition of shock. There has been some discussion surrounding the criteria used to diagnose hypotension. The primary difficulty lies in the involvement of a therapeutic element in the definition, since hypotension requires immediate intervention with fluids and vasoactive agents.

The issue of fluid requirements is already quite complex, since increased fluid requirements may reflect the persistence of hemodynamic instability and/or increased fluid losses. On the other hand, transient hypotension responding rapidly to fluid challenge may not fit the definition of circulatory shock.

The degree of severity of the hypotension is obviously influenced by the vasoactive agents administered to the patient. Much imprecision surrounds the commonly used term "inotropic agents." A "vasopressor" agent is selected to increase vascular tone and thus arterial pressure while an "inotropic" agent is used to increase myocardial contractility. The use of a low dose of dopamine for renal purposes further complicates this issue, although the routine use of low doses of dopamine "to protect the kidneys" has recently been seriously challenged [22]. Vasopressor agents such as dopamine and norepinephrine can also exert potent inotropic effects, but their overall effects on ventricular function result from a combination of afterload-increasing and inotropic effects. We could thus call these agents "inoconstricting" agents. On the other hand, the increase in cardiac output is usually greater with dobutamine, which does not increase ventricular afterload and is today considered the inotropic agent of reference. Newer agents such as dopexamine or phosphodiesterase inhibitors are sometimes called "inodilators" for their combined inotropic and afterload-reducing effects. Vasodilators are generally avoided in shock, although they are sometimes used in a judicious attempt to improve blood flow when hypotension is not severe. According to Goris and Boekhorst [8], the association of arterial hypotension and the use of nitroglycerin could fit the definition of cardiac failure.

It is surprising to find reference to signs of tissue underperfusion in only one article [18]. Circulatory shock is rapidly associated with altered perfusion of the organs, so that the definition should include some signs of decreased tissue perfusion, such as oliguria, altered mentation or altered skin perfusion (Table 1).

Heart Failure

It is also important to separate the terms ventricular failure from dysfunction or myocardial depression. Cardiac failure refers to an inadequate pump function, resulting in an insufficient blood flow to the tissues. Ventricular dysfunction reflects an alteration in the relation between the ventricular output or stroke volume and the ventricular preload. Ventricular preload is best assessed by measurements of ventricular end-diastolic volume, although ventricular filling pressures are often used as a substitute. The ejection fraction, the ratio of the stroke volume to ventricular end-diastolic volume, is usually used as an indicator of ventricular function. Importantly, ventricular function is influenced not only by contractility, but also by afterload and to some extent by preload [23]. In ventricular dysfunction as in failure, the ventricular end-diastolic volume is enlarged and the right atrial pressure increased, resulting in venous congestion. Thus, ventricular dilation can allow the maintenance of stroke volume by the Frank-Starling mechanism in the presence of ventricular dysfunction, but this compensatory mechanism is exhausted in the presence of failure. Simultaneous measurements of cardiac output and right ventricular ejection fracture (RVEF) can be very helpful in distinguishing ventricular dysfunction from failure.

Myocardial depression refers to a reduction in contractility. Myocardial depression is commonly present in severe sepsis and septic shock, and is primarily attributed to the influence of various mediators. The severity of myocardial depression has been directly related to the severity of sepsis [24]. Yet the cardiac output may remain normal or high, as the same mediators are involved in the reduction in the left ventricular afterload associated with the peripheral vasodilation, which facilitates left ventricular outflow and thus increases venous return. Thus, in many critically ill patients, myocardial depression and even cardiac dysfunction may be present, but cardiac failure is not reached. For instance, acute respiratory distress syndrome (ARDS) is usually associated with an alteration in right ventricular function, which primarily results from the development of pulmonary hypertension, representing an increase in right ventricular afterload. In severe cases, a reduction in myocardial contractility may also contribute, as a result of an insufficient blood supply to the right ventricle or the release of cardiodepressant substances.

Increased Cardiac Output or Decreased Systemic Vascular Resistance

In a number of studies, cardiovascular dysfunction is assimilated with low systemic vascular resistance (SVR), but since SVR is basically the ratio of blood pressure over cardiac output, and since hypotension is already included in the definition of shock, then a low SVR is basically equivalent to a high cardiac output, which is a characteristic rather than an ominous complication of severe sepsis. In patients with sepsis or multiple organ failure, the development of a low cardiac output unresponsive to fluids is usually a terminal event, so that defining cardiovascular dysfunction by a low cardiac output is probably too restrictive. In the presence of septic shock, a lower SVR is associated with poorer prognosis [24, 25].

Specific Diagnoses

Other complications such as myocardial infarction, tamponade and endocarditis should be considered as disease processes as such and should probably not be listed as signs of cardiovascular dysfunction or failure in the critically ill. Myocardial infarction is a rare complication in severe sepsis, probably because the coronary blood flow is usually preserved in these conditions [26]. Arrhythmias are neither sensitive nor specific signs of cardiovascular complications.

Conclusions

Circulatory shock is a common cause of organ dysfunction/failure. It can be considered as a cause of organ dysfunction/failure rather than as a part of the syndrome. Hypotension is an important sign of shock, but circulatory shock is more complex. For practical purposes, shock can be defined by arterial hypotension associated with signs of tissue hypoperfusion (Table 2).

Table 2. Definition of circulatory shock

1.	Arterial hypotension (mean arterial pressure <65 mmHg or systolic arterial pressure <90 mmHg) or vasopressor dependency
2.	Signs of altered organ perfusion: Elevated lactate level (2 mEq/l) Oliguria (20 ml/h) Acute alteration in mental status Impaired skin perfusion

Beyond this definition of shock, it is difficult to define cardiovascular dysfunction. An elevated cardiac output and/or a low systemic vascular resistance is an important sign of sepsis and is usually present in multiple organ dysfunction/failure, but it should not be considered as a sign of cardiovascular dysfunction or failure. On the other hand, a low cardiac output due to cardiac failure is a rare, terminal event in septic patients.

References

1. Borzotta AP, Polk HC (1983) Multiple system organ failure. *Surg Clin North America* 63: 315-336
2. Faist E, Baue A, Ditmer H et al. (1983) Multiple organ failure in polytrauma patients. *J Trauma* 23: 775-787
3. Pine RW, Wertz MJ, Lennard ES et al. (1983) Determinants of organ malfunction or death in patients with intra-abdominal sepsis. *Arch Surg* 118: 242-249
4. Bohnen J, Boulanger M, Meakins JL et al. (1983) Prognosis in generalized peritonitis. *Arch Surg* 118: 285-290
5. Bell RC, Coalson JJ, Smith JD et al. (1983) Multiple organ system failure and infection in adult respiratory distress syndrome. *Ann Intern Med* 99: 293-298
6. Knaus WA, Draper EA, Wagner DP et al. (1985) Prognosis in acute organ-system failure. *Ann Surg* 202: 685-693

7. Knaus WA, Draper EA, Wagner DP et al. (1985) APACHE II: a severity of disease classification system. Crit Care Med 13: 818-829
8. Goris RJA, Boekhorst TPS (1985) Multiple-organ failure. Arch surg 120: 1109-1115
9. Carrico CJ, Meakins JL, Marshall JC et al. (1986) Multiple-organ-failure syndrome. Arch Surg 121: 196-208
10. Bihari D, Smithies M, Gimson A et al. (1987) The effects of vasodilation with prostacyclin on oxygen delivery and uptake in critically ill patients. N Engl J Med 317: 397-403
11. Marshall JC, Christou NV, Horn R et al. (1988) The microbiology of multiple organ failure. Arch Surg 123: 309-315
12. DeCamp MM, Demling RH (1988) Posttraumatic multisystem organ failure. JAMA 260: 530-534
13. Tran DD, Groeneveld ABJ, Vander Meulen J et al. (1990) Age, chronic disease, sepsis, organ system failure, and mortality in a medical intensive care unit. Crit Care Med 18: 474-479
14. Moore F, Moore E, Poggetti R et al. (1991) Gut bacterial translocation via the portal vein: a clinical perspective with major torso trauma. J Trauma 31: 629-638
15. Ruokonen E, Takala J, Kari A et al. (1991) Septic shock and multiple organ failure. Crit Care Med 19: 1146-1151
16. Pinsky MR, Vincent JL, Deviere J et al. (1993) Serum cytokine levels in human septic shock: relation to multiple-systems organ failure and mortality. Chest 103: 565-575
17. Hebert PC, Drummond AJ, Singer J et al. (1993) A simple multiple system organ failure scoring system predicts mortality of patients who have sepsis syndrome. Chest 104: 230-235
18. Fagon JY, Chastre J, Novara A et al. (1993) Characterization of intensive care unit patients using a model based on the presence or absence of organ dysfunctions and/or infections: the ODIN model. Intensive Care Med 19: 137-144
19. Marik PE (1993) Gastric intramucosal pH. A better predictor of multiorgan dysfunction syndrome and death than oxygen-derived variables in patients with sepsis. Chest 104: 225-229
20. Sauaia A, Moore FA, Moore EE et al. (1994) Early predictors of postinjury multiple organ failure. Arch Surg 129: 39-45
21. Bone RC, Fisher CJJ, Clemmer TP et al. (1989) Sepsis syndrome: a valid clinical entity. Methylprednisolone Severe Sepsis Study Group [see comments]. Crit Care Med 17: 389-393
22. Vincent JL (1994) Renal effects of dopamine: may our dream ever come true? (Editorial). Crit Care Med 22: 5-6
23. Robotham JL, Takala M, Berman M et al. (1991) Ejection fraction revisited. Anesthesiology 74: 172-183
24. Vincent JL, Gris P, Coffernils M et al. (1992) Myocardial depression characterizes the fatal course of septic shock. Surgery 111: 660-667
25. Groeneveld AB, Nauta JJ, Thijs LG (1988) Peripheral vascular resistance in septic shock: its relation to outcome. Intensive Care Med 14: 141-147
26. Dhainaut JF, Huyghebaert MF, Monsallier JF et al. (1987) Coronary hemodynamics and myocardial metabolism lactate, free fatty acids, glucose, and ketons in patients with septic shock. Circulation 75: 533-541

Challenges of the Concept of Supranormal Oxygen Delivery in Patients with Sepsis: Evidence Against Tissue Hypoxia but for Impaired Oxygen Metabolism in Sepsis

P. Boekstegers, K. Werdan

Introduction

The existence of a "pathological oxygen uptake supply dependency" in sepsis has been inferred from experimental and clinical studies [1-8], which have suggested that oxygen consumption is linearly related to oxygen delivery over an abnormally wide range of oxygen delivery [3-5]. From their observations several authors concluded that a "covert tissue hypoxia" or a "tissue oxygen debt" may exist in patients with sepsis. Together with the assumption of an increased point of critical oxygen delivery in sepsis [1-3], this has been the main argument for increasing oxygen delivery to supranormal levels in sepsis [9-14]. Furthermore, the finding of increased serum lactate levels in patients with sepsis [9, 15] seemed to support the assumption of tissue hypoxia in sepsis and, thus, the concept of supranormal oxygen delivery to prevent tissue hypoxia.

Recent experimental and clinical studies, however, have challenged these basic assumptions of the concept of supranormal oxygen delivery: First, there is evidence that the pathological oxygen uptake supply dependency in patients with sepsis is the result of a mathematical coupling error [16-18]. Because in the earlier studies the thermodilution technique and the Fick equation were used to calculate both oxygen delivery and oxygen consumption, the two components of the regression analysis shared the same variable and its associated error in measurement [19]. Such a mathematical coupling error may lead to an artificial linear relationship between oxygen delivery and oxygen consumption [19]. Using two independent measurements for determination of oxygen delivery and oxygen consumption and, thereby, avoiding the mathematical coupling error, recent studies failed to demonstrate a pathological oxygen uptake supply dependency [18, 20, 21].

Second, an increased point of critical oxygen delivery in sepsis was not observed in a clinical study which, for the first time, actually determined the point of critical oxygen delivery in patients with sepsis [22]. Both patients with sepsis and nonseptic patients showed physiological relationships between oxygen delivery and oxygen consumption [22].

Third, a number of experimental and clinical studies showed that increased tissue or plasma levels of lactate did not necessarily imply tissue hypoxia in sepsis [23-26]. Changes in metabolic pathways such as a decrease in the proportion of active pyruvate dehydrogenase activity may lead to lactic acidosis without evidence of tissue hypoxia. A reversal of lactic acidosis was possible using dichloroacetate for stimulation of pyruvate dehydrogenase complex in septic models [27]. Interestingly, in patients with sepsis, treatment with dicholoracetate improved lactic acidosis without a change in oxygen delivery or oxygen consumption [28].

From these observations the existence of a clinically relevant tissue hypoxia or a covert oxygen debt in patients with sepsis may be doubted. Evidence against cellular hypoxia in sepsis has also come from recent studies in rats with sepsis although sensitive methods for the detection of cellular hypoxia such as in vivo phosporus 31 nuclear magnetic resonance spectroscopy, [18F]fluoromisonidazole and microfluorometric enzymatic techniques were used [29]. The authors concluded that cellular hypoxia may not be the major pathophysiological abnormality in sepsis [29] and, thus, the role of cellular hypoxia and bioenergetic failure in sepsis should be reevaluated [30].

Because direct evidence for tissue hypoxia in patients with sepsis would be of crucial importance with regard to the concept of supranormal oxygen delivery, we determined the oxygen partial pressure distribution within skeletal muscle using polarographic measurements. This paper summarizes the main results of our studies in patients with sepsis [31-33], providing evidence against tissue hypoxia but for impaired oxygen metabolism within skeletal muscle.

Methods

Two different methods were used to determine skeletal muscle pO_2. For intermittent measurement of pO_2 distribution a rapidly responding polarographic needle electrode with a diameter of 350 μm was moved forward stepwise in the muscle as described in detail elsewhere [32]. For continuous measurement of skeletal muscle pO_2, flexible and smooth polarographic catheters (diameter, 650 μm) were used. The pO_2 sensitive area (about 32 mm^2) of the catheter was completely inserted into the muscle. Before and after each measuring period of 96 h the pO_2 catheters were calibrated. For correction of the pO_2 data, the temperature within the biceps muscle was measured simultaneously and linear drift of the pO_2 catheter was assumed [32].

Study Groups and Results

In the first study [31] skeletal muscle pO_2 was compared in patients with sepsis ($n=20$), patients with limited infection ($n=10$) and patients with cardiogenic shock ($n=10$). Apparently skeletal muscle pO_2 was not critically reduced in patients with sepsis, but was more than twice as high as in patients with cardiogenic shock (Fig. 1). Because skeletal muscle pO_2 was measured once and for a short period only, tissue hypoxia might have been missed in these patients. Using intermittent and continuous measurements, however, in a second study in 67 patients with sepsis, the initial results were confirmed and extended [32]. Skeletal muscle pO_2 in patients with sepsis was related to severity of sepsis (Fig. 2): it increased as the state of sepsis increased in severity, and a decrease of abnormally high skeletal muscle pO_2 was associated with recovery from sepsis (Figs. 2, 3).

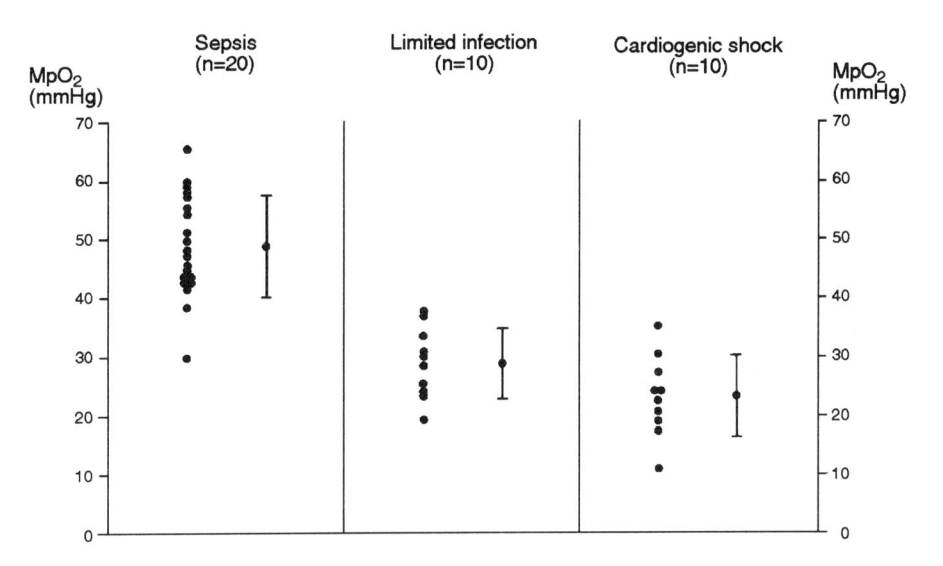

Fig. 1: Mean skeletal muscle pO₂ (MpO₂) determined by needle electrodes in 20 patients with sepsis, 10 patients with limited infection and 10 patients with cardiogenic shock (for details see [31])

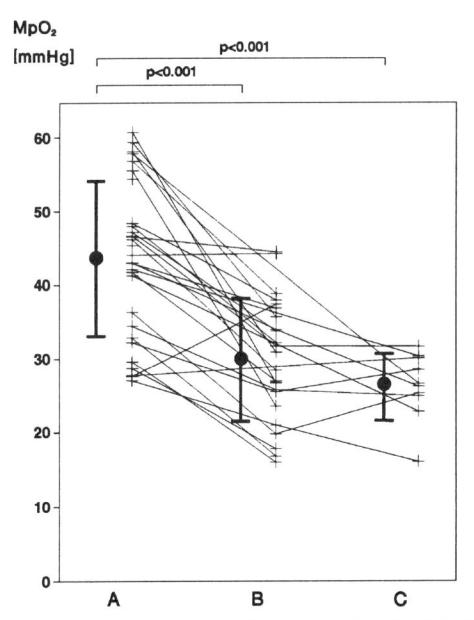

Fig. 2: Serial intermittent determination of skeletal muscle pO₂ (MpO₂) in 28 patients with sepsis during seven consecutive days. A, days of septic state; B, days of intermediate state; C, days of nonseptic state. Values for each patient and the mean (± SD) of each state are given (for details see [32])

MpO₂ [mmHg] (catheter)

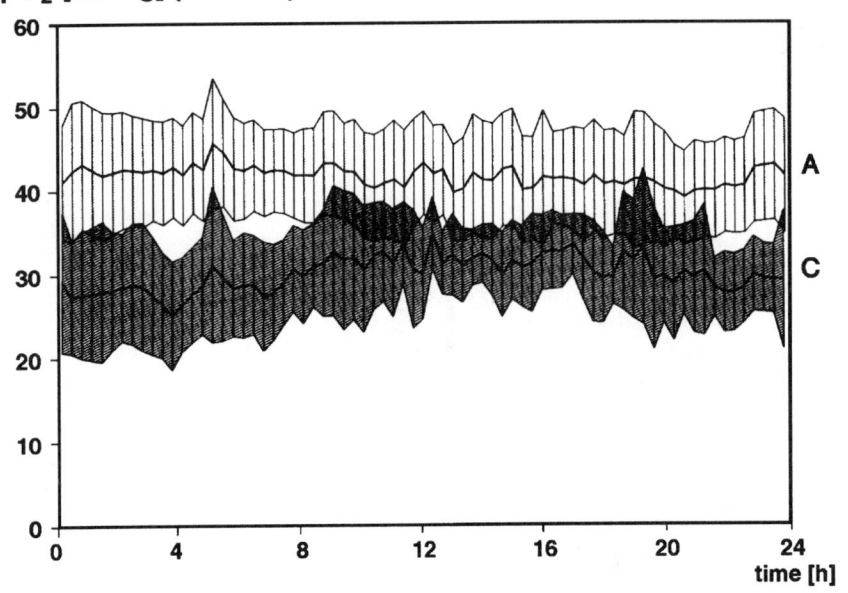

Fig. 3: Continuous measurement of skeletal muscle pO₂ (MpO₂) (catheter) in 13 patients with sepsis. Pooled data of 24-h measurements (replicated observations per patient were reduced by taking the mean). A, days with septic state; C, days with nonseptic state. Data are shown as means ±95% confidence interval (for details see [32])

In a third study of 20 patients with sepsis [33], skeletal muscle pO_2 was continuously measured after intravenous administration of anti-TNFα-antibody. Before administration of anti-TNFα-antibody mean skeletal muscle pO_2 was abnormally high, with a mean of 44±11 mmHg. Taking all the patients into consideration, mean skeletal muscle pO_2 decreased from 44 to 36 mmHg ($P = 0.006$) within 24 h after the first administration of the anti-TNFα-antibody. In the patients ($n=11$, group A) showing a decrease in mean skeletal muscle pO_2 of more than 5 mmHg (range 7-19 mmHg) (Fig. 4), this was associated with a decrease in interleukin-6 serum levels (Δ -280 pg/ml), in APACHE II scores (Δ -4.4 points) and in Elebute scores (Δ -3.2 points) within 7 days. However, no change in interleukin-6 serum levels, APACHE II scores or Elebute scores was observed in the patients ($n=9$, group B) without a decrease of skeletal muscle pO_2 by more than 5 mmHg within the first 24 h after administration of anti-TNFα-antibody (Fig. 4). The latter patients also had a worse clinical outcome: 28-day mortality was 7 of 9 patients in group B but 2 of 11 patients in group A.

Discussion

Although intermittent or continuous measurements of skeletal muscle pO_2 were performed in a total of 107 patients with sepsis, no periods of tissue hypoxia were observed except in the very final hypodynamic state of severe sepsis [32]. It has to be stressed that all patients were studied after or during adequate volume replacement and during catecholamine treatment if required. Furthermore, at inclusion into the study each patient showed the characteristic cardiovascular pattern of sepsis with hypotension despite normal or elevated cardiac output resulting in a decrease in systemic vascular resistance [34]. Because of the elevated cardiac output, oxygen delivery was consecutively increased to a mean of 450-600 ml/min per square meter in our patients. These levels of oxygen delivery were higher than normal but were still far below the levels (600-800 ml/min per square meter) which have been suggested to avoid or improve tissue hypoxia in sepsis if following the concept of supranormal oxygen delivery [9,10,13,14]. Although skeletal muscle may not be representative for other organs such as the kidney or the gut, our data, which show no skeletal muscle hypoxia in patients with severe sepsis without supranormal oxygen delivery, argue against the necessity of this kind of treatment on the basis of direct determinations of tissue pO_2. Indirect measures of tissue oxygenation, however, such as gastric pH [35] or serum lactate [15], if pathologically changed in patients with sepsis do not necessarily indicate a critical reduction in tissue oxygenation. Because lactic acidosis may be induced by metabolic changes in sepsis [26, 28] without evidence for tissue hypoxia, these measurements cannot prove a tissue oxygen debt in patients.

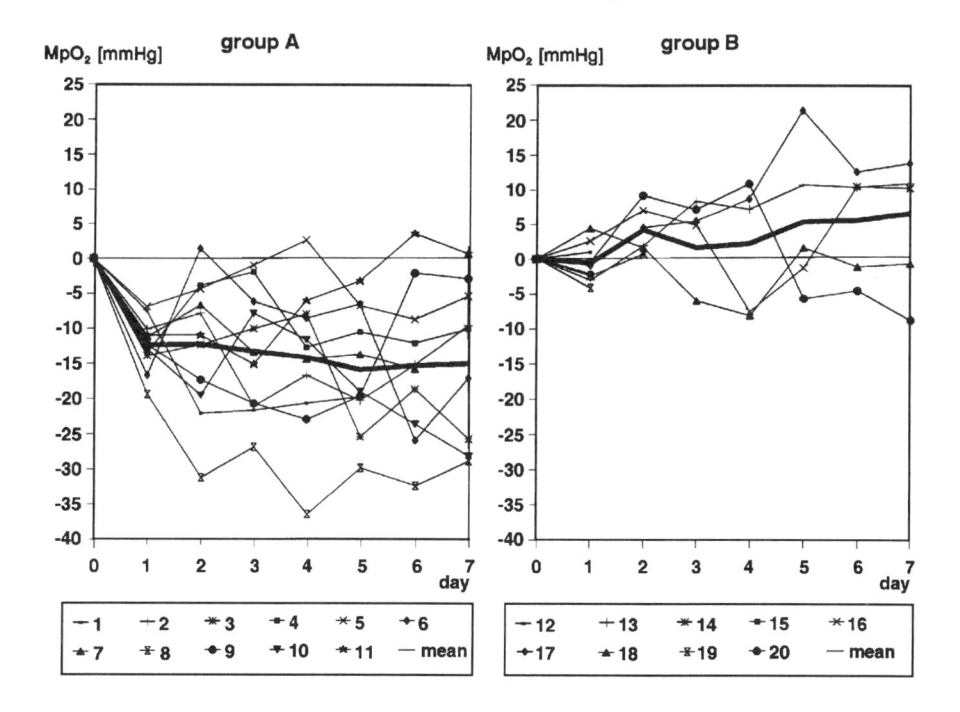

Fig. 4: Change in skeletal muscle pO_2 (MpO_2) after administration of anti-TNFα-antibody (day 1 to day 5). Group A (n=11) with decrease in MpO_2 >5 mmHg within 24 h, group B (n=9) with no decrease of MpO_2 >5mmHg within 24 h. Individual patients are indicated by different symbols. Mean of group A and B are indicated by the continuous line (for details see [33])

Controversial results have been reported as to whether supranormal oxygen delivery improves survival in patients with sepsis [8-10, 12-14, 36]. The conflicting data may in part result from methodological problems because of the presence of the mathematical coupling error [16-18, 37] existing in many of the studies. More recent studies, however, also failed to demonstrate a beneficial effect of increasing oxygen delivery to supranormal oxygen delivery by the inotropic agent dobutamine in patients with sepsis [13, 14]. From a meta-analysis of 40 studies in this field [38], the authors also concluded that their study failed to identify either an optimal or a critical value of oxygen delivery or oxygen consumption in critically ill patients.

Obviously, the concept of supranormal oxygen delivery and pathological oxygen uptake supply dependency in sepsis - though very attractive at the beginning - failed to be convincing in clinical practice. Because there is also increasing evidence that the basic assumptions of this concept might have been misleading, the pathophysiological abnormalities of oxygen metabolism in sepsis have been started to be reevaluated [30, 39].

If tissue hypoxia is not the major pathophysiological abnormality in sepsis, cell death and organ dysfunction are likely to result from a primary metabolic disorder. Although this theory was proposed by Siegel et al. more than 10 years ago [40], the role of metabolic dysfunction in sepsis is still poorly defined. With the identification of the pathophysiological importance of cytokine mediated injury in sepsis (TNFα, interleukin-1, interleukin-6, interleukin-8) [41-46], there has been growing interest in cytokine-mediated metabolic dysfunction in sepsis in recent years [47-52].

Our clinical observations showing that skeletal muscle pO_2 increased in relation to the severity of the stage of sepsis (Figs. 2, 3) suggest that oxygen utilization within tissue decreased with deterioration of sepsis, thereby increasing skeletal muscle pO_2 [32]. Because a decrease in skeletal muscle pO_2 was associated with a decrease of interleukin-6 serum levels and improvement of sepsis after administration of anti-TNFα-antibody in patients with severe sepsis, a change of skeletal muscle oxygenation might reflect a change in cytokine induced dysfunction of oxygen metabolism. In cell cultures and animal models cytokines such as TNFα, interleukin-1 and γ-interferon have been shown to change mitochondrial substrate metabolism leading to reduced oxygen consumption within hours [47, 49, 51, 52]. These effects were mediated either by a certain cytokine alone [51] or by synergism of cytokines [47, 52]. The activity of mitochondrial enzymes such as the pyruvate dehydrogenase decreases in sepsis [23-25], and complex I and II activities of the mitochondrial respiratory chain are inhibited [52]. Because the activity of these enzymes can be restored within hours [24, 49], abnormalities of mitochondrial substrate metabolism might have been effectively counteracted by anti-TNFα-antibody administration in the patients with sepsis showing a decrease in skeletal muscle pO_2 within 24 h (Fig. 4). Furthermore, there is evidence from determination of oxygen consumption within skeletal muscle (results not shown) that oxygen consumption increased in patients recovering from sepsis after administration of anti-TNFα-antibody.

In summary, tissue oxygen partial pressure measurements in skeletal muscle provide evidence against tissue hypoxia but for reduced oxygen metabolism in patients with sepsis. A disturbed oxygen metabolism which may be induced at the mitochondrial level, apparently cannot be counteracted by supranormal oxygen transport to tissue. Therefore, other strategies aiming to improve cytokine mediated injury such as cytokine antibodies or cytokine receptor antagonists [33, 53-57] may be required to prevent or reverse metabolic dysfunction and multiple organ failure in sepsis.

References

1. Samsel RW, Nelson DP, Sanders WM, Wood LDH, Schumacker PT (1988) Effect of endotoxin on systemic and skeletal muscle O_2 extraction. J Appl Physiol 65: 1377-1382
2. Nelson DP, Beyer C, Samsel RW, Wood LDH, Schumacker PT (1987) Pathological supply dependence of O_2 uptake during bacteremia in dogs. J Appl Physiol 63: 1487-1492
3. Nelson DP, Samsel RW, Wood LDH, Schumacker PT (1988) Pathological supply dependence of systemic and intestinal O_2 uptake during endotoxemia. J Appl Physiol 64: 2410-2419
4. Bredle DL, Samsel RW, Schumacker PT, Cain SM (1989) Critical O_2 delivery to skeletal muscle at high and low PO_2 in endotoxemic dogs. J Appl Physiol 66: 2553-2558
5. Gutierrez G, Pohil RJ (1986) Oxygen consumption is lineary related to O_2 supply in critically ill patients. J Crit Care 1: 45-53
6. Wolf YG, Cotev S, Perel A, Manny J (1987) Dependence of oxygen consumption on cardiac output in sepsis. Crit Care Med 15: 198-203
7. Rackow EC, Astiz ME, Weil MH (1988) Cellular oxygen metabolism during sepsis and shock. The relationship of oxygen consumption to oxygen delivery. JAMA 259: 1989-1993
8. Bihari D, Smithies M, Gimson A, Tinker J (1987) The effects of vasodilation with prostacyclin on oxygen delivery and uptake in critically ill patients. N Engl J Med 317: 397-403
9. Vincent JL, Roman A, deBacker D, Kahn RJ (1990) Oxygen uptake/supply dependency. Effects of short-term dobutamine infusion. Am Rev Respir Dis 142: 2-7
10. Tuchschmidt J, Fried J, Astiz M, Rackow E (1992) Elevation of cardiac output and oxygen delivery improves outcome in septic shock. Chest 102: 216-220
11. Shoemaker WC, Appel PL, Kram HB, Waxman K, Lee TS (1988) Prospective trial of supranormal values of survivors as therapeutic goals in high-risk surgical patients. Chest 94: 1176-1186
12. Silverman HJ, Slotman G, Bone RC, Maunder R, Hyers TM, Kerstein MD, Ursprung JJ and the Prostaglandin E_1 Study Group (1990) Effects of prostaglandin E_1 on oxygen delivery and consumption in patients with the adult respiratory distress syndrome. Results from the prostaglandin E_1 multicenter trial. Chest 98: 405-410
13. Hayes MA, Yau EH, Timmins AC, Hinds CJ, Watson D (1993) Response of critically ill patients to treatment aimed at achieving supranormal oxygen delivery and consumption. Chest 103: 886-895
14. Hayes MA, Timmins AC, Yau E, Palazzo M, Hinds CJ, Watson D (1994). Elevation of systemic oxygen delivery in the treatment of critically ill patients. N Eng J Med 330: 1717-1722
15. Bakkar J, Coffernils M, Leon M, Gris, P, Vincent JL (1991) Blood lactate levels are superior to oxygen-derived variables in predicting outcome in human septic shock. Chest 99: 956-962
16. Archie JP (1981) Mathematic coupling of data. Ann Surg 193: 296-303
17. Stratton HH, Feustel PJ, Newell JC (1987) Regression of calculated variables in the presence of shared measurement error. J Appl Physiol 62: 2083-2093
18. Vermeij CG, Feenstra BWA, Bruining HA (1990) Oxygen delivery and oxygen uptake in postoperative and septic patients. Chest 98: 415-420
19. Cain SM (1994) A current view of oxygen supply dependency. In: Reinhart K, Eyrich K, Sprung C (eds.) Sepsis: Current perspectives in pathophysiology and therapy. Springer, Berlin, Heidelberg, New York
20. Wysocki M, Besbes M, Roupie E, Brun-Buisson C (1992) Modification of oxygen extraction ratio by change in oxygen transport in septic shock. Chest 102: 221-226

21. Annat G, Viale JP, Percival C, Froment M, Motin J (1986) Oxygen delivery and uptake in the adult respiratory distress syndrome. Lack of relationship when measured independently in patients with normal lactate concentrations. Am Rev Respir Dis 133: 999-1001
22. Ronco JJ, Fenwick JC, Tweeddale MG, Wiggs BR, Phang PT, Cooper DJ, Cunningham KF, Russel JA, Walley KR (1993) Identification of the critical oxygen delivery for anaerobic metabolism in critically ill septic and nonseptic humans. JAMA 270: 1724-1730
23. Vary TC, Siegel JH, Nakatani T, Sato T, Aoyama H (1986) Effect of sepsis on activity of pyruvate dehydrogenase complex in skeletal muscle and liver. Am J Physiol 250: E634-E640
24. Vary TC, Siegel JH, Tall BD, Morris JG, Joyce AS (1988) Inhibition of skeletal muscle protein synthesis in septic intra-abdominal abscess. J Trauma 28: 981-988
25. Vary TC, Martin LF (1993) Potentiation of decreased pyruvate dehydrogenase activity by inflammatory stimuli in sepsis. Circ Shock 39: 299-305
26. Curtis SE, Cain SM (1992) Regional and systemic oxygen delivery/uptake relations and lactate flux in hyperdynamic, endotoxin-treated dogs. Am Rev Respir Dis 145: 348-354
27. Vary TC, Siegel JH, Placko R, Tall BD, Morris JG (1989) Effect of dichloroacetate on plasma and hepatic amino acids in sterile inflammation and sepsis. Arch Surg 124: 1071-1077
28. Stacpoole PW, Wright EC, Baumgartner TG, Bersin RM, Buchalter S, Curry SH, Duncan CA, Harman EM, Henderson GN, Jenkinson S, Lachin JM, Lorenz A, Schneider SH, Siegel JH, Summer WR, Thompson D, Wolfe CL, Zorovich B, the Dichloroacetate-Lactic Acidosis Study Group (1992) A controlled clinical trial of dichloracetate for treatment of lactic acidosis in adults. N Engl J Med 327: 1564-1569
29. Hotchkiss RS, Rust RS, Dence CS, Wasserman TH, Song SK, Hwang DR, Karl IE, Welch MJ (1991) Evaluation of the role of cellular hypoxia in sepsis by the hypoxic marker $[^{18}F]$fluoromisonidazole. Am J Physiol 261: R965-R972
30. Hotchkiss RS, Karl IE (1992) Reevaluation of the role of cellular hypoxia and bioenergetic failure in sepsis. JAMA 267: 1503-1510
31. Boekstegers P, Weidenhöfer S, Pilz G, Werdan K (1991) Peripheral oxygen availability within skeletal muscle in sepsis and septic shock: comparison to limited infection and cardiogenic shock. Infection 19: 317-323
32. Boekstegers P, Weidenhöfer S, Kapsner T, Werdan K (1994) Skeletal muscle partial pressure of oxygen in patients with sepsis. Crit Care Med 22: 640-650
33. Boekstegers P, Weidenhöfer S, Zell R, Holler E, Kapsner T, Redl H, Schlag G, Kaul M, Kempeni J, Werdan K (1994) Changes in skeletal muscle PO_2 after administration of anti-TNFα-antibody in patients with severe sepsis: comparison to interleukin-6 levels, Apache II, and elebute scores. Shock 1: 246-253
34. Parker ME, Shelhamer JH, Natanson C, Alling DW, Parrillo JE (1987) Serial cardiovascular variables in survivors and nonsurvivors of human septic shock: heart rate as an early predictor of prognosis. Crit Care Med 15: 923-929
35. Gutierrez G, Palizas F, Doglio G, Wainsztein N, Gallesio A, Pacin J, Dubin A, Schiavi E, Jorge M, Pusajo J, Klein F, Roman ES, Dorfman B, Shottlender J, Giniger R (1992) Gastric intramucosal pH as a therapeutic index of tissue oxygenation in critically ill patients. Lancet 339: 195-199
36. Russell JA, Ronco JJ, Lockhat D, Belzberg A, Kiess M, Dodek PM (1990) Oxygen delivery and consumption and ventricular preload are greater in survivors than in nonsurvivors of the adult respiratory distress syndrome. Am Rev Respir Dis 141: 659-665
37. Dantzker DR, Foresman B, Gutierrez G (1991) Oxygen supply and utilization relationships. Am Rev Respir Dis 143: 675-679

38. Steltzer H, Hiesmayr M, Mayer N, Krafft P, Hammerle AF (1994) The relationship between oxygen delivery and uptake in the critically ill: is there a critical or optimal therapeutic value? Anaesthesia 49: 229-236
39. Bone RC (1992) Abnormal cellular metabolism in sepsis. JAMA 267: 1518-1519
40. Siegel JH, Cerra FB, Coleman B, Giovannini I, Shetye M, Border JR, McMenamy RH (1979) Physiological and metabolic correlations in human sepsis. Surgery 86: 163-193
41. Natanson C, Eichenholz PW, Danner RL, Eichacker PQ, Hoffman WD, Kuo GC, Banks SM, MacVittie TJ, Parrillo JE (1989) Endotoxin and tumor necrosis factor challenges in dogs simulate the cardiovascular profile of human septic shock. J Exp Med 169: 823-832
42. Schirmer JW, Schirmer JM, Fry DE (1989) Recombinant human tumor necrosis factor produces hemodynamic changes characteristic of sepsis and endotoxemia. Arch Surg 124: 445-448
43. Tracey KJ, Lowry SF, Fahey TJ, Albert JD, Fong Y, Hesse D, Beutler B, Manogue K, Calvano S, Wei H, Ceramy A W, Shires GT (1987) Cachectin/tumor necrosis factor induces lethal shock and stress hormone responses in the dog. Surg Gynecol Obstet 164: 415-422
44. Beutler B, Milsark IW, Cerami AC (1985) Passive immunization against cachectin/tumor necrosis factor protects mice from the lethal effect of endotoxin. Science 229: 869-871.
45. Möller A, Emling F, Blohm D (1990) Monoclonal antibodies to human tumour necrosis factor alpha: in vitro and in vivo application. Cytokine 2: 162-169
46. Okusawa S, Gelfand JA, Ikejima T, Conolly RJ, Dinarello A (1988) Interleukin 1 induces a shock-like state in rabbits. J Clin Invest 81: 1162-1172
47. Tredget EE, Yu YM, Zhong S, Burini R, Okusawa S, Gelfand JA, Dinarello CA, Young VR, Burke JF (1988) Role of interleukin 1 and tumor necrosis factor on energy metabolism in rabbits. Am J Physiol 255: E760-E768
48. Taylor DJ, Faragher EB, Evanson JM (1992) Inflammatory cytokines stimulate glucose uptake and glycolysis but reduce glucose oxidation in human dermal fibroblasts in vitro. Circ Shock 37: 105-110
49. Schulze-Osthoff K, Bakker AC, Vanhaesebroeck B, Beyaert R, Jacob WA, Fiers W (1992) Cytotoxic activity of tumor necrosis factor is mediated by early damage of mitochondrial functions. Evidence for the involvement of mitochondrial radical generation. J Biol Chem 267: 5317-5324
50. Mela-Riker L, Bartos D, Viessis AA, Widener L, Muller P, Trunkey DD (1992) Chronic hyperdynamic sepsis in the rat. II. Characterization of liver and muscle energy metabolism. Circ Shock 36: 83-92
51. Eizirik DL (1988) Interleukin-1 induced impairment in pancreatic islet oxidative metabolism of glucose is potentiated by tumor necrosis factor. Acta Endocrinol (Copenh) 119: 321-325.
52. Geng Y, Hansson GK, Holme E (1992) Interferon-γ and tumor necrosis factor synergize to induce nitric oxide production and inhibit mitochondrial respiration in vascular smooth muscle cells. Circ Res 71: 1268-1276
53. Fisher CJ, Opal SM, Dhainaut JF, Stephens S, Zimmerman JL, Nightingale P, Harris SJ, Schein RMH, Panacek EA, Vincent JL, Foulke GE, Warren EL, Garrard C, Park G, Bodmer MW, Cohen J, Van der Linden C, Cross AS, Sadoff JC and the CB0006 sepsis syndrome study group (1993) Influence of an anti-tumor necrosis factor monoclonal antibody on cytokine levels in patients with sepsis. Crit Care Med 21: 318-327
54. Boekstegers P, Weidenhöfer S, Zell R, Pilz G, Holler E, Ertel W, Kapsner T, Redl H, Schlag G, Kaul M, Kempeni J, Stenzel R, Werdan K (1994) Repeated administration of a $F(ab')_2$ fragment of an anti-tumor necrosis factor α antibody in patients with severe sepsis: effects on the cardiovascular system and cytokine levels. Shock 1: 237-245

55. Ohlsson K, Björk P, Bergenfeldt M, Hagemann R, Thompson RC (1990) Interleukin-1 receptor antagonist reduces mortality from endotoxin shock. Nature 348: 550-552
56. Lesslauer W, Tabuchi H, Gentz R, Brockhaus M, Schlaeger EJ, Grau G, Piguet P, Pointaire P, Vassalli P, Loetscher H (1991) Recombinant soluble tumor necrosis factor receptor proteins protect mice from lipopolysaccharide-induced lethality. Eur J Immunol 21: 2883-2886
57. Fisher CJ, Dhainaut JFA, Opal SM, Pribble JP, Balk RA, Slotman GJ, Iberti TJ, Rackow EC, Shapiro MJ, Greenman RL, Reines HD, Shelly MP, Thompson BW, LaBrecque JF, Catalano MA, Knaus WA, Sadoff JC (1994) Recombinant human Interleukin 1 receptor antagonist in the treatment of patients with sepsis syndrome. JAMA 271: 1836-1843

Hemorrhagic Shock Severely Impairs Liver Function

A.E. Barber, W.J. Millikan, H. Illner, L. Montalvo, L. Griffith, G.T. Shires

Introduction

Hemorrhagic shock following trauma or gastrointestinal bleeding remains a major cause of morbidity and mortality. The hepatic dysfunction attendant to hemorrhagic shock has not been well characterized. The low tolerance of cirrhotic subjects to hemorrhagic shock has been attributed to their decreased hepatic reserve [1]. Tumor necrosis factor (TNF) is elevated in human cirrhotic subjects, but few data are available in the cirrhotic rat [2]. The role of cytokines in septic shock has been well characterized and therapeutic interventions based on modulating cytokine flux in sepsis are currently being evaluated [3]. However, little data regarding cytokine interactions in hypovolemic shock are available. The present study was designed to assess changes in quantitative liver function, liver blood flow, and TNF following resuscitation from severe hemorrhagic shock in normal and cirrhotic rats.

Methods

Production of Cirrhosis

Cirrhosis was produced in male Sprague-Dawley rats (average weight, 250 g) using the method of Proctor and Chatamra [4]. After 2 weeks of phenobarbital induction (35 mg/dl in drinking water taken at libitum), animals were gavaged with carbon tetrachloride on a weekly basis. Phenobarbital was continued as before. Cirrhosis was produced in 8 - 10 weeks as manifested by onset of ascites. The characteristic liver injury of cirrhosis was confirmed by histology from liver biopsies at the time of further studies.

Liver Blood Flow/Liver Function

Low-dose galactose clearance (GLC) was measured in order to approximate liver blood flow [5]. Galactose elimination capacity (GEC) was determined by measuring plasma galactose concentration on serial samples drawn during the zero order portion of the plasma disappearance curve following an intravenous galactose bolus (500 mg/kg body weight) [6]. Functional hepatocyte mass (FHM) served to normalize liver function to tissue weight and was defined as GEC divided by liver weight. Values were obtained prior to, and following, shock and resuscitation.

Tumor Necrosis Factor

Baseline TNF was measured from plasma samples by a modified flow cytometric WEHI cell bioassay [7]. Serial blood samples were drawn at baseline and at shock for TNF analysis.

Hemorrhagic Shock

Serial blood samples were withdrawn to reduce blood pressure to 50 ±5 mmHg. This level of hypotension was maintained until skeletal muscle transmembrane potential E_m depolarized by 25%, defining onset of shock [8]. Animals were then resuscitated with three times the volume of shed blood with Ringer's lactate solution. Resuscitation restored blood pressure and E_m to preshock levels. Animals were considered survivors if they were alive following resuscitation.

Data Analysis

Comparisons were made using Student's t-test for matched pairs for pre- and postshock values. Differences between controls and cirrhotic within specific experimental groups, change in variables were evaluated by using Student's t-test for two independent sample means. Significance was considered at $p < 0.05$.

Results

Preliminary Experiments

TNF levels were significantly greater at baseline in cirrhotic animals than controls ($p < 0.05$). Functional hepatic mass was greater ($p < 0.05$) in normal than in cirrhotic rats. These preliminary studies demonstrated that the methods previously reported by Proctor could reproducibly yield cirrhosis; and, further, that methods to measure galactose kinetics previously published for human subjects [9] could be extrapolated to control and cirrhotic rats.

Hemorrhagic Shock Experiments

Hepatic Blood Flow. Shock produced a significant ($p < 0.05$) decrease in GLC in both control and cirrhotic rats (Fig. 1). The decrement in GLC was similar in both study groups.
Hepatic Function. Changes in hepatic function (GEC, FHM) are depicted in Figs. 2 and 3. Shock was associated with significant decreases in GEC and FHM despite resuscitation ($p<0.05$). The change in net GEC was greater ($p < 0.05$) in cirrhotic animals. However, the change in FHM was similar in the two groups.
Circulating TNF. Elevations of plasma TNF were observed in both control and cirrhotic animals. The increase was significant ($P < 0.05$) in cirrhotic animals (Fig. 4).
Survival. Cirrhotic animals tolerated shock poorly, with only 71% surviving to the end of resuscitation. This is significantly different from the control groups, which exhibited a 91% survival ($p < 0.05$).

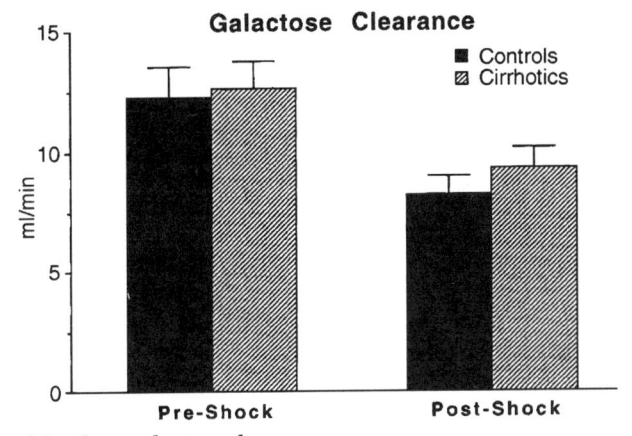

Fig. 1: Effect of shock on galactose clearance

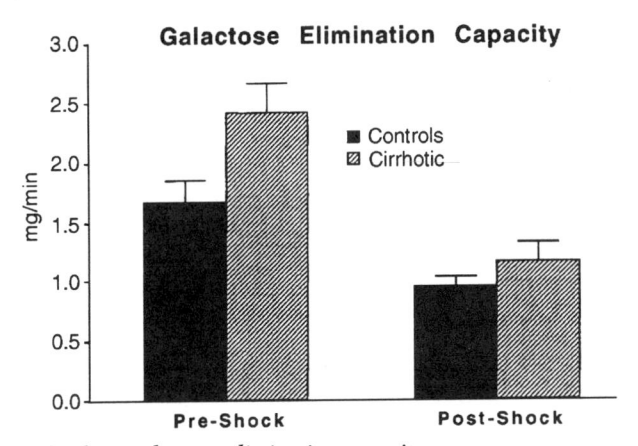

Fig. 2: Effect of shock on galactose elimination capacity

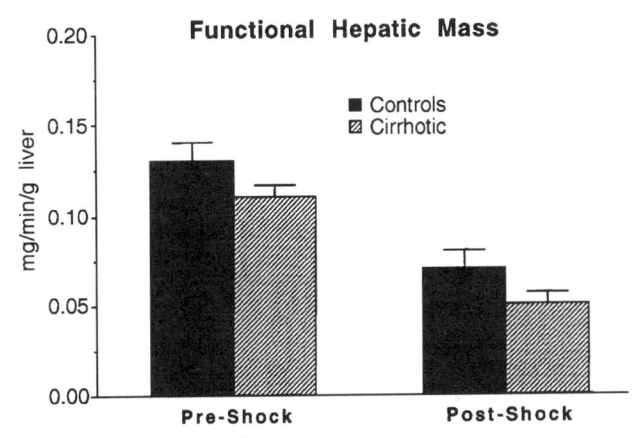

Fig. 3: Effect of shock on functional hepatic mass

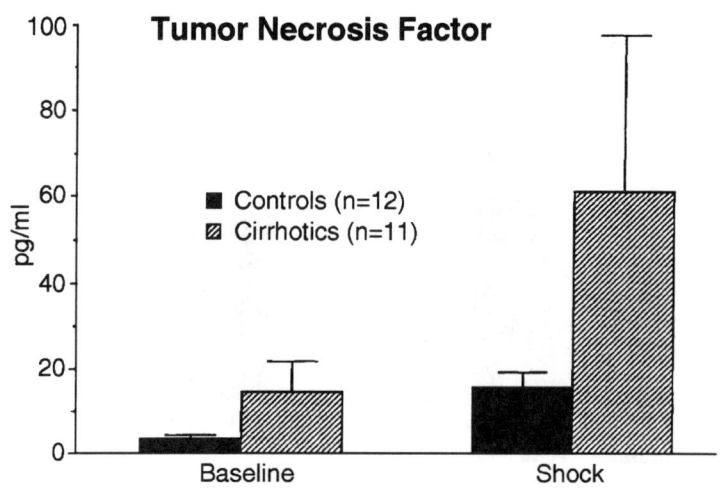

Fig. 4: Effect of mass on tumor necrosis factor

Discussion

Quantitative liver function and blood flow determinations were used to monitor the physiologic effects of hemorrhagic shock in normal and cirrhotic rats. Hemorrhagic shock produced a significantly greater mortality in cirrhotic rats than in controls despite restoration of blood pressure and skeletal muscle membrane potential following resuscitation with Ringer's lactate solution. The results documented in this animal model mimic clinical observations in cirrhotic human subjects. The decrease in survival in cirrhotics in spite of restitution of hepatic blood flow, suggesting the role of factors other than hypoperfusion, contributes to mortality. The production of cirrhosis resulted in lower functional hepatocyte mass, implying that a minimal FHM per body weight may be necessary for survival. Another possible difference between the two study groups was that cirrhotic animals were usually larger and older than controls. Further experiments with age-matched control animals could be carried out to clarify this.

Although there is an abundance of data detailing cytokine flux and the pathophysiologic role of endotoxin in TNF dynamics in septic models, there are very little data regarding TNF changes after hemorrhagic shock. These data clearly show hemorrhagic shock is accompanied by a rise in TNF in cirrhotic animals and defines the need for further studies to define the possible etiologic role of bacterial translocation and endotoxin in the cirrhotic animals subject to hemorrhagic shock.

References

1. Vierling JM (1984) *Epidemiology and clinical course of liver diseases: identification of candidates for hepatic transplantation.* Hepatology 4(1): 845-945
2. Khoruts A, Stahnke L, McClain C et al. (1991) *Circulating tumor necrosis factor, interleukin-1 and interleukin-6 concentration in clinic alcoholic patients.* Hepatology 13: 267-276

3. Barber AB, Coyle SM, Marano MA, Fischer E et al. (1993) GLucocorticoid therapy alters hormonal and cytokine responses to endotoxin in man. J Immunol 150: 1999-2006
4. Proctor E, Chatamra K (1982) High yield micronodular cirrhosis in the rat. Gastroenterology 83: 1183-1190
5. Henderson JM, Kutner MA, Bain RP (1982) First order clearance of plasma galactose: the effect of liver disease. Gastroenterology 83: 1090-1096
6. Tygstrup N (1966) Determination of the hepatic elimination capacity of galactose by single injection. Scand J Clin Lab Invest [Suppl] 92: 118-124
7. Wang P, Ayala A, Zheng BA, Zhou M et al (1991) Differential alterations in plasma IL-6 and TNF levels following trauma and hemorrhage. Am J Physiol 260: R167-R171
8. Cunningham JN Jr., Shires GT, Wagner Y (1971) Cellular transport defects in hemorrhagic shock. Ann Surg 70: 215-221
9. Millikan WJ Jr., Henderson JM, Stewart MT, Warren WD et al. (1989) Change in hepatic function, hemodynamics, and morphology after liver transplant. Ann Surg 209: 513-524

Mechanisms of Gut Barrier Failure

E.A. Deitch, N. Cruz

Background/Significance

It is now clear that the intestinal mucosa has a physiologic role as a local defense barrier that prevents bacteria and endotoxin normally present within the intestinal lumen from escaping and reaching extraintestinal tissues and organs and that loss of intestinal barrier function may play a role in the development of systemic infection or multiple organ failure in selected patients [1, 2]. Although not fully mechanistically understood, the phenomenon of bacteria crossing the mucosal barrier and invading extraintestinal tissues has been termed bacterial translocation [3]. Our initial interest in experimentally investigating the phenomenon of bacterial translocation was based on the clinical observation that trauma victims, burn patients and patients developing multiple organ failure relatively frequently develop life-threatening bacteremias with enteric organisms in the absence of an identifiable focus of infection [1, 2]. Therefore, the goal of our previous work has largely been to investigate the relationships between the gut microflora, systemic host defenses, and injury in an attempt to delineate the mechanisms by which bacteria contained within the GI tract can translocate to cause systemic infections [4].

These studies indicate that, although bacterial translocation can be induced in a variety of animal models, one or more of three basic pathophysiologic conditions appear to be necessary for bacterial translocation to occur. These are: (1) disruption of the ecologic balance of the normal indigenous microflora, resulting in bacterial overgrowth with gram-negative enteric bacilli, (2) impaired host immune defenses, and (3) physical loss of the mucosal barrier [4]. These same conditions are commonly observed in the critically ill or injured patient at risk of developing enteric bacteremias or multiple organ failure. These patients frequently have experienced major blood loss or a hypotensive episode; they are usually immunocompromised and the antibiotic, medication, or dietary regimens they receive may disrupt the normal ecology of the gut flora, resulting in subsequent overgrowth by certain members of the indigenous microflora or colonization with exogenous pathogens.

Yet, in spite of the rapid progress being made in this area, little is known of the exact mechanisms by which bacteria cross the intestinal mucosal barrier to reach the lamina propria. Although bacterial translocation is a complex physiologic process, the process of translocation can be conceptualized as occurring through a series of distinct steps, the first step being bacterial association and subsequent penetration through the mucus layer such that the bacteria come into direct contact with the intestinal epithelial cells. The second step is the passage of bacteria across the epithelial cell barrier to the submucosal space. The route of bacterial translocation across the epithelial barrier may occur via a paracellular (between the cells) or transcellular (through the cells) process in conditions where the mucosal barrier is intact or through gaps in this barrier when the mucosa is injured.

Clarification of the physiology of intestinal barrier function and the pathophysiology of bacterial translocation has been hampered by the lack of adequate experimental models and the limitations of in vivo systems. Consequently, we have developed an in vitro cultured epithelial monolayer system, utilizing the Caco-2 cell line, in order to begin to investigate the mechanisms of bacterial translocation and the physiology of bacterial-enterocyte interactions.

Caco-2 Cell Model

Caco-2, as well as several other intestinal cell lines (HT29, and T84 cell lines), forms polarized monolayers and has brush borders [5]. Caco-2 cells were chosen over these other intestinal cell lines since, of these cell lines, the Caco-2 cell line most closely mimics normal intestinal epithelium. For example, in addition to forming well-polarized monolayers that are joined by tight junctions, the microvilli in the Caco-2 cell line are well developed and contain disaccharidases and peptidases typical of normal small intestinal villous cells. In contrast, unlike Caco-2 cells, T84 cells do not form well-developed brush borders and fail to express microvillar membrane hydrolases, while the HT29 cell line does not show polarity or differentiated characteristics of intestinal cells under standard culture conditions [6]. Thus, although the Caco-2 cell line originally was derived from a human colonic adenocarcinoma cell line it has developed the ability to differentiate into ileal enterocyte-like cells, which are similar to human enterocytes. That is, when grown in vitro only Caco-2 cells spontaneously develop a polarized monolayer with intact tight junctions and manifest typical brush border microvilli on the apical membrane which contain high levels of brush border associated enzymes [5, 7].

There are several advantages to using a cultured epithelial monolayer model system. Since the system is physiologically simple and is relatively easy to manipulate, the performance of basic cellular and mechanistic studies is facilitated. Furthermore, since the cultured intestinal monolayer does not contain goblet cells, studies of epithelial cell function are not confounded by the presence of mucus. Although Caco-2 cells have been used by other investigators to study bacterial-enterocyte interaction, this work has been limited largely to pathogenic bacteria in a one compartment model system. In this regard, our Caco-2 cell model system, which is illustrated in Fig. 1, is more physiologically relevant in that the Caco-2 cells are grown on a porous 3-µm membrane in the upper compartment of a two compartment system, thereby allowing the passage of bacteria across the epithelial monolayer to be quantitated.

In this in vitro model of bacterial translocation, the Caco-2 cells were grown as a polarized monolayer on semipermeable membranes in bicameral chambers (Transwell, 3µm-pore, Costar, Cambridge, MA). The formation of a sealed monolayer of Caco-2 cells was monitored by measurements of the transepithelial electrical resistance (TEER) with a Millicell electrical resistance system (Millipore EVOM-6, World Precision Instruments). The integrity of the monolayer is a reflection of the TEER; as this number rises the tight junctions between the cells become stronger and permeability of the monolayer decreases [7]. The Caco-2 cells were used in experiments only after the TEER had risen above 130

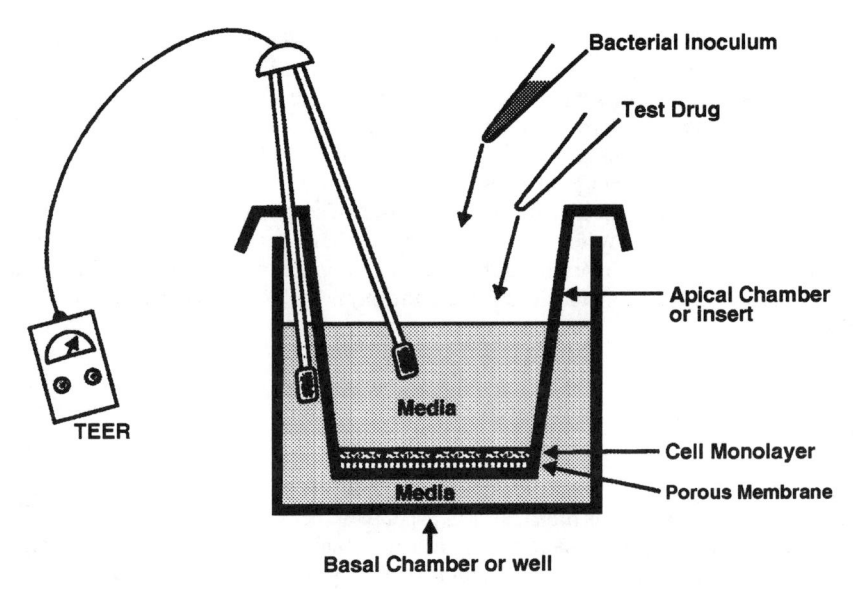

Fig. 1: Schematic illustration of the Caco-2 in vitro model. Caco-2 cells were grown over a 3-%m porous membrane. TEER was measured with an ohmeter by placing electrodes in each chamber

ohms·cm^2. This number was based on permeability studies done with the probes dextran blue (2 x 106 daltons) and phenol red (500 daltons), since at a TEER of 130 ohms cm^2 the Caco-2 monolayer is sealed and tight junction integrity is established [8]. Typically 12-15 days of culture are needed to reach such a TEER. During this period the cells differentiate and become polarized with abundant microvilli on the apical surface. Once the Caco-2 monolayer was ready, bacterial translocation across the Caco-2 monolayer was measured by culturing samples obtained from the basal well compartment of the Transwell system at various times after inoculating the apical chamber with bacteria (Fig. 1).

In the first group of experiments [8], the ability of a nonpathogenic gram-negative bacterium (*E. coli* C25) to cross the Caco-2 monolayer was serially tested after addition of the following amounts of bacteria to the apical chamber: 10^2, 10^4, or 10^6 colony-forming units (CFU). As illustrated in Fig. 2, the magnitude of *E. coli* C25 translocation was both dose dependent and time dependent, since, as the bacterial inoculum placed in the apical compartment was increased, the number of bacteria crossing the monolayer increased. In fact *E. coli* C25 translocation was observed as early as 10 min after inoculation of the Caco-2 monolayer with the higher doses of bacteria. However, a threshold bacterial challenge level was necessary to observe translocation, since at an *E. coli* inoculum of 10^2 bacteria translocation was rarely observed. The passage of *E. coli* C25 across the Caco-2 monolayer did not appear to be associated with disruption of the tight junctions or loss of integrity of the monolayer, since the TEER values did not decrease over the 3-h experimental period.

It is currently unknown whether the strains of bacteria that are recovered from the organs in animal models of translocation or from the blood of patients with occult (gut-associated) bacteremias are more efficient translocators than other strains because of an increased ability to cross the mucosal barrier or because of an increased ability to survive once they have reached the submucosal space or other host tissues. Consequently, we investigated the

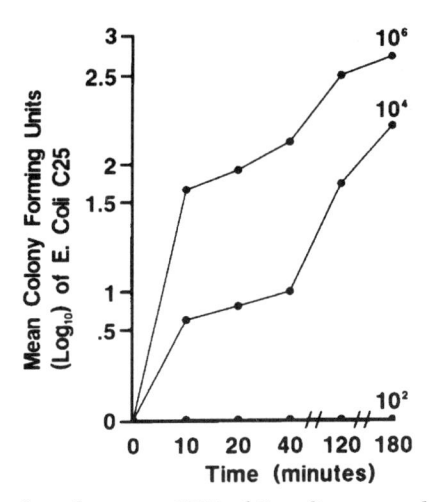

Fig. 2: These results reflect the mean CFU of E. coli recovered from the basal well. A minimum of ten monolayers for each bacterial concentration (10^2, 10^4, 10^6) were run on at least two separate occasions

question of whether various organisms of the indigenous GI flora translocate at the same rate or whether certain species are especially adept at crossing the mucosal barrier using the Caco-2 monolayer system. Based on the results of this study [8], gram-negative enteric bacilli are better translocators than gram-positive cocci and that obligate anaerobes, such as *B. fragilis*, are very poor translocators (Table 1). These Caco-2 monolayer results are consistent with our previous work in germ-free mice monoassociated with different strains of bacteria, in which a similar hierarchy of bacterial translocation with gram-negative enteric bacilli being the best translocators, gram-positive cocci being intermediate and strict obligate anaerobes being the worst translocators was observed [9]. Thus, it appears that the strains of bacteria (gram-negative enterics) that are most commonly cultured in vivo are better able to successfully cross the intestinal epithelial barrier in vitro.

Table 1: Incidence and magnitude of bacterial translocation (BT) across the Caco-2 monolayer 180 min after bacterial challenge with 10^6 bacteria

Bacteria	Magnitude of BT (Log_{10} CFU)	Incidence of BT (10^6 CFU)
S. aureus	1.3±0.5	100%
S. facialis	1.8±1.0	83%
C. freundii	2.4±0.5*	100%
E. aerogenes	1.6±1.4	67%
E. coli	4.1±0.1**	100%
B. fragilis[a]	0.3±0.6***	17%

*p <0.01 vs. *S. aureus* and *B. fragilis*; **$p < 0.001$ vs. all other groups; ***$p < 0.01$ vs. all other groups.

Having shown that bacteria will translocate across the Caco-2 monolayer when tested at physiologically relevant bacterial concentrations (10^4-10^7 CFU/ml), we next began to investigate the cellular events involved in the process of translocation [10]. Specifically, the possibility that the Caco-2 cells play an active role in the translocation process was tested. To determine whether inert particles would cross the Caco-2 monolayer, Caco-2 monolayers were incubated with 1-μm red fluorescent beads for 180 min. At the end of the 3-h experiment, the quantity of fluorescent beads recovered from the basal chamber was measured using a hemocytometer under a fluorescent microscope. When the 1.0-μm fluorescent beads were added to the apical chambers at inocula of 1×10^5 or 1×10^7 beads per insert, 4.23±2.08 and 5.35±0.33 $\log_{10}$ beads were recovered at 180 min respectively ($n=6$ membranes/dose). These results were consistent with the concept that Caco-2 cells play an active role in the translocation process, since inert beads translocated across the Caco-2 monolayers. Bead passage across the Caco-2 monolayers was not associated with a decrease in TEER, indicating that tight junction integrity was maintained.

Next we tested the ability of a microtubule inhibitor (nocodazole), a microfilament inhibitor (phalloidine), and an inhibitor of oxidative metabolism (sodium azide) to modulate *E. coli* translocation across the Caco-2 monolayer. Pretreatment of the Caco-2 monolayers with an inhibitor of oxidative metabolism (sodium azide) had no significant effect on the number of bacteria translocating across the monolayer. In contrast, bacterial translocation was decreased in the Caco-2 cell monolayers pretreated with either the microtubule inhibitor nocodazole or the microfilament inhibitor phalloidine (Fig. 3). In order to verify that the test drugs were not affecting the viability of the *E. coli*, inocula of 10^7 bacteria were exposed to each of the test drugs at the concentrations used in the above described experiments. The nocodazole and phalloidine-induced decreases in bacterial translocation did not appear to be related to a direct drug effect on bacterial viability or growth, since bacterial growth did not appear to be adversely affected by the presence of any of the test drugs.

Because Caco-2 cells are polarized with microvilli present only on the apical membrane, we tested the polarity of bacterial translocation by measuring bacterial passage across the Caco-2 monolayer 3 h after adding *E. coli* to either the apical or basal chamber. Since the carbonated porous filters (3.0-μm pores) on which the Caco-2 monolayers were grown could impose a barrier to the passage of bacteria (1 μm diameter), bacterial movement across the carbonate filter was measured in a similar manner. Measurements were made only at the 3-h time point to give adequate time for equilibrium between the chambers to be established. Studies on the polarity of bacterial translocation by the Caco-2 cells revealed that translocation occurred in both directions but was 25-fold greater across the apical than basal membrane of the Caco-2 cells ($p < 0.01$). This difference in polarity-based bacterial passage did not appear to be related to either the mechanical construction of the Transwell system or to the presence of the polycarbonate membrane filter, since there was no difference between the magnitude of passage across the Transwell system in either direction in the absence of a Caco-2 monolayer.

Since in vivo endotoxin has been reported to increase intestinal permeability by causing loss of tight junction integrity [11], the effect of endotoxin on Caco-2 monolayer tight junction integrity as measured by TEER was quantitated. Endotoxin, even in doses as high as 1 mg/ml, did not affect monolayer TEER values. This was true whether the endotoxin was placed in the apical or basal chambers. These results suggest that the endotoxin-induced increase in intestinal permeability observed after the in vivo administration is not due to a direct effect of endotoxin on tight junction integrity and instead may be mediated by other factors, such as cytokines or products of activated immunoinflammatory cells. These endotoxin results also argue against the possibility that the passage of *E. coli* across the Caco-2 monolayer was secondary to an endotoxin-induced loss of tight junction integrity and a subsequent increase in the permeability of the Caco-2 monolayer.

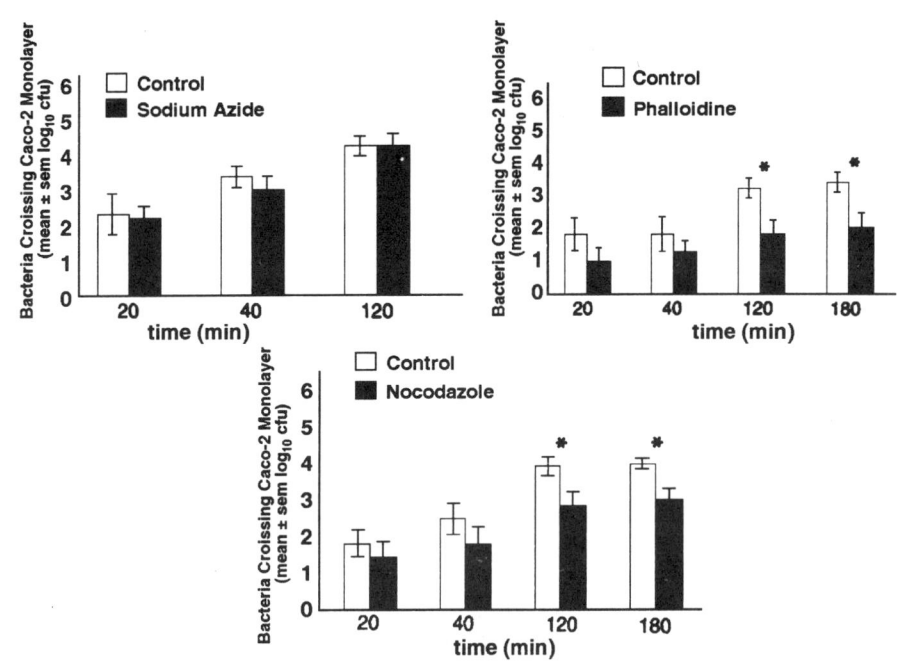

*Fig. 3: Caco-2 monolayers were pretreated with 1.0 mM sodium azide for 30 min, 10 mg/ml nocodazole for 60 min or 10 mM phalloidine for 30 min prior to E. coli C25 challenge. *p<0.05 drug vs. control*

Thus, based on results documenting that several strains of bacteria will translocate across the Caco-2 monolayer and that 1-μm inert fluorescently labeled latex beads also translocate across the Caco-2 monolayer, it appears likely that epithelial cell uptake of bacteria is important in the translocation process. This concept that epithelial cells play an active role in the transport of bacteria across the monolayer was supported by the observation that the microtubule inhibitor, nocodazole, and the actin filament stabilizer, phalloidine, decrease the magnitude of bacterial translocation. These results further imply that the transport of *E. coli* across the Caco-2 cell is at least partly microtubule and microfilament dependent. That cytoskeletal components are important in the movement of bacteria within cells has been previously documented. For example, *Listeria monocytogenes* has been shown to spread intracellularly and infect adjacent cells by interacting with host cell microfilaments [12), while *Shigella flexneri* has been shown to move along actin cables towards the nucleus of fibroblasts in an organelle-like fashion [13]. In fact, as reviewed by Findlay [14], there is increasing evidence that pathogenic bacteria, such as *Salmonella*, *Shigella*, *Vibrio cholerae*, *Campylobacter*, and enterotoxigenic *E. coli* cross eukaryotic cells in a transcellular fashion and that de novo microfilament assembly is required for passage.

The above described results indicating that the Caco-2 cells are actively involved in bacterial translocation across the monolayer are consistent with increasing evidence that the entry of bacteria into host cells is initiated by bacterial binding to surface receptors on the surface of the host cell [14, 15]. In fact, the adhesion of bacteria to their target cells is not only recognized as a prerequisite for infectivity in vivo but also is recognized as the initial event that precedes the colonization and infection of host tissues [14]. For example, in the pathogenesis of most natural bacterial infections, adhesion of the microorganisms to the mucosal surfaces of the respiratory, gastrointestinal, or urogenital mucosa precedes infection [14, 16]. The ability of bacteria to adhere and thereby colonize mucosal surfaces appears to be largely a receptor-mediated process in which bacterial adhesins bind to epithelial cell receptors. For numerous bacteria, viruses, and protozoa, it has been established that specific lectin-carbohydrate interactions generally mediate microorganism-epithelial cell recognition and adhesive interactions. For example, the receptors on the epithelial cell membrane for gram-negative bacteria are generally composed of carbohydrates and for many species of bacteria, including the Enterobacteriaceae, the receptor appears to reside in the monosaccharide, mannose [14, 17]. For this reason, receptor-mediated, gram-negative bacterial adhesion can be competitively inhibited by high levels of mannose. In addition to mannose-sensitive receptors, there are also mannose-resistant receptors on the cell membrane, which belong to the integrin family [15]. Since certain of these integrin (mannose-resistant) receptors can be competitively inhibited with the tripeptide Arg-Gly-Asp (RGD) or fibronectin [15], the role of integrin receptors in the translocation process can be assessed by competitive inhibition assays. Thus, by using mannose, RGD, or fibronection as competitive inhibitors, it is possible to begin to test whether bacterial passage in the Caco-2 system is mediated by mannose-sensitive or resistant (integrin family) receptors. Thus, the next group of experiments were carried out to investigate the role of integrin and mannose receptors [18].

The addition of mannose to the apical compartment, in which the bacterial inoculum was placed, reduced the incidence and magnitude of bacterial passage across the Caco-2 monolayer (Fig. 4). At a mannose concentration of 6 mg/ml, this reduction in bacterial passage was limited to the early 40-min time point and was lost after 180 min of culture. However, at concentrations of 12 mg/ml and 25mg/ml, mannose's protective effect against bacterial translocation persisted throughout the 180-min test period (Fig. 4). As has been observed previously [8, 9], the transepithelial resistance (TEER) of the control Caco-2 monolayers increased by about 20% over the 180-min experimental period (Fig. 4c). In contrast, the TEERs of the Caco-2 monolayers incubated with 12 mg/ml or 25 mg/ml mannose decreased during this time period (Fig. 4c). Treatment of the Caco-2 monolayers with RGD, a competitive inhibitor of the integrin $_1$-receptor, had no significant effect on the Caco-2 monolayer resistance or number of bacteria translocating across the monolayer at the three doses tested. Fibronectin, which also binds to the integrin $_1$-receptor, was associated with a modest but significant increase in *E. coli* passage across the Caco-2 cell monolayers. This increase in bacterial translocation across the fibronectin-treated Caco-2 monolayers was not associated with any alterations in transepithelial monolayer resistance.

These studies suggest that BT in the Caco-2 system is mediated by lectin but not integrin receptor inteactions and that intestinal mucin contributes to the barrier function of the monolayer. The mechanism by which mannose reduced *E. coli* translocation across the Caco-2 monolayer most likely is by competing with the *E. coli* for mannose-specific receptors on the apical membrane of the Caco-2 cells. This concept is consistent with a large body of work documenting that type 1 fimbriae or common pili, which are major adhesins of Enterobacteriaceae, mediate attachment to eukaryotic cells by binding to mannose residues expressed on the surface of epithelial cells [14] and that polarized intestinal cell lines, including Caco-2 cells, express apical membrane receptors that bind a number of bacteria including *E. coli* [19, 20]. The failure of mannose to completely block bacterial *E. coli* translocation is not surprising, since most bacteria display a number of adhesins. For example, at least nine distinct adhesins have been described for *E. coli*, which predominately recognize carbohydrates on the surface of eukaryotic cells [21]. Other commonly recognized residues on eukaryotic glycoconjugates besides mannose are galactose and sialic acid.

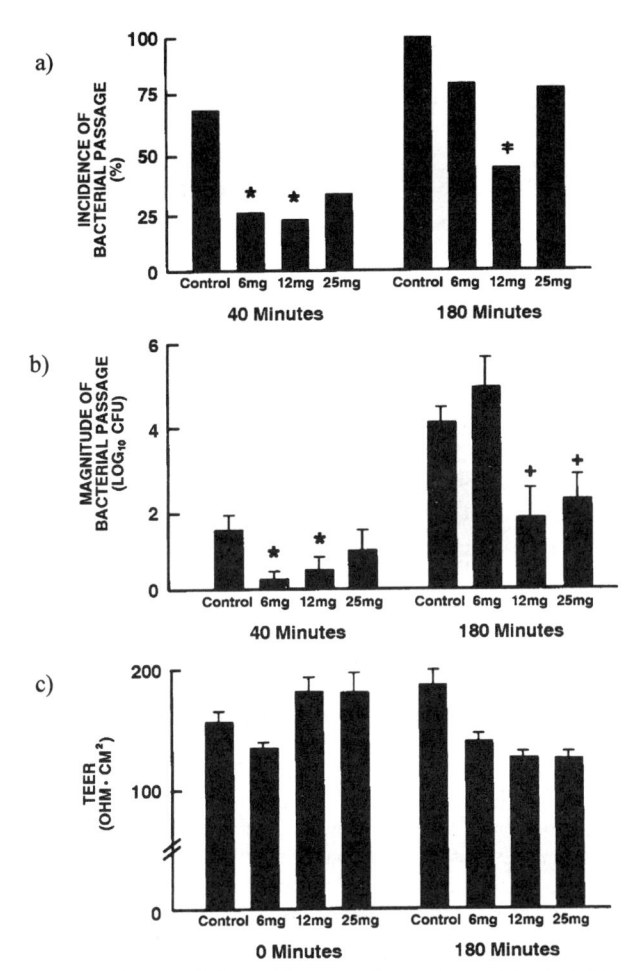

*Fig. 4:a)-c) Mannose decreased the incidence and magnitude of bacterial translocation across the Caco-2 monolayer. *$p<0.05$ vs. control; #$p<0.01$ vs. control; +$p<0.05$ vs. control and 6 mg mannose. TEER values of the control Caco-2 monolayers increased ($p<0.05$), while TEERs of the Caco-2 monolayers exposed to 12 mg or 25 mg mannose decreased ($p<0.05$)*

We investigated the ability of purified intestinal mucin to modulate bacterial passage across the Caco-2 monolayer next [18], since in vivo the intestinal mucus layer is an important barrier which slows the penetrance of particles and the mucus layer has been proposed to act as a mechanical barrier limiting microorganisms present in the intestinal lumen from reaching and colonizing epithelial surfaces [22, 23]. To test the general protective effect of the mucus layer, the monolayers were pretreated with purified mucin. Forty minutes after bacterial inoculation, the number of bacteria crossing the Caco-2 monolayers treated with purified mucin at doses of 1 mg/ml or 5 mg/ml was reduced. However, this reduction was not significant. When the concentration of mucin was raised to 8 mg/ml, the magnitude of bacterial passage across the monolayer was significantly reduced at both 40 and 180 min (Fig. 5a). Transepithelial resistance levels of the mucin-treated monolayers did not significantly change during the 180-min experimental procedure (Fig. 5b).

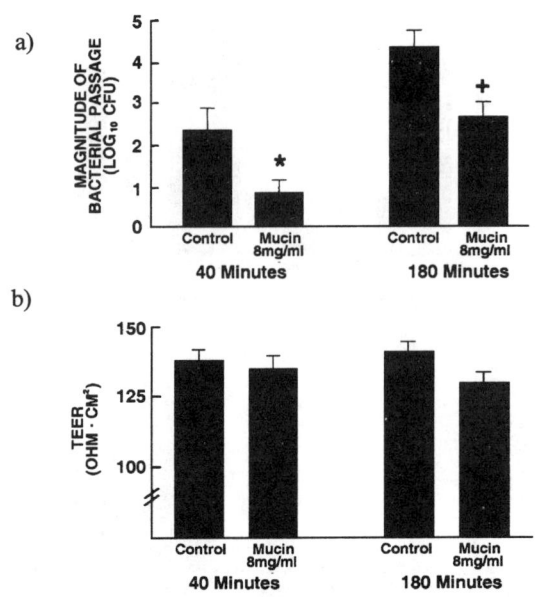

Fig. 5: a), b). Mucin at a dose of 8 mg/ml decreased bacterial translocation across the Caco-2 monolayer (*p <0.03; $^+$p <0.004), but had no effect on TEER

To our knowledge, the observation that purified mucin decreases the rate of *E. coli* bacterial translocation across the Caco-2 monolayer is the first direct experimental evidence that the mucin component of the mucus gel inhibits the ability of nonpathogenic bacteria to successfully cross an intestinal monolayer. The exact mechanism by which the mucin decreased *E. coli* passage across the Caco-2 monolayer cannot be answered by this study. However, some of the carbohydrate moieties on the mucin molecule mimic certain epithelial membrane glycoproteins that are recognized by some bacterial adhesins [24]. The fact that mucins have been documented to bind to the mannose-sensitive type 1 pili of *E. coli* [24] plus our results that mannose decreases *E. coli* translocation across the Caco-2 monolayer adds further support to the concept that lectin-mediated *E. coli* adherence to the Caco-2 cell is an important factor in the translocation process. In summary, these studies suggest that lectin-mediated bacterial adhesion to the apical surface of the Caco-2 cell is involved in the translocation of *E. coli* in this system and that intestinal mucin contributes to the barrier function of the monolayer.

Since intestinal epithelial cells have receptors that recognize bacterial antigens and in some circumstances are actively involved in bacterial internalization, the aim of the next group of experiments was to test the hypothesis that intestinal epithelial cells possess bactericidal capabilities [25]. To test this hypothesis, the bactericidal activity of two intestinal cell lines (IEC-18 and Caco-2) was measured using *S. aureus*, *P. aeruginosa*, and *E. coli* as test organisms. To determine the relative bactericidal efficacy of these two intestinal cell lines, their ability to ingest and kill bacteria was compared against neutrophils (PMN) using a standard in vitro bactericidal assay. To determine the role of superoxide, hydrogen peroxide, and nitric oxide in Caco-2-mediated bactericidal activity, in separate experiments, superoxide dismutase (SOD), catalase, or the nitric oxide synthase inhibitor, N^G-nitro-L-arginine methyl ester (L-NAME), was added to the culture medium.

The IEC-18 and Caco-2 cells as well as the PMNs killed *S. aureus* and *P. aeruginosa* but not *E. coli* ($p < 0.05$). In fact, when tested in serum-free medium, the IEC-18 and Caco-2 cells killed a greater percentage of bacteria than the PMNs ($p < 0.05$) (Fig. 6). The addition of the antioxidant SOD significantly reversed the bactericidal activity of both Caco-2 cells and neutrophils for *P. aeruginosa* and *S. aureus*, while catalase had no effect. Nitric oxide inhibition by L-NAME had no effect on bactericidal active cells. These results indicate that intestinal epithelial cells can function as "nonprofessional" phagocytes and kill certain strains of bacteria. Additionally, the mechanisms involved in the killing of *P. aeruginosa* and *S. aureus* by the Caco-2 cells appear similar to the PMNs to the extent that bactericidal activity appeared to be oxidant but not nitric oxide mediated in both the Caco-2 cell line and the neutrophils.

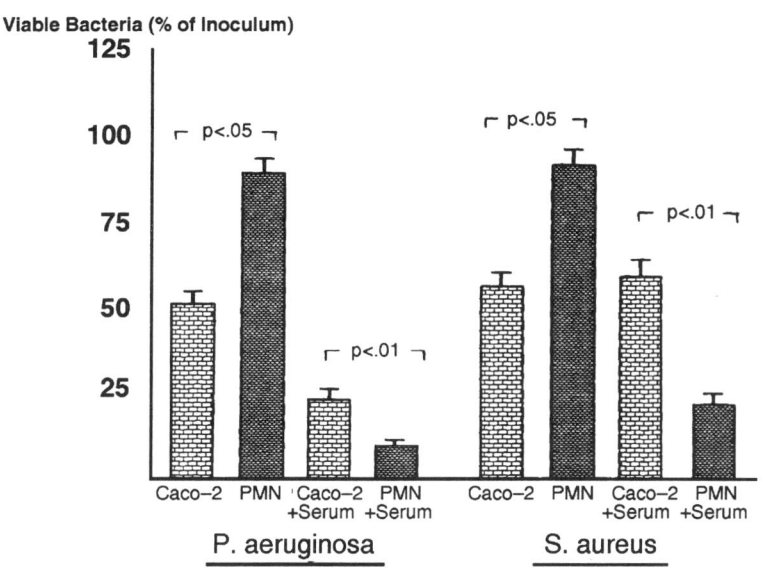

Fig. 6: Comparison of bactericidal activity of Caco-2 cells vs. PMNs. In the absence of serum, the percentage of viable bacteria was greater in the bacterial suspensions containing PMNs than Caco-2 cells, while in the presence of serum the PMN-containing suspensions had greater bactericidal activity.

Conclusions

Although this in vitro model has several attractive features, it does differ from the normal intestinal environment. For example, the normal gut is peristaltic, contains goblet cells, mucus, secretory immunoglobulins, a complex bacterial flora, as well as other factors. Thus, although this model system is providing important insights into the underlying mechanisms of the translocation process, some caution must be exercised in directly applying results obtained in this system to the more complex intestinal environment. Nonetheless, since the in vivo study of intestinal epithelial function is confounded by the geometric complexity and cellular heterogeneity that characterize this epithelium, the ability to study transport across impermeable, polarized, cultured monolayers composed of a single species of epithelial cells provides a unique opportunity to study the basic biology of bacterial-enterocyte interactions.

References

1. Deitch EA (1990) The role of intestinal barrier failure and bacterial translocation in the development of systemic infection and multiple organ failure. Arch Surg 125: 403-404
2. Deitch EA (1992) Multiple organ failure: pathophysiology and potential future therapies. Ann Surg 216: 117-134
3. Berg RD, Garlington AW (1979) Translocation of certain indigenous bacteria from the gastrointestinal tract to the mesenteric lymph nodes and other organs in gnotobiotic mouse model. Infect Immun 23: 403-411
4. Deitch EA (1990) Bacterial translocation of the gut flora. J Trauma 30: s184-s190
5. Pinto M, Robine-Leon S, Appay MD, Redinger M, Triadoo N, Dussaulx E, Laoroix B, Simmon-Assman P, Hatten K, Fogh J, Zweibaum A (1983) Enterocyte like differentiation and polarization of the human colon carcinoma cell line caco-2 in culture. Biol Cell 47: 323-330
6. Neutra M, Louvard D (1989) Differentiation of intestinal cells in vitro. In: Malin KS, Valentich JD (eds.) Functional epithelial cells in culture. Liss, New York, pp. 363-398
7. Hidalgo IJ, Raub TJ, Borchardt RT (1989) Characterization of the human colon carcinoma cell line (caco-2) as a model system for intestinal epithelial permeability. Gastroenterology 96: 736-749
8. Cruz N, Qi L, Alvarez X, Deitch EA (1994) Bacterial translocation is bacterial species dependent: results using the caco-2 intestinal cell line. J Trauma 36: 612-616
9. Steffen EK, Deitch EA, Berg RD (1988) Comparison of the translocation rate of various indigenous bacteria from the gastrointestinal tract of euthymic and athymic gnotobiotic mice. J Infect Dis 157: 1032-1038
10. Cruz N, Alvarez X, Berg RD, Deitch EA (1994) Bacterial translocation across enterocytes: results of a study of bacterial-enterocyte interactions utilizing Caco-2 cells. Shock 1: 67-72
11. Walker RI, Porvaznik MJ (1978) Disruption of the permeability barrier (zonula occludens) between intestinal epithelial cells by lethal doses of endotoxin. Infect Immunol 21: 655-658
12. Mounier J, Ryter A, Rodon MC, Sansonetti PJ (1990) Intracellular and cell to cell spread of Listeria monocytogenes involves interactions with f-actin in the enterocytelike cell line caco-2. Infect Immun 58: 1048-1058
13. Wick MJ, Madara JL, Fields BN, Normark SJ (1991) Molecular cross talk between epithelial cells and microorganisms. Cell 67: 651-659
14. Finlay BB, Falkow S (1989) Common themes in microbial pathogenicity. Microbiol Rev 53: 210-230
15. Isberg RR (1991) Discrimination between intracellular uptake and surface adhesion of bacterial pathogens. Science 252: 934-938
16. Hoepelman AM, Tuomanen EI (1992) Consequences of microbial attachment: directing host cell functions with adhesins. Infect Immun 60: 1729-1733
17. Beachey EH (1981) Bacterial adherence: adhesion-receptor interactions mediating the attachment of bacteria to mucosal surfaces. J Infect Dis 143: 325-345
18. Cruz N, Alvarez X, Specian RD, Berg RD, Deitch EA Lectin but not integrin receptors are involved in bacterial translocation across the Caco-2 cell monolayer (submitted)
19. Michaud AD, Aubel D, Chauviere G, Rich C, Bourges M, Servin S, Joly B (1990) Adhesion of enterotoxigenic Escherichia coli to the human colon carcinoma cell line caco-2 in culture. Infect Immun 58: 893-902
20. Elsinghorst EA, Kopecko DJ (1992) Molecular cloning of epithelial cell invasion determinants from enterotoxigenic Escherichia coli. Infect Immun 60: 2409-2417

21. *Gbarah A, Gahmberg CG, Ofek I, Jacobi U, Sharon N (1991) Identification of the leukocyte adhesion molecules CD11 and CD18 as receptors for type 1-fimbriated (mannose specific) Escherichia coli. Infec Immun 59: 4524-4530*
22. *Freter R, Jones GW (1983) Models for studying the role of bacterial attachment in virulence and pathogenesis. Rev Infect Dis 5: s647-s658*
23. *Savage D (1984) Overview of the association of microbes with epithelial surfaces. Microecol Therapy 14: 169-182*
24. *Specian RD, Oliver MG (1991) Functional biology of intestinal goblet cells. Am J Physiol 260: c183-c193*
25. *Deitch EA, Haskel Y, Cruz N, Xu D, Kvietys PR (1995) Caco-2 and IEC-18 intestinal epithelial cells exert bactericidal activity through an oxidant-dependent pathway. Shock 5: 345-350*

Postischemic Gut Serves as a Priming Bed for Circulating Neutrophils That Provoke Multiple Organ Failure

E.E. Moore, F.A. Moore, R.J. Franciose, F.J. Kim

Global Study Hypothesis

Postinjury multiple organ failure (MOF) is typically produced by multiple insults (two-hit model), which can be characterized as priming (systemic inflammatory response) and activation (secondary event). Activated neutrophils (PMNs), and their interaction with other components of the inflammatory cascade, play an integral role in the pathogenesis of MOF. Postinjury gut ischemia/reperfusion (I/R), secondary to splanchnic hypoperfusion, generates a local inflammatory environment which primes circulation PMNs that, when activated, provoke distant organ injury.

Study Background: Gut I/R Provokes Systemic Inflammation

Postinjury MOF appears to result from unbridled systemic inflammation [1]. MOF became the predominant cause of delayed mortality in the surgical intensive care unit (ICU) in the mid-1970s when life support capabilities began to prolong survival beyond that previously imagined [2, 3]. Early epidemiologic studies concluded that MOF was a fatal expression of uncontrolled infection [4]. Consequently, for the ensuing decade, clinical investigation and basic mechanistic research focused on how the initial progressive cascade of MOF. Early clinical work supported overwhelming infection as a unified concept for the pathogenesis of MOF. But this experience was derived from urban trauma centers in the United States representing ICU population of predominantly gunshot wounds complicated by secondary abdominal abscesses. Where intestinal perforations could not be implicated, bacterial analysis of nosocomial infections suggested the gut was the occult source [5]. Indeed extensive branch research, employing a variety of rodent models, produced compelling evidence suggesting bacterial/endotoxin translocation was a common event in the stressed patients [6-8]. In the mid 1980s, however, several European groups, representing trauma centers managing blunt multisystem injuries, made the cogent observation that most of their patients developed MOF without an identifiable source of infection or antecedent bacteremia [9. 10]. Our clinical study, failing to confirm bacterial translocation in the portal blood of severely injured patients developing MOF, supported these findings [11]. Collectively, these studies and other contemporary reports have redirected MOF investigation toward elucidating the mechanisms promoting diffuse inflammation, i.e., the systemic inflammatory response syndrome (SIRS) that appears to render the injured patient at risk for MOF. Further, while an initial massive insult can precipitate severe SIRS evolving directly into MOF (one-hit model), the more likely clinical scenario is sequential insults (two-hit model) in which the inflammatory system is primed to respond to a secondary activating stimulus. Priming may result from the by-products of overt tissue disruption or secondary via mediators released following protracted shock. The gut is particularly vulnerable to hypoperfusion following multisystem trauma because of disproportionate splanchnic vasoconstriction in response to injury stress. Moreover, unrecognized flow-dependent oxygen consumption may produce ongoing mesenteric ischemia in the patient judged adequately resuscitated by standard measures [12]. In our ICU studies, we have found that severely injured patients unable to consume supranormal levels of oxygen (>150 ml/min/m^2) within 12 h, despite maximal resuscitative efforts, are at high risk for developing MOF [13].

Study Background: Primed Neutrophils Mediate Organ Failure

Although a number of inflammatory cascades have been incriminated in the pathogenesis of MOF, diffuse PMN-mediated tissue injury remains an attractive unifying concept [14]. The PMN is uniquely equipped to promote inflammation as well as cytotoxicity via oxygen-dependent (NADPH oxidase) and -independent (digestive enzymes) mechanisms. Regulated adhesion, stimulation, and migration of PMNs through the endothelium are recognized as crucial steps in acute inflammation [15]. Induction and control of these events involve the expression and interaction of adhesion molecules on both endothelium and PMNs [16]. Coordinated interaction of these cellular elements leads to appropriate host defense against infection and facilitates repair of injured tissue; whereas derangement of these regulatory processes may lead to widespread systemic inflammation resulting in MOF. Several classes of adhesion molecules have been implicated in acute inflammation. Early responses include endothelial expression of selectin molecules and membrane-bound platelet-activating factor (PAF) with affinity for specific molecules and receptors on the PMN. A secondary adhesion event involves the interaction of a family of inducible surface glycoproteins expressed by the PMN (CD11a/CD18 and CD11b/CD18, B$_2$ integrins) and their ligand counterparts expressed by endothelium (intracellular adhesion molecules, ICAM 1 and 2). Interruption of these CD11/CD18 - ICAM interactions with specific monoclonal antibodies has been shown to reduce tissue I/R injury and organ dysfunction following hemorrhagic shock in animal models. While neutrophil adhesion is a necessary step, the priming and activation events in the PMN may play critical roles in determining cytotoxicity. A conspicuous mechanism through which PMNs produce tissue injury is the stimulated elaboration and release of reactive oxygen metabolites. Several chemoattractants such as formyl-methionyl-leucyl-phenylalanine (fMLP), complement-derived C5a, leukotriene B4, interleukin-8, and PAF stimulate the respiratory burst [17]. PMN O$_2$-generation is believed to occur via the NAPHH oxidase system, but the precise signaling pathways and secondary events involved in priming and activation remain ill defined. During this process, activated protein kinase C(PKC) translocates to the membrane, where phosphorylation of various assembled protein components of the NADPH oxidase system appears important for O_2-generation [18, 19].

Study Hypothesis: Priming Followed by Activation Results in MOF

Our working hypothesis was that gut ischemia/reperfusion (I/R) primes the systemic inflammatory cascade, and an activating stimulus, during this vulnerable period, results in distal organ injury. For this purpose, we developed a sequential insult rodent model in which (a) the priming event consisted of superior mesenteric arterial (SMA) clamping for 45 min followed by 6 h reperfusion and, then (b) activation was induced with low-dose endotoxin (2.5 mg/kg) [20]. In brief, adult mature Sprague-Dawley rats (350-499 g) were anesthetized and via a midline laparotomy the SMA was occluded at the aortic origin. After 45 min of intestinal ischemia, the arterial clamp was removed, the laparotomy incision closed, and the animals allowed to awake. (The 45-min clamp time was based on preliminary work which demonstrated this relatively brief period of ischemia resulted in 100% survival, and, moreover, did not alter the intestinal mucosa by histologic examination.) Six hours after SMA reperfusion, the study animals were administered low-dose endotoxin (*Salmonella typhimurium*), 2.5 mg/kg. (The 2.5-mg/kg dose was based on previous work showing that it did not produce lung leak.) Eleven and a half hours after the lipopolysaccharide (LPS), the animals were reanesthetized, the laparotomy reopened, and ^{125}I-albumin injected into the inferior vena cava (IVC); 30 min later blood samples were obtained and the lung harvested following Kreb-Henseleit solution washout. Animals were divided into four study groups; 45 min postlaparotomy (LAP) was the control for gut I/R, while saline injection 6 h later was the control for endotoxin (LPS). Thus, the study groups were: (1) LAP plus saline, (2) I/R plus saline. (3) LAP plus LPS, and (4) I/R plus LPS. Lung injury as measured by ^{125}I-albumin lung uptake was calculated as the ratio of ^{125}I lung count to ^{125}I blood counts. Pulmonary inflammation was determined by myeloperoxidase (MPO) activity in homogenized lung tissue and histologic examination with hematoxylin and eosin staining. Gut ischemia of 45 min followed by 18 h of reperfusion did not increase lung albumin leak compared with the laparotomy alone and, similarly, endotoxin alone had no adverse effect (Fig. 1). Gut I/R alone did not promote PMN localization in the lung compared with controls but, interestingly, low-dose LPS did increase lung MPO activity (Fig. 2). The sequential insults, gut I/R plus endotoxin (ETX), increased pulmonary PMN sequestration, produced lung ^{125}I-albumin leak, and resulted in a 40% mortality (Fig. 3). In sum, a relatively brief period of gut I/R primed the systemic inflammatory response such that low-dose endotoxin exposure during this vulnerable period resulted in MOF. Furthermore, gut I/R stimulated PMNs to sequester in the lung and the arrival of PMNs correlated temporally with endothelial dysfunction. Conversely, the mere presence of increased PMNs was insufficient to produce lung injury. This observation was consistent with our previous work in hemorrhagic shock [21].

Study Hypothesis: Gut I/R Primes Circulating PMNs

Our hypothesis was that gut I/R provoked distal organ injury via a mechanism that involved priming of circulating PMNs in the reperfused mesenteric bed. PMN priming was determined by superoxide (O^2-) generation stimulated by fMLP. PMNs were isolated by plasma-

Pulmonary Capillary Leak

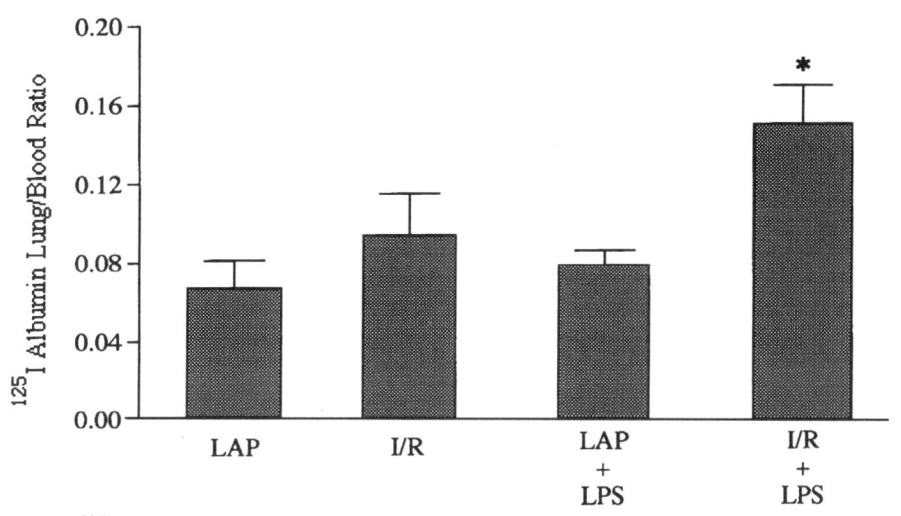

Fig. 1: ^{125}*I-albumin lung/blood ratio at 18 h reperfusion: (1) sham laparotomy (LAP), (2) 45 min intestinal ischemia (I/R), (3) LAP plus endotoxin (LPS) 6 h later, and (4) I/R plus LPS 6 h later.* *$p < 0.05$ compared with LAP, I/R, and LAP + LPS

Lung Myeloperoxidase

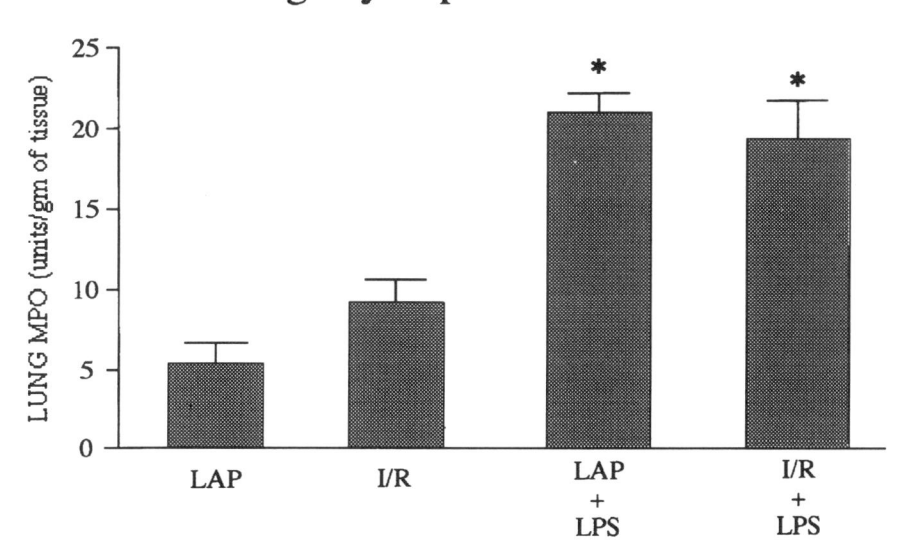

Fig. 2: Lung myeloperoxidase at 18 h reperfusion: (1) sham laparotomy (LAP), (2) 45 min intestinal ischemia (I/R), (3) LAP plus endotoxin (LPS) 6 h later, and (4) I/R plus LPS 6 h later. *$p < 0.05$ compared with LSP, I/R, and LAP + LPS

Animal Mortality

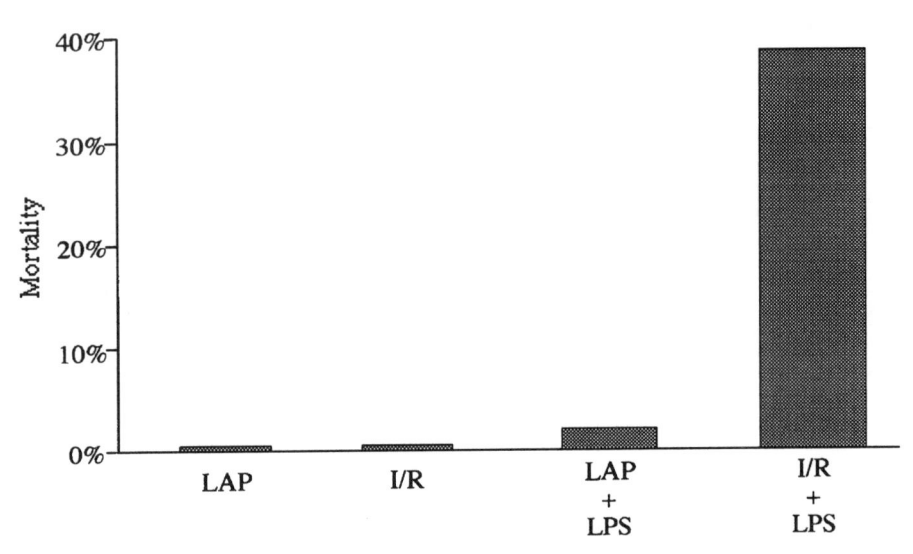

Fig. 3: Mortality at 18 h reperfusion: (1) sham laparotomy (LAP), (2) 45 min intestinal ischemia (I/R), (3) LAP plus endotoxin (LPS) 6 h later, and (4) I/R plus LPS 6 h later. *p<0.05 compared with LSP, I/R, and LAP + LPS

Percoll gradients and O^2-generation measured by superoxide dismutase (SOD)-inhibitable cytochrome C reduction. In our I/R model, described above, circulating PMNs became primed at 2 h reperfusion [21, 22]. Pursuing our hypothesis that priming occurred in the intestinal circulation, we determined PMN priming at 90 min reperfusion in the mesenteric inflow (aorta = SMA). At this time point there was significant priming among the PMNs exiting the gut contrasted to no evidence of priming at entry (Fig. 4). In sum, PMN priming in the reperfused gut preceded systemic priming, indicating the gut, following I/R, acted as a priming bed for circulating PMNs.

Study Hypothesis: Gut I/R Induced PMN

Our next series of experiments focused on potential mechanisms responsible for PMN priming following gut I/R. In view of the ongoing debate regarding the pathologic role of bacterial translocation [11], we proposed that priming occurred independent of endotoxin. In fact, we were surprised to find that (1) plasma endotoxin levels were not different in the gut I/R than in sham laparotomy groups (Fig. 5) and (2) endotoxin levels were highest during early mesenteric ischemia and did not rise with subsequent reperfusion [24]. Furthermore, the elimination of endotoxin by pretreatment with the E_5 monoclonal antibody had no impact on PMN priming following gut I/R (Fig. 6).

Neutrophil Priming (O_2^-)

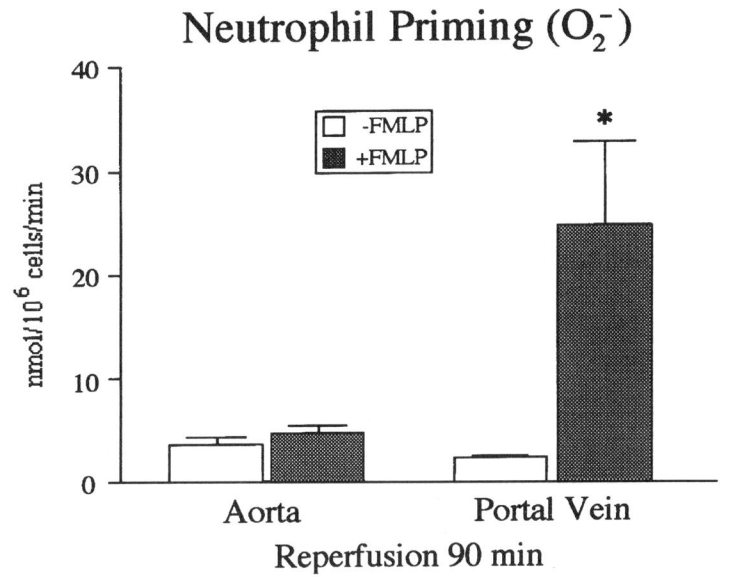

*Fig. 4: Primed state of PMNs isolated from aorta and portal vein following 45 min intestinal ischemia and 90 min reperfusion. PMN priming was defined by SOD-inhibitable superoxide generation with and without the activating stimulus FMLP. *$p < 0.05$*

Plasma Endotoxin

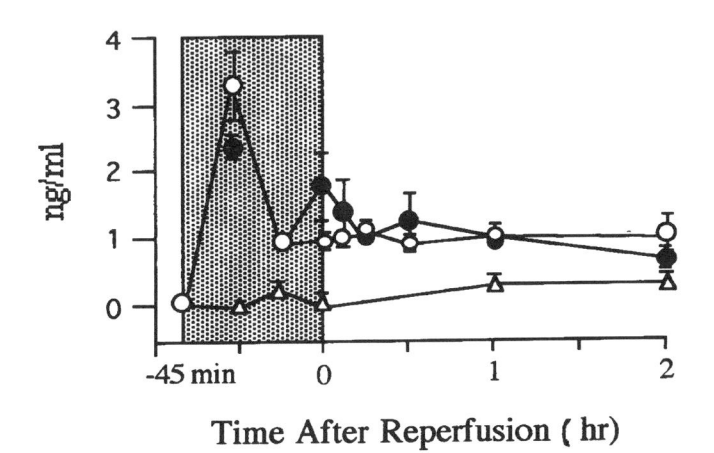

Fig. 5: Plasma endotoxin in animals: (1) 45 min of gut ischemia followed by 2 h reperfusion (○), (2) sham laparotomy (●), and (3) gut I/R with E_5 antiendotoxin antibody pretreatment (△)

Neutrophil Priming (O_2^-)

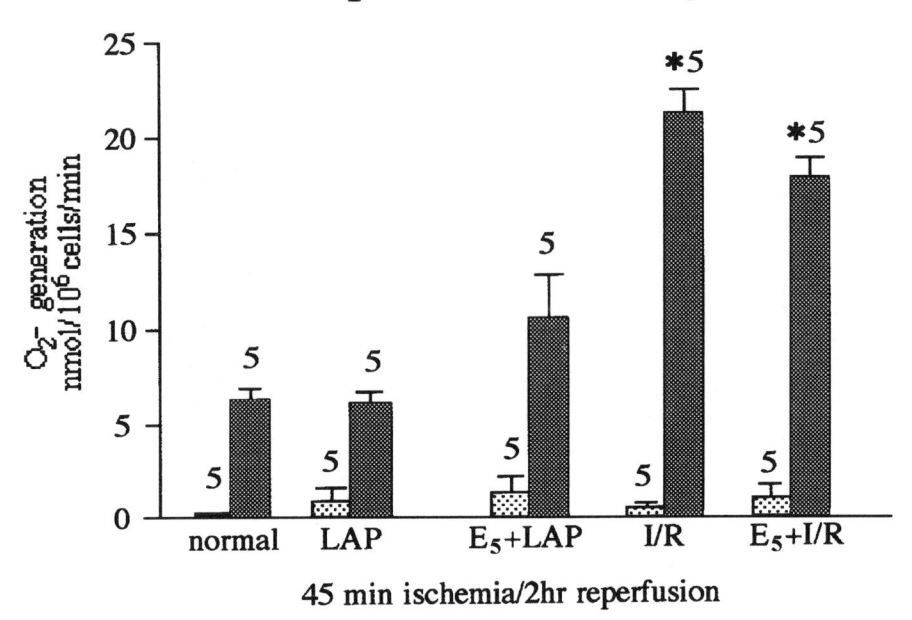

*Fig. 6: Superoxide (O_2^-) generation by PMNs harvested from animals: (1) normal, (2) sham laparotomy (LAP), (3) E_5 antiendotoxin antibody pretreatment (E_5 + LAP), (4) 45 min of gut ischemia followed by 2 h reperfusion (I/R) and, (5) E_5-pretreated gut I/R (E_5 + I/R). PMNs were activated with fMLP (-) *p <0.05 compared with normal, LAP, and E_5 LAP*

Study Hypothesis: Gut I/R Induced PMN Priming Involves Intestinal PLA_2 Activation

At this time in our evolving understanding of PMN priming in the animal model, we identified platelet-activating factor (PAF) as a mediator of PMN priming in burn and trauma patients [25, 26]. We also began to characterize PAF priming in isolated PMNs, and developed a human umbilical vein culture (HUVEC) to study the role of endothelial PAF receptors in priming PMNs [16]. In considering the potential source of PAF, phospholipase A_2 (PLA_2) became a prime suspect in view of its established capacity of generate PAF. PLA_2 is a family of *sn-2* acylhydrolases that are involved in a number of inflammatory processes, and this enzyme is highly concentrated in gut mucosa [26, 27]. Activated PLA_2 cleaves the *sn-2* acyl bond of phospholipids, yielding equimolar amount of fatty acids and lysophospholipids. Free fatty acid in the form of arachidonic acid serves as primary substrate for eicosanoids, while lysophospholipids are directly cytotoxic and, remodeled, yield PAF. The details of PLA_2 activation remain unclear but differences in substrate preference and phosphorylation control are known [28]. Given their obligate calcium dependence, the accumulation of cytosolic calcium during ischemia could be a mechanism for activation. In addition, serotonin, thrombin and bradykinin produced during ischemia may stimulate PLA_2 through receptor-operated pathways [29, 30]. Furthermore, reperfusion may sustain or augment PLA_2 activity through reactive oxygen metabolites generated following reoxygenation [31]. Thus, our hypothesis was that gut I/R promotes distal organ injury by serving as a priming bed for circulating PMNs via a PLA_2-dependent mechanism.

Employing our standard gut I/R model, we studied intestinal PLA_2 activity and temporally correlated this with PMN priming and lung leak. PLA_2 activity was assessed in a segment of distal small bowel by the release of ^{14}C-labeled oleic acid from a parent phospholipid. Interestingly, PLA_2 became activated during ischemia and this activity was sustained throughout reperfusion (Fig. 7). PMNs began to accumulate in the gut at 30 min, as reflected in MPO levels, and circulating PMNs manifested evidence of priming at 1 h. Lung 125I leak was first evident at 2 h. To further pursue the mechanistic role of gut PLA_2 activation, quinacrine (10 mg/kg) was administered i.v. prior to application of the SMA clamp. Quinacrine (mepacrine) is a synthetic acridine derivation, structurally related to primaquine and used clinically as an antimalarial agent. The pharmacology of its antimalarial efficacy is not known, but quinacrine is believed to inhibit PLA_2 activity by altering substrate-enzyme interaction. Using our standard gut I/R protocol PLA_2 inhibition abrogated (1) gut PLA2 activation, (2) PMN accumulation in the gut, (3) systemic PMN priming, (4) lung PMN sequestration, and (5) lung injury. Preemptying gut PLA_2 activation, prior to mesenteric ischemia, supported our contention that this enzyme is a proximal step in the pathogenesis of distant organ injury after splanchnic hypoperfusion. Clinical application of this therapy in the trauma arena, however, would be limited if administration had to precede the development of shock. Consequently, we delivered quinacrine after ischemia to ascertain its effectiveness during early resuscitation. Despite the activation of PLA_2 during ischemia, blockade at the time of reperfusion effectively deactivated the enzyme and this prevented the ensuing cascade of gut PMN sequestration, systemic PMN priming, lung PMN accumulation, and lung injury (Fig. 8). In further studies we found that PLA_2 inhibition was protective within the 1st h of reperfusion but, therefore, was completely ineffective [32]. Most recently, we have investigated the role of PMN integrin receptors in this process. CD11b/CD18 receptor blockade with a monoclonal antibody (IB6) attenuated lung injury but did not alter intestinal PMN localization or systemic PMN priming following gut I/R. We believe these findings are consistent with our previous in vitro work demonstrating PAF priming of PMNs is independent of CD11b/CD18 adhesion, although this receptor becomes expressed concurrently with priming [16]. Our more recent in vitro studies, in fact, suggest priming and CD18 expression are regulated via disparate signal transduction pathways [33].

Conclusion

In sum, we believe this series of in vivo studies suggests that intestinal ischemia/reperfusion can provoke remote organ injury via the pathogenic sequence; (1) gut PLA_2 activation, (2) gut PMN accumulation, (3) PMN priming in the reperfused mesenteric bed (perhaps via PAF), (4) PMN sequestration in distal organs, and (5) organ failure following a secondary activation event (Fig. 9).

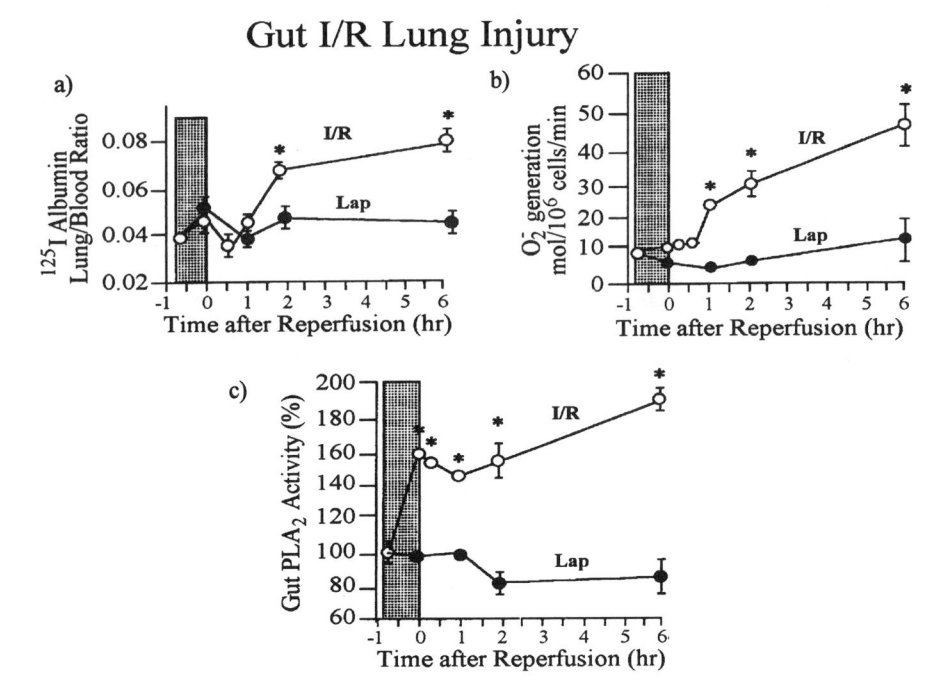

Fig. 7: a) Gut PLA$_2$ activity during 45 min intestinal ischemia/6h reperfusion (I/R) vs. sham laparotomy (LAP); b) circulating PMN priming I/R vs. LAP; c. ^{125}I-labeled albumin lung/blood ratio I/R vs. LAP. *p <0.05 I/R compared with LAP

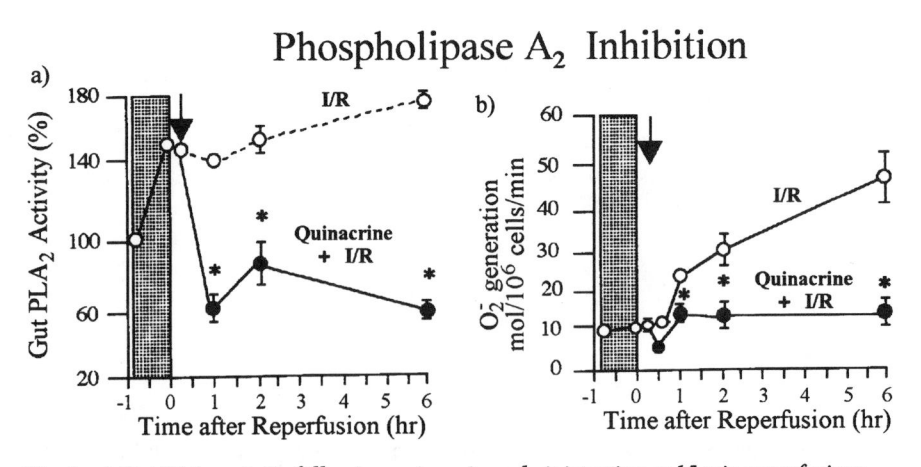

Fig. 8: a) Gut PLA$_2$ activity following quinacrine administration at 15 min reperfusion; b) circulating PMN priming following quinacrine. *p <0.05 I/R compared with I/R with saline

Sequence of Pathophysiology – In Vivo

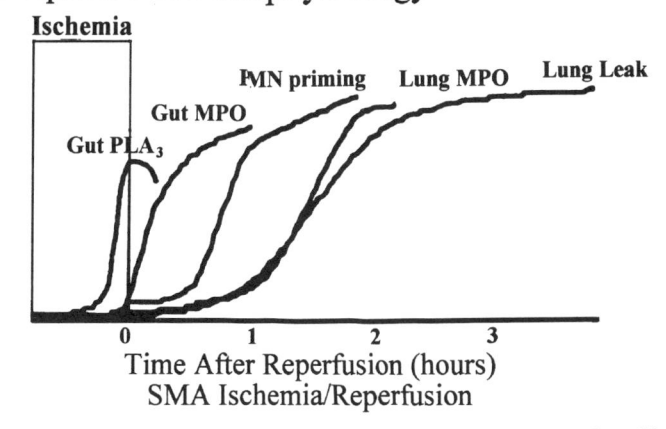

Fig. 9: Proposed mechanistic sequence in the pathogenesis of gut I/R induced lung injury. The reperfused mesenteric circulation serves as a priming bed for circulating PMNs that provoke distant organ injury following secondary activation

References

1. Moore FA, Moore EE, Read RA (1993) Postinjury multiple organ failure: role of extrathoracic injury and sepsis in adult respiratory distress syndrome. New Horizons 1: 538-549
2. Baue AE (1975) Multiple, progressive, or sequential systems failure. Arch Surg 110: 779-781
3. Eiseman B, Beart R, Norton L (1977) Multiple organ failure. Surg Gynecol Obstet 144: 323-326
4. Fry DE, Pearlstein L, Fulton RL et al. (1980) Multiple system organ failure: the role of uncontrolled infection. Arch Surg 115: 136-140
5. Marshall JC, Christow NV, Horn R et al. (1988) The microbiology of multiple organ failure. Arch Surg 123: 309-315
6. Alexander J, MacMillan B, Stinnet J et al. (1980) Beneficial effects of aggressive protein feeding in severely burned children. Ann Surg 192: 505-518
7. Baker JW, Deitch EA, Berg RD et al. (1990) Hemorrhagic shock induces bacterial translocation from the gut. J Trauma 28: 896-906
8. Herndon DN, Ziegler ST (1993) Bacterial translocation after thermal injury. Crit Care Med 21: 550-561
9. Faist E, Baue AE, Dittmer H et al. (1983) Multiple organ failure in polytrauma patients. J Trauma 23: 775787
10. Goris JA, Boekhoerst TP, Nuytinck JK et al. (1985) Multiple organ failure. Arch Surg 120: 1109-1115
11. Moore FA, Moore EE, Poggetti et al. (1991) Gut bacterial translocation via the portal vein: a clinical perspective with major torso trauma. J Trauma 31: 629-638
12. Shoemaker WC, Appel PL, Kram HB (1988) Tissue oxygen debt as a determinant of lethal and nonlethal postoperative organ failure. Crit Care Med 16: 1117-1129
13. Moore FA, Haevel LB, Moore EE et al.(1992) Incommensurate oxygen consumption in response to maximal oxygen availability predicts MOF. J Trauma 33: 58-67

14. Anderson BO, Brown JM, Harken AH (1991) Mechanism of neutrophil-mediated tissue injury. J Surg Res 52: 170-178
15. Schleiffenbaum B, Moser R, Patarroyo M et al. (1989) The cell surface glycoprotein mac-1 (CD11b/CD18) mediates neutrophil adhesion and modulates degranulation independently of its quantitative cell surface expression. J Immunol 142: 3537-3544
16. Read RA, Moore EE, Moore FA et al. (1993) PAF induced PMN superoxide production does not require PMN-EC adhesion. Surgery 114: 308-313
17. Walter BAM, Hagenlocker BE, Ward PA (1991) Superoxide responses to formyl-methionyl-leucyl-phenylalanine in primed neutrophils. J Immunol 146: 3124-3131
18. O'Flaherty JT, Jacobson DP, Redman JF, Rossi AG (1990) Translocation of protein kinase C in human polymorphonuclear neutrophils. Regulation by cystolic Ca^{2+}-independent and Ca^{2+}-dependent mechanisms. J Biol Chem 265: 9146-9152
19. Thelen M, Dewald B, Baggiolini M (1993) Neutrophil signal transduction and activation of the respiratory burst. Phys Rev 73: 797-820
20. Koike K, Moore FA, Moore EE et al. (1992) Endotoxin after gut ischemia/reperfusion causes irreversible lung injury. J Surg Res 52: 656-662
21. Anderson BO, Moore EE, Moore FA et al. (1991) Hypovolemic shock promotes neutrophil sequestration in lungs by a xanthine oxidase-related mechanism. J Appl Physiol 71: 1862-1865
22. Koike K, Moore EE, Moore FA et al. (1992) Phospholipase A_2 inhibition decouples lung injury from gut ischemia-reperfusion. Surgery 112: 173-180
23. Franciose RJ, Moore EE, Moore FA et al. (1993) Postischemic gut is the priming bed for PMNs. Surg Forum 44: 142-144
24. Koike K, Moore EE, Moore FA et al. (1994) Gut ischemia/reperfusion produces lung injury independent of endotoxin. Crit Care Med 22: 1438-1444
25. Pitman JM, Anderson BO, Poggetti RS et al. (1991) Platelet activating factor may mediate neutrophil priming following clinical burn and blunt trauma. Surg Forum 40: 108-111
26. Longhurst JC, Benham RA, Rendig SV (1992) Increased concentration of leukotriene B4 but not thromboxane B2 in intestinal lymph of cats during ischemia. Am J Physiol 262: H1482-H1485
27. Otamiri T, Lindahl M, Tagesson C (1988) Phospholipase A2 inhibition prevents mucosal damage associated with small intestine ischemia in rats. Gut 29: 489-494
28. Lin LL, Wartmann M, Lin AY et al. (1993) $cPLA_2$ is phosphorylated and activated by MAP kinase. Cell 72: 269-278
29. Kajiyama Y, Murayama T, Kitamura Y et al. (1990) Possible involvement of different GTP-binding proteins in noradrenaline- and thrombin-stimulated release of arachidonic acid in rabbit platelets. Biochem J 270: 69-75
30. Kaya H, Patton GM, Hong SL (1989) Bradykinin-induced activation of phospholipase A_2 is independent of the activation of polyphosphoinositide-hydrolyzing phospholipase C. J Biol Chem 264: 4972-4977
31. Au AM, Chan PH, Fishman RA (1985) Stimulation of phospholipase A2 activity by oxygen-derived free radicals in isolated brain capillaries. J Cell Biochem 27: 449-453
32. Koike K, Moore EE, Moore FA et al. (1995) Gut phospholipase A2 mediates neutrophil priming and lung injury after mesenteric ischemia-reperfusion. Am J Physiol 268: 6397-6403
33. Kim EJ, Moore FA et al. (1994) Disparate signal transduction in neutrophil CD18. Adhesion receptor expression versus priming for superoxide generation. Surgery 116: 262-267

Section 3:

Spectrum of Immuno- and Molecular Diagnostics

Use of Neopterin for the Monitoring of Cell-Mediated Immune Response In Vivo

D. Fuchs, A. Gruber, C. Murr, G. Reibnegger, H. Wachter

Introduction

Cell-mediated immunity (CMI) plays an important role in the control of infections with viruses, intracellular bacteria and parasites. CMI is also strongly involved in the pathogenesis of autoimmune diseases, and it mediates rejection in allograft recipients. In addition, CMI is critical for the development and the control of malignant disorders. The central cellular components of CMI are T-lymphocytes and antigen-presenting cells such as monocytes/macrophages. However, properly functioning CMI not only depends on the presence of these cells but also on intense interaction and communication between the cells being established via the release of soluble mediators, the so-called cytokines. One of the primary steps stimulated during CMI is the activation of a subclone of CD4+ T-lymphocytes, namely Th1 cells, which is characterized by the release of specific cytokines, interleukin-2 (IL-2) and interferon-gamma (IFN-γ) (Fig. 1). The functional response of CMI strictly depends on these cytokines since, among other activities, IL-2 is needed to achieve clonal expansion and further activation of T-cells, and IFN-γ is a potent activator of monocytes/macrophages inducing cytotoxicity.

Monitoring of specific cytokines could be anticipated to be a reliable method for monitoring CMI in patients. However, the situation is complicated by the short biological half-life of cytokines which may immediately bind to specific receptors present either on target cells or circulating as their soluble forms. In addition, the concentrations of one cytokine would only allow a crude estimate of the CMI status because biological effects of one specific cytokine are very often influenced by other cytokines relased in parallel. Thus, the concentration of a certain cytokine provides only limited insight into the web of concerted actions between immunocompetent cells and cytokines. Therefore, biologically more inert products released during CMI are of interest for examination of the immune status.

Immunologic Background of Neopterin

Increased concentrations of neopterin were first described to occur in patients with malignancies and with virus infections [1]. In vitro investigations applying the mixed lymphocyte reaction demonstrated that activation of T-lymphocytes was involved in the production of increased amounts of neopterin [2]. Finally, it has been demonstrated that large amounts of neopterin are released by human monocytes/macrophages upon stimulation with T-cell-derived IFN-γ [3] (Fig. 2). Although other cytokines have less or no potential to induce neopterin formation directly, it was found that, e.g., tumor necrosis factor-alpha (TNF-α) is capable of enhancing neopterin output by macrophages prestimulated with IFN-γ [4]. Thus, neopterin changes seen in patients appear to reflect the concerted actions of a variety of cytokines on the population of macrophages stimulated with IFN-γ (Fig. 2). In summary, endogenously released IFN-γ is a prerequisite for neopterin formation but IFN-γ concentrations in patients do not necessarily correlate with neopterin levels in a linear fashion for the reasons mentioned above.

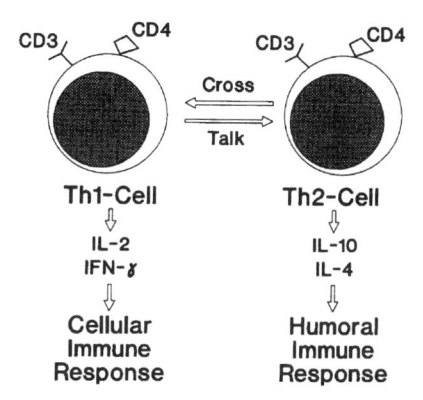

Fig. 1: Activation of cell-mediated immunity via Th1-cells. Stimulated Th1-cells release interleukin-2 (IL-2) and interferon-γ (IFN-γ) which are both required for cellular immune response, whereas interleukin-4 (IL-4) and interleukin-10 (IL-10) released by Th2-cells support humoral immunity. Both types of immune response interfere with each other

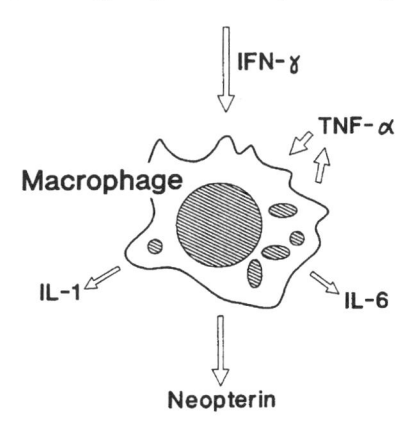

Fig. 2: Neopterin production by human monocytes/macrophages upon stimulation with interferon-gamma (IFN-γ). Other cytokines such as tumor necrosis factor-alpha (TNF-α) but not interleukin-1 (IL-1) or interleukin-6 (IL-6) may amplify the amount of neopterin produced in a synergistic manner

Enhanced formation of neopterin is biochemically linked to the induction of GTP cyclohydrolase I, the key enzyme of pteridine biosynthesis, by IFN-γ. Due to differences in the constitutive repertoire of enzymes in cells, human macrophages are unique in producing large amounts of neopterin and almost no other pteridine derivatives [5], whereas in cell cultures of other cells of human origin as well as of cells originating from other species, e.g., murine monocytes/macrophages, only small amounts of neopterin can be detected upon stimulation. Instead, excessive amounts of biopterin derivatives including 5,6,7,8-tetrahydrobiopterin are formed (Fig. 3).

In agreement with the results obtained in vitro, increased amounts of neopterin can be detected not only in patients with virus infections and certain malignant diseases (see above) but also in patients suffering from autoimmune disorders or from rejections crises after allograft transplantations [6]. Likewise, immunostimulatory therapy with cytokines activating the T-cell/macrophage interplay causes an increase in neopterin levels.

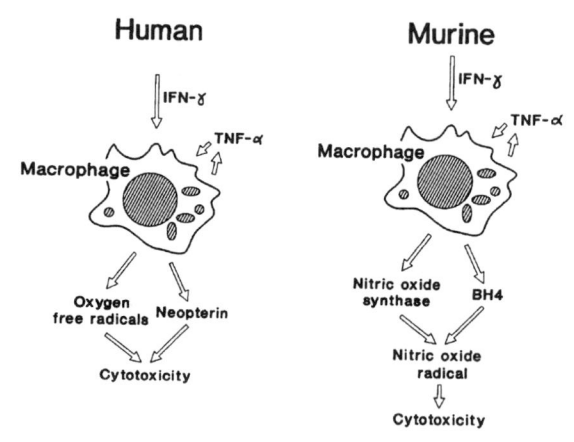

Fig. 3: Cytotoxicity of activated macrophages may be mediated by distinct biochemical pathways in human and murine cells, both involving pteridine derivatives. Human macrophages stimulated by interferon-gamma (IFN-γ) and tumor necrosis factor-alpha (TNF-α) produce large amounts of neopterin (but almost no biopterin derivatives), which is able to amplify cytotoxicity by oxygen free radicals (e.g., O_2^-, OH^-). Murine macrophages produce excess 5,6,7,8-tetrahydrobiopterin (BH4) which is cofactor of nitric oxide synthase, and is thus required for cytotoxicity mediated by nitric oxide radical

Oxygen Free-Radicals and Neopterin

Besides their potential to relase cytokines such as TNF-α or IL-1 upon activation, macrophages are potent cytotoxic effector cells. Stimulation of these cells by IFN-γ induces priming for the so-called oxidative burst, which preferentially includes the peoduction of a variety of oxidizing agents such as hydrogen peroxide and superoxide-anion (Fig. 3). Interestingly, the amount of neopterin released by human monocytes/macrophages stimulated with IFN-γ correlates to the capacity of these cells to produce peroxide upon stimulation with, e.g., phorbol esters, which indicates an association between neopterin concentrations and the killing capacity of cells [7]. Enhanced neopterin concentrations in humans allow the assumption that radicals are produced in parallel.

Recent data suggest that neopterin itself may have a role in the killing mechanisms of activated macrophages which employ oxygen free radicals. It was found that neopterin is able to enhance radical-mediated effector functions as it is measurable by enhanced light-output using the luminol-dependent chemiluminescence triggered by hydrogen peroxide and chloramine-T. Similarly, addition of neopterin enhanced the bactericidal potential of hydrogen peroxide in vitro [8]. It is particularly interesting that the enhancing effects of neopterin could be demonstrated only at a pH value higher than 6.5 and in the presence of chelated iron [9].

Because only human macrophages produce relevant amounts of neopterin, these findings suggest a specific discrepancy between the killing repertoire of human macrophages and macrophages from other species. In contrast to, e.g., murine macrophages, cytokine-inducible nitric oxide synthase (NOS) has not been demonstrated in human macrophages so far. It appears that the relative deficiency of tetrahybiopterin in human macrophages is linked with this observation, because optimal induction of NOS depends on the pteridine cofactor (Fig. 3). On the one hand, endogenously released neopterin by the human macrophage, together with oxygen free-radicals formed in parallel, may replace effects which are mediated by nitric oxide-radicals in macrophages from other species [10]. One the other hand, neopterin could probably enhance effects mediated by nitric oxide-radical relased from other sources such as endothelial cells in humans.

Measurement of Neopterin

Significant disease-associated changes of neopterin concentrations are know to occur in a variety of body fluids, most studies having been performed using serum and urine but also cerebrospinal fluid, synovial fluid or amniotic fluid [11]. In specimens with a high protein content such as serum, immunoassays like commercially available RIA and ELISA assay are the methods of choice. HPLC using C18 reversed phase material is preferentially used for urine measurements.

Neopterin in Infections and Autoimmune Disorders

The highest neopterin concentrations in urine and blood have been documented in patients suffering from acute infections with viruses, e.g., hepatitis, cytomegalovirus, Epstein-Barr virus and human immunodeficiency virus (HIV). During the acute phase of infections, neopterin concentrations rapidly increase, usually reaching a peak before antibody seroconversion becomes measurable. Neopterin concentrations normalize thereafter except in patients with HIV infection, where more than three quarters of individuals remain with increased neopterin levels even in the asymptomatic phase of infection [6]. Neopterin concentrations reveal prognostic information, higher levels being associated with more rapid disease progression. As in virus infections, infections by intracellular bacteria or parasites are associated with increased neopterin levels, whereas acute bacterial infections are not associated with high neopterin levels [11].

In autoimmune disease such as rheumatoid arthritis or systemic lupus erythematosus, high neopterin concentrations have been described correlating to the extent and the activity of the disease. Follow-up of patients during treatment shows an association between amelioration of the disease and decreasing neopterin concentrations [11].

Neopterin for Prognosis in Malignancies

Neoplastic diseases may be associated with a varying incidence of increased neopterin levels depending on the type and location of the malignant process [12]. The highest neopterin concentrations (and more than 80% of patients with increased levels) are found preferentially in patients suffering from hematological neoplasias such as chronic myelogenous leukemia or non-Hodgkin's lymphoma. Moderate frequencies of increased neopterin levels (approximately 50% of patients with increased levels) were seen in patients with gynecological neoplasias (ovarian cancer, cervical cancer) and cancers of the urogenital tract (prostate cancer, bladder cancer). A low frequency of increased neopterin levels is known to be the rule in patients with breast cancer or with head and neck cancer. In several studies of patients with cancer, a strong predictive power has been demonstrated for neopterin levels. Although a correlation usually exists between neopterin changes and the stage of the disease, the prognostic value of neopterin levels for predicting survival has been shown to be at least partly independent of stage.

Correlations of Neopterin with Other Immune Parameters

Several investigations in, e.g., patients with cancer, patients with virus infections and patients after allograft transplantation revealed significant correlations between neopterin concentrations and serum levels of IFN-γ [13]. However, for measurements of IFN-γ concentrations it has always been necessary to use more sensitive tests than bioassays, because circulating IFN-γ levels, although markedly elevated in patients compared with healthy controls, are low compared with those in in vitro studies.

There are correlations between neopterin and other serum soluble markers of immune activation. Usually the correlation is strongest for soluble receptors of TNF-α (sTNF-Rs) and β 2-microglobulin [14], but there are also correlations to, e.g., soluble IL-2 receptors and soluble intercellular adhesion molecule type 1 (sICAM-1). However, the data may point to a somewhat closer relationship between the interaction of IFN-γ and TNF-α on the macrophages to induce changes of neopterin and of, e.g., sTNF-Rs. In contrast to neopterin, the formation of β_2-microglobulin, sICAM-1 and also sTNF-Rs is less specific for a certain cell type.

Immunodeficiency and Increased Neopterin

Increased neopterin concentrations are usually found in clinical conditions which are know to be linked with immunodeficiency such as virus infections and certain types of tumors. This at first glance surprising parallelism between signs of immune activation and diminished function of cellular immunity may give a hint that chronic stimulation of immune cell in patients is involved in the loss of immunocompetence [13]. In fact, it was shown in patients with HIV infection that a higher degree of CMI activation (as measured by neopterin concentrations) was associated with reduced replicative capacity of T cells upon secondary stimulation with soluble antigens. This was even true in the early asymptomatic phase of infection [15]. The data imply that activation signals are likely to be involved in the induction of tolerance and apoptosis. It is interesting to note that one important mechanism triggering cells for programmed cell-death involves endogenously formed radicals [16, 17]. Thus, high concentrations of neopterin due to CMI activation could increase the rate of apoptosis by enhancing the biological effects of endogenous radicals.

Future Aspects

Measurements of neopterin allow a sensitive examination of the activated CMI in humans. With the data generated so far, a variety of aspects can be discussed under a new light. Especially the finding of an inverse correlation between T-cell functional response in vitro and activation of CMI in vivo may lead to a new rational for pathogenetic processes being involved in a variety of chronic disorders. In addition, due to its biochemical background and its potential role in radical-mediated processes, neopterin measurements may provide some further understanding of the role of endogenous radicals in the development of diseases.

Acknowledgement

This work was financially supported by the Austrian Ministry for Science and Research "Sektion Forschung."

References

1. Wachter H, Hausen H, Grassmayr K (1979) Erhöhte Ausscheidung von Neopterin im Harn von Patienten mit malignen Tumoren und mit Viruserkrankungen. Hoppe Seylers Z Physiol Chemie 360: 1957-1960
2. Fuchs D, Hausen H, Huber C et al. (1982) Pteridinausscheidung als Marker für alloantigen-induzierte Lymphozytenproliferation. Hoppe Seylers Z Physiol Chem 363: 661-664
3. Huber C, Batchelor JR, Fuchs D et al. (1984) Immune response-associated production of neopterin - Release from macrophages primarily under control of interferon-gamma. J Exp Med 160: 310-316
4. Werner Felmayer G, Werner ER, Fuchs D, Hausen A, Reibnegger G, Wachter H (1989) Tumor necrosis factor-alpha and lipopolysaccharide enhance interferon-induced tryptophan degradation and pteridine synthesis in human cells. Biol Chem Hoppe Seyler 370: 1063-1069
5. Werner ER, Werner-Felmayer G, Fuchs D et al. (1990) Tetrahydrobiopterin biosynthetic activities in human macrophages, fibroblasts, THP-1 and T 24 cells. GTP-cyclohydrolase I is stimulated by interferon-gamma, 6-pyruvoyl terahydropterin synthase and sepiaterin reductase are constitutively present. J Biol Chem 265: 3189-3192
6. Fuchs D, Hausen A, Reibnegger G, Werner ER, Dierich MP, Wachter H (1988) Neopterin as a marker for activated cell-mediated immunity: application in HIV infection. Immunol Today 9: 150-155
7. Nathan CF (1986) Peroxide and pteridine: a hypothesis on the regulation of macrophage antimicrobial activity by interferon-gamma. In: Gresser I, Vilcek J (eds.) Interferon vol. 7. Academic, London, pp. 124-143
8. Weiss G, Fuchs D, Hausen A et al. (1993) Neopterin modulates toxicity mediated by reactive oxygen and chloride species. FEBS Lett 321: 89-92
9. Murr C, Fuchs D, Gössler W et al. (1994) Enhancement of hydrogen peroxide-induced luminol-dependent chemiluminescence by neopterin depends on the presence of iron chelator complexes. FEBS Lett 338: 223-226
10. Fuchs D, Murr C, Reibnegger G et al. (1994) Nitric oxide synthase and antimicrobial armature of human macrophages. J Infect Dis 169: 224

11. Wachter H, Fuchs D, Hausen A et al. (1991) Neopterin - biochemistry, methods, clinical application. de Gruyter, Berlin
12. Reibnegger G, Fuchs D, Fuith LC et al. (1991) Neopterin as a marker of cell-mediated immunity: application in malignant disease. Cancer Detect Prevent 15: 483-490
13. Fuchs D, Malkowsky M, Reibnegger G, Werner ER, Forni G, Wachter H (1989) Endogenous release of interferon-gamma and diminished response of peripheral blood mononuclear cells to antigenic stimulation. Immunol Lett 23: 103-108
14. Zangerle R, Gallati H, Sarcletti M et al. (1994) Increased serum concentrations of soluble tumor necrosis factor receptors in HIV-infected individuals are associated with immune activation. J Acquir Immune Defic Syndr 7: 79-85
15. Fuchs D, Shearer GM, Boswell RN et al. (1990) Increased serum neopterin in patients with HIV-1 infection is correlated with reduced in vitro interleukin-2 production. Clin Exp Immunol 80: 44-48
16. Buttke TM, Sandstrom PA (1993) Oxidative stress as a mediator of apoptosis. Immunol Today 15: 7-10
17. Fuchs D, Gruber A, Überall F et al. (1994) Oxidative stress and apoptosis. Immunol Today 15: 496

Interleukin-2 Receptor as a Useful Tool for Diagnosis and Treatment of Autoimmune, Infectious and Malignant Diseases in Clinical Medicine and Immunopathology: Comparison with Other Markers of Immune Activation and Therapeutical Consequences

G.P. Tilz, E. Faist, F. Schreiber, U. Demel, D. Demel, H. Becker, J. Schafhalter, H. Wachter, L. Kenner, D. Fuchs

Introduction

This is a report of our experience of the application of the soluble interleukin-2 receptor assay (SILA). The test was initially standardized using monoclonal antibodies (mAbs) from Andreas and Barbara Ziegler (Berlin) and later using the Bender assay (T Cell Sciences).

A large variety of cytokines interact during cellular activation, and these can be quantitated by biological and immunochemical assays. After considerable experience of investigating the half-life and sensitivity of these mediators, we decided to look at the more stable molecules such as the receptors. Of these the SIL2R plays a central role, interacting with the appropriate cytokine during the daily processes of immunoregulation. Our group has quantitated SIL2R using ELISA with standardized monoclonal antibodies. This assay has become a useful tool for clinicians in the assessment of the stage of immune function and activation in a variety of disorders and to enable more light to be shed on the diagnosis, prognosis and course of a variety of diseases (Table 1).

Materials and Methods

All the assays indicated in Table 2 were performed using sandwich ELISAs with standardized reagents from the manufacturer Bender, Vienna. The sera from patients were examined immediately or after a short storage period. Samples from healthy individuals were used as controls. Patients with different types of blood cell dyscrasia, autoimmune or inflammatory diseases, infections, transplantations and neurologic disorders were investigated. The immune function was also studied using SILA and other assays.

Table 1: Experiences with the soluble IL2R assay (SILA) in clinical situations. Clinical relevance and therapeutic consequences are discussed in the text

Pathological entity	Disease
Malignant diseases	Leukemias
	Lymphomas
	Solid tumors
Infections	AIDS
	Malaria
	Hepatitis
	CMV
	EBV
Autoimmunity	SLE
	Rheumatoid arthritis
	Hashimoto thyreoiditis
	Different types of vasculitis
	Accelerated sclerosis (some)
	Sarcoidosis) (some)
Transplantations	Kidney
	Heart

Table 2: Comparison of the various assays useful for the assessment of cellular activation in human serum. All these cell activation parameters have been quantified in our laboratory and the normal ranges give are in accordance with international standards

Parameter	IL-2-R	TNF-α	CD 23	T8	ICAM 1
Normal range	575-919 IU	1.5-4.2 IU	15-250 IU	138-533 IU	300 $^+$

IL-2-R = 55 kDa antigen; TNF-α = 60 kDa antigen; CD 23 = 43 kDa antigen; T8 = 32 kDa antigen (membrane glycoprotein); ICAm = 55 kDa single chain glycoprotein for the intercellular adhesion molecule 1.

Results

Our panel of serum laboratory tests for the assessment of cellular immune activation along with the normal ranges for these tests is shown in Table 2. Tests on immune complexes, complement levels, immunoglobulins, neopterin, $_2$-microglobulin and a variety of autoantibodies are also underway in our laboratories.

Pathological findings were as follows: regardless of the peripheral T-cell count in malignancies the SILA indicated total tumor volume or its interaction with the lymphoid tissue. We therefore considered Tac expression and release into the peripheral blood to be a useful marker for the follow-up of *hairy cell leukemia* (HCL), which in itself is not very leukemogenic but more infiltrative.

The SILA predicted recurrence and relapse in preclinical situations in patients with HCL and some *chronic lymphocytic leukemias* (CLLs). We also used it in patients with *Hodgkin's disease*, where the amount of SIL2R is an indicator of the amount of tumor. Even in *chronic myelocytic leukemia* (CML) patients, the SILA gave impressive results, since the Tac antigen is present in the blastic phase cells and consequently appears in the peripheral blood as an indicator of immaturity and mass and, hence, of poor prognosis. In contrast, stable CML and *myeloma* do not express increased amounts of SIL2R. In Hodgkin's disease the results of the SILA again correlated with the preclinical state of recurrence, while stable remission was SILA negative. All *T-cell lymphomas* and most *B-cell malignancies* were SILA positive in our experience.

In patients suffering from solid tumors we were able to show equally high SILA titers in the case of enormous tumor masses and hence a poor prognosis. These results underline the importance of hopelessly activated immune system to compete with malignancy. Our experience is confined to *tumors of the pancreas, colon* and *lung*, where the malignant cells examined were CD25-negative cells surrounded by tumor-infiltrating CD-25-positive cells. In *AIDS* the SILA again indicated a poor prognosis and disease progression, which was in accordance with our experience with neopterin, which represents an additional marker of disease activity in *infections* such as *AIDS* and high-risk *malaria*. In patients with *chronic hepatitis B* the e antigen-positive subgroup appeared to be more elevated than the a subgroup, and in acute viral infection regardless of hepatitis B or hepatitis C SILA titers were greatly elevated, only returning to normal when the disease subsided. Cytomegalovirus and Epstein-Barr virus infections also caused a major increase in SILA titers.

In *autoimmune diseases* our findings were similar since autoimmunity is not an exception to the rule that high SILA titers are correlated with the activity index. In our experience with *systemic lupus erythematosus* and *RA* patients, pleural and synovial determinations complete the usefulness of the differential diagnosis and disease activity, since gouty and metabolic processes were constantly negative in our laboratory. With *multiple sclerosis* we found the same principle of immune activation to hold true for progressive disease in contrast to quiescent situations, which were indicated by a negative SILA. With *vasculitis* and accelerated *sclerosis* we interpreted increased SILA titers as being indicative of the presence of immune mechanisms detrimental to the host. This picture was characteristic of our patients with *Kawasaki syndrome* and also some of those with *Winiwarter-Bürger* disease. SILA and T8 assays should also be performed before *graft rejection*, although the degree of renal damage may make interpretation difficult, which is also complicated if infection, especially viral, cannot be ruled out. In patients with *bile disease* we found the SILA to give a positive result in patients suffering from malignancies, whereas in patients with *inflammatory bile disease* SILA values were not noticeably different from normal. In some of our patients with *sarcoidosis*, increased SILA and sodium dismutase values were correlated with extension of the lymph nodes involved although the results obtained so far are still to preliminary to enable us to give precise information about the correlation of both markers with this disease.

Conclusion

In summary, the SILA assay represents a very useful indicator in the diagnosis, prognosis, course and successful treatment of a variety of clinical disorders. Irrespective of specificity, increased SILA levels are correlated with the number of immune cells involved in the process and hence the magnitude of the clinical burden. Since new immunotherapeutic approaches are available for a variety of disease entities, assessment of immune function is particularly important before and during the protocol to monitor the reaction of the patient to these new methods of immune intervention (Fig. 1). The SILA, neopterin, T8 and soluble TNF receptors are all particularly useful in providing answers to the clinical questions posed once the diagnosis has been made. Although these markers appear to be highly correlated in some situations, they reflect different aspects of immunoregulation because of the different signals and cell types involved in their production.

- antigen
- APC
- T cell
- B cell
- Plasmocytes

ICAM
Neopterin, TNF
IL 2 R, T8
beta 2 m, CD 23
Immunoglobulin antibodies

CELLULAR ACTIVATION

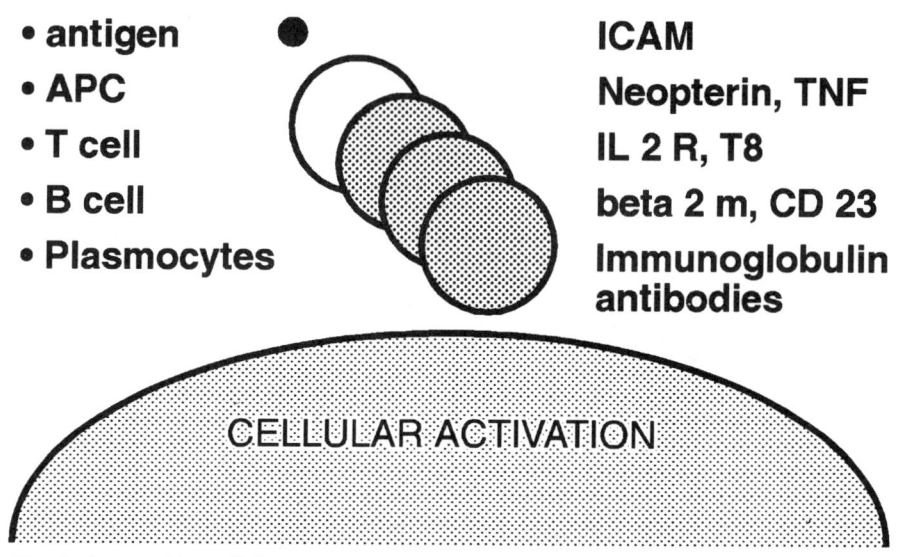

Fig. 1: Approach to cellular activation at the different levels quantified by our assays. The more the activation progresses, the broader the polyimmunotherapy that is applied

References

1. Diez-Ruiz A, Tilz GP, Zangerle R, Baier-Bitterlich G, Wachter H, Fuchs D (1995) Soluble receptors for tumor necrosis factor in clinical laboratory diagnosis. Eur J Haematol (in press)
2. Fuchs D, Hausen A, Reibnegger G, Werner ER, Dierich MP, Wachter H (1988) Neopterin as a marker for activated cell-mediated immunity. Immunol Today 9: 150-155
3. Samsonov MY, Tilz GP, Egorova O, Reibnegger G, Balabanova RM, Nassonov EL, Nassonova VA, Wachter H, Fuchs D (1995) Serum soluble markers of immune activation and disease activity in systemic lupus erythematosus. Lupus 4: 29-32
4. Tilz GP, Domej W, Diez-Ruiz A, Weiss G, Brezinschek R, Brezinschek HP, Hüttl, Wachter H, Fuchs D (1993) Increased immune activation during and after physical exercise. Immunobiology 188: 194-202

Soluble Tumor Necrosis Factor Receptors

H.Denz

Introduction

Tumor necrosis factor alpha (TNF), a pleiotropic cytokine produced mainly by mononuclear phagocytes, plays a key role in a number of immunologically mediated reactions. Its effect is provided by specific cell surface receptors. Two types of TNF receptors (TNF-R), called p55, TNF-R type I, and p75, TNF-R type II, have been identified [4]. Both receptors exist in soluble form and represent fragments of the extracellular domain of the cell-bound TNF-R [9]. Soluble TNF-Rs (sTNF-Rs) are able to block the cytotoxic effect of TNF, acting as a negative feedback mechanism (Aderka, 1991). On the other hand, sTNF-Rs enhance and stabilize some of the effects of TNF, e.g., growth of B-CLL cells [2]. These effects are seen with low concentrations of sTNF-Rs, whereas high concentrations show inhibiting effects.

Soluble TNF Receptors in Nonmalignant Diseases

Significantly increased concentrations of sTNF-Rs have been described in a number of inflammatory disorders (Table 1). Foley et al. described enhanced levels in patients with sarcoidosis, tuberculosis and Crohn's disease [6]. Increased levels of sTNF-Rs p55 and p75 were found in 85% and 95% of HIV-infected patients respectively. The extent of the increase sTNF-R p75 was greater in more advanced HIV infection pointing to a correlation with the course of the disease. A strong correlation was found between sTNF-Rs p75 and markers of cellular immunoactivation such as $_2$-microglobulin and urinary neopterin and a less strong correlation with interferon gamma [10].

Soluble TNF-Receptors in Malignant Disorders

In several tumor cell lines soluble forms of the TNF-Rs are produced continuously [7]. Based on these data sTNF-Rs were determined in patients with various tumors. Enhanced levels were found in patients with cancer of colon, breast, pancreas, stomach, lung, etc. [1] (Table 1). Higher

Table 1: Disorders with enhanced levels of sTNF-Rs

1. Inflammatory disorders
    a) Sarcoidosis
    b) Tuberculosis
2. Infectious disorders
    a) Bacterial: tuberculosis
    b) Viral: HIV infection
3. Malignant disorders
    a) Solid tumors: cancer of breast, pancreas, stomach, lung etc.
    b) Hematological: non-Hodgkin's lymphomas, Hodgkin's disease, multiple myeloma
4. Others
    a) Immunotherapy (IL-2, IFN, TNF, etc.)

concentrations were found in patients with a more advanced stage of disease. The sera of patients showed significant inhibition of the cytocidal effect of TNF.

Our group determined concentrations of sTNF-Rs in patients with hematological disorders [5]. Fifty patients suffering from non-Hodgkin's lymphoma ($n=35$), Hodgkin's disease ($n=10$) and multiple myeloma ($n=5$) were analyzed. Compared with healthy controls, significantly elevated concentrations of sTNF-Rs were found (2.68 vs. 1.23 ng/ml, P 0.0001). A significant correlation between sTNF-R P55 and neopterin concentrations was found ($r = 0.544, P$ 0.001). Patients with weight loss showed higher sTNF-R p55 concentrations than patients with stable weight. These data point to a possible association between signs of immunoactivation and the development of weight loss and cachexia in patients with hematological disorders.

Soluble TNF Receptors Under Immunostimulatory Therapy

Treatment with immunomodulatory substances includes therapy with interleukin-2 (IL-2), interferon (IFN), TNF and muramyltripeptide. This form of therapy leads to stimulation of the immune system, measurable by enhanced levels of neopterin and $_2$-microglobulin [3, 8]. Landmann et al. [8] found that immunotherapy induces not only enhanced concentrations of TNF, but simultaneously elevates those of both types of soluble TNF-Rs. Eleven patients with well-advanced metastatic cancer were studied during three different regimens of immunotherapy with IL-2 and/or IFN. There was a significant relationship between TNF and sTNF-Rs p55 and p75 in two of the three groups of patients. The increase in sTNF-Rs parallels or exceeds that of TNF and may influence the immunomodulatory effects of TNF during cytokine therapy.

Conclusions

Enhanced concentrations of both types of sTNF-Rs can be found not only in inflammatory diseases, but also in a variety of malignant disorders. Their physiological role has not yet been elucidated, they seem to act as a negative feedback, attenuating TNF effects. The close correlation with neopterin and $_2$-microglobulin concentrations and the association with weight loss point to the fact that they represent another sign of endogenous immunoactivation. The findings confirm that immunoactivation takes place in many malignant disorders and that this activation leads to exactly the same changes as those seen in inflammatory disorders. Further studies will help to shed more light on the pathophysiology of the puzzling network of cytokines.

References

1. Aderka D, Engelmann H, Hornik V, Skornick Y, Levo Y, Wallach D, Kushtai G (1991) Increased serum levels of soluble receptors for tumor necrosis factor in cancer patients. Cancer Res 51: 5602-5607
2. Aderka D, Engelmann H, Maor Y, Brakebusch C, Wallach D (1992) Stabilization of the bioactivity of tumor necrosis factor by its soluble receptors. J Exp Med 175: 323-329
3. Aulitzky WE, Tilg H, Herold M, Berger M, Vogel W, Judmaier G, Gastl G, Mull B, Flener R, Wiegele J, Pichler E, Denz H, Böheim E, Aulitzky WK, Huber C (1988) Enhanced serum levels of beta-2-microglobulin, neopterin, and interferon gamma in patients treated with recombinant tumor necrosis factor alpha. J Interferon Res 8: 655-664
4. Brockhaus M, Schoenfeld H-J, Schlaeger E-J, Hunziker W, Lesslauer W, Loetscher H (1990) Identification of two types of tumor necrosis factor receptors on human cell lines by monoclonal antibodies. Proc Natl Acad Sci USA 87: 3127-3131
5. Denz H, Orth B, Weiss G, Gallati H, Herrmann R, Huber P, Wachter H, Fuchs D (1993) Serum soluble tumour necrosis factor receptor 55 is increased in patients with haematological neoplasias and is associated with immune activation and weight loss. Eur J Cancer 29A: 2232-2235
6. Foley N, Lambert C, McNicol M, Johnson N, and Rock GAW (1990) An inhibitor of the toxicity of tumour necrosis factor in the serum of patients with sarcoidosis, tuberculosis and Crohn's disease. Clin Exp Immunol 80: 395-399
7. Hohmann HP, Remy R, Brockhaus M, van Loon APGM (1989) Two different cell types have different major receptors for human tumor necrosis factor (TNF alpha). J Biol Chem 264: 14927-14934
8. Landmann R, Keilholz U, Scheibenbogen C, Brockhaus M, Gallati H, Denz H, Bargetzi M, Ludwig C (1994) Increase of soluble TNF-receptors and TNF-alpha in serum during immunotherapy with rIL-2 and/or rIFN-alpha. J Immunol Immunother, (in press)
9. Olsson I, Lantz M, Nilsson E, Peetre C, Thysell H, Grubb A (1989) Isolation and characterization of a tumor necrosis factor binding protein from urine. Eur J Haematol 42: 270-275
10. Zangerle R, Gallati H, Sarcletti M, Weiss G, Denz H, Wachter H, Fuchs D (1994) Serum concentrations of soluble tumor necrosis factor receptors in HIV infected individuals are associated with immune activation. J AIDS 7: 79-85

Procalcitonin: A New Innovative Marker for Sepsis and Very Severe Inflammatory Diseases

C. Bohuon, M. Assicot

In 1984, analytical studies using monoclonal antibodies (Mabs) were initiated in order to develop a new ultraspecific and sensitive assay to measure calcitonin (CT) [1], which is an excellent marker for the diagnosis of a rare and sometimes transmissible tumor of the C thyroid cells (MCT). During this research, many Mabs against various parts of the precursor of CT, procalcitonin (ProCT), were also found. These Mabs were produced after immunization of mice with synthetic peptides bound to tetanus toxin, and have shown extraordinary analytical usefulness in "molecular dissection." As an example of this progress some of these Mabs were able to specifically recognize the prolinamide C-terminal part of the calcitonin molecule as well as the proline-glycine terminal part (of the calcitonin glycine molecule) [2]. Studies of patients with MTC have shown that the increase in CT precursor (ProCT) was correlated with an increase in CT. In 1992, a study was initiated for the study of burn patients, which again found an increase in only the intact molecules of ProCT (116 AA) in some patients. However, there was a clear connection between ProCT and an infection which was not always dependent on lung injury. As a result of these findings other areas required testing with ProCT in order to determine whether ProCT was increased only as a result of systemic reaction from the body against a trauma such as a burn or whether it was a sign of the body's attempt to fight infection. As a result, the study of ProCT was immediately extended to test young children with various kinds of meningitis. All the children with bacterial meningitis were found to have a highly increased ProCT levels. This increase was much higher than in the burned patients, probably as a result of the systematic antibiotic therapy which was given to them. In these children ProCT was only increased in blood but not in the cerebral spinal fluid. Another finding was that ProCT was only increased in the children with bacterial meningitis and not in those with viral meningitis, where ProCT was only slightly increased [3]. As a result of these further findings, other clinical studies have been develop to test ProCT and its value not only as a bacterial infection indicator but also as a new innovative marker of sepsis. In order to test ProCT accurately, a new sensitive and specific luminometric sandwich assay has been developed (LUMItest PCT, Brahms Diagnostica, Berlin, FRG).

Two studies, in collaboration with Prof. Dandona's group (Buffalo, USA) and Prof. Eberhardt's group (Freiburg, FRG), were conducted, in which endotoxin from *Salmonella Abortus suis* was injected by bolus (i.v.), 4 ng/kg, to both normal volunteers and patients with advanced cancer. In both studies, ProCT was present 3 h after the injection, with a subsequent steady increase to reach a plateau at 24 h after injection. ProCT levels were still high the following day in cancer patients who had received one injection per day. ProCT showed a steady decrease after the 2nd day in these patients, but was still measurable on the 3rd day. These findings correlated very well with the results obtained with TNF within the same patients population.

In contrast to cytokines (such as TNF, IL-6), ProCT was observed to have a very long half-life in blood, which is very important in the diagnosis of bacterial infections such as bacterial sepsis. It is also of interest since CT itself has a relatively short half-life (about 10 min). This may be due to the fact that ProCT binds to proteins giving them an apparently high molecular weight and thus causing them to last longer than cytokines. This large molecular weight could also be the reason for the absence of transfer across the blood-brain barrier as well as the absence of any proteolytic cleavage in the blood.

The initial research conducted on ProCT found that in many normal subjects the amount of ProCT was less than 10 pg/ml in comparison with a mean "normal value" established from 500 blood donors of around 40 pg/ml. Consequently, we may consider a value of higher than 200 pg/ml to be abnormal. In fact, the values observed in the patients with bacterial meningitis and septicemias were always higher than 10 000 pg/ml. In nearly all of the sepsis patients tested, the quantity of ProCT was greater than 1000 pg/ml. In contrast, patients with viral infections generally had low values of ProCT (1000 pg/ml).

Since the recent discovery of ProCT and its role as a sepsis marker, we currently have only preliminary data from various kinds of infection. However, it is clear that patients with viral infections including those who are HIV positive, even in advanced stages of the disease, still do not show a major increase in ProCT in their blood. In addition, we found that in the nonseptic inflammatory diseases, such as rheumatoid arthritis, rectocolitis, Crohn's disease, cirrhosis, Kahler's disease, and various metastatic cancers, the majority of patients show normal or a very low decrease in ProCT values. However, in these patients C-reactive protein is generally high, demonstrating the existence of inflammation.

The following are preliminary data for ProCT as measured in other infectious diseases.

1. A significant correlation was found between ProCT and severity of disease according to Bone score (Dr. Zeni, Table 1 [5]).
2. Very high amounts of ProCT were found in patients with gram-negative septicemia, especially patients with melioidosis where we found values of more than 100 000 pg/ml (Prof. Smith, Figure 1 [6]).
3. High values were also observed in malaria patients with *P. falciparum* and *P. vivax*. In eight studies in collaboration with Profs. Gendrel and Davies, ProCT was found to be very high in the patients with the most severe forms of malaria [7].
4. A very good correlation was found with tumor necrosis factor (TNF) and also with IL-6 and CRP. The more rapid increase in ProCT levels than CRP levels explains the discrepancy found in some of the patients.
5. However, we currently have no data from the other parasite diseases such as leishmaniosis or schistosomiasis.

Curiously enough the exact site of ProCT production is still unknown. However, thyroid cells as well as macrophages, granulocytes, lymphocytes, hepatocarcinoma and endothelial cells can be excluded (data found in our in vitro studies) as not producing ProCT. The greatest difficulty lies in the absence of an animal model since the antibodies produced against human ProCT are not able to react with rat or rabbit ProCT. Some of the histochemical results found in the literature indicate that lung or pancreatic cells could be candidates. The possible physiological or pathological role of ProCT is also an interesting question. Another difficulty arises because pure ProCT molecules are very difficult to synthesize, making it difficult to conduct pharmacological studies. Does ProCT have a role in the cytokine cascade or in the endocrine activity? One very important fact about ProCT is that it is a promising new marker for patients with infective diseases. Detailed studies are now needed to verify these initial stimulating and interesting findings.

Table 1: Serum procalcitonin levels on admission in septic and nonseptic patients

Group	No of patients	Procalcitonin mean (ng/ml)±SEM
S+	22 (15%)	0.12±0.04
S-	96 (66.2%)	2.36±0.59
SS	19 (13.2%)	37.1±16.4
SC	8 (5.6%)	44.8±22.0

S-, no sepsis; S+, sepsis; SS, severe sepsis; SC, septic shock

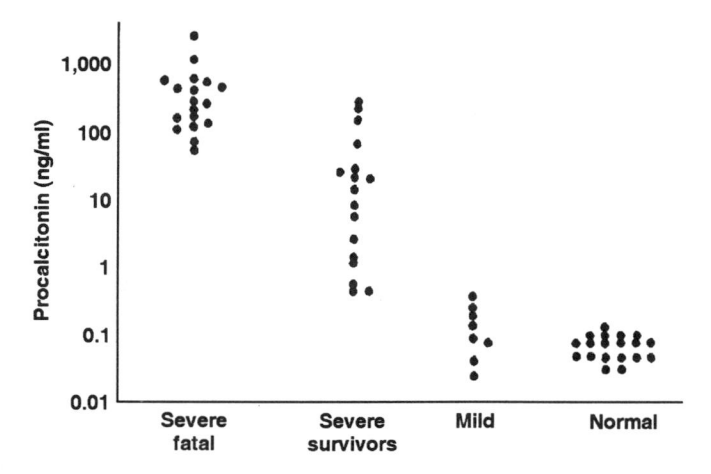

Fig. 1: Serum procalcitonin levels in septic and nonseptic patients

References

1. Motte P, Vauzelle P, Gardet P et al. (1980) Construction and clinical validation of a sensitive and specific assay for serum mature calcitonin using monoclonal antipeptide antibodies. Clin Chem Acta 174: 35-54
2. Motte P, Vauzelle P, Alberici G et al. (1987) Utilization of synthetic peptides for the study of calcitonin and biosynthetic precursors for calcitonin. Nucl Med Biol 14(4): 289-294
3. Assicot M, Gendrel D, Carsin H et al. (1993) High serum procalcitonin concentrations in patients with sepsis and infection. Lancet 541: 515-518

4. Dandona P, Nix D, Wilson MF et al. (1994) Procalcitonin increase following endotoxin injection in normal subjects. J Clin Endocrinol Metab 79(6): 1605-1609
5. Zeni F, Viallon A, Assicot M et al. (1995) Serum procalcitonin in sepsis: Relation to severity and cytokines (TNF, IL-6, IL-8) (Abstract) Clin Intensive Care 5 Suppl 2
6. Smith M, Suputtamongkol Y, Chaowagul W et al. (1995) Serum procalcitonin in melioidosis. Clin Infect Dis 20: 641-645
7. Davis T, Assicot M, Bohuon C et al. (1994) Serum procalcitonin concentrations in acute malaria. Trans Roy Soc Trop Med Hyg 88: 670-673

Early Diagnosis of Sepsis by Rapid Measurement of C3a/C3 Plasma Levels

S.Stöve, H.Hartmann, A.Klos, W.Bautsch, J.Köhl

Introduction

Sepsis is by definition a systemic inflammatory response of the body to infection caused by bacteria, fungi, viruses and parasites. Numerous proinflammatory mediators are involved in the pathogenesis of the sepsis syndrome and can be detected in enhanced amounts in different body fluids. These mediators include the cytokines tumor necrosis factor-α (TNF-α), interleukin-1 (IL-1) or Il-6 as well as active fragments from the clotting cascade, the kallikrein and the complement systems [1, 5, 7, 17].

One of the earliest events in sepsis is activation of the complement system, either by the classical or the alternative pathway. Beside the bacterial opsonization by C3-split products and bacterial lysis by the membrane attack complex (C5b-9) the proinflammatory anaphylatoxins C3a, C4a, C5a and C5adesArg are generated by proteolytic cleavage of C3, C4, and C5. These polypeptides are responsible for a series of inflammatory reactions, including activation of neutrophils, basophils, mast cells, eosinophils and monocytes and macrophages, and result in release of pharmacologically active mediators (for review see [6, 12]). C5a is one of the most potent chemotaxins and promotes neutrophil aggregation and adherence to endothelial cells. Stimulation of the oxidative metabolism in PMN leads to the release of reactive oxygen intermediates. Taken together these events lead to increased vascular permeability, contraction of smooth muscle and, finally, to tissue destruction.

Due to the early activation of complement in sepsis, anaphylatoxin plasma levels should be elevated prior to the clinical syndrome at the very beginning of sepsis. Based on this hypothesis, plasma levels of complement components C3, C3a/C3adesArg and C5a/C5adesArg in 20 septic and ten critically ill patients from a medical intensive care unit were evaluated. Two questions were addressed: (1) Does determination of complement components allow differentiation between septic patients and critically ill patients at risk for sepsis at the very beginning of the syndrome? (2) Are these parameters of prognostic value for clinical outcome?

Material and Methods

Patients

Thirty patients from the medical intensive care unit (ICU) of the Medical School Hannover entered the study. Sepsis was diagnosed according to the criteria given by the ACCP/SCCM consensus conference [2]. A minimum of four of the following criteria had to be fulfilled for the diagnosis of sepsis: (1) clinical signs of a focal infection; (2) temperature >38°C or <36°C; (3) heart rate >90 beats/min; (4) respiratory rate >20 breaths/min or $PaCo_2$ <32 mmHg; (5) leukocyte count >12000 cells/ml^3 or <4000 cells/ml^3. In addition one ore more of the following criteria of inadequate organ perfusion was required: (1) hypoxemia (P_aO_2/F_iO_2 ≤280); (2) elevated plasma lactate >2.5 mM/l; (3) oliguria (<0.5 ml/kg body weight for at least 1 h in patients with catheters). The clinical diagnosis of sepsis was confirmed in all but one patient by evidence of bacteria, fungi or parasites in blood culture, bronchoalveolar lavage (BAL) (≥10^5/ml) or section material. According to the aforementioned criteria 20 of 30 patients (age range 14 - 64; 13 men and 7 women) were considered to be septic. The remaining ten patients (age range 21 - 78; 7 men and 3 women) were considered septic at their admission to the ICU by clinical criteria, which means that they fulfilled a maximum of three sepsis criteria (most often fever, leucocytosis or tachycardia), without signs of inadequate organ perfusion. Microbiological examination of blood, BAL or section material revealed no pathogenic organisms. Underlying diseases of control patients were autoimmune thrombocytopenia (n=1), cholecystitis (n=1), Crohn's disease (n=1), polytrauma (n=1), liver transplantation (n=1), gastrointestinal bleeding (n=1), diabetes (n=2) or cardial surgery (n=2).

Collection of Blood

Patients were monitored for 10 days. During this observation period 17 blood samples were taken. The first sample was drawn on admission (T0) to the ICU. The following six samples (T1-T5) were obtained every 8 h and from T6-T13 (day 3-7) every 12 h. The last 3 days (days 8-10), blood was taken once daily. Blood samples were collected in 2.5 ml K-EDTA Monovettes (Sarstedt) from arterial catheters, centrifuged for 10 min at 1200 x g and stored in triplicates at -70°C until tested.

Complement Assays

The plasma levels of C3, C3a/C3adesArg and C5a/C5adesArg were determined by the ABICAP C3a, C3 and C5a sandwich-type assay [10], based on neoepitope specific antibodies, which recognize C3a/C3adesArg or C5a/C5adesArg but not the respective parent molecules C3 or C5, eliminating separation of C3 or C5 prior to the assay. Due to the combination of column chromatography with immunoanalysis results are obtained in 20-25 min.

Statistical Analysis

Data are given as mean ±1 S.D. Significance level was determined by Student's t test; p values <0.05 were accepted as significant.

Results

Pneumonia was diagnosed most frequently as the underlying disease within the septic group ($n = 11$; 55%). Other patients had severe endocarditis ($n=3$; 15%), catheter-related infection ($n=3$; 15%), meningitis ($n=1$), malaria ($n=1$) or peritonitis ($n=1$) (Table 1). Gram-positive bacteria were more often isolated from BAL or blood culture ($n=10$; 50%) than gram negative bacteria ($n=7$; 35%). Other microorganisms isolated were fungi ($n=2$) and in one case *Plasmodium falciparum* ($n=1$) (Table 1). Mortality within the septic group was 55%. In the control group all patients survived.

Table 1: Microorganisms isolated from blood culture or bronchoalveolar lavage (BAL)

a) Microorganisms isolated from BAL or blood	Number	%	Died	%
Gram positive bacteria	10	50	5	25
Gram negative bacteria	7	35	5	25
Fungi	2	10	1	5
Parasites	1	5	-	-
Σ	20	100	11	55
b) Underlying diseases of patients from the septic group.				
Pneumonia	11	55	8	40
Endocarditis	3	15	2	10
Catheter-related infection	3	15	-	-
Meningitis	1	5	-	-
Malaria	1	5	-	-
Peritonitis	1	5	1	5

C3a Plasma Levels

During the study period at the ICU, plasma levels of all patients, either from the control or the septic group, were markedly increased (5-10-fold) compared to healthy volunteers (Table 2). The highest levels within the septic group were found during the first 32 h after clinical onset of sepsis and were significantly ($P<0.05$) different from the control group (Fig. 1). C3a levels of septic survivors and septic non-survivors were equal during the first 32 h after onset of sepsis. However, C3a values of septic non survivors remained high (≥ 800 ng/ml) until they died. In contrast, C3a values of septic survivors steadily declined and were indistinguishable from the control group at day 4 after onset of sepsis (Fig. 2).

C3 Plasma Levels

All patients included in the study had an approximately 50% reduction of their C3a levels at T1-T4 (Table 2.) compared to healthy volunteers (1.95 ± 0.29 mg/ml vs. $0.86 - 1.19$ ng/ml). Although the C3 plasma levels increased in both groups during the observation period, they did not reach the C3 levels of healthy individuals. At T 16 (day 10) C3 plasma levels were 1.67 ± 0.59 within the septic group and 1.35 ± 0.95 within the control group.

Table 2: Plasma C3a, C3a/3 and C5a levels. a) Plasma values taken 0-3 h (T0), 8 h (T1), 16 h (T2), 24 h (T3), and 32 h (T4) after clinical onset of sepsis. C3a/C3 ratios determined from C3a and C3 plasma values. * $p<0.05$, Student's t test

C3a values (ng/ml)	T0	T1	T2	T3	T4
Septic patients	1181±1085*	1217±1090*	1062±805*	1089±730*	1091±856*
Nonseptic patients	449±220*	487±218*	457±186*	470±233*	498±206*
Septic survivors	1023±847	1125±896	991±714	1020±731	981±699
Septic nonsurvivors	1310±1297	1293±1294	1120±925	1137±795	1190±1031
Healthy persons	86±29				
C3a/C3 ratio (ng/ml)/(mg/ml)					
Septic patients	2669±4765*	2622±3692*	3396±7339*	2873±5243*	2593±4592*
Nonseptic patients	488±225*	537±215*	562±305*	527±446*	574±545*
Septic survivors	2137±2760	2362±3227	2320±3065	2351±3202	1884±2605
Septic nonsurvivors	3056±5928	2978±4463	4178±9422	3254±6474	3161±5809
Healthy persons	44±13				
C3 values (mg/ml)					
Septic patients	0.86±0.52	0.86±0.55	0.85±0.62	0.86±0.62	0.87±0.62
Nonseptic patients	0.99±0.53	1.00±0.53	1.00±0.64	1.13±0.64	1.19±0.88
Healthy persons	1.95±0.29				
C5a values (ng/ml)					
Septic patients	6.88±2.72	6.45±2.73	6.18±2.50	5.85±2.31	5.94±1.49
Nonseptic patients	5.90±1.72	6.58±1.55	5.91±1.77	6.29±1.76	5.73±1.90
Healthy persons	3.6±2.5				

C3a/C3 ratio

At T1-T4 (0-32 h) C3a/C3 ratios of septic patients were significantly higher then in control patients ($P<0.05$). Great interpatient differences occurred (Table 2; Fig. 3) within the septic group, ranging from 350 to 8084. In the control group, C3a/C3 ratios were found to be between 150 and 1000. Septic non-survivors exhibited higher C3a/C3 ratios than septic survivors did during the first 32 h after onset of sepsis (not significant; Fig. 4).

C5a Values

A comparison of the C5a values from either the control group, the septic group or even healthy persons did not reveal any differences (Table 2).

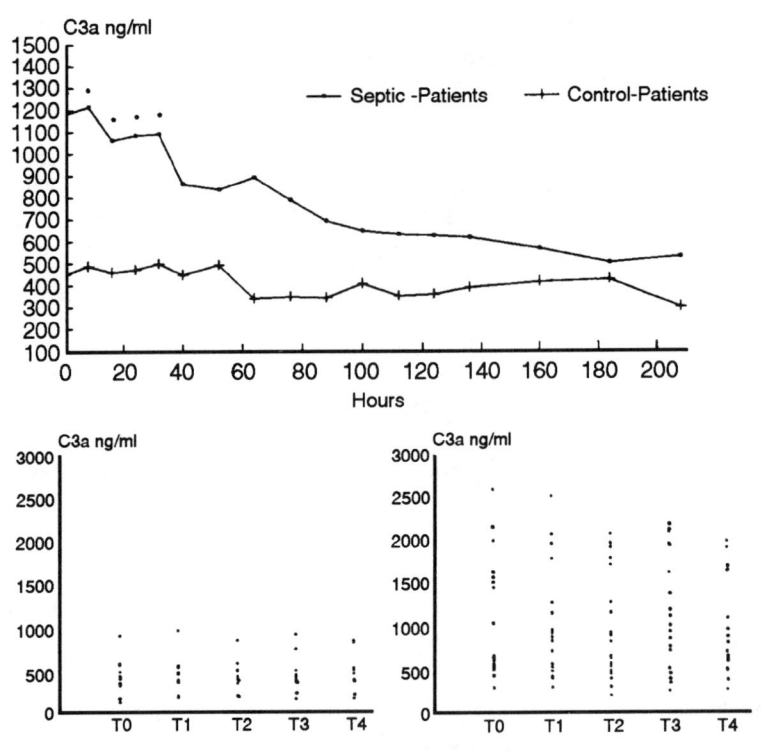

Fig. 1: C3a plasma values from septic patients and control patients during a 10 day observation period at the ICU. Upper right, C3a plasma levels of control patients at T0-T4 are plotted. Below, C3a levels of septic patients are given

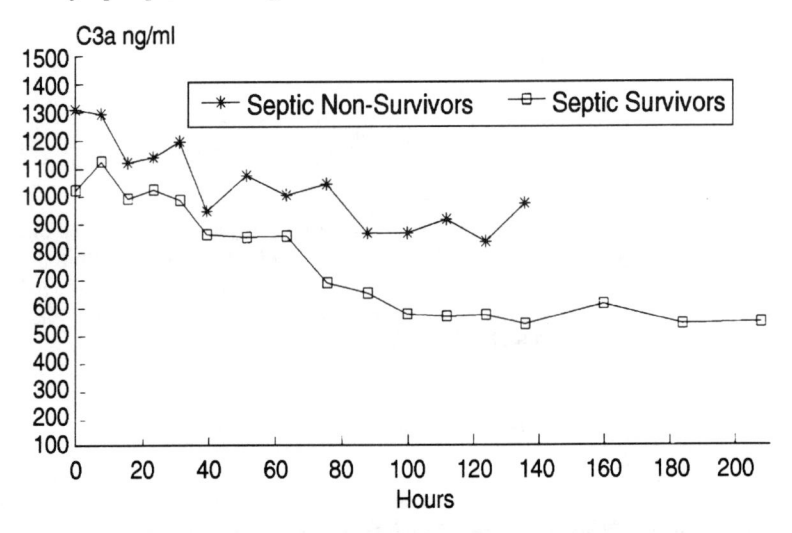

Fig. 2: C3a plasma levels of septic survivors and septic nonsurvivors

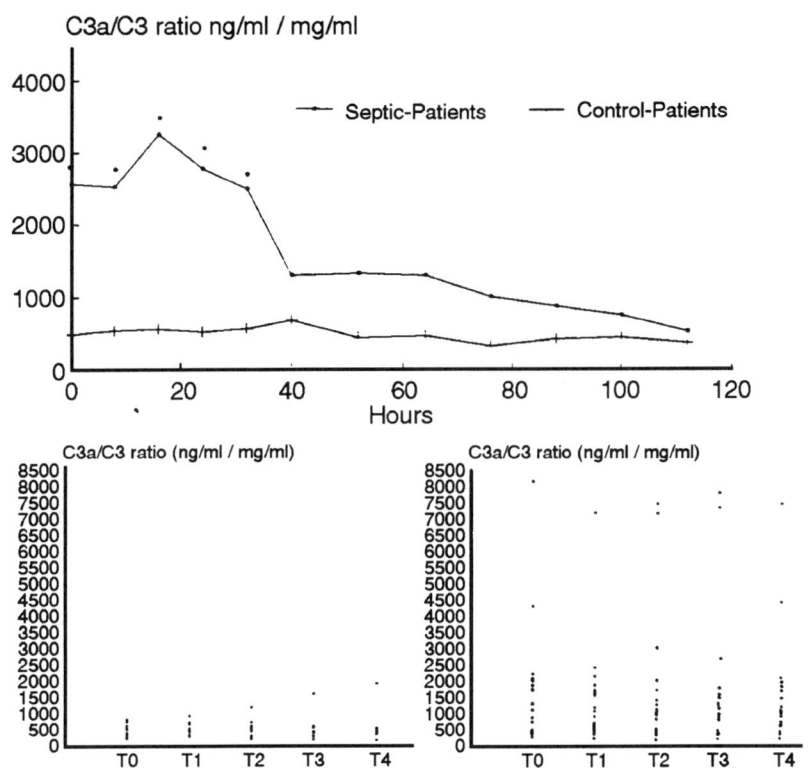

Fig. 3: C3a/C3 ratios from septic patients and control patients. Upper right, C3/C3 ratios of control patients at T0-T4 are plotted. Below, C3a/C3 ratios of septic patients are given.

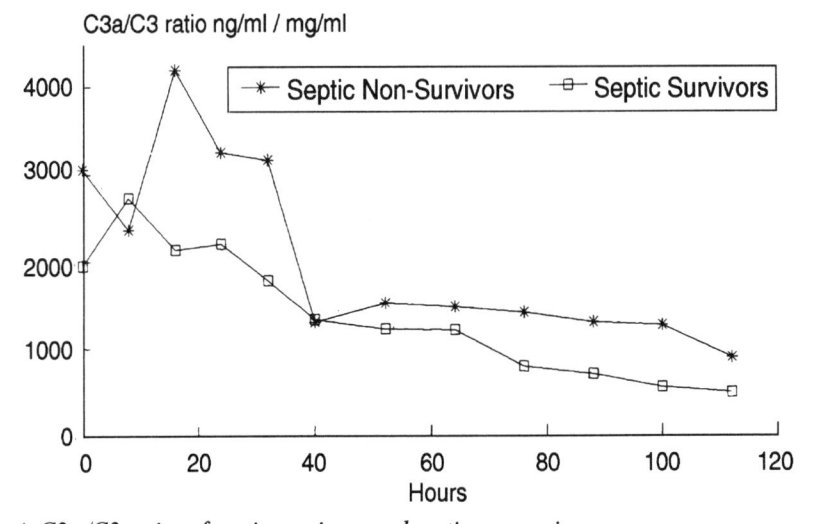

Fig. 4: C3a /C3 ratios of septic survivors and septic nonsurvivors.

Discussion

Our preliminary results indicate that C3a and the C3a /C3 ratio can be used to differentiate between septic patients and critically ill patients at risk for sepsis but not having yet developed sepsis syndrome. As both parameters are markedly elevated when sepsis is clinically apparent, C3a and C3a/C3 ratio are most likely elevated prior to clinical signs of sepsis, too. In the literature, a variety of studies, either with similar or contrasting results exists. Slotman et al. [15] found increased C3a plasma levels in a group of patients with septic shock as well as in a normotensive, nonseptic group. However, their data are average values from a 10 day observation period, not reflecting C3a values at onset of sepsis. Weinberg et al. [18] assessed C3adesArg values from patients with suspected septicemia within 24 h of admission to the hospital and found elevated plasma levels in comparison to healthy control persons. In contrast, no differences were reported between plasma levels from patients with documented bacteremia or patients with negative blood cultures. Elevated C3adesArg plasma levels in septic patients on admission to the ICU have also been reported by Heidemann et al. [11]. Hack et al. [7] found a significant difference between C3adesArg plasma levels of critically ill and septic patients on admission to the ICU, although much lower C3adesArg plasma concentrations were determined. This may be due to the different assays used for measuring C3adesArg values.

In our study C3 plasma levels in septic and control patients were decreased by approximately 50% compared to healthy individuals. This observation is in contrast to observations made by McCabe [14] and Fearon [3]. They found normal C3 plasma levels in septic patients. Only in case of septic shock or severe sepsis associated with death were C3a plasma levels significantly reduced. However, in a recent study, Gardinali et al. [4] described decreased C3 plasma levels in all septic patients on admission to the ICU. Furthermore they reported a significant difference between septic survivors and nonsurvivors. This difference could not be observed in our study.

In addition to C3a and C3 plasma levels, we assessed C3a/C3 ratios. This parameter has been shown previously to serve as a predictive marker for early diagnosis of ARDS in polytrauma patients [20]. In a recent study by Gardinali [4] the predictiveness of this parameter was shown for clinical outcome in sepsis, too. Our data revealed that the C3a/C3 ratio can be used, as can C3a alone, to differentiate between septic and critically ill patients. In contrast, no significant difference was found between septic survivors and septic nonsurvivors during the first 32 hours after clinical onset of sepsis. In comparison to data by Gardinali et al., the C3a/C3 ratios in our study showed greater interpatient differences, which may be attributable to differences in the underlying diseases of the study groups. Gardinali et al. studied surgical patients most often with peritonitis or infected pancreatic necrosis, whereas the most frequent underlying disease in our patients was pneumonia. It is conceivable that severe abdominal infections lead to a more profound and homogenous complement activation than pneumonia. In fact, bacteremia is present in up to 75% of patients with primary peritonitis [19] but only in 20%-30 % of patients with bacterial pneumonia.

Assessment of C5adesArg plasma levels did not lead to identification of any differences between patients at the ICU or healthy individuals. In previous studies Langlois [13] and Weinberg [18] reported a significant increase in C5adesArg plasma levels either in septic or ARDS patients. In contrast there are other reports on either normal [16] or only slightly elevated [9, 15] C5a plasma levels in septic patients. The main reason for difficulties in measuring elevated C5a plasma levels during complement activation is that, in contrast to C3adesArg which lacks C3a receptor binding on phagocytic cells, both C5a and C5adesArg interact with the C5a receptor and are rapidly cleared from plasma. In summary, we have shown that C3a plasma levels and C3a/C3 ratio can be used to differentiate between septic patients and patients at risk for sepsis. In contrast, neither of the parameter predicts clinical outcome at the onset of sepsis. Monitoring of C3a plasma levels may be useful to follow up on therapeutical progress. C3 plasma levels are markedly reduced in critically ill patients with or without sepsis. C5a plasma levels are within the normal range.

Due to the conflicting results of various studies dealing with complement activation in case of sepsis, multicenter studies with increased patient numbers are essential to obtain reliable data on the role of complement cleavage products (e.g C3a/C3adesArg, C4a, C5a/desArg and C5b-9 complex) in the diagnosis of sepsis.

References

1. Beutler B, Cerami A (1987) The endogenous mediator of endotoxin shock. Clin Res 35: 192
2. Bone RC, Balk RA, Cerra FB, Dellinger AM, Fein AM, Knaus WA, Schein MH, Sibbald WJ, et al. (1992) ACCP/SCCM consensus conference: definitions for sepsis and organ failure and guidelines for the use of innovative therapies in sepsis. Chest 101: 1644
3. Fearon DT, Ruddy S, Schur PH, McCabe WR (1975) Activation of the properdin pathway of complement in patients with gram-negative bacteremia. N Engl J Med 292: 937
4. Gardinali M, Padalino P, Vesconi S, Calcagno A, Ciappellano S, Conciato L, Chiara O, Agostini A, Nespoli A (1992) Complement activation and polymorphonuclear neutrophil leukocyte elastase in sepsis: Correlation with severity of disease. Arch Surg 127: 1219
5. Girardin E, Grau GE, Dayer J-M, Roux-Lombard P, J5 study group, Lambert P-H (1988) Tumor necrosis factor and interleukin 1 in the serum of children with severe infectious purpura. N Engl J Med 319: 397
6. Goldstein IM (1988) Complement: biologically active products. In: Gallin JI, Goldstein IM, Snyderman R (eds.) Inflammation: Basic principles and clinical correlations. Raven, New York, pp. 55.
7. Hack CE, Nuijens JH, Felt-Bersma RJF, Schreuder WO, Eerenberg-Belmer AJM, Paardekooper J, Bronsveld W, Thijs LG (1989) Elevated plasma levels of the anaphylatoxins C3a and C4a are associated with a fatal outcome in sepsis. Am J Med 86: 20
8. Hack CE, de Groot ER, Felt-Bersma RJF, Nuijens JH, Strack van Schijndel RJM, Eerneberg-Belmer AJM, Tijs LG, Aarden LA (1989) Increased plasma levels of interleukin-6 in sepsis. Blood 74: 1704
9. Hammerschmidt DE, Weaver L-J- Hudson LD, Craddock PR, Jacobs HS (1980) Association of complement activation and elevated plasma-C5a with adult respiratory distress syndrome. Lancet 1: 947
10. Hartman H, Lübbers B, Casaretto M, Bautsch W, Klos A, Köhl J (1993) Rapid quantification of C3a and C5a using a combination of chromatographic and immunoassay procedures. J Immunol Methods 166: 35
11. Heidemann M, Norder-Hansson B, Mollnes TE (1988) Terminal complement complexes and anaphylatoxins in septic and ischemic patients. Arch Surg 123: 645
12. Köhl J, Bitter-Suermann D (1993) Anaphylatoxins. In: Whaley K, Loos M, Weiler JM (eds.) Complement in health and disease. Kluwer Academic, Dordrecht, pp. 295
13. Langlois PF, Gawryl MS (1988) Accentuated formation of the terminal C5b-9 complex in patient plasma precedes development of the adult respiratory distress syndrome. Am Rev Respir Dis 138: 368

14. McCabe WR (1973) Serum complement levels in bacterimia due to gram-negative organisms. N Engl J Med 288: 21
15. Slotmann GJ, Burchard KW, Williams JJ, DArezzo A, Yellin SA (1988) Interaction of prostaglandins, activated complement and granulocytes in clinical sepsis and hypotension. Surgery 99: 744
16. Vogt W (1986) Anaphylatoxins: possible roles in disease. Complement 3: 177
17. Waage A, Halstensen A, Espevik T (1987) Association between tumor necrosis factor in serum and fatal outcome in patients with meningococcal disease. Lancet I: 355-357
18. Weinberg PF, Matthay MA, Webster RO, Roskos KV, Goldstein IM, Murray JF (1984) Biologically active products of complement and acute lung injury in patients with the sepsis syndrome. Am Rev Respir Dis 130: 791
19. Wilcox CM, Dismukes WE (1987) Spontaneous bacterial peritonitis: A review of pathogenesis, diagnosis and treatment. Medicine 66: 447
20. Zilow G, Sturm JA, Rother U, Kirschfink M (1990) Complement activation and the prognostic value of C3a in patients at risk of adult respiratory distress syndrome. Clin Exp Immunol 79: 151

Endotoxin: Does Its Detection Provide Diagnostic Benefit?

T.J. Novitsky

Introduction

The *Limulus* amebocyte lysate (LAL) test for endotoxins has been studied in clinical situations since 1970. For various reasons the assay has never been seen as clinically useful for the diagnosis of endotoxemia and sepis. Indeed, no way of validating the LAL bioassay in clinical situations exists, since no direct means of measuring endotoxin has yet been found. With the recent interest in antiendotoxin therapies, however, there is renewed interest in LAL as the most rapid, specific, and sensitive assay currently available. Even so, the assay needs to be standardized and consistent results shown in multicenter trials. Once this is accomplished, the more difficult clinical question "Does the presence (or level) of endotoxin have clinical significance?", can be addressed.

The Assay

In 1970 Levin et al. [50] demonstrated the ability of an in vitro assay made from a lysate of blood cells (amebocytes) obtained from the North American horseshoe crab, *Limulus polyphemus*, to detect endotoxin in human blood (plasma and serum). This technique employed chloroform to remove substances from the plasma that interfered with the assay. The extraction process took up to 60 min, while the assay itself required 24 h to achieve a sensitivity of 0.5 ng endotoxin/ml. Even so these authors concluded: "The technique should have application for clinical and experimental studies of endotoxin and endotoxemia." In subsequent studies on patient plasma, Levin et al. [49, 51] demonstrated that the *Limulus* amebocyte lysate assay, or LAL assay as it has come to be called, was extremely specific for endotoxin and could be used as an indirect method for detecting the presence of gram-negative bacteria. Levin et al. [49] also showed that administration of antibiotics did not interfere with the LAL reagent to cause false-negative results. After a study involving 281 patients [51], the authors concluded: "The Limulus test permits correlation of endotoxemia, with or without bacteremia, and many of the pathophysiologic alterations that have been presumed to result from its biological effects." The original work of Levin has been confirmed by numerous studies [6, 8, 9, 16, 17, 22, 28, 31, 33, 34, 38-40, 53, 55, 56, 61, 62, 65, 66, 87, 88, 90, 91]. Several of these investigators employed various modifications of the assay in an attempt to improve the sensitivity of the LAL. The original assay [50] is referred to as the gel clot method. This is a serological type assay which is based on the formation of a solid gel in the presence of endotoxin. This assay is quite subjective and relatively insensitive (0.3 EU/ml, based on a current commercially available LAL reagent sensitivity of 0.03 EU/ml and a 1:10 dilution of plasma/serum to overcome assay inhibition). Most of the studies prior to 1980 used the gel-clot LAL method, often with extended incubation times (up to 24 h) to increase sensitivity (although none of these studies achieved much more than a 0.5 EU/ml sensitivity).

In 1977, a chromogenic method was introduced [58]. This assay is faster and more sensitive (0.05 EU/ml, based on an LAL reagent sensitivity of 0.005 EU/ml and a 1:10 dilution of plasma/serum to overcome assay inhibition) and is objective - the color developed in response to the presence of endotoxin is read in a spectrophotometer or microplate reader. Since 1981, the majority of studies employing LAL on blood have been performed using various modifications of the chromogenic assay [3, 5, 6, 8, 14, 16, 20-22, 27, 47, 56, 57, 59, 60, 62, 75, 83, 85-88, 90, 91, 94]. Tamura et al. [85] described a further modification of the chromogenic assay which employs the diazo derivative of the *para*-nitroanilide chromophore. Thus, a magenta color is produced with a strong extinction at 540-550 nm rather than a yellow color with a weak extinction at 405 nm. This assay removes interference due to sample color (due to hemolysis) and also increases the sensitivity and reproducibility of the assay.

A turbidimetric modification of the LAL assay has also been used in a few studies but has never gained popularity for clinical use [19, 31, 32, 67].

It is unlikely that the sensitivity of the assay (all methods) itself will increase significantly, as the ubiquitous presence of low levels of endotoxin in reagents and supplies used to conduct the test are already close to the detection limit of the test. In addition, the "normal" background of circulating endotoxin in human plasma is currently thought to be around the existing detection limit of 0.05 EU/ml.

Removal of Plasma Interference

No less important than the assay itself is the extraction method for removing plasma interference (inhibition). Levin et al. originally demonstrated that inhibitors (of the LAL test) existed in human plasma and serum. These inhibitors act on endotoxin by binding to the molecule and rendering it unable to activate LAL. The net effect of these inhibitors is at worst a negative test, but in most cases a lowering of the actual amount of endotoxin detected. Thus, in the presence of inhibitors it is possible to have endotoxin, and even culturable gram-negative bacteria, and a negative LAL test (false negative). It has always been the aim of investigators to improve the clinical usefulness of the LAL test by not only improving the sensitivity of the LAL reagent itself, but also by improving the sensitivity of the assay through the removal of the inhibitors present in plasma or serum. The removal of plasma/serum inhibitors has therefore been a topic of considerable interest and research. Several methods have been described including solvent (chloroform extraction), pH shift/acid extraction, capture/recovery (bead assay), dilution/heating and combinations of these [15, 39, 51, 60, 65, 71].

The chloroform extraction method was originally described by Levin et al. [51] and was used in a number of studies [9, 10, 17, 24, 26, 33, 34, 38, 49, 50, 55, 61, 73, 82, 93]. Its major drawback is that it is time consuming. The method also requires some care in recovering the entire layer containing the endotoxin, while excluding any chloroform which, if present, could inhibit the LAL test per se.

A very interesting method of separating the LAL inhibitors from the LAL assay was reported by Harris and Feinstein in 1977 [40]. These authors used a polymer bead to absorb endotoxin directly from heparinized blood samples. The bead was then washed free of blood components and incubated directly with LAL. For reasons not entirely clear, this method never became popular and was only used in one other published study [39]. To Harris and Feinstein's credit, however, they were the first to extract whole blood.

One of the first studies to employ heat to remove plasma inhibitors was that by Cooperstock et al. in 1975 [15]. Heating coupled with dilution in water or saline, rapidly became the method of choice, having been used in a large number of studies up to the present [3, 5, 8, 14, 16, 22, 32, 36, 45, 56, 57, 59, 62, 64, 77, 79, 87-91] ([94] dilution only, no heat]). Although heating is easy to accomplish, it is difficult to control precisely. Furthermore, in spite of a recent study [71], there seems to be no consensus in the literature as to the ideal time/temperature regime.

Reinhold and Fine [65] described a pH shift which denatured plasma euglobulins to allow complete recovery of endotoxin. The pH shift method was used in a number of early studies [13, 17, 52, 53, 66]. In the last several years improvements using acid or base extraction have appeared [27, 60, 86]. In 1991, Tamura et al. [85] described an acid/detergent extraction of whole blood, allowing the most complete recovery of endotoxin (and removal of LAL inhibitors) to date. Of all the methods described to date, acid extraction is the most precise and also the least time consuming. It is also recognized that non-endotoxin activators of the LAL test are also normally present in blood, notably serine proteases (e.g., factor X). Fortunately, all of the methods used to eliminate inhibitors of LAL also inactivate blood serine proteases.

Nature of the Sample (Specimen)

Although recent studies [85] indicate that whole blood is the ideal sample for recovering endotoxin, all studies but three [23, 39, 40] used plasma as a starting material. Most recent studies [3, 5, 8, 14, 20, 21, 26, 27, 31, 32, 55-57, 59, 62, 75, 83, 85-91, 94], however, do use platelet rich plasma since Das et al. in 1973 [17] found appreciable endotoxin associated with platelets. Although Sakon et al. [75] found no difference in the recoveries of endotoxin from either platelet-rich or platelet-poor plasma, his results suggested that "...the measurement of endotoxin concentration of whole blood seems to be clinically more important than that of PRP or PPP..."

In a recent paper, Tamura et al. [85] described a method for the extraction of whole blood. Surprisingly, no one in the 22 years since Levin first used the LAL test to detect endotoxin in blood has tried to extract whole blood (not counting the unsuccessful attempt by Harris and Feinstein [39] with the "bead" extraction or du Moulin et al. [23], who attempted to recover bacteria from lysed blood and detect them with LAL. All published work (as far as my search has found] has used either plasma or serum. Sakon et al. [75] presents an excellent case for starting with whole blood rather than plasma since endotoxin has a propensity for sticking to blood cells. The use of a chemical extraction of whole blood accomplishes two things: (1) the extraction can be precisely controlled and (2) more endotoxin could be collected for assay (thus increasing the sensitivity of the test and possibly finding more "true positives").

Other studies also support the use of extracted whole blood. Pearson [63] in his book, *Pyrogen, Endotoxins, LAL Testing, and Depyrogenation* states: "Although Braude et al. [7] did not find erythrocyte-associated labeled endotoxin, the recent work of Abdelnoor et al. [1], Hawiger et al. [41], Washida [92], Maxie and Valli [54], Herring et al. [42], Fritze and Doering [35], and Rubenstein et al. [74] has confirmed the intense association of labeled endotoxin with the buffy coat. Taken together, these studies strongly indicate that the sensitivity of the LAL assay for circulating LPS could be enhanced significantly, not only by using the platelet-rich plasma suggested by Das et al. [17], but also by including monocytes and leukocytes in the test sample. Indeed, whole blood would provide the ideal test sample, because the data of Maxie and Valli [54] suggest sensitivity could be increased by approximately 10% due to erythrocyte-associated LPS.

A further piece of evidence to support a whole blood extraction procedure has been published by Sakon et al. [75]. These authors show that binding of endotoxin to blood components can vary according to the species of endotoxin, with *Salmonella* endotoxin binding better than *E. coli*. Thus even the finding of Braude et al. [7], who used a labeled *E. coli* endotoxin, is not contradicted. Recently, however, Roth et al. [72] reported very little binding of endotoxin to platelets in either human or rabbit blood. Unfortunately, these experiments were done with highly purified endotoxins in ex vivo experiments. From all the in vivo studies that have preceded Roth et al. [72], it is almost certain that any in vitro or ex vivo studies using highly purified endotoxin will result in a partitioning that is quite different from that in clinical endotoxemia or even experimentally induced endotoxemia.

For more detailed reviews of the clinical applications of LAL prior to 1985 see Pearson [63] and Jorgensen [46]. This review covers the pertinent literature up to October 1993.

Clinical Significance of Endotoxin

Although the LAL test has been successfully used by the pharmaceutical industry to ensure a lack of pyrogenic amounts of endotoxin in parenteral drugs, biologics, and devices since 1977 when it was approved for such use by the US Food and Drug Administration, the use of LAL as a diagnostic for endotoxemia and/or gram-negative bacterial sepsis has yet to be approved. The reasons for this and a description of a new and improved LAL diagnostic for sepsis form the basis of the remainder of this paper. A discussion of endotoxin's clinical significance has been ongoing in the literature beginning shortly after Levin's initial studies were published [12, 29, 30, 37, 48, 68, 81]. In early studies, a lack of correlation between circulating endotoxin and gram-negative bacteremia was regarded as a "false-positive test." One specific problem centered on the occurance of circulating endotoxin in the absence of viable bacteria in patients with cirrhosis or fulminant hepatic failure [36, 45, 64, 89, 93]. It is now generally accepted that when liver function is impaired, endotoxins, which are normally eliminated in the liver, can enter the peripheral circulation. These endotoxins most likely enter the circulation from the gut. On the other hand, some patients with documented gram-negative bacteremia showed no detectable endotoxin. This latter problem may be a function of assay sensitivity, but more likely it is the ability of the patient to eliminate endotoxin. It is well known that the LAL assay cannot detect less than 100 *E. coli*/ml under optimal conditions. In a recent review, Hoffman and Natanson [43] examined the role of endotoxin in septic shock. After reviewing both animal and human data they found that although endotoxin was sufficient to cause many if not all of the symptoms of septic shock, other toxins and bacteria themselves were often sufficient to cause physiologic dysfunction similar to septic shock. These authors were also not able to establish a direct cause and effect relationship between endotoxin levels and the clinical outcome of septic shock. One of the problems with animal models when examining the effects of endotoxin is that the endotoxin is delivered in a single dose or bolus. This may be likened to the initial reaction a patient would encounter in the early stages of infection but is hardly realistic. Studies that provide continuous delivery of endotoxin may be of more value [43]. In addition, some of the transient manifestations of endotoxemia, e.g., fever, may actually help in fending off infection. In a healthy animal, for example, endotoxin is cleared quite rapidly from the system, even though many of the so-called toxic effects of endotoxin are exhibited. It is very likely that humans would vary in their ability to detoxify endotoxin, perhaps explaining the lack of correlation between endotoxemia and clinical outcome. In another recent study, Casey et al. [11] found that the average level of endotoxin was higher in patients diagnosed with sepsis than in critically ill patients without sepsis and normal controls. When endotoxin was combined with cytokine levels (scores) and compared with mortality, a positive correlation was evident ($P < 0.001$).

The LAL test itself has not been without problems. In 1973 Stumacher et al. [82] described the limitations of the *Limulus* assay for the detection of endotoxin in blood; and in 1975 Elin et al. [26] dismissed outright the clinical usefulness of the *Limulus* test for the diagnosis of endotoxemia. These papers and others effectively prevented official clinical acceptance of the LAL test for the diagnosis of endotoxemia, and/or gram negative-sepsis.

There were several reasons for the "lack of clinical usefulness" of the LAL test. First and foremost, all of the studies used a positive blood culture of gram negative bacteria as the "gold" standard. Thus, a positive LAL test in the absence of culturable gram-negative bacteria was counted as a "false positive." Likewise, the presence of culturable gram-positive bacteria coupled with a positive LAL test was counted as a "false positive." In the absence of an equally (to the LAL assay) sensitive independent test for endotoxin, there was no way of knowing whether these tests were indeed "false" for endotoxemia. It is now generally recognized that if prediction of the presence of viable, circulating gram negative bacteria is the purpose of the LAL test, then indeed the test "lacks clinical usefulness". In the study by Elin et al. [26] several technical factors also influenced a negative conclusion. First, these authors used a very insensitive "homemade" gel clot LAL reagent (0.1 ng/ml, equivalent to 1.0 EU/ml). In an attempt to increase sensitivity, the LAL was incubated for up to 24 h. The LAL currently available is capable of good reproducibility at 0.005 EU/ml in under 30 min. Second, these authors used plasma (heparinized) stored in polypropylene tubes. Apart from the fact that some endotoxin may have been missed in the cellular fraction of blood because only plasma was tested, heparin is a known inhibitor of the LAL test [84] and is often highly contaminated with endotoxin. It is also now known that most polypropylene strongly adsorbs endotoxin and thus makes a poor storage container [70]. Third, a time-consuming and technically difficult chloroform extraction procedure was used to remove plasma inhibitors. Although Elin et al. showed a positive correlation between documented gram-negative septicemia and a positive LAL test ($P < 0.005$, Yates modification of the chi-square test), the authors concluded: "This study has demonstrated... a positive test had limited clinical utility. Since about two hours are needed to obtain and process the blood sample... positive tests required more than four hours of incubation... this considerable delay... compromises the possible value... in emergency situations. Furthermore, two of eight patients with a positive test... were ambulatory, which means... test cannot be equated with severe endotoxemia.

Finally there has been much discussion in the literature on the reactivity of LAL to glucans [63, 69]. Although there is evidence that LAL can detect *Candida* in plasma, the amount of glucan required to trigger the LAL test is from 100- to 1000-fold higher than that of endotoxin. With the incidence of all fungemias lower than 5% of all positive blood cultures, and given the other clinical indications of fungemia, it is unlikely that the LAL test will be significantly influenced (increased false positivity) by the presence of glucan (i.e., fungemia) in blood samples.

SepTest

In order to standardize the LAL test as a diagnostic bioassay for endotoxin, a new kit has been recently prepared. It is being tested in a multicenter trial. The kit, SepTest, is based on a diazo-coupled chromogenic LAL assay (Pyrochrome, Associates of Cape Cod, Mass, USA) an acid extraction chemistry, and all the necessary accessories for performing the test (Table 1). The chromogenic assay was selected because it is sensitive and quantitative. It is also similar in nature to ELISA-type assays which are very familiar to clinical laboratories. Reading is accomplished with any commercially available microplate reader. The diazo modification of the test was chosen to increase the sensitivity and reproducibility, make the test more visual (to prevent mistakes), and overcome interference from background color due to hemolysis. Acid extraction was chosen since it works well with whole blood (which was chosen to increase the amount of endotoxin available for detection). Acid extraction is also easier to control than heating. All the accessories that are necessary to prevent the accidental contamination of the sample with endotoxin were also included in the kit (e.g. microplate, pipette tips, non-shedding gloves). Collection in relatively endotoxin-free EDTA vacuum collection tubes is recommended for obtaining blood samples.

Table 1. SepTest methodology and kit composition

1. Collect blood in a purple-top tube (EDTA)[a]
2. Remove 100 µl blood and add to 400 %l nitric acid/Triton X-100
3. Mix and incubate 5 min at 37°C
4. Centrifuge 5 min at 3300 rpm
5. Remove 200 µl clear supernatant and neutralize with equal volume NaOH
6. Ass 50 µl neutralized sample to prepared microplate along with controls
7. Dilute sample and standard
8. Add 50 µl Pyrochrome to each sample, sample dilution, standard, and control
9. Mix plate and incubate at 37°C for 30 min
10. Add 50 µl reagent #1 (HC1/sodium nitrate), mix
11. Add 50 µl reagent #2 (amonium sulfamate), mix
12. Add 50 µl reagent #3 (NEDA), mix
13. Read at 540 nm in microplate reader

Total time from collection of blood to readout = 1 h; [a]Collection tube not included in SepTest kit

SepTest is currently undergoing in an eight-center clinical trial in the United States. This trial is part of a larger trial on sepsis in general. It is anticipated that at least 50 septic patients and 100 controls will be enrolled in the SepTest study (Table 2). The results of the study will be used to support a Product License Amendment for use of SepTest as an endotoxin test in blood.

Table 2. Enrollment criteria for SepTest multicenter trial[a]

All four of the following in the preceding 24 h
● Clinical evidence of infection (i.e., + blood culture in previous 48 h or suspected site of infection) or receiving nonprophylactic antibiotic for treatment of infection
● Respiration >20/min or ventilated mechanically
● Pulse >90/min, or on beta-blocker, or completely paced
● Temperature >38.3°C or <35.6°C
and at least one of the following in preceding 24 h
☐ PaO_2 ≤75 mmHg or FIO_2 ≥40 without intubation; Pa/FIO_2 ≤280 with intubation
☐ Lactate above normal or unexplained acidosis
☐ Oliguria
☐ Systolic blood pressure ≤90 mmHg or sustained drop in blood pressure ≤40 mmHg in presence of fluid challenge and absence of antihypertensive agents
☐ Systemic vascular resistance <800 dynescm^5
☐ Elevated prothrombin or partial prothrombin time above normal, or platelets <100 000/mm^3
☐ Acutely altered mental status without other explanation, e.g., recent stroke
Blood draw for SepTest must be made within 6 h of a patient meeting these criteria

[a] Essentially sepsis definition from Bone [4]

References

1. Abdelnoor AM, Kassem H, Bikhazi AB, Nowotny A (1980) *Effect of gram-negative bacteria lipopolysacchride-derived polysaccharides, glycolipids, and lipopolysaccharides on rabbit and human platelets in vitro.* Immunobiology 157: 145-153
2. Bayston KF, Cohen J (1990) *Bacterial endotoxin and current concepts in the diagnosis and treatment of endotoxaemia.* J Med Microbiol 31: 73-83
3. Behre G, Schedel I, Nentwig B, Wörmann B, Essink M, Hiddemann W (1992) *Endotoxin concentration in neutropenic patients with suspected gram-negative sepsis: Correlation with clinical outcome and determination of anti-endotoxin core antibodies during therapy with polyclonal immunoglobulin M-enriched immunoglobulins.* Antimicrob Agents Chemother 36: 2139-2146
4. Bone RC (1991) *The pathogenesis of sepsis* Ann Int Med 115: 457-469
5. Brandtzaeg P, Oktedalen O, Kierulf P, Opstad PK (1989) *Elevated VIP and endotoxin plasma levels in human gram-negative septic shock.* Regulatory Peptides 24: 37-44
6. Brandtzaeg P, Bryn K, Kierulf P, Ovstebo R, Namork E, Aase B, Jantzen E (1992) *Meningococcal endotoxin in lethal septic shock plasma studied by gas chromatography, mass-spectrometry, ultracentrifugation, and electron microscopy.* J Clin Invest 89: 816-823

7. Braude AI, Carey FJ, Zalesky M (1955) Studies with radioactive endotoxin. II. Correlation of physiologic effects with distribution of radioactivity in rabbits injected with lethal dose of E. coli endotoxin labeled with radioactive sodium chromate. J Clin Invest 34: 858-866
8. Büller HR, ten Cate JW, Sturk A, Thomas LL (1985) Validity of the endotoxin assay in post surgical patients. In: Bacterial endotoxins: structure, biomedical significance, and detection with the Limulus amebocyte lysate test. Liss, New York, pp. 405-416
9. Butler T, Levin J, Cu DQ, Walker RI (1973) Bubonic plague: detection of endotoxemia with the Limulus test. Ann Intern Med 79: 642-646
10. Butler T, Bell WR, Levin J, Linh NN, Arnold K (1978) Typhoid fever. Studies of blood coagulation, bacteremia, and endotoxemia. Arch Intern Med 138: 407-410
11. Casey LC, Balk RA, Bone RC (1993) Plasma cytokine and endotoxin levels correlate with survival in patients with sepsis syndrome. Ann Intern Med 119: 771-778
12. Catchpole BN (1974) Limulus assay for gram-negative endotoxin (Letter). Lancet 2: 225
13. Clumeck N, Lauwers S, Kahn A, Mommens M, Butzler JP (1977) Apport du test limule au diagnostic des endotoxinemies et des meningites a germes gram-negatif. (Contribution of the "Limulus test" to the diagnosis of endotoxemias and meningitis due to gram-negative bacteria) Nouv Presse Med 6: 1451-1454
14. Cohen J, McConnell JS (1984) Observations on the measurement and evaluation of endotoxemia by a quantitative Limulus lysate microassay. J Infect Dis 150: 916-924
15. Cooperstock MS, Tucker RP, Baublis JV (1975) Possible pathogenic role of endotoxin in Reye's syndrome. Lancet 1: 1272-1274
16. Danner RL, Elin RJ, Hosseini JM, Wesley RA, Reilly JM, Parillo JE (1991) Endotoxemia in human septic shock. Chest 99: 169-175
17. Das J, Schwartz AA, Folkman J (1973) Clearance of endotoxin by platelets: role in increasing the accuracy of the Limulus gelation test and in combating experimental endotoxemia. Surgery 74: 235-240
18. Demonty J, De Graeve J (1982) Release of endotoxic lipopolysaccharide by sensitive strains of Escherichia coli submitted to the bactericidal action of human serum. Med Microbiol Immunol 170: 265-277
19. Ditter B, Becker KP, Urbaschek R, Urbaschek B (1983) Quantitativer Endotoxin-Nachweis Automatisierter, kinetischer Limulus-Amobozyten-Lysat-Mikrotiter-Test mit Messung probenabhängiger Interferenzen. Arzneim-Forschung 33: 681-687
20. Dofferhoff ASM, Nijland JH, De Vries-Hospers HG, Mulder POM, Weits J, Bom VJJ (1991) Effects of different types and combinations of antimicrobial agents on endotoxin release from Gram-negative bacteria: an in-vitro and in-vivo study. Scand J Infect Dis 23: 745-754
21. Dofferhoff ASM, Bom VJJ, De Vries-Hospers HG, Van Ingen J, Vd Meer J, Hazenberg BPC, Mulder POM, Weits J (1992) Patterns of cytokines, plasma endotoxin, plasminogen activator inhibitor, and acute-phase proteins during the treatment of severe sepsis in humans. Crit Care Med 20: 185-192
22. Dolan SA, Riegle L, Berzofsky R, Cooperstock M (1987) Clinical evaluation of the plasma chromogenic limulus assay. In: Detection of bacterial endotoxins with the Limulus amebocyte lysate test. Liss, New York, pp. 405-429
23. Du Moulin GC, Lynch SE, Hedley-Whyte J, Broitman SA (1985) Detection of gram-negative bacteremia by Limulus amebocyte lysate assay: evaluation in a rat model of peritonitis. J Infect Dis 151: 148-152
24. Elin RJ (1979) Clinical utility of the Limulus test with blood, CSF and synovial fluid. In: Biomedical applications of the horseshoe crab (Limulidae). Liss, New York, pp. 279-292

25. Elin RJ, Hosseini J (1985) Clinical utility of the limulus amebocyte lysate (LAL) test. In: Bacterial endotoxins: structure, biomedical significance, and detection with the Limulus amebocyte lysate test. Liss, New York, pp. 307-324
26. Elin RJ, Robinson RA, Levine AS, Wolff SM (1975) Lack of clinical usefulness of the Limulus test in the diagnosis of endotoxemia. N Engl J Med 293: 521-524
27. Endo S, Inada K, Inoue Y, Kuwata Y, Suzuki M, Yamashita H, Hoshi S, Yoshida M (1992) Two types of septic shock classified by the plasma levels of cytokines and endotoxin. Circ Shock 38: 264-274
28. Feldman S, Pearson TA (1974) The Limulus test and gram-negative bacillary sepsis. Am J Dis Child 128: 172-174
29. Fine J (1972) Endotoxaemia in man Lancet 2: 181
30. Fine J (1974) Limulus assay for gram-negative endotoxin. Lancet 1: 1295
31. Fink PC, Grunert JH (1984) Endotoxemia in intensive care patients: a longitudinal study with the Limulus amebocyte lysate test. Klin Wochenschr 62: 986-991
32. Fink PC, Lehr L, Urbaschek RM, Kozak J (1981) Limulus amebocyte lysate test for endotoxemia: investigations with a femtogram sensitive spectrophotometric assay. Klin Wochenschr 59: 213-218
33. Fossard DP, Kakkar VV (1974) The Limulus test in experimental and clinical endotoxaemia. Br J Surg 61: 798-804
34. Fossard DP, Kakkar VV, Elsey PA (1974) Assessment of Limulus test for detecting endotoxaemia Br Med J 2: 465-468
35. Fritze E, Doering P (1959) Der transport eines markierten endotoxins im blust 2. Gesamte Exp Med 132: 334-336
36. Fulenwider JT, Sibley C, Stein SF, Evatt B, Nordlinger BM, Ivey GL (1980) Endotoxemia of cirrhosis: an observation not substantiated. Gastroenterology 78: 1001-1004
37. Fumarola D (1975) The Limulus test and gram-negative bacillary sepsis. Am J Dis Child 129: 644
38. Garibaldi RA, Allman GW, Larsen DH, Smith CB, Burke JP (1973) Detection of endotoxemia by the Limulus test in patients with indwelling urinary catheters. J Infect Dis 128: 551-554
39. Harris NS, Feinstein R (1977) Relationship of endotoxemia with clinically defined gram-negative septicemia. Surg Forum 28: 23-25
40. Harris NS, Feinstein R (1977) A new Limulus assay for the detection of endotoxin. J Trauma 17: 714-718
41. Hawiger J, Hawiger A, Timmons S (1975) Endotoxin sensitive membrane component of human platelets. Nature 256: 125-127
42. Herring WB, Herion JC, Walker RI, Palmer JC (1963) Distribution and clearance of circulating endotoxin. J Clin Invest 42: 79-87
43. Hoffman WD, Natanson C (1993) Endotoxin in septic shock. Anesth Analg 77: 613-624
44. Hurley JC (1992) Antibiotic-induced release of endotoxin: a reappraisal. Clin Infect Dis 15: 840-854
45. Jacob AI, Goldberg PK, Bloom N, Degenshein GA, Kozinn PJ (1977) Endotoxin and bacteria in portal blood. Gastroenterology 72: 1268-1270
46. Jorgensen JH (1986) Clinical applications of Limulus amebocyte lysate test In: Clinical aspects of endotoxin (Handbook of endotoxin, vol 4) Elsevier, Amsterdam
47. Kinsey SE, Machin SJ (1988) Endotoxemia in neutropenic patients. Lancet 2: 345
48. Levin J (1973) Endotoxin and endotoxemia. N Engl J Med 288: 1297-1298
49. Levin J, Poore TE, Zauber NP, Oser RS (1970) Detection of endotoxin in the blood of patients with sepsis due to gram-negative bacteria. N Engl J Med 283: 1313-1316

50. Levin J, Tomasulo PA, Oser RS (1970) Detection of endotoxin in human blood and demonstration of an inhibitor. J Lab Clin Med 283: 903-911
51. Levin J, Poore TE, Young NS, Margolis S, Bell WR (1972) Gram-negative sepsis: detection of endotoxemia with the Limulus test. With studies of associated changes in blood coagulation, serum lipids, and complement. Ann Intern Med 76: 1-7
52. Magliulo E, Scevola D, Fumarola D, Vaccaro R, Burberi S (1976) Clinical experience in detecting endotoxemia with the Limulus test in typhoid fever and other Salmonella infections. Infection 4: 21-24
53. Martinez-G LA, Quintiliani R, Tilton RC (1973) Clinical experience on the detection of endotoxemia with the Limulus test. J Infect Dis 127: 102-105
54. Maxie MG, Valli VEO (1974) Studies with radioactive endotoxin. III. Localization of 3H-labelled endotoxin in the formed elements of the blood and detection of endotoxin in calf blood with the Limulus amebocyte lysate. Can J Comp Med 38: 383-390
55. McCartney AC, Banks JG, Clements GB, Sleigh JD, Tehrani M, Ledingham IM (1983) Endotoxaemia in septic shock: clinical and post mortem correlations. Intens Care Med 9: 117-122
56. McCartney AC, Piotrowicz BI, Edlin SE, Ledingham IM (1987) Evaluation of the chromogenic limulus lysate assay in septic shock. In: Detection of bacterial endotoxins with the Limulus amebocyte lysate test. Liss, New York, 459-474
57. McCartney AC, Robertson MRI, Piotrowicz BI, Lucie NP (1987) Endotoxaemia, fever and clinical status in immunosuppressed patients: a preliminary study. J Infect 15: 201-206
58. Nakamura S, Morita T, Iwanaga S, Niwa M, Takahashi K (1977) A sensitive substrate for the clotting enzyme in horseshoe crab hemocytes. J Biochem 81: 1567-1569
59. Nitsche D, Kriewitz M, Rossberg A, Hamelmann H (1987) The quantitative determination of endotoxin in plasma samples of septic patients with peritonitis using the chromogenic substrate and its correlation with the clinical course of peritonitis. In: Detection of bacterial endotoxins with the Limulus amebocyte lysate test. Liss, New York, 417-429
60. Obayashi T, Kawai T, Tamura H, Nakahara C (1982) New Limulus amoebocyte lysate test for endotoxaemia (Letter). Lancet 1: 289
61. Oberle MW, Graham GG, Levin J (1974) Detection of endotoxemia with the Limulus test: preliminary studies in severely malnourished children. J Pediatr 85: 570-573
62. Pearson FC, Dubczak J, Weary M, Bruszer G, Donohue G (1985) Detection of endotoxin in the plasma of patients with gram-negative bacterial sepsis by the Limulus amoebocyte lysate assay. J Clin Microbiol 21: 865-868
63. Pearson FC III (1985) Pyrogens. Endotoxins, LAL testing, and depyrogenation. Dekker, New York
64. Prytz H, Holst-Christensen J, Korner B, Liehr H (1976) Portal venous and systemic endotoxaemia in patients without liver disease and systemic endotoxaemia in patients with cirrhosis. Scand J Gastroenterol 11: 857-863
65. Reinhold RB, Fine J (1971) A technique for quantitative measurement of endotoxin in human plasma. Proc Soc Exp Biol Med 137: 334-340
66. Reinhold RB, Caridis DT, Fine J (1972) Diagnosis of clinical endotoxemia. J Reprod Med 8: 335-339
67. Remillard JF, Gould MC, Roslansky PF, Novitsky TJ (1987) Quantitation of endotoxins in products using the LAL kinetic turbidimetric assay. In: Detection of bacterial endotoxin with the Limulus amebocyte lysate test. Liss, New York, pp. 197-210
68. Roberts RS, Tech B, Tech M (1985) Designs for the evaluation of the endotoxin assay as a diagnostic test. In: Bacterial endotoxins, structure, biomedical significance, and detection with the Limulus amebocyte lysate test. Liss, New York, pp. 433-450

69. Roslansky PF, Novitsky TJ (1991) Sensitivity of Limulus amebocyte lysate (LAL) to LAL-reactive glucans. J Clin Microbiol 29: 2477-2483
70. Roslansky PF, Dawson ME, Novitsky TJ (1991) Plastics, endotoxins, and the limulus amebocyte lysate test. J Parenter Sci Technol 45: 83-87
71. Roth RI, Levin FC, Levin J (1990) Optimization of detection of bacterial endotoxin in plasma with the Limulus test. J Lab Clin Med 116: 153-161
72. Roth RI, Levin FC, Levin J (1993) Distribution of bacterial endotoxin in human and rabbit blood and effects of stroma-free hemoglobin. Infect Immun 61: 3209-3215
73. Rowe MI, Buckner DM, Newmark S (1975) The early diagnosis of gram-negative septicemia in the pediatric surgical patient. Ann Surg 182: 280-286
74. Rubenstein HS, Fine J, Coons AH (1962) Localization of endotoxin in the walls of the peripheral vascular system during lethal endotoxemia. Proc Soc Exp Biol Med 111: 458-461
75. Sakon M, Tachiyama G, Kambayashi J, Ohsiro T, Mori T (1986) Studies on blood sample preparation for clinical endotoxin assay. Thromb Res 43: 361-365
76. Schedel I, Dreikhausen U, Nentwig B, Höckenschnieder M, Rauthmann D, Balikcioglu S, Coldewey R, Deicher H (1991) Treatment of gram-negative septic shock with an immunoglobin preparation: a prospective, randomized clinical trial. Crit Care Med 19: 1104-1113
77. Scheifele DW, Melton P, Whitchelo V (1981) Evaluation of the Limulus test for endotoxemia in neonates with suspected sepsis. J Pediatr 98: 899-903
78. Schmeichel CJ, McCormick D (1992) Septic shock - what do physicians want. Biotechnology 10: 264-267
79. Shenep JL, Mogan KA (1984) Kinetics of endotoxin release during antibiotic therapy for experimental gram-negative bacterial sepsis. J Infect Dis 150: 380-388
80. Shenep JL, Flynn PM, Barrett FF, Stidham GL, Westenkirchner DF (1988) Serial quantitation of endotoxemia and bacteremia during therapy for gram-negative bacterial sepsis. J Infect Dis 157: 565-568
81. Sibbald WJ (1976) Bacteremia and endotoxemia: a discussion of their roles in the pathophysiology of gram-negative sepsis. Heart Lung 5: 765-771
82. Stumacher RJ, Kovnat MJ, McCabe WR (1973) Limitations of the usefulness of the limulus assay for endotoxin. N Engl J Med 288: 1261-1264
83. Sturk A, Janssen ME, Muylaert FR, Joop K, Thomas LLM, ten Cate JW (1987) Endotoxin testing in blood. In: Detection of bacterial endotoxins with the Limulus amebocyte lysate test. Liss, New York, pp. 371-385
84. Sullivan JD Jr, Watson SW (1975) Inhibitory effect of heparin on the Limulus test for endotoxin. J Clin Microbiol 2: 151
85. Tamura H, Tanaka S, Obayashi T, Yoshida M, Kawai T (1991) A new sensitive method for determining endotoxin in whole blood. Clin Chi 200: 35-42
86. Tamura H, Tanaka S, Obayashi T, Yoshida M, Kawai T (1992) A new sensitive microplate assay of plasma endotoxin. J Clin Lab Anal 6: 232-238
87. Thomas LLM, Sturk A, Kahle LH, ten Cate J (1981) Quantitative endotoxin determination in blood with a chromogenic substrate. Clin Chim Acta 116: 63-68
88. Thomas LL, Sturk A, Buller HR, ten Cate JW, ten Cate H, Spijker RE (1984) Comparative investigation of a quantitative chromogenic endotoxin assay and blood cultures. Am J Clin Pathol 82: 203-206
89. Trinchet JC, Jupeau A, Hornstein M, Beaugrand M, Ferrier JP, Hecht Y (1981) La recherche d'endotoxines par le test Limule dans le liquide d'ascite des cirrhotiques a-t-elle un intérêt? Résultats de 110 tests (Are endotoxins present in cirrhotic ascitic fluid? Results of 110 tests). Gastroenterol Clin Biol 5: 1103-1107

90. Van Deventer SJH, Pauw W, ten Cate JW, Janssen ME, Büller HR, Sturk A (1987) Clinical evaluation in febrile patients of an optimized endotoxin assay in blood. In: Detection of bacterial endotoxins with the Limulus amebocyte lysate test. Liss, New York, pp. 489-499
91. Van Deventer SJH, ten Cate JW, Büller HR, Sturk A, Pauw W (1988) Endotoxaemia: an early predictor of septicaemia in febrile patients. Lancet I: 605-608
92. Washida S (1978) Endotoxin receptor site. I. Binding of endotoxin to platelets. Acta Med Okayama 32: 159-223
93. Wilkinson SP, Arroyo V, Gazzard BG, Moodie H, Williams R (1974) Relation of renal impairment and haemorrhagic diathesis to endotoxaemia in fulminant hepatic failure. Lancet 1: 521-524
94. Wortel CH, Von der Möhlen MAM, van Deventer SJH, Sprung CL, Jastremski M, Lubbers MJ, Smith CR, Allen IE, ten Cate JW (1992) Effectiveness of a human monoclonal anti-endotoxin antibody (HA-1A) in gram-negative sepsis: relationship to endotoxin and cytokine levels. J Infect Dis 166: 1367-1374

Acute-Phase Proteins in SIRS

F. Stüber, F.U. Schade, J. Schröder, F. Bokelmann, M. Petersen, J. Seifert

Introduction

The systemic inflammatory response syndrome (SIRS) still presents a challenge concerning its early diagnosis, therapy and prognosis [1]. Frequently, patients show long courses of the disease due to advanced symptomatic treatment of acute respiratory distress syndrome (ARDS) and multiple organ dysfunction. Therefore, evaluation of inflammatory and disease activity has become more important.

C-reactive protein (CRP) is a well established acute phase protein in rheumatoid arthritis and lupus erythematosus. Recent reports suggest induction of CRP by interleukin-6 (IL-6), a cytokine involved in the mediator cascade of SIRS. On the other hand, tumor necrosis factor alpha (TNFα) is a very early released mediator in SIRS capable of inducing the mediator cascade that evokes shock and multiple organ failure. TNFα is removed very rapidly from the circulation. In addition, soluble TNF receptors (sTNF-R$_{55}$, sTNF-R$_{75}$) are released into the circulation in the acute-phase response [2]. This study examines the prevalence and the kinetics of five acute-phase proteins (CRP, IL-6, TNFα, sTNF-R$_{55}$, sTNF-R$_{75}$) in patients suffering from SIRS.

Methods

Eighteen patients entered the study after diagnosis of SIRS and fulfilled the criteria of severe sepsis [1]. Blood samples were drawn every 6 h during the first 2 days and every 12 h thereafter. CRP was measured in a routine turbimetric assay (Boehringer-Mannheim). IL-6 was detected by a biological assay using the IL-6 dependent B-cell line B13/29. Detection of TNFα was performed with an ELISA system using a monoclonal antibody for TNFα. Free TNFα as well as complexed TNF molecules were measured. Soluble TNF receptors were measured by an enzyme linked immunobinding assay (Dr. Gallati, Hoffmann La Roche). This assay detected free soluble TNF receptors exclusively.

Results

The mean APACHE II score was 22.6 ± 6 in the 18 patients. Ten patients had peritonitis and four patients were suffering from necrotizing pancreatitis. Other diagnoses were mediastinitis, and hemorrhagic shock with subsequent SIRS and severe sepsis (Table 1). CRP levels were elevated (> 10 mg/l) in all patients at all time points. CRP values did not differ significantly in patients with (133.2 ± 39.6 mg/l) or without (117.1 ± 31.1) multiple organ dysfunction syndrome (MODS) and between survivors (128,8133,7) and nonsurvivors (137.5 ± 41.9). In contrast, IL-6 was detectable in only 84/211 serum samples. It was elevated in patients with MODS but not in patients without MODS (Table 2). IL-6 levels were correlated especially with pulmonary dysfunction and severity of ARDS (Fig. 1). TNFα levels were elevated in patients with MODS. In contrast to IL-6, the kinetics of TNFα showed no clear correlation with the clinical course of the disease. Patients with consistently high TNF serum levels had a poor prognosis (Table 2). CRP, IL-6 and TNFα did not correlate with each other. In contrast, levels for both sTNF-R$_{55}$ and sTNF-R$_{75}$ showed a positive correlation ($r=0.6$). Patients could be divided into two groups on the basis of sTNFR$_{55}$ and sTNFR$_{75}$ values: The group with higher soluble TNF receptor levels showed increasing values in the course of the disease combined with a poor prognosis (Fig. 2). The group with lower levels of soluble TNF receptor consisted of patients surviving MODS or without MODS.

Table 1: Characteristics of 18 patients with SIRS

Patient	APACHE II score	MODS	Outcome	ARDS (Morel)	Diagnosis
1	21	C,P,K,L	Survivor	3-4	Peritonitis
2	16	C,P,K,L	Survivor	3-4	Peritonitis
3	14	No	Survivor	-	Hemorrhagic shock
4	9	No	Survivor	-	Peritonitis
5	17	No	Survivor	-	Peritonitis
6	20	C,P,K,L	Nonsurvivor	4	Peritonitis
7	19	C,P,K,L	Survivor	3	Septicemia
8	25	C,P,K	Nonsurvivor	4	Peritonitis
9	15	No	Survivor	-	Peritonitis
10	27	C,P,K,L	Nonsurvivor	3-4	Pancreatitis
11	26	C,P,K,L	Nonsurvivor	4	Mediastinitis
12	30	C,P,K	Nonsurvivor	4	Peritonitis
13	17	No	Survivor	-	Peritonitis
14	27	C,P,K	Nonsurvivor	-	Pancreatitis
15	24	C,P,K	Nonsurvivor	4	Peritonitis
16	29	C,P,K	Nonsurvivor	3-4	Pancreatitis
17	36	C,P,K	Nonsurvivor	3-4	Pancreatitis
18	30	C,P,K	Nonsurvivor	-	Peritonitis

MODS, Multiple organ dysfunction; C, cor; P, pulmo; K, kidney; L, liver

Table 2: Acute phase proteins in SIRS: correlation with multiple organ dysfunction and outcome

	Total	Survivors	Nonsurvivors	MODS	No MODS
CRP (mg/l)[a]	131.6 ± 37.9	128.8 ± 33.7	137.5 ± 41.9	133.2 ± 39.6	117.1 ± 31.1
IL-6 (pg/ml)[b]	2307	1554	3814	2731	60
Range of pos. samples	10-8900	10-8900	60-8300	60-8900	10-60
TNFα (pg/ml)[b]	292	91	456	366	21
Range of pos. samples	10-3300	10-240	10-3300	10-3300	10-180
sTNF-R55[a]	14.2 ± 8.4	10.2±5.7	17±9	158±8.6	7.3±1.6
sTNF-R75[a]	15.4 ± 8.8	11.7±4.4	18±10.0	16.2±9.4	11.8±4

[a]Mean ± SD. [b]Median of pos. samples

A.K., 67 yrs, peritonitis, ARDS, MODS (patient 6)

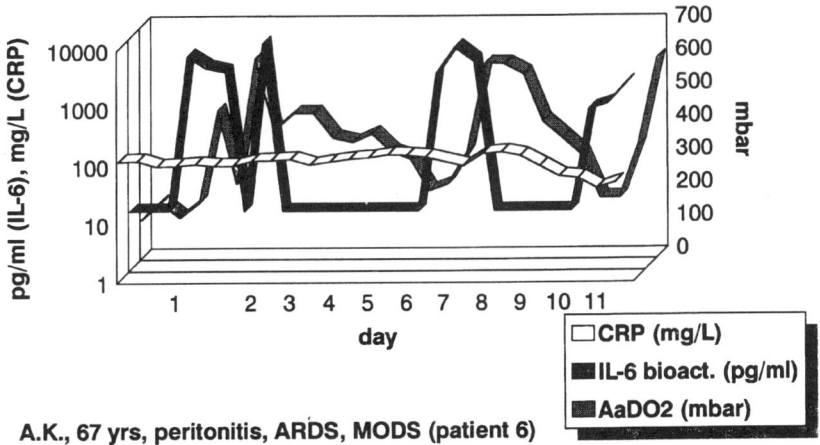

Fig. 1: IL-6 and CRP in MODS: kinetics of IL-6 and CRP

A.K., 67 yrs., peritonitis, ARDS, MODS (patient 6)

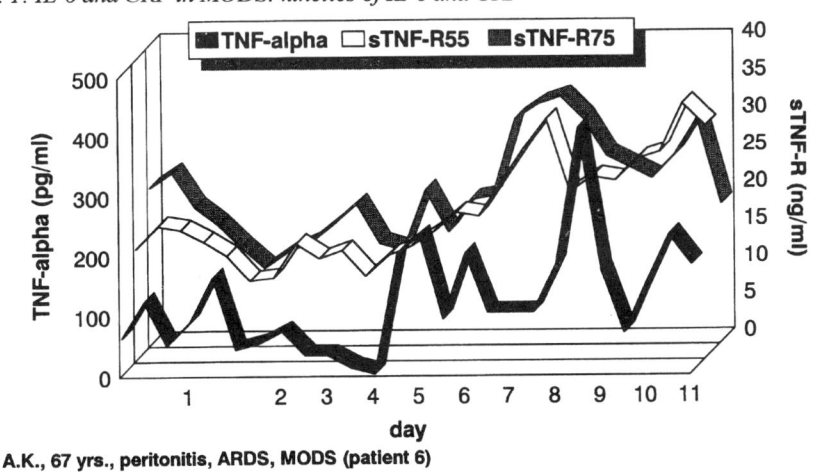

Fig. 2: TNFα and soluble TNF receptors in MODS: kinetics of TNFα, sTNF-R55 and sTNF-R75

Discussion

IL-6 and CRP levels show a positive correlation in rheumatoid arthritis [3]. IL-6 is a cytokine induced by primary mediators of SIRS, e.g., TNFα or IL-1β. There is evidence for induction of CRP by IL-6 [4]. Our results indicate that they are not correlated in SIRS. CRP levels are elevated in all states of SIRS. The kinetics of CRP levels do not adequately indicate development of multiple organ failure and outcome. In contrast, elevated IL-6 levels seem to indicate multiple organ failure and ARDS. IL-6 is released during single phases of high inflammatory activity that may occur with high frequency. This explains the sustained high levels of CRP induced by IL-6 in SIRS. These findings agree with the study by Takemoto et al. [5], who demonstrated the importance of IL-6 levels in septic patients with hematological disorders in contrast to CRP and endotoxin. TNFα kinetics show no clear pattern, but consistently high levels indicate poor prognosis. TNFα peaks did not correlate with changes in the inflammatory activity of SIRS as closely as IL-6. Clearance of TNFα from the circulation could be facilitated by soluble TNF receptors. The ELISA assay employed for TNF measurement in this study also detected free (biologically active) and complexed TNFα molecules so that we could not estimate the bioactivity and levels of free TNF-α.

Soluble TNF-R behaves as acute phase proteins. Serum levels were elevated in all patients suffering from SIRS. As sTNF-R are able to block TNF bioactivity and TNF binding to membrane bound receptors [6], these proteins can act as immunomodulators in vivo. Increasing levels of soluble TNF receptors may indicate contraregulatory mechanisms in response to high and toxic levels of TNFα in patients who do not survive SIRS [7].

In conclusion, CRP and TNFα do not adequately monitor the course of SIRS. In contrast, IL-6 correlates with MODS and episodes of high disease activity. Increasing sTNF-R levels may indicate poor prognosis.

References

1. *ACCP/SCCM Consensus Conference (1992) Definitions for sepsis and organ failure and guidelines for the use of innovative therapies in sepsis. Crit Care Med 20: 864-874*
2. *Girardin E, Roux-Lombard P, Grau GE et al. (1992)Imbalance between tumor necrosis factor-alpha and soluble TNF receptor concentrations in severe meningococcaemia. Immunology 76: 20-23*
3. *Metsarinne KP, Nordstrom DC, Kontinnen YT et al. (1992) Plasma interleukin-6 and renin substrate in reactive arthritis, rheumatoid arthritis, and systemic lupus erythematosus. Rheumatol Int 12(3): 93-96*
4. *Ganapathi MK, Rzewnicki D, Samols D et al. (1991) Effect of combination of cytokines and hormones on serum amyloid A and c-reactive protein in Hep 3B cells. J Immunol 147(4): 1261-1265*
5. *Takemoto Z, Kanamaru A, Kakishita E et al. (1992) Interleukin-6 in hematological disorders with septic shock. Rinsho Ketsueki 33(6): 838-840*
6. *Adolf GR, Fruhbeis B (1992) Monoclonal antibodies to soluble human TNF receptor (TNF binding protein) enhance its ability to block TNF activity. Cytokine 20: 724-726*
7. *Van Zee KJ, Kohno T, Fischer E, Rock CS, Moldawer LL, Lowry SF (1992) TNF soluble receptor protect against excessive TNF alpha during infection and injury. Proc Natl Acad Sci (USA) 89: 4845-4849*

Early Recognition of Sepsis Using IL-6, TNF, Elastase, and CRP

A. Gaitzsch, R. Lefering, D. Weber, S. Sauerland, M.L. Dangel, D. Rixen, P. Fink

Introduction

Many investigators have described elevated levels of cytokines and other mediators [4, 5] in patients who have sepsis, or in the early postoperative period. However, there are no known parameters which can be used to predict sepsis in advance, for example, on the day before onset. We therefore conducted a prospective observational study in patients with a high risk for sepsis in order to evaluate the usefulness of certain mediators for predicting sepsis before its clinical manifestation.

Patients and Methods

For the study period of one year, we included all our polytraumatized patients and those having undergone a major vascular or abdominal surgery and closely observed them until death, discharge, or the patient's refusal to continue the study. C-reactive protein (CRP) elastase, and the cytokines interleukin 6 (IL-6) and tumor necrosis factor (TNF) were analyzed in plasma and serum samples every day. For the determination of cytokine levels we used enzyme-amplified sensitivity immunoassays (Medgenix, Ratingen). The day of trauma event and the following day were excluded from the analysis in order to assess only stabilized patients. The description of early trauma response was not the primary aim of this investigation.

A patient was classified as having sepsis when at least four of the following seven clinical criteria were fulfilled:
1. Temperature > 38.9°C or < 35.5°C
2. Heart rate > 100 beats/min
3. Respiration > 28 breaths/min or $PaCO_2$ < 32 mmHg or mechanically ventilated
4. Blood pressure > 90 mmHG
5. Thrombocytes < 100 000/mm^3

6. Leukocytes > 15 000/mm^3 or < 3000/mm^3 or > 20% immature cells
7. Obvious septic focus (positive blood culture or reoperation)

We also considered the fact that these signs can be masked by drugs. This definition of "systemic sepsis" was first introduced by the Veterans Administration [2] for their sepsis trials.

Results

A total of 142 patients were included and 40 of them belonged to the group of trauma patients. Compared to the whole population, the trauma patients were younger (42 vs. 56 years, range 15-75 years) with a greater proportion of male patients (71% vs. 64%). Five patients died in the trauma group (12%). The severity of trauma was documented by the injury severity score (mean, 30 points) and the trauma score (mean, 13.8 points). About half of the patients had systemic sepsis, for at least 1 day. The consensus definition for "sepsis" [1], which requires a proven source of infection, would have missed some severely ill patients, while SIRS criteria [1] would apply to two-third of our patients (Fig. 1).

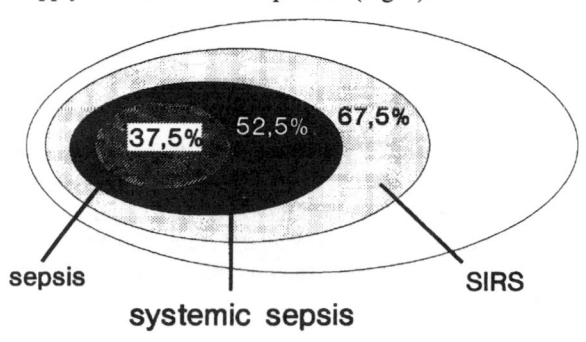

Fig. 1: Incidence of sepsis, systemic sepsis and systemic inflamatory response syndrome (SIRS) among 40 polytraumatized patients (100%). The definition of sepsis and SIRS was according to the consensus conference of the American College of Chest Physicians/Society of Critical Care Medicine [1], and the systemic sepsis was as defined by the Veterans Administration [2]. A patient was assigned to one of the groups if the respective criteria were fulfilled at least for one day, where the day of trauma and the following day were excluded

On 150 days, patients had less than four of the clinical signs listed above, while on 53 days patients had systemic sepsis. Comparing the mean levels of mediators on all these days when patients had no systemic sepsis with when patients had sepsis revealed significantly increased values for all four mediators. Mean CRP levels were 190 vs. 125 mg/l (p=0.001); elastase, 142 vs. 101 µg/l (p=0.05); IL-6, 659 vs. 234 ng/l (p=0.001) and TNF, 41 vs. 17 ng/l (p=0.05). This comfirms the results from other investigators [4, 5].

We attempted to ascertain whether mediator levels measured on a certain day gave predictive information about the patient's status the following day. Therefore, from the patient data we selected those days on which no sepsis was present and also not present the following day, from which we calculated mean values. The same procedure was used for those days when no sepsis was present but when the patient became septic the day after. We found 132 days where the patient was not septic on that day or the day after. The mean CRP level from those days was 121 mg/l (Fig. 2a). On 18 days, a nonseptic patient was septic on the following day. On these days the mean CRP level was found to be 160 mg/l, which is significantly higher. During sepsis these values remained at an increased level (mean, 199 mg/l) and there was a slight decrease at the end of a septic period (Fig. 2a). Elastase showed a remarkable increase on the day before sepsis (92 vs. 168 ng/l), but this difference was not significant due to some very high values in both groups (Fig. 2b). IL-6 (Fig. 2c) and TNF levels (Fig. 2d) show patterns similar to those of CRP. The mean levels of both cytokines were increased on the day before sepsis, and even more increased during sepsis. But in all cases the variability of the values was so great that a single parameter could not be used as a valid predictor for sepsis.

Discussion

Although there are many publications describing the course of levels of mediators during sepsis, there is a lack of information about the period before the onset of sepsis. This period can only be investigated by continuous observation of all patients at risk for sepsis. The clinical course of the trauma patients in this study was very heterogeneous. Some recovered quickly, some slowly, some had an early septic period, and some developed systemic sepsis 2 weeks after trauma. Drawing conclusions from these individual courses is difficult. The definition of systemic sepsis used in this study may be regarded as a type of score describing the patients' severity of illness. The approach of calculating a mean value for days and not for patients reflects much better the situation in an ICU where some patients require much more attention than others. The number of days that each patient contributes to the bars shown in Fig. 2 may vary, but the total number of patients is sufficiently large to avoid the effect of one mean value being dominated by a single patient. Unfortunately, the absolute values of all four mediators showed great variations. Elastase, which seems to be the optimal parameter for early recognition of sepsis when looking only at the mean values, was not even significant. Threshold analysis revealed no more than a 50% correct prediction of systemic sepsis on the following day. In general, however, the extremely elevated levels of each of the four mediators considered in this study are good indicators of the deterioration of the clinical status of the patient.

Conclusion

The definition of systemic sepsis is a useful tool for the classification of severely ill patients. All patients with a proven bacteremia were covered by this definition. Regarding the early recognition of sepsis, our data show that the values of CRP, elastase, IL-6, and TNF - on average - are already increased on the day before sepsis. The large variability, even in nonseptic patients, limits the clinical validity of a single parameter. We are hopeful, however, that the combination of these parameters with clinical measurements, also with regard to dynamic changes, will be able to be used to define at least a subgroup of patients at high risk of subsequent sepsis.

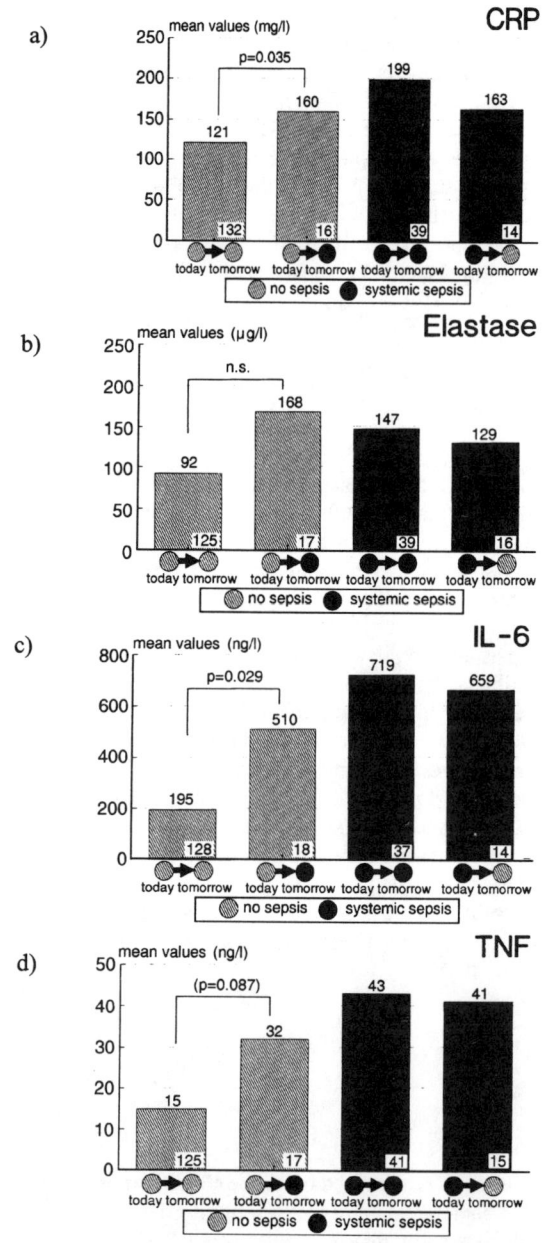

Fig. 2: Mean levels of a) CRP, b) elastase, c) IL-6 and d) TNF according to the presence of sepsis on the measurement day and the following day. The number within each bar indicates the number of days from which the mean values were calculated. Systemic sepsis was defined according to the criteria of the Veterans Administration [2]. P values were calculated using the unpaired two-sided t-test.

References

1. American College of Chest Physicians/Society of Critical Care Medicine Consensus Conference (1992) Definition for sepsis and organ failure and guidelines for the use of innovative therapies in sepsis Crit Care Med 20: 864-874
2. Veterans Administration Systemic Sepsis Cooperative Study Group (1987) Effect of high-dose glucocorticoid therapy on mortality in patients with clinical signs of sepsis. N Engl J Med, 317: 659-665
3. Spitzer IA (1993) Interleukins in sepsis. In: Neugebauer E, Holaday JW (eds.) Handbook of mediators in septic shock. CRC, Boca Raton, pp. 279-290
4. Tracey KJ, Cerami A (1993) Tumor necrosis factor (cachectin) in septic/endotoxic shock. In: Neugebauer E, Holaday JW (eds.) Handbook of mediators in septic shock. CRC, Boca Raton, pp. 291-308
5. Pinsky MR, Vincent J-L, Devierce J, Alegre M, Kahn RJ, Dupont E (1993) Serum cytokine levels in human septic shock. Chest 103: 565-575.

Acute-Phase Response Predicts Complications After Trauma Better than Protease Inhibitors or Collagen Precursor

Å. Lasson, J. Göransson, K. Jönsson

Introduction

Early diagnosis of complications after trauma is imperative to decrease morbidity and mortality after both major accidental trauma and surgical trauma. The three main surgical hazards after major surgical trauma today are bacterial complications, cardiopulmonary failure and deep venous thrombosis and its complications. Modern anesthesiology and intensive care treatment have minimized the risks of cardiopulmonary failure, and various prophylactic regimens have lowered the risk of fatal pulmonary embolism. However, local bacterial complications and septicemia still remain dangerous postoperative complications with high morbidity and mortality. Thus, major efforts must be made to discover and to treat these bacterial complications as early as possible, to prevent multiple organ failure at a later stage [4]. Today most local bacterial complications may be quite accurately diagnosed using sophisticated modern radiological examinations, e.g., computerized tomography, nuclear magnetic resonance and ultrasonography; and bacterial septicemia can be diagnosed using repeated blood cultures. However, the main problem remains the identification of those patients who need these examinations and their identification early enough for successful treatment.

The aim of the present study was to analyze whether complications after surgical trauma of varying extents could be diagnosed earlier using preoperative or daily postoperative measurements of various plasma proteins than by using clinical signs of complications.

Materials and Methods

Plasma was taken preoperatively from 286 patients undergoing surgery for cancer ($n=208$) or benign disease ($n=78$). Another 83 patients were studied with daily samples for 7 days. These 83 patients were operated on for breast cancer ($n=17$), pulmonary cancer ($n=11$), colorectal cancer ($n=43$), duodenal ulcer ($n=5$) or coxarthrosis ($n=7$).

Electroimmunoassay was used to quantitate C-reactive protein (CRP), C1-esterase inhibitor, α_2-macroglobulin, antithrombin III and albumin, using antisera prepared in our laboratory. Functional levels of the C1-esterase inhibitor were determined using chromogenic peptide substrates (Pharmacia, Sweden). Procollagen III peptide was determined using a commercial RIA kit (Behringwerke AG, Germany). Patient data concerning postoperative course and routine blood chemistry tests were collected retrospectively from patient records.

Results

Preoperative

High preoperative CRP levels indicated an increased risk of developing postoperative complications (Fig. 1). This was true for almost all the different diagnostic groups studied, as depicted in Fig. 2. There was no difference found between complicated and uncomplicated cases regarding the levels of C1-esterase inhibitor (Fig. 3) or α_2-macroglobulin and antithrombin III (results not shown).

Postoperative

CRP behaved like a fast-reacting acute-phase protein. Peak levels were reached on the 2nd day, and returned to normal levels within 7 days in uncomplicated cases (Fig. 4). Continuing high levels, or a second increase of the CRP level, were seen in severe infectious complications requiring treatment (Fig. 5). These changes were seen 1-3 days before any clinical signs or symptoms of developing complications were seen (results not shown). The C1-esterase inhibitor behaved like a slow-reacting acute-phase protein (Fig. 6). There was a difference between functional and quantitative levels, especially in complicated cases and in patients undergoing extensive surgery (Fig. 6). This difference was, however, not statistically significant. Procollagen III peptide also increased like a slow-reacting acute-phase protein (Fig. 7). There were some slight differences, although not significant, between complicated and uncomplicated cases (Fig. 7). α_2-Macroglobulin decreased in parallel to hemoglobin and albumin after surgery (Fig. 8). The decrease was proportional to the extent of the surgical trauma (Fig. 8). There were no significant differences between complicated and uncomplicated cases (results not shown).

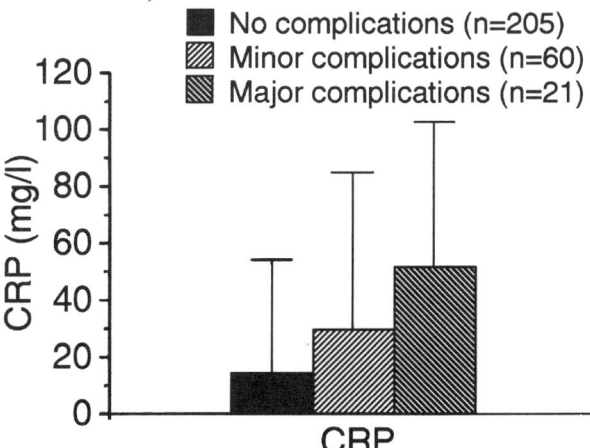

Fig. 1: Preoperative plasma CRP levels in 286 patients related to the postoperative course

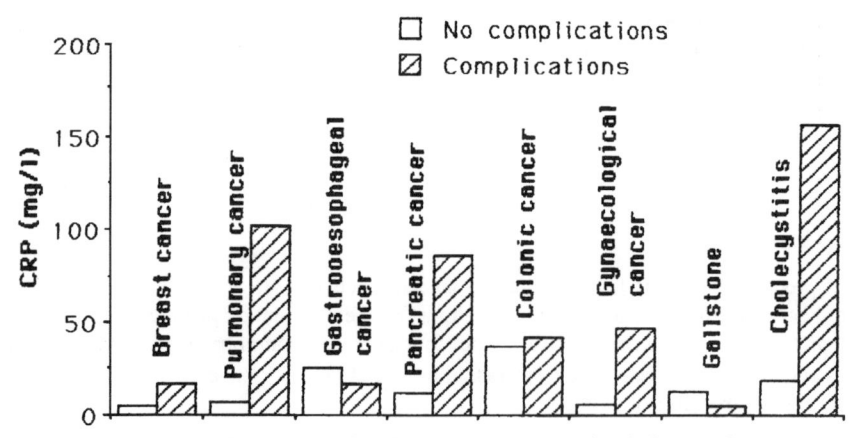

Fig. 2: Preoperative plasma CRP levels in 286 patients, divided according to surgical diagnosis and related to the postoperative course

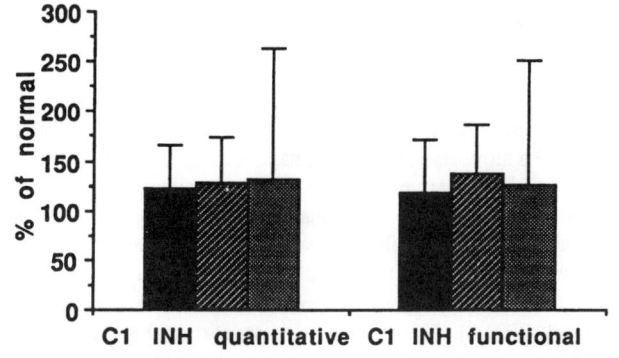

Fig. 3: Preoperative plasma levels of C1-esterase inhibitor (quantitative and functional levels) in 286 patients related to the postoperative course (groups = Fig. 1)

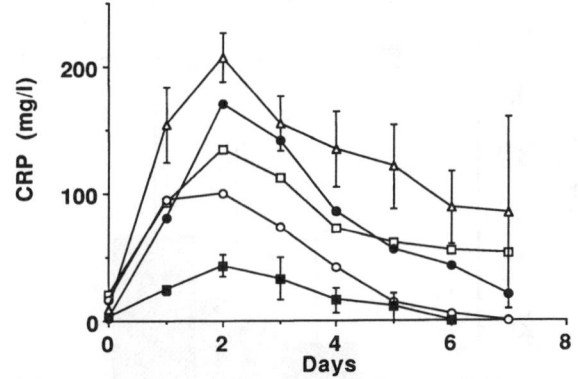

Fig. 4: Plasma CRP levels in 83 patients operated on with mastectomy (■, n=17), proximal gastric vagotomy (○, n=5), pulmonary resection (△, n=11), total hip replacement (●, n=7) and colorectal resection (□ n=43)

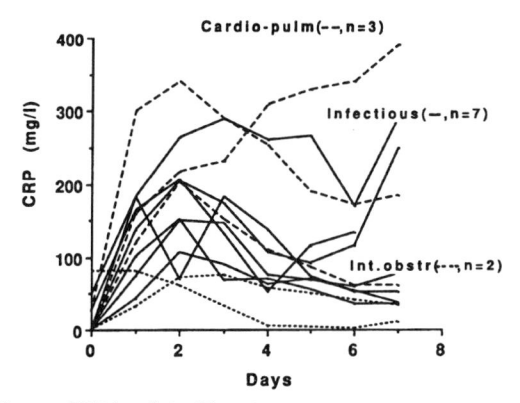

Fig. 5: Individual plasma CRP levels in 12 patients experiencing postoperative complications

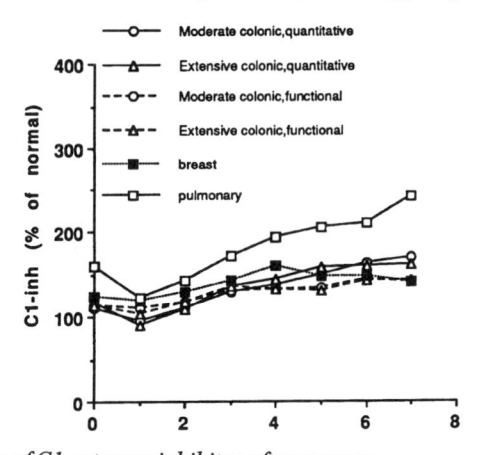

Fig. 6: Plasma levels of C1-esterase inhibitor after surgery

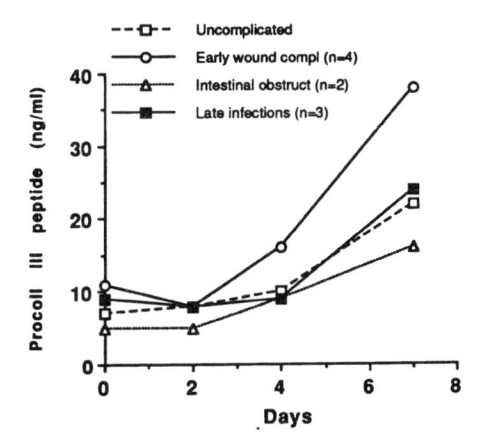

Fig. 7: Procollagen III peptide levels in complicated and uncomplicated colorectal resections

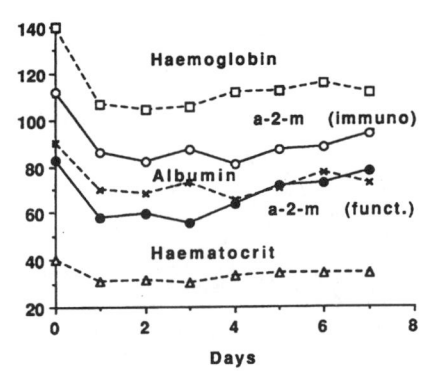

Fig. 8: Quantitative and functional levels of α_2-macroglobulin after colorectal resection

Discussion

This study has shown that complications after surgical trauma of varying extents can be diagnosed earlier using preoperative as well as daily postoperative measurements of some plasma proteins than by using clinical signs of complications. The acute-phase protein CRP predicts complications better than plasma protease inhibitors or procollagen precursor. High preoperative plasma CRP levels indicate an increased risk of postoperative complications. Daily monitoring of plasma CRP levels may predict complications 1-3 days earlier than clinical signs.

The findings that the peak CRP level is proportional, also using statistical comparisons, to the extent of the operative trauma (Fig. 1), is in agreement with some reports on operative and other types of trauma, although a few studies do not show this graded response. In the normal, uncomplicated postoperative patient, the CRP levels rapidly decreased after the second postoperative day to reach normal levels (< 10 mg/l) within the 7-day study period. In contrast to these findings, continued high levels, or a second increase in CRP levels, were seen in the presence of postoperative complications (Fig. 2). This is in agreement with other studies on serial postoperative CRP measurements [3, 8], also after emergency operations for peritonitis [6]. It is of great clinical importance that this rise in CRP mostly precedes the clinical diagnosis of the complication by 1-3 days, as we showed earlier for complications occurring after operations for peritonitis [6] and during the course of acute pancreatitis [1]. Neither the CRP level nor the pattern of changes could, however, discriminate between local/general or infectious/noninfectious complications. This is in agreement with earlier studies, and is quite logical, since CRP is an unspecific, acute-phase protein produced in the liver [9]. The differences found may partly be explained by our earlier data indicating that the "tumor burden" is important for the CRP response [7], in agreement with some other recent studies of CRP levels in malignant disease and their relationship to the stage/spread of the tumor [2]. Another explanation is that patients with high preoperative CRP levels have a more "active disease," as indicated by the findings for patients with cholecystitis (Fig. 2), where the high CRP levels seen in patients developing complications also coincided with a more active inflammatory state of the cholecystitis.

None of the plasma protease inhibitor could be used to predict postoperative complications using neither preoperative (Fig. 3) nor daily postoperative measurements (Figs. 6 and 8). Although differences existed between complicated and uncomplicated cases, the differences were not statistically significant and did not precede the clinical signs. In contrast to earlier reports [10], where the high-molecular-weight α_2-macroglobulin showed unchanged postoperative levels, in this study it decreased after surgery (Fig. 8). The decrease was proportional to the extent of the trauma and was probably caused by a number of peri- and postoperative, events, i.e., accumulation of α_2-macroglobulin in wounded tissues, consumption of the inhibitor, redistribution and hemodilution.

Although anastomotic complications could theoretically be identified by increased levels of procollagen precursors [5], in this study procollagen III peptide, we found no "clinically useful" difference between complicated and uncomplicated cases (Fig. 7). Patients developing complications had higher plasma levels during the postoperative course, but the increase did not precede the clinical diagnosis of complications.

In conclusion, a raised CRP level pre- as well as postoperatively is a quite specific biochemical marker of (any kind) of postoperative complications after elective surgery. The rise in CRP usually precedes the clinical suspicion/diagnosis of postoperative complications by 1-3 days, and may thus facilitate an earlier diagnostic awareness, making early, aggressive therapy possible. In malignant disease a raised preoperative CRP or a continued elevation of CRP after the first postoperative week may indicate metastatic spread or massive local growth. Since measurement of CRP can be done cheaply (US $4 for ordinary analysis) using a commercially available antiserum and can be analyzed using nephelometry in most hospital laboratories on a continuous 24-h basis, it fulfills many requirements for a useful "screening" test for this purpose.

Acknowledgements

This investigation was supported by grants from The Medical Faculty, University of Lund, the Påhlsson Foundation, Crafoord Foundation and the Swedish Society for Medical Research.

References

1. Berling R, Lasson Å, Axelsson L, Hjelmqvist B, Ohlsson K (1990) Plasma CRP levels in the prediction of complications during acute pancreatitis. Surg Res Commun 8: 241-249
2. Büchler M, Malfertheiner P, Uhl W, Beger HG (1987) C-reaktives Protein als Entzündungs- und Nekrosemarker in der Gastroenterologie. Med Klin 82: 180-185
3. Crockson RA, Payne CJ, Ratcliff AP, Soothill JF (1966) Time sequence of acute phase reactive proteins following surgical trauma. Clin Chim Acta 14: 435-441
4. Fry DE (1988) Multiple system organ failure. Surg Clin North Am 68: 107-122
5. Jiborn H, Ahonen H, Zederfeldt B (1980) Healing of experimental colonic anastomoses. Am J Surg 139: 406-413
6. Lasson Å, Delshammmar M, Ohlsson K (1988) Severity scoring and prediction of complications in peritonitis. Surg Res Commun 3: 327-334

7. Lasson Å, Berling R, Göransson J (1992) Plasma CRP-levels in the diagnosis of postoperative complications. Surg Res Commun 12: 203-211
8. Mustard RA, Bohnen JMA, Haseeb S, Kasina R (1987) C-reactive protein levels predict postoperative septic complications. Arch Surg 122: 69-73
9. Pepys MB, Baltz ML (1983) Acute phase proteins with special reference to C-reactive protein and related proteins (Pentaxins) and serum amyloid A protein. Adv Immunol 34: 141-211
10. Werner M, Odenthal D (1967) Serum protein changes after gastrectomy as a model of acute phase reaction. J Lab Clin Med 70: 302-308

Lidocaine Metabolite Formation: An Indicator of MOF After Multiple Trauma

U. Lehmann, M. Oellerich, G. Regel, D. Pape

Introduction

Polytraumatized patients who initially do not die from hemorrhagic shock or severe head injury are at danger from developing multiple organ failure (MOF), which is associated with high lethality. A major part of the pathogenesis of MOF is liver dysfunction. Static or dynamic tests can be used for an assessment of hepatic function. Traditional static tests only indirectly test liver function by measurement of the concentration of an endogenous substance, e.g., enzyme or metabolite, at a single point of time. On the other hand, dynamic tests are a measure of actual performance, the dimension of time being considered in addition. Instead of serum concentrations, turnover rates are measured. The functional state of the liver is reflected by the clearance of test substances or the formation kinetics of drug metabolites. The prognostic value of the MEGX test (based on the formation of the lidocaine metabolite monoethylglycinexylide, MEGX) still has to be proved for polytraumatized patients who are at risk of developing MOF.

Methods and Patients

The severity of injury of the polytraumatized patients was determined by the Hannover Polytrauma Score (PTS) [1] and the Injury Severity Score (ISS) [2]. The modified Multiple Organ Failure Score of Goris et al. [3] was used to classify the patients into one group with (+MOF) and one group without MOF (-MOF). The criteria used to establish the severity of each case of specific organ failure were those described by Goris et al. [3] with the exception of the liver, for which only serum bilirubin values were considered since increased aspartate aminotransferase (AST) activities are also observed after muscle damage.

The MEGX liver function test was carried out as previously described [4]. Blood specimens for MEGX determination were taken before and 15 min after administration of an i.v. bolus of lidocaine (1 mg/kg BW) injected over about 2 min. MEGX values were determined in serum by a fluorescence polarization immunoassay (Abbott Laboratories, Chicago, Ill.,

USA). Serial determinations were performed on the first 3 days and then every 2nd day after trauma and were compared with conventional liver function tests: serum concentrations of aspartate aminotransferase (AST), alanine aminotransferase (ALT), glutamate dehydrogenase (GLDH), cholinesterase (CHE), γ-glutamyl transferase (γ-GT), alkaline phosphatase (AP), clotting factor V (FV) and total bilirubin. The significance of differences between groups (+MOF/-MOF) was calculated for unpaired data using Mann-Whitney's U-test. The null hypothesis was rejected for $P < 0.05$.

Results

Of the 28 patients investigated, 10 patients developed MOF and 18 patients did not. Of the MOF group, 8 patients died between the 7th and the 35th day after trauma, whereas all patients without MOF survived. One patient from the +MOF group was excluded because he developed MOF induced by sepsis beginning on the 6th day after trauma. Severity of injury was significantly different between the groups (Table 1.) MEGX test values from both groups were in the normal range on the 1st day, and in the MOF group the test values decreased markedly between the 1st and 2nd day, remaining low to the 11th day (Fig. 1). The test values of the two surviving patients of the MOF group normalized during intensive therapy on day 28 and day 39, respectively. The median of the test values in the -MOF group was between 65 and 77 µg/l and corresponded to the test values of healthy volunteers (72 µg/l). Table 2 lists the median values of the MEGX test and the other liver function tests.

Table 1: Severity of injury (PTS, ISS). Both scores indicate a significantly higher severity of injury in the +MOF group

	+MOF	-MOF
PTS	51 ± 13	38 ± 8
ISS	32 ± 8	26 ± 5

Table 2: Median values of the MEGX test and other liver function tests. Shading indicates differences between the +MOF and -MOF groups

	Day 1		Day 2		Day 3		Day 5		Day 7		Day 9		Day 11	
+MOF/-MOF	+	-	+	-	+	-	+	-	+	-	+	-	+	-
MEGX (µg/l)	77	68	20	77	22	67	26	56	24	69	18	65	19	70
Bilirubin (µmol/l)	30	19	27	15	33	21	52	17	160	18	199	28	247	36
g-GT (U/l)	11	10	18	11	17	12	20	28	22	72	61	82	104	85
AP (U/l)	57	58	59	79	72	86	126	104	148	151	247	199	292	279
GLDH (U/l)	48	7	40	4	31	3	12	3	9	4	7	6	9	6
AST (U/l)	99	49	87	44	80	36	27	19	24	18	34	27	25	20
ALT (U/l)	115	28	68	30	54	21	32	15	26	14	32	19	30	24
CHE (U/l)	3070	2910	2825	2760	2460	2430	2222	2025	1825	1715	1410	1725	1180	1530
FV (%)	44	76	52	90	60	100	62	100	45	100	82	100	85	100

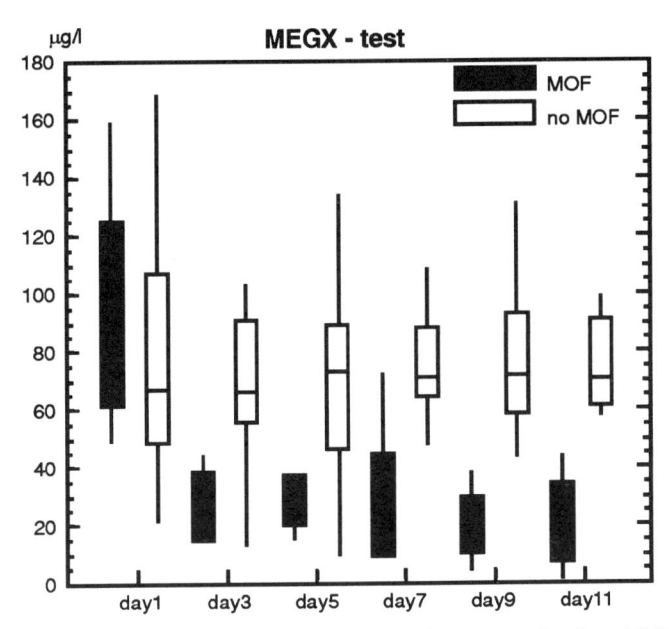

*Fig. 1: MEGX concentration in serum on days 1 - 11 after trauma for the +MOF and -MOF groups. Horizontal bar indicates the median. **Whiskers** represent scatter at that point of time. **Boxes** delimit the 25th and 75th percentiles*

Discussion

The significantly increased injury severity score of the +MOF group indicates the influence of the extent of trauma causing MOF. Bilirubin levels increased significantly on the 5th day after trauma in the +MOF group as a sign of diminished excretory liver function. Initially there was a slight and on day 5 a steep increase in bilirubin levels. These values might have been influenced by hemolyses or the absorption of hematoma. It may be helpful to measure separately conjugated and unconjugated bilirubin to differentiate the components.

Cholestasis was seen in both groups after the 7th day but there were no significant differences. The continuously rising AP levels in the two groups indicated the healing process of the fractures. Significantly elevated values of GLDH, from days 1 to 5, and of ALT, from days 3 to 7, indicated greater liver cell damage in the +MOF group. These differences can be explained by the greater proportion of severe abdominal injuries associated with liver trauma in the +MOF group (44%) than in the -MOF group (17%). Only initially were the values clearly elevated and they normalized on the subsequent days. Early after trauma AST levels were increased in both groups, falling continuously on the following days. This can be explained by traumatization of the musculature releasing the AST enzyme. CHE levels decreased continuously in both groups, indicating a diminished synthesis performance of the liver.

Clotting factor V was impaired on days 1 - 9 in the +MOF group, indicating diminished protein synthesis of the liver. This parameter is in principle suitable for estimation of protein synthesis, because it has a halflife of 5-6 h. Substitution of clotting preparations, however, e.g., fresh frozen plasma, influenced the measurement of this parameter.

In comparison to the other biochemical parameters of liver function, the MEGX test showed the greatest discrimination between patients with and without MOF on the 3rd day after trauma. If an MEGX value of 30 µg/l is chosen as a cutoff point, the corresponding sensitivity and specificity are 89% and 94%, respectively.

In conclusion the MEGX test may serve as an early indicator of multiple organ failure in the absence of overt biochemical abnormalities in multiple trauma patients.

References

1. Oestern HJ, Tscherne H, Sturm JA, Nerlich M (1985) Klassifizierung der Verletzungsschwere. Unfallchirurg 88: 465-472
2. Baker SP, O'Neil B (1976) The injury severity score: an update. J Trauma 16: 882-885
3. Goris RFA, Bekhorst TPA, Nuytinck JKS, Gimbrere JSF (1985) Multiple organ failure: generalized autodestructive inflammation. Arch Surg 120: 1109-1115
4. Oellerich M, Raude E, Burdelski M, Schulz M, Schmidt FW, Ringe B et al. (1987) Monoethylglycinexylidide formation kinetics, a novel approach to assessment of liver function. J Clin Chem Clin Biochem 25: 845-853

Assessment of Free Radical Production by Electron Spin Resonance Spectroscopy During the Ischemia-Reperfusion Phenomenon: From Animal Models to Clinical Investigation

J. Pincemail, J.O. Defraigne, C. Franssen, O. Detry, D. Serteyn, G. Hartstein, M. Meurisse, M. Lamy, M. Limet

Introduction

Under physiological conditions, 98% of oxygen is consumed at the level of the mitochondrial respiratory chain and directly reduced to water, via the cytochrome oxidase complex. However, under some conditions, fundamental oxygen ($^3O_2$) can be reduced step by step, electron by electron, giving rise to the formation of intermediate oxygen species, including superoxide anion radical ($O_2^{\bullet-}$), hydroxyl radical ($OH^\bullet$), hydrogen peroxide (H_2O_2) and singlet oxygen ($^1O_2$). Free radical species are characterized by the presence of an unpaired electron in their electronic structure, which confers them a high instability and therefore a great reactivity with many biological substrates. In this way, activated oxygen species have a high toxicity since they can promote DNA scission and base modification, inactivate plasma proteins, cross-link membrane proteins and induce lipid peroxidation in the membrane (for a review, see [2]).

For several years it has been asserted that oxygenated free radical species may be critically involved in human health and disease. One area that has received enthusiastic interest in clinical medicine is that of reoxygenation injury or ischemia reperfusion, a phenomenon accepted as making a major contribution to organ dysfunction in trauma, shock and sepsis but also in cardiovascular diseases and organ transplantation. Ischemia phenomenon or hypoperfusion will trigger a cascade of biochemical events (abnormalities in mitochondrial electron transport, calcium accumulation, endothelium dysfunction, xanthine oxidase activation, release of iron acting as a powerful free radical reaction catalyst), resulting in increased oxygen free radical production on reperfusion with oxygen [37]. Increased eicosanoid biosynthesis, attracting and activating macrophages and granulocytes, hemoglobin oxidation, and endotoxemia are also responsible for increasing accumulation in free radical activity.

In Vivo Free Radical Evidence

One basic problem in the transposition of biochemistry and pharmacology of reactive oxygen species to the ischemia-reperfusion phenomenon in clinical medicine is the fact that their detection in vivo always remains a difficult challenge. The main techniques which have been described for analysis of oxidative stress in biological samples are: detection of lipid peroxidation by-products (malondialdehyde, 4-hydroxynonenal, ethane, pentane) and oxidized proteins, consumption of endogenous defenses against oxygen toxicity (glutathione, vitamin E, ubiquinone), salicylate trapping or improvement of organ function by antioxidant therapy, including the administration to animals of substances capable of scavenging free radicals or limiting their production (superoxide dismutase, allopurinol, desferrioxamine, lazaroids, etc.). Recently, in vivo chemiluminescence techniques have been proposed but their application is difficult because capturing emitted light photons is hindered by tissue.
All the evidence provided by these studies, however, remains indirect and, therefore, the exact role played in vivo by free radicals in inducing tissue injury during ischemia-reperfusion remains largely hypothetical. Efforts have been made recently to establish in a way as direct as possible the formation of free radicals in biological samples as complex as blood, plasma or tissue with the use of electron spin resonance (ESR) spectroscopy, the technique of choice for detecting free radicals.

Short ESR Principles (for Detailed Information, see [20])

Electron spin resonance spectroscopy is a physical method able to evidence the absorption energy due to the interaction for the unpaired electron present in the free radical with a magnetic field produced by a magnet in the laboratory. Because the electron has a magnetic moment (μ), it behaves as a bar magnet when placed in a magnetic field. Two states of lowest (μ is aligned with the magnetic field) and highest (μ is aligned against the magnetic field) energies are defined (Zeeman effect, Fig. 1). The two states are labeled by the projection of the electron spin Ms, on the direction of the magnetic field. In the absence of magnetic field,

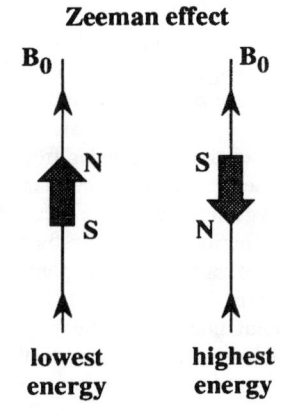

Fig. 1: Minimal and maximal energy orientations of the moment of the electron (μ) regarding an external magnetic field (B_0)

the two spin states have the same energy and are therefore indistinguishable. However, by increasing the magnetic field, the energies of the two spin states are split into Ms = +1/2 (high-energy state) and Ms = -1/2 (low-energy state). As the energy difference (ΔE) between the two spin states is directly proportional to a frequency by the equation $\Delta E = h\nu$, a single spectrum of energy absorption can be observed by applying electromagnetic radiation of known frequency (ν) generated by a klystron (Fig. 2).

The height of the signal taken as the first derivative spectrum will be directly proportional to the concentration of free radical present in the analyzed sample (Fig. 2). The unpaired electron is also very sensitive to the nuclei of neighboring atoms (hydrogen, oxygen, nitrogen) so that the single ESR absorption signal due to the electron will be split into additional signals. Therefore, some information can be given about the molecular structure of the sample.

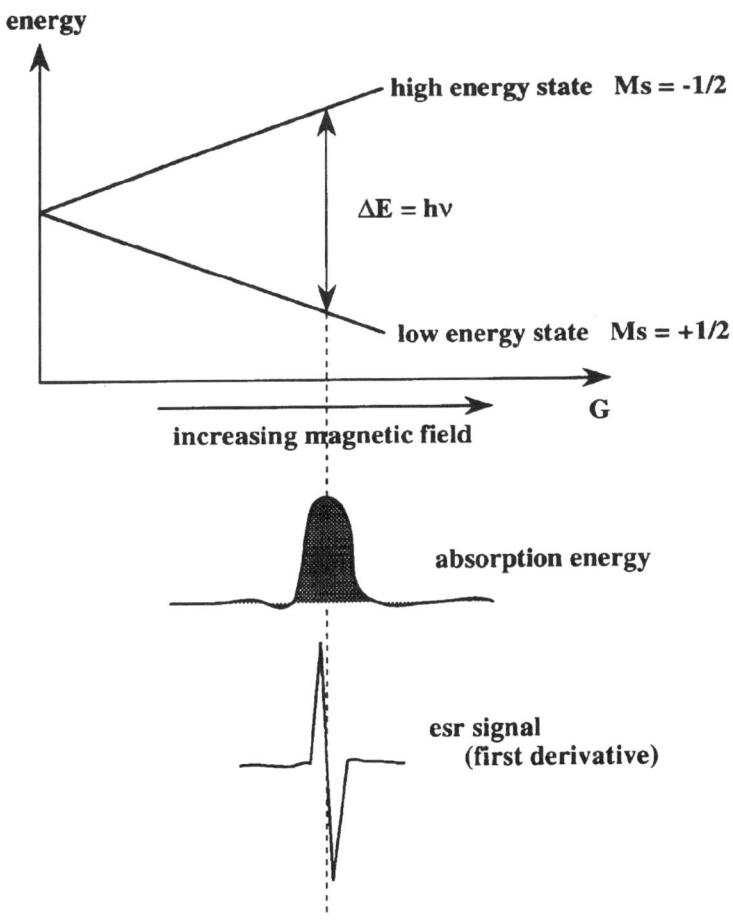

Fig. 2: As a function of the external magnetic field, the energies of the two spin states (Ms = +1/2 and Ms = -1/2) can be split with an energy difference given by the relation $\Delta E = h\nu$. Application of electromagnetic radiation of frequency equal to ν will induce an energy absorption between both states that can be visualized as the first derivative

Spin-Trapping Technique

Spin-trapping agents are, however, often required in ESR measurements to increase the half-life of in vivo generated free radicals. Such agents can react with transient free radicals to form more stable radicals (spin adducts) that can be detected, identified and eventually quantitated. Numerous spin-trapping agents are available (non-exhaustive list): 5,5-dimethyl-1-pyrroline 1-oxide (DMPO),-phenyl-*N-tert*-butyl nitrone (PBN), 2-methyl-2-nitrosopropane (MNP), pyridyl-N-oxide-tert-butyl nitrone (POBN), 2,2,6,6-tetramethylpiperidine-1-oxyl (TEMPO), and 2-ethyl-2,5,5-trimethyloxazolidine (OXANOH). Spin-trapping agents behave with some specific affinity for free radicals: DMPO is useful for trapping superoxide anion or hydroxyl radical (Fig. 3) while PBN, a lipophilic agent, preferentially reacts with lipid radicals (Fig. 3).

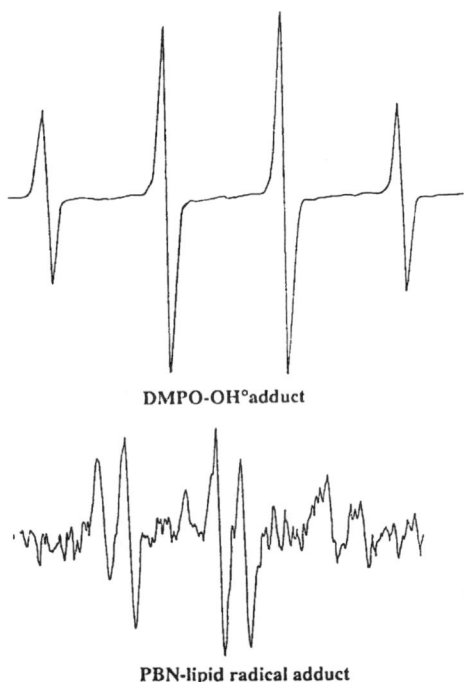

Fig. 3: ESR spectra of DMPO-OH• and PBN-lipid radical spin adduct

Other Free Radicals

Some radicals can be detected in biological samples by ESR without using spin-trap agents. Ascorbyl radical is one such radical since the free electron can be delocalized on the whole molecule, giving rise to a very stable free radical species that can be easily evidenced at room temperature in tissue or plasma (Fig. 4). Nitric oxide (NO•), recognized as endothelial-derived release factor (EDRF), is a free radical which binds firmly to hemoglobin (Hb) to form a stable species •NOHb [23], the ESR spectrum of which can be obtained at 77°K.

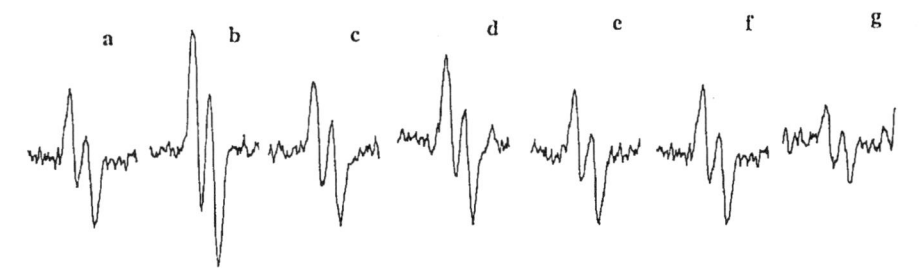

Fig. 4: Time course of ascorbyl radical during human kidney transplantation. Spectrum a, blood sample taken from the renal artery just prior to graft reperfusion. Spectra b-g, blood samples taken from the renal vein immediately, 5, 10, 15, 20 and 30 min after graft reperfusion, respectively. After collection, blood samples were immediately spun (1000 g, 5 min) and a 1-ml aliquot of plasma was added to 1 ml dimethysulfoxide (DMSO). Samples were frozen on ice until ESR analysis, which was performed within 30 min of the collection of the last blood sample.

ESR Animal Studies on Ischemia Reperfusion

Heart

Reperfusion of ischemic myocardium is recognized as potentially beneficial because mortality is directly related to infarct size, and the latter is related to the severity and duration of ischemia. However, the restoration of coronary artery blood flow by methods such as thrombolytic agents or coronary artery bypass is associated with extension of injury that is additive to that produced by ischemia alone.

With or without (freezing technique) using spin traps, several ESR studies [1, 14, 16, 22, 27, 34, 44, 50, 51, 56] with isolated hearts provided direct evidence that cardiac ischemia and reperfusion are associated with increased free radical generation. With the freezing technique, Rao et al. [40] observed increased ESR signals in myocardial tissue after 15 min of ischemia in open-chest dogs. However, it is likely that ESR signals observed at 77°K arose from electron transfer centers of the respiratory chain and could not be attributed to the appearance of oxygen free radicals [52]. In very elegant studies, Bolli et al. [3] and recently Li et al. [25] provided indisputable proof that free radicals were generated since, after intracoronary infection of spin-trap PBN, these authors were able to detect ESR signals within the coronary venous effluent in open-chest or conscious dogs submitted to 15 min of coronary occlusion and reperfusion. The production of free radicals assigned as lipidic radicals started within seconds after reperfusion to reach a maximum value after 5 min, confirming in vitro observations. After this initial burst, the production of free radicals decreased but persisted for up to 3 h after reflow. In these dog models, administration of PBN was significantly correlated with an improvement of postischemic recovery of function, likely due to the free radical scavenging activity of PBN. In other ESR studies, Bolli et al. [4, 5] showed that infusion of antioxidant agents (superoxide dismutase, N-(2-mercaptopropionyl)-glycine, desferrioxamine) before but not after the reperfusion were able to markedly inhibit free radical production but also to improve postischemic myocardial dysfunction. An experiment with desferrioxamine, an iron chelator, emphasized the pathogenic role of iron-catalyzed free radical reaction in heart ischemia-reperfusion injury [6].

Kidney

After aortic infusion of PBN, we provided the first ESR evidence that renal ischemia for 60 min followed by subsequent reperfusion for 10 min in rabbit provoked the appearance of signals in the renal venous effluent [36]. The ESR signals were consistent with a nitroxy-radical adduct resulting from the spin-trapping of PBN of either oxygen- or carbon-centered lipidic radicals, in agreement with Bolli's study. The intensity of free radical production was related to the duration of ischemia ESR signals [13]. Regarding the time course of in vivo free radical production, a weak intensity signal was generally observed within the 3rd minute after reperfusion, then its intensity progressively increased to form a well-defined asymmetric signal after 10 min of reperfusion [39]. Similar to in the heart, this observation indicates that a burst of free radical production took place in the early phase after restoration of flow in the ischemic kidney and is in line with a recent study by Haraldsson et al. [17], who used OXANOH as another spin-trapping agent. The same group [31] also evidenced that i.v. administration of superoxide dismutase, as the free radical destroyer, before ischemia and before reperfusion prevented 85% of the radical formation seen in control animals.

Brain

The lipid peroxidation process induced by massive free radical production is thought to play a key role in central nervous system (CNS) injury and stroke (e.g., ischemia). Indeed, the brain is particularly sensitive to oxygen radical damage because of the high levels of polyunsaturated lipids, a poor antioxidant defense and the presence of an elevated concentration of nonbinding iron [19].

Lange et al. [24] demonstrated in pig the production of carbon-centered free radicals in the efflux during ischemia after infusion of PBN through ventriculocisternal perfusion. In the gerbil pretreated with PBN, Oliver et al. [32] reported the presence of ESR spectra in the lipid extract of cortical homogenates after a transient occlusion (10 min) of both common carotid arteries followed by 60 min of reperfusion. Interestingly, PBN administration, presumably by its radical scavenging properties, could also partially prevent protein oxidation in the brain and protect from loss of glutamine synthetase activity, which is very sensitive to free radical activity. Such protective action of PBN in ischemia-reperfusion injury of brain was later confirmed since it has been shown that PBN administration could reduce the damage to the hippocampal CAI pyramidal cell layer observed 5 days postischemia in rat [9] and could also significantly attenuate hydroxyl radical production in gerbil as assessed by ESR [41].

Recently, Zini et al. [55] detected extracellular free radicals during brain ischemia and reperfusion by intracerebral microdialysis coupled to the spin-trapping technique. Using POBN as the spin-trapping agent, they found in striatal perfusate samples of rats subjected to four-vessel occlusion a radical adduct during ischemic insult, the intensity of which was significantly increased during the first 30 min of reperfusion. These findings are in agreement with a recent study by Phillis and Sen [33], who monitored in a similar model of brain ischemia the release of free radicals from cerebral hemispheres using a cortical cup technique in conjunction with POBN. These authors also demonstrated that animal pretreatment with oxypurinol (40 mg/kg i.p.), a xanthine oxidase inhibitor, could practically abolish free radical production.

Nitric oxide radical is thought to be implicated in the development of ischemic brain injury. Using ESR, Tominaga et al. [48] recently demonstrated the potentiation of NO• production during rat cerebral ischemia. In order to increase the life span of NO• in tissue, they used a spin-trapping technique which consisted of separately administering diethyldithiocarbamate (DETC) and iron, both molecules forming a complex in vivo which can trap NO•.

Intestine and Gut

Intestine is a particularly sensitive target organ for hypoperfusion damage since the mucosa loses its integrity and allows access to the circulation for microorganisms and toxins. Moreover, intestine is extremely rich in xanthine dehydrogenase that can be converted within a few seconds of ischemia into the free radical generating xanthine oxidase [28].
Nilsson et al. [30] evidenced free radical formation with ESR technology during 2 h of intestinal ischemia in the cat at a blood flow < 5 ml/min per 100 g, followed by 30 min reperfusion. Using OXANOH, which reacts with in vivo free radicals to form OXANO• radical, they found that the burst of free radical production which occurred within the first minutes after reperfusion could be significantly prevented by manipulating intestinal blood flow at 8-15 ml/min per 100 g or by inhibiting xanthine oxidase with allopurinol. Recently, Sonoda et al. [45] were able to evidence ESR signals of PBN adducts in the gastric mucosa subjected to ischemia-reperfusion.

Liver

Both storage and reperfusion injury are strongly associated with organ transplantation. Following cold storage of liver in University of Wisconsin (UW) solution during 48 h at +4°C, Gao et al. [15] transplanted the organ into rat and reperfused with oxygenated blood containing PBN. Under these experimental conditions, they were able to detect strong ESR signals and assigned to lipidic radicals in blood samples collected from the suprahepatic vena cava since the beginning of reperfusion. Such free radical production was associated with liver damage as evidenced by increase in serum glutamic oxaloacetic transaminase (SGOT). However, if liver was rinsed after the cold storage and just prior to transplantation with Carolina rinse solution, which contains antioxidants (allopurinol, desferrioxamine), no ESR signal could be detected at reperfusion. Such a decrease in free radical formation was associated with a significant improvement in survival of liver graft and reduction in the release of SGOT.
In a similar ESR study, Takeuchi et al. [46] studied free radical production after in vivo reperfusion of a canine heart-lung transplant immersed in UW solution and preserved for 4 h at =4°C. In blood samples taken from the pulmonary vein and placed in tubes containing PBN as spin trap, they were able to evidence an ESR signal after 60 min of reperfusion, the intensity of which could be significantly reduced by a prostacyclin analog infused from 10 min before to 15 min after the onset of reperfusion.

Muscle

Hypotension during general anesthesia is considered triggering factor of equine postanesthetic myopsitis (EPAM), but local factors, such as a dramatic increase in the intracompartmental muscle pressure, could also play a prominent role. Existence of ischemic-reperfusion phenomena related to the generation of free radicals in experimental EPAM has been recently provided by ESR spectroscopy associated with the use of PBN as spin-trap agent [42].

Endotoxemia and Sepsis

Because of the gross hemodynamic instability and changes in microcirculatory perfusion, ischemia-reperfusion phenomena are thought to occur during septic states. ESR investigations using (MeO$_3$) PBN as spin trap have been conducted to detect endotoxin-induced free radical generation in rat liver [7] and rabbit lung [29]. In a primate model receiving DMPO as spin trap, Lloyd et al. [26] recently demonstrated that infusion of *E. coli* resulted in he appearance of ESR-detectable free radicals in liver and blood lipid extracts. Exogenously administered tumor necrosis factor (TNF) led to an increase in the intensity of the ESR signals, suggesting that this molecule plays a key role as a central mediator of tissue injury during sepsis and septic shock. In another model of endotoxin shock in rat, Westenberger et al. [54] detected in blood ESR a free radical signal assigned as the nitric oxide (NO$^\bullet$) adduct of hemoglobin.

ESR Clinical Investigations

Except for ascorbyl radical and NO$^\bullet$ detection [8, 53], direct transposition to humans of these ESR methods is not possible since spin-trap agents must be infused at a high concentration not devoid of toxicity. However, this problem can be solved with a noninvasive spin-trapping technique consisting of drawing blood samples into syringes containing a sterile spin-trap agent (ex vivo reaction). In the field of ischemia-reperfusion, an initial application of this technique was made by Coghlan et al. [10], who showed increased free radical production after reperfusion of infarcting tissue in a road traffic injured man undergoing delayed repair of a transected aorta. The same authors [11] also evidenced ESR signals in PBN-treated blood taken from the coronary sinus of patients undergoing percutaneous transluminal coronary angioplasty, an ideal model of myocardial ischemia-reperfusion. As only small ESR signals could be detected during ischemia, the authors concluded that reperfusion was the necessary condition for significant radical detection.

Using DMPO as the spin-trapping agent, Culcasi et al. [12] also evidenced increased DMPO-OH$^\bullet$ formation in the coronary sinus blood drawn from patients subjected to cardiopulmonary bypass (CBP) in the first 20 min following aortic declamping. With PBN, Tortolani et al. [49] demonstrated a biphasic profile of free radical production in the coronary sinus blood with an initial burst 5 - 10 min after heart reperfusion followed by a second maximum at 25 min. We confirmed that CPB is well associated with free radical production since we evidenced the appearance of a characteristic spectrum of a stable lipid-based radical spin adduct of PBN in the peripheral blood of similar patients, in parallel to strong vitamin E consumption [18].

During human kidney transplantation, we recently provided direct initial evidence of a growing free radical production in PBN-treated blood samples drawn from the renal vein immediately after the graft reperfusion [38]. Such direct evidence was associated with the decrease in plasma vitamin E, an index of the lipoperoxidation phenomenon, and the increase in plasma myeloperoxidase, a marker of leukocyte activation, a great source of free radical generation.

In addition to noninvasive spin-trapping, the ESR detection in plasma of ascorbyl free radical, which is directly dependent on the ascorbate concentration, has been proposed as another reliable indicator of free-radical-mediated ischemic and postischemic injury [35, 43]. Pilot studies in our patients undergoing renal transplantation indicate that the ascorbyl radical signal intensity shows a large tendency to increase immediately after the restoration of blood flow in the graft (Fig. 4).

From all these ESR studies in humans, it can be concluded that a burst of free radical production takes place in the early phase (within a few minutes) after restoration of flow into the organ, in agreement with data obtained from animal studies.

Conclusion

The use of reliable markers for free radical generation in clinical situations in which ischemia-reperfusion states occur is becoming more and more a necessity. Due to its direct visualization of the phenomenon, there is no doubt that the use of electron spin resonance spectroscopy to detect free radicals in clinical studies will strongly increase in the near future. Cost, size, manipulation of the device but also time between the taking of blood and ESR analysis are considered to be the factors limiting its use in clinical routine. During open-chest surgery in man, we are, however, able to obtain before end of surgery data about the time course of ascorbyl free radical production in the coronary sinus after declamping the aorta. In this way, surgeons can establish a possible correlation between free radical production and clinical parameters.

Moreover, by its ability to provide an integrated measure of free radical production over a given period (e.g., in controlled ischemia-reperfusion), this methodology can delineate the production over time of free radicals. This should afford interesting data in order to clarify our knowledge as to the exact role played by free radicals in ischemic and postischemic injury but also in the protective mechanisms of antioxidant agents (allopurinol, vitamin E, desferrioxamine, lazaroids, etc.).

A final point that must be brought to light is that, like other techniques of free radical determination, the use of ESR spectroscopy is not without its pitfalls. Many suspect interpretations of the results are possible since the appearance of an ESR signal could sometimes be related to a non free radical process (for review see [47]). As an example, DMPO spin trap in the presence of iron gives an ESR signal which is indistinguishable from the signal due to the reaction of DMPO with hydroxyl radical. Well-defined control conditions but also a profound knowledge of ESR spectroscopy are therefore required. The development of ESR spectroscopy coupled with electrospray ionization mass spectrometry and liquid chromatography will also be helpful in providing better comprehensive information about the structures of the radical adduct and avoiding false interpretations of ESR signals [21].

References

1. *Arroyo CM, Kramer JH, Dickens BF et al. (1987) Identification of free radicals in myocardial ischemia/reperfusion by spin trapping with nitrone DMPO. FEBS Letters 221: 101-104*
2. *Bast A, Goris RJA (1989) Oxidative stress. Biochemistry and human disease. Pharm Weekbl 11: 199-206*
3. *Bolli R, Patel BS, Jeroudi M et al. (1988) Demonstration of free radical generation in "stunned" myocardium of intact dogs with the use of the spin trap alpha-phenyl-N-tert-butyl nitrone. J Clin Invest 82: 476-485*

4. Bolli R, Jeroudi M, Patel BS et al. (1989a) Direct evidence that oxygen-derived free radicals contribute to postischemic myocardial dysfunction in the intact dog. Proc Natl Acad Sci USA 86: 4695-4699
5. Bolli R, Jeroudi M, Patel BS et al. (1989b) Marked reduction of free radical generation and contractile dysfunction by antioxidant therapy begun at the time of reperfusion. Circ Res 65: 607-622
6. Bolli R, Patel BS, Jeroudi MO et al. (1990) Iron-mediated radical reactions upon reperfusion contribute to myocardial "stunning". Am J Physiol 259: H1901-1911
7. Bracket DJ, Lai EK, Lerner MR et al. (1989) Spin trapping of free radicals produced in vivo in heart and liver during endotoxemia. Free Rad Res Commun 7: 3-6
8. Cantilena LR, Smith RP, Kruszyna H et al. (1992) Nitric oxide hemoglobin in patients receiving nitroglycerin as detected by electron paramagnetic resonance spectroscopy. J Lab Clin Med 120: 902-907
9. Clough-Helfman C, Phillis JW (1991) The free radical trapping agent N-tert-butyl--alpha-phenylnitrone (PBN) attenuates cerebral ischaemic injury in gerbils. Free Rad Res Commun 15: 177-186
10. Coghlan JG, Flitter WD, Isley CD et al. (1991a) Reperfusion of infarcted tissue and free radicals. Lancet 338: 1145
11. Coghlan JG, Flitter WD, Holle AE et al. (1991b) Detection of free radicals and cholesterol hydroperoxides in blood taken from the coronary sinus of man during percutaneous transluminal coronary angioplasty. Free Rad Res Commun 14: 409-417
12. Culcasi M, Pietri S, Carrière I et al. (1993) Electron-spin-resonance study of the protective effects of Ginkgo biloba extract (EGb 761) on reperfusion-induced free-radical generation associated with plasma ascorbate consumption during open-heart surgery in man. In: Ferradini C, Deroy-Lefaix MT, Christen Y (eds.) Advances in Ginkgo biloba extract research, vol 2. Ginkgo biloba extract (EGb 761) as a free radical scavenger. Elsevier, Paris, pp. 153-162
13. Defraigne JO, Pincemail J, Franssen C et al. (1993) In vivo free radical production after cross-clamping and reperfusion of the renal artery in the rabbit. Cardiovasc Surg 1: 343-349
14. Flaherty JT, Weisfeldt ML (1988) Reperfusion injury, Free Rad Biol Med 5: 409-419
15. Gao W, Currin RJ, Lemasters JJ et al. (1992) Reperfusion rather than storage injury predominates following long-term (48 h) cold storage of grafts in UW solution: studies with Carolina rinse in transplanted rat liver. Transp Int 5: S329-S335
16. Garlick PB, Davies MJ, Hearse DJ et al. (1987) Direct detection of free radicals in the reperfused rat heart using electron spin resonance spectroscopy. Circ Res 61: 757-760
17. Haraldsson G, Nilsson U, Bratell S et al. (1992) ESR-measurement of production of oxygen radicals in vivo before and after renal ischemia in the rabbit. Acta Physiol Scand 146: 99-105
18. Hartstein G, Pincemail J, Deby-Dupont G et al. (1993) Evidence for free radical formation during cardiopulmonary bypass in man. Anesthesiology 79(3A): 140 (abstract)
19. Halliwell B (1992) Reactive oxygen species and the central nervous system. In: Packer L, Prilipko L, Christen Y (eds.) Free radicals in the brain. Springer, Berlin, Heidelberg, New York, pp. 21-40
20. Hoff AJ (1989) Advanced EPR: applications in biology and biochemistry. Elsevier, Amsterdam
21. Iwahashi H, Parker CE, Mason RP et al. (1992) Combined liquid chromatography/electron paramagnetic resonance spectrometry/electrospray ionization mass spectrometry for radical identification. Anal Chem 1: 2244-2252
22. Kramer JH, Arroyo CM, Dickens BJ et al. (1987) Spin-trapping evidence that graded myocardial ischemia alters post-ischemic superoxide formation. Free Rad Biol Med 3: 153-159

23. Kruszyna H, Kruszyna R, Smith RP et al. (1987) Red blood cells generate nitric oxide from directly acting, nitrogenous vasodilators. Toxicol Appl Pharmacol 91: 429-438
24. Lange DG, Kirsch JR, Helfaer M et al. (1990) In vivo model of ischemia/reperfusion induced free-radical formation in CNS of pigs using spin-traps and electron paramagnetic resonance techniques. Free Rad Biol Med 9: 97 (abstract)
25. Li X-Y, McCay PB, Zughaib M et al. (1993) Demonstration of free radical generation in the "stunned" myocardium in the conscious dog and identification of major differences between conscious and open-chest dogs. J Clin Invest 92: 1025-1041
26. Lloyd SS, Chang AK, Taylor FT et al. (1993) Free radicals and septic shock in primates: the role of tumor necrosis factor. Free Rad Biol Med 14: 233-242
27. Maupoil V, Rochette L (1988) Evaluation of free radical and lipid peroxide formation during global ischemia and reperfusion in isolated perfused rat heart. Cardiovasc Drugs Ther 2: 615-621
28. McCord JM (1985) Oxygen-derived free radicals in post-ischemic tissue injury. N Engl J Med 312: 159-163
29. Murphy PG, Myers DS, Webster NR et al. (1991) Direct detection of free radical generation in an in vivo model of acute lung injury. Free Rad Res Commun 15: 167-176
30. Nilsson UA, Lundgren O, Haglind E et al. (1989) Radical production during in vivo intestinal ischemia and reperfusion in the cat. Am J Physiol 257: G409-G414
31. Nilsson UA, Haraldsson G, Bratell S et al. (1993) ESR-measurement of oxygen radicals in vivo after renal ischemia in the rabbit. Effects of pretreatment with superoxide dismutase and heparin. Acta Physiol Scand 147: 263-270
32. Oliver CN, Sarke-Reed PE, Stadtman ER et al. (1990) Oxidative damage to brain proteins, loss of glutamine synthetase activity, and production of free radicals during ischemia/reperfusion-induced injury in gerbil brain. Proc Natl Acad Sci USA 87: 5144-5147
33. Phillis JW, Sen S (1993) Oxypurinol attenuates hydroxyl radical production during ischemia/reperfusion injury of the rat cerebral cortex: an ESR study. Brain Res 628: 309-312
34. Pietri S, Culcasi M, Cozzone PJ (1989) Real-time continuous-flow spin trapping of hydroxyl radical in the ischemic and post-ischemic myocardium. Eur J Biochem 186: 163-173
35. Pietri S, Culcasi M, Stella L et al. (1990) Ascorbyl free radical as a reliable indicator of free-radical-mediated myocardial ischemic and post-ischemic injury. Eur J Biochem 193: 845-854
36. Pincemail J, Defraigne JO, Franssen C et al. (1990) Evidence of in vivo free radical generation by spin trapping with alpha-phenyl-N-tert-butyl nitrone during ischemia-reperfusion in rabbit kidneys. Free Radic Res Commun 9: 3-6
37. Pincemail J, Deby-Dupont G, Lamy M (1992) Biochemical alterations in ischemia and reperfusion. In: Vincent JL (ed.) Yearbook of intensive care and emergency medicine. Springer, Berlin, Heidelberg, New York, pp. 104-114
38. Pincemail J, Defraigne JO, Franssen C et al. (1993) Evidence for free radical formation during human kidney transplantation. Free Rad Biol Med 15: 343-348
39. Pincemail J, Detry O, Philippart C et al. (1995) Diaspirin crosslinked hemoglobin: absence of increased free radical generation following administration in a rabbit model of renal ischemia and reperfusion. Free Rad Biol Med 19: 1-9
40. Rao PS, Cohen MV, Mueller HS (1983) Production of free radicals and lipid peroxides in early experimental myocardial ischemia. J Mol Cell Cardiol 15: 713-716
41. Sen S, Phillis JW (1993) Alpha-phenyl-tert-butyl-nitrone (PBN) attenuates hydroxyl radical production during ischemia-reperfusion injury of rat brain: an EPR study. Free Rad Res Commun 19: 255-265

42. Serteyn D, Pincemail J, Mottard E et al. (1994) Myopathie postanesthésique équine (MPAE): une approche directe pour la mise en évidence des phénomènes radicalaires. Can J Vet Res 58: 303-312
43. Sharma MK, Buettner GR, Kerber RE (1992) Ascorbyl free radical as a real-time marker of oxidative myocardial stress: an electron paramagnetic resonance study. J Am Coll Cardiol 19, 1A
44. Shuter SL, Davies MJ, Garlick PB, et al. (1990) Studies on the effects of antioxidants and inhibitors of radical generation on free radical production in the reperfused rat heart using electron spin resonance spectroscopy. Free Rad Biol Med 9: 223-232
45. Sonoda M, Asakuno G, Matsuki M et al. (1993) Radical trapping by PBN during reperfusion in rabbit gastric mucosa. Free Rad Res Commun 19: S185-S191
46. Takeuchi K, Suzuki S, Kako N et al. (1992) A prostacyclin analogue reduces free radical generation in heart-lung transplantation. Ann Thorac Surg 54: 327-332
47. Tomasi A, Iannone A (1993) ESR spin-trapping artifacts in biological models. In: J Reuben, LJ Berliner (eds.) Biological magnetic resonance, vol 13: EMR of paramagnetic molecules. Plenum, New York, pp. 353-384
48. Tominaga T, Sato S, Ohnishi T et al. (1993) Potentiation of nitric oxide formation following bilateral carotid occlusion and focal cerebral ischemia in the rat: in vivo detection of the nitric oxide radical by electron paramagnetic resonance spin trapping. Brain Res 614: 342-346
49. Tortolani A, Powell SR, Misik V et al. (1993) Detection of alkoxyl and carbon-centered free radicals in coronary sinus blood from patients undergoing elective cardioplegia. Free Rad Biol Med 14: 421-426
50. Tosaki A, Blasig IE, Pali T et al. (1990) Heart protection and radical trapping by DMPO during reperfusion in isolated working rat hearts. Free Rad Biol Med 8: 363-372
51. Tosaki A, Bagchi D, Pali T et al. (1993) Comparisons of ESR and HPLC methods for the detection of OH$^\bullet$ radicals in ischemic/reperfused hearts. Biochem Pharmacol 45: 961-969
52. van der Kraai J, Koster JF, Hagen WR (1989) Reappraisal of the e.p.r. signals in (post)-ischemic cardiac tissue. Biochem J 264: 687-694
53. Wennmalm A, Lanne B, Peterson A-S (1990) Detection of endothelial-derived relaxing factor in human plasma in the basal state following ischemia using electron paramagnetic resonance spectrometry. Anal Biochem 187: 359-363
54. Westenberger U, Thanner S, Ruf HH et al. (1990) Formation of free radicals and nitric oxide derivative of hemoglobin in rats during shock syndrome. Free Rad Res Commun 11: 167-178
55. Zini I, Tomasi A, Grimaldi R et al. (1992) Detection of free radicals during brain and reperfusion by spin trapping and microdialysis. Neurosci Lett 138: 279-282
56. Zweier JL, Flaherty JT, Weisfeldt ML (1987) Direct measurement of free radical generation following reperfusion of ischemic myocardium. Proc Natl Acad Sci USA 84: 1404-1407

Gene Cloning I: Preparation of DNA Libraries

C.W. Schweinfest, M.W. Graber, X.-K. Zhang, P.G. Vanek, D.K. Watson

Introduction

The often stated long-range goal of much molecular biological research is to impact human disease through improved diagnostics and improved therapeutic modalities. Genetic-based diseases such as sickle cell anemia, thalassemia, muscular dystrophy, and cystic fibrosis have been obvious targets for "molecular medicine". More complex diseases such as cancer initiation and progression are also subject to analysis for diagnosis and possible therapeutic intervention by the molecular biologist. Finally, somatic diseases such as atherosclerosis, hypertension, and Alzheimer's disease (of which there are also familial versions) are becoming candidates for intervention by molecular medicine. In addition, the tools of the molecular biologist are appropriate for the basic researcher studying stress-induced gene expression (such as the heat shock gene, hsp 70), the regulation of the nitric oxide synthetase gene and its products, or the induction of cytokines and growth factors as a result of trauma or injury.

Cloning allows the investigator to make a large supply of a purified gene (or its cDNA) and a large supply of that gene's protein product. The purified gene can be used to study how that gene's expression is regulated during physiological alterations of cells. It can also be used as a diagnostic reagent to assess changes in the level of expression of the gene or to assess mutations in diseased tissue. Recently, genes have been used therapeutically to treat adenosine deaminase (ADA) deficiency [5] and to induce an immunological reaction against tumor cells [27]. Another application for a cloned gene (or cDNA) is to make large quantities of protein. This protein, in turn, can be used for structure/function analyses or as an antigen to generate antibodies useful for diagnostic or therapeutic applications. The protein itself may also be useful therapeutically as in the use of human insulin and human clotting factor. In this paper, and in the one that follows ("Gene Cloning II: Screening and Sequencing of Genes"), we will discuss the means by which cDNAs and genes are isolated, amplified, and identified; we will also discuss the strategies and methods for cloning cDNA and genomic DNA, for finding specific genes, and for characterizing those genes. While far from comprehensive, these papers should give the investigator wishing to use a molecular biological approach a basis for understanding the approaches that may be used.

cDNA Cloning

cDNA is the reverse transcribed product of mRNA, so cDNA cloning is typically employed in order to study a gene that is expressed in a particular cell type. This may mean a tissue or a cell line that is the object of an investigator's experiments, but it may also refer to cells which the investigator has perturbed in a very specific way (e.g., heat shock stress, activated T or B cells).

mRNA Purification

cDNA library construction requires that the mRNA template be of the highest quality. This means that great care must be taken to eliminate all possible sources of RNase contamination from the laboratory: all glassware should be baked (200°C for several hours), all nonbakable materials should be treated with 0.1% diethylpyrocarbonate (DEPC) and then autoclaved, as should all solutions which do not contain reactive amines or imines, all nontreatable solutions should be autoclaved; and all nonautoclavable solutions should be made up in DEPC-treated water. Since skin is a major source of RNase, gloves should be worn at all times and should be changed frequently.

Total RNA is prepared using one of the guanidinium salt-based methods [7, 8]. If desired, there are also protocols for specific isolation of nuclear RNA [29], cytoplasmic RNA [4], polysomal RNA [10], or membrane-bound polysomal RNA [24]. Polyadenylated RNA is then purified by affinity chromatography using oligo(dT) attached to a matrix [2]. Traditionally, this has involved oligo(dT) attached to cellulose, however, recent innovations have produced oligo(dT) attached to magnetic beads [20]. mRNA purified through two to three cycles of binding to and elution from oligo(dT) is pure enough to serve as template for cDNA synthesis. Purified mRNA may be further enriched by size selection on sucrose gradients in the presence of the denaturant methylmercury hydroxide [36]. An optional test of the quality of the mRNA is in vitro translation in one of the commercially available mRNA translation kits. The mRNA should be able to direct the synthesis of an array of different sized proteins, including high molecular weight species (200kDa).

cDNA synthesis

The most widely used strategy to create cDNA libraries (see Fig. 1) is synthesis based on the method of Gubler and Hoffman [16] and insertion into a modified λ-phage vector. Synthesis can be initiated at the 3' end of the mRNA template by using an oligo(dT) oligonucleotide primer or can be initiated at random locations along the mRNA by use of random hexamer oligonucleotide to prime first-strand synthesis. The latter approach usually results in a cDNA library of smaller insert sizes, however, it may overcome the problem of creating a library with a relative paucity of 5' ends caused by mRNA secondary structure that causes premature termination of reverse transcription.

All cDNA syntheses utilize reverse transcriptase to synthesize the first strand of cDNA. For directional cloning, it is useful to incorporate a restriction endonuclease site into the primer for subsequent use in cloning the cDNA into the vector. Typically, we utilize the λZAP system (see below), in which the oligo(dT) primer also contains an *XhoI* site. This *XhoI* site will be cleaved later on. First-strand synthesis is then conducted in the presence of deoxyadenosine, deoxyguanosine, and deoxythymidine triphosphate (dATP, dGTP, dTTP) as well as 5-methyl-dCTP (deoxycytidine triphosphate). Second-strand synthesis proceeds without 5-methyl-dCTP (dCTP is used); therefore, the double-stranded cDNA is methylated only on

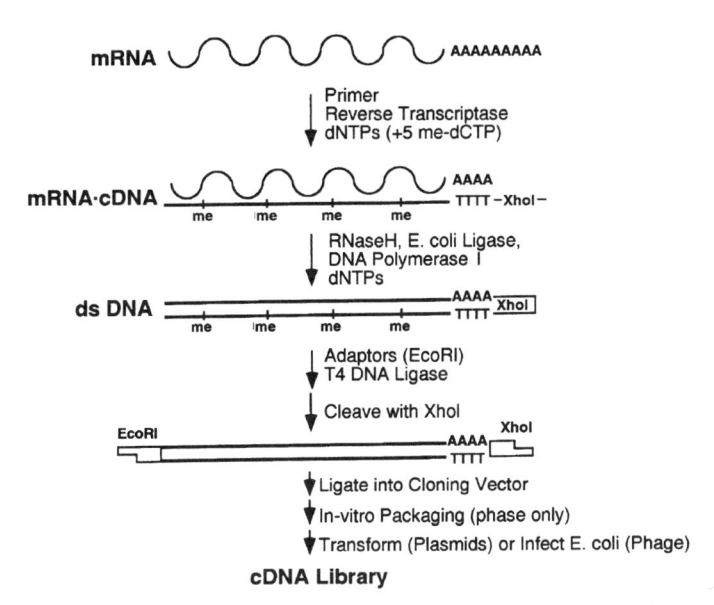

Fig. 1: cDNA synthesis. A basic scheme for synthesizing directional cDNA libraries is shown. mRNA is reverse transcribed into cDNA (first strand) with Moloney murine leukemia virus reverse transcriptase. Second-strand synthesis is accomplished with E. coli DNA polymerase I. EcoRI adaptors are added, and the cDNA is cleaved with XhoI, ligated into a cloning vector and introduced into E. coli. ds, double-stranded; 5me-dCTP, 5-methyl-deoxycytidine triphosphate; NTP, nucleoside triphosphate

its first strand (i.e., it is hemi-methylated). This hemimethylation renders all internal *Xho*I sites uncleavable; however, the *Xho*I site in the primer remains unmethylated and cleavable. Adaptors (short, partially double-stranded oligonucleotides with one blunt end and one restriction endonuclease-cleaved end) for a different restriction endonuclease site such as *Eco*RI are ligated onto the cDNA. The cDNA is then cleaved with *Xho*I which cuts only the 3' (primer) site. The cDNA can now be directionally cloned into the *Eco*RI and *Xho*I sites of the vector. Other restriction site combinations can be used for directional cloning provided their cognate enzymes are unable to cleave hemi-methylated DNA. At least ten other common restriction enzymes show this behavior [28]. For single-site cloning, the strategy for protecting internal sites is a little different. After synthesis of the double-stranded cDNA using oligo(dT) as a primer, a methyltransferase enzyme such as *Eco*RI methylase is used to methylate both strands of its cognate restriction site. Non-methylated linkers (uncleaved double-stranded oligonucleotides) are ligated onto the cDNA ends, and digested, and the cDNA is cloned into the vector. High-quality cDNA libraries typically yield 10^7-10^8 plaque forming units (pfu) per μg insert cDNA.

cDNA Cloning Vectors

The choice of a cloning vector for your cDNA depends, in part, on the intended use of the library. However, most cDNA libraries today are inserted into lambda phage-based vectors.

Lambda vector-based libraries offer several advantages over plasmid-based libraries: (a) more clones (hence a more complete library) per microgram of DNA are generated in lambda vectors than in plasmids; (b) lambda-based libraries are easier to store and handle; (c) lambda libraries are more convenient to screen; and (d) cDNA up to 12 kbp are easily cloned. One scenario in which it may be more convenient to generate a plasmid-based cDNA library would be if its purpose is to transfect the entire library into tissue culture cells for subsequent expression and possible phenotype selection. Here, plasmid DNA is a better format for transfection than phage DNA. In this case, the system of Okayama and Berg [30], in which the cDNA is cloned directly into a plasmid that also acts as a primer for cDNA synthesis, is most convenient. The cloned DNA is then expressed in the transfected cells under the direction of the SV40 virus promoter. A novel lambda vector, ZAP Express (Stratagene), allows for cloning into lambda and expression in *Escherichia coli* under control of the *lacZ* promoter while also permitting conversion to a plasmid form for transfection into mammalian cells and expression under control of the constitutive cytomegalovirus (CMV) promoter.

Some of the most commonly used lambda-based cDNA cloning vectors are listed in Table 1. These vectors have several features worth noting. These are all insertion vectors in which packaging does not require an insert. On the other hand, replacement vectors (used for cloning larger, genomic DNA) must contain insert DNA between the vector arms in order to be efficiently packaged in their protein coats. The vectors shown in Table 1 lack this feature, and therefore it is possible to package a vector lacking insert DNA. As a result, the investigator must adopt a strategy to minimize the production of such "useless" phage. Vectors λgt10, λgt11 and λZAPII all utilize single-site cloning (an *Eco*RI site). Therefore, the arms are digested with *Eco*RI, and then treated with calf intestine alkaline phosphatase. This removes an essential phosphate group from the 5' end of the *Eco*RI site. As a result, the two arms cannot ligate together by themselves, but rather require the presence of these phosphate groups at the 5' ends of the cDNA inserts to permit ligation. A second strategy is to perform directional cloning. Directional cloning is achieved by digestion of the vector at two noncompatible restriction sites (two sites that cannot be ligated to each other) and removal of the small piece of DNA between the sites following digestion. This prevents the two phage arms from ligating directly to each other. Only the insert cDNA can provide the appropriate compatible ends for ligation to the arms, and only this ligated product is packageable as a viable phage particle. Another advantage to directional cloning is that it minimizes the possibility of producing jumbled cDNA inserts. With single site (nondirectional) cloning, two non-contiguous DNA fragments may ligate together (A-A:A-A) as a single insert. While this usually does not occur in any given clone, it can happen. Directional cloning would require the much less likely probability of three fragments ligating in such a way as to produce a clonable insert (A-B:B-A:A-B). Below, we consider some attributes of specific lambda cDNA cloning vectors.

λgt10

This vector contains a single *Eco*RI cloning site located in the gene for the lambda repressor *cI*. Insertion of cDNA into the *Eco*RI site interrupts the repressor gene. Compared to the turbid plaques produced by lambda with an intact repressor gene (cI^+), cI^- phages yield a clear plaque morphology. Therefore, non-recombinant plaques (cI^+ genotype) have a turbid morphology. However, even these nonrecombinants can be eliminated by plating the phage on an *E. coli* strain carrying the high frequency of lysogeny (*hfl*) mutation such as C600*Hfl*. This strain completely suppresses plaque formation in cI^+ phages.

Table 1: cDNA cloning vectors

Vector	Insert capacity (kbp)	Directional cloning	Protein expression (promoter)	In vivo plasmid excision	References (commercial source)
λgt10	0-7.6	No	No	No	Huynh et al. [21] (Stratagene, Gibco BRL, Promega)
λgt11	0-7.2	No[a]	Yes (*lacZ*)	No	Huynh et al. [21] (Stratagene, Gibco BRL, Promega)
λ22A	0-8.2	No	Yes (*lacZ*)	No	Han and Rutter [17] (Gibco BRL)
λZAPII	0-10	Yes	Yes (*lacZ*)	Yes	Short et al. [37] (Stratagene)
Uni ZAP XR	0-10	Yes	Yes (*lacZ*)	Yes	Short et al. [37] (Stratagene)
ZAP Express	0-12	Yes	Yes (*lacZ*, CMV)	Yes	Alting-Mees et al. [1] (Stratagene)
λpCEV27	0-8	Yes	Yes (M-MLV)	No[b]	Miki et al. [25]
λSHlox	0-8	Yes	No	Yes	Palazzolo et al. [31] (Novagen)
λEXlox	0-8	Yes	Yes (T7)	Yes	Palazzolo et al. [31] (Novagen)
λZiplox	0-7	Yes	Yes (*lacZ*)	Yes	D'Alessio et al. [13] (Gibco BRL)
pJuFo	0-7	Yes	Yes (*lacZ*)	-	Crameri and Suter [12]

CMV, cytomegalovirus; M-MLV, Moloney murine leukemia virus.
[a]Gibco BRL and Promega make a modified λgt11 with a *Not*I-*Sfi*I directional cloning site.
[b]Plasmid can be rescued be digestion, circularization, and transformation into *E. coli*.

λgt11/λgt22A

*Eco*RI cloning site in this vector is located in the inducible (with isopropylthiogalactopyranoside, IPTG) *lacZ* gene. cDNAs inserted into this vector have a one in six chance of being expressed as a fusion product with the product of *lacZ*, β-galactosidase. The odds are one in six because the cDNA may insert in one of two orientations, each with three possible open reading frames. There is no genetic selection to favor recombinants over non-recombinants. The repressor is temperature sensitive (*cI857*), therefore lytic phage growth is performed at 42°C (the nonpermissive temperature) whereas subsequent protein induction is performed at 37°C. λgt22A (Gibco BRL) is a variant of λgt11 in which the *Eco*RI site has been replaced by a multiple cloning site (*Not*I, *Xba*I, *Spe*I, *Sal*I, *Eco*RI) to permit directional cloning.

λZAP

These versatile vectors allow for both nondirectional and directional cDNA cloning, depending on whether the vector is digested with a single or two non-compatible restriction enzymes. They all contain a multiple cloning site to allow for directional cloning. The ZAP vectors (Stratagene) are distinguished by the inclusion of a 3-kbp linear plasmid within the phage DNA. The plasmid contains the cloning sites flanked by the RNA polymerase promoters T3 and T7 and is bordered by signals which direct the in vivo excision of the plasmid (plus its cDNA insert). The excision is under the control of genes supplied by a helper phage. The helper phage permits the excised plasmid to be packaged and secreted as a single-stranded DNA virus or to be selected as a double-stranded plasmid by plating bacteria in the presence of ampicillin. All the λZAP are capable of expressing protein from the cloned DNA under the control of *lacZ*. ZAP Express also contains the CMV promoter 5' to the insert cDNA as well as the selectable marker kanamycin. This permits the excised plasmid to be used as a mammalian cell transfection/expression vector selectable in the drug G418. ZAP Express has also been engineered from λZAP to contain more unique cloning sites in the multiple cloning site region.

Another system designed to shuttle between prokaryotic and eukaryotic hosts has been described [25]. As with λZAP, cDNA is constructed in a lambda-plasmid composite vector. However, rather than use in vivo excision, the lambda form of the library is transfected directly into mammalian hosts and selected for by expressing the SV40-driven *neo* gene in the presence of the drug G418. G418-resistant clones are screened or selected for the desired phenotype caused by expression of the cDNA insert under control of the Moloney murine leukemia virus (M-MLV) promoter. Plasmids from these G418-resistant clones are rescued from mammalian cells by digestion of their genomic DNA at the lambda-plasmid junctions and reintroduced back into *E. coli*.

cre-lox Vectors

As with the ZAP vectors, the *cre-lox*-based vectors (λSHlox, λEXlox, λZiplox) are distinguished by the ability to excise a plasmid containing the cDNA insert in vivo. However, the mechanism used to accomplish this is quite different. The plasmid component of these lambda vectors is bordered by two 34bp *loxP* sites from the bacteriophage P1. When these λ-phages are infected into *E. coli* hosts carrying P1 lysogens, the P1-encoded recombinase, *cre*, excises the plasmid plus cDNA insert by recognizing the *loxP* sites. The plasmid also contains a gene to permit selection on ampicillin. λSHlox and λEXlox each contain a multiple cloning site (*Eco*RI, *Sac*I, *Hind*III, *Apa*I) flanked by a T7 and an SP6 polymerase promoter. However, the λEXlox vector also contains a short reading frame from the T7 gene 10 located 5' to the multiple cloning site, which creates a fusion protein with the cDNA insert. The T7 gene 10-cDNA fusion product is induced with IPTG in cells harboring a T7 polymerase gene under *lacZ* control. In λZIPlox, the *lacZ* promoter drives expression of the cDNA insert directly. Furthermore, the level of *cre* recombinase is automatically reduced following excision due to the inclusion of an *incA* site on the excised plasmid. This site interferes with the P1 origin of replication on the host-borne plasmid (pZIP) which carries the *cre* recombinase gene. As a result, when the bacteria divide, the pZIP and *cre* recombinase are diluted out. The excised plasmid with the cDNA is selected with ampicillin. The *cre-lox* method of in vivo excision does not involve a single-stranded DNA intermediate.

Surface Display Libraries

A novel cDNA library system has been recently described [12] wherein the expressed protein products of the insert cDNA are displayed on the surface of a filamentous phage. The phage (M13) is produced by infection of *E. coli* harboring a directional cDNA library in the phagemid vector pJuFo with a helper phage required to package single-stranded phagemid DNA into phage particles. The phage particles carry the expressed cDNA product as a Fos fusion protein inducible under *lacZ* control. The Fos fusion protein is covalently bound to a second fusion protein also encoded by the phagemid, Jun-pIII, which is similarly under *lacZ* control. Protein pIII is a viral coat protein which causes this fusion product to localize to the phage surface. The Fos and Jun moieties of the two fusion products interact by means of their leucine zipper motifs, and disulfide bridges which form upon this interaction make the binding covalent. The phages bearing the expressed cDNA product on their surface are selected by "panning," i.e., sticking the phages to a bound antibody, binding protein, or nucleic acid. The bound phages are then released and reinfected into *E. coli* for use in subsequent rounds. Phagemids containing the desired cDNA at a starting ratio of $1:10^7$ can be purified through four rounds of panning.

Subtractive cDNA Libraries

Subtractive cDNA libraries are enriched for clones of mRNA expressed at higher levels in one cell type or tissue relative to a second cell type or tissue. This allows the investigator to isolate and identify differentially expressed genes for which there is no a priori knowledge. A detailed review of this subject has been recently published [35] however, a discussion of the concept and its application is warranted.

All subtractive cDNA hybridizations work by mixing the nucleic acids of the two cell types being compared (as cDNA-cDNA mixtures or mRNA-cDNA mixtures), allowing the homologous species to hybridize to one another, removing those hybridized or "in common" species and either cloning the remaining "unique" species or using it to probe for such species. One strategy for producing subtractive cDNA libraries is depicted in Fig. 2. In this case, an enrichment for sequences preferentially expressed in carcinoma is shown. cDNA library construction itself is conventional, utilizing the λZAP system because this system can produce the single-stranded DNA used in the hybridization. As indicated in the figure, the use of directional cloning such that the two libraries contain their inserts in opposite orientations to one another assures that only interlibrary hybridization will occur. This results in a two-fold increase in the efficiency of the hybridization. Also note that, in this example, biotinylation of the driver cDNA (the cDNA used in molar excess) permits removal of interlibrary hybrids as well as unhybridized driver cDNA by employing an avidin-affinity matrix. As a result, the unbound cDNA is enriched for sequences present in the carcinoma cells, but not in the normal (driver) cells.

There are many variations to the subtractive hybridization/cloning theme. If the tissue source is not limited, mRNA (as driver) and first-strand cDNA (as target) may be used instead of cDNA libraries [40]. Also, matrix-bound libraries have been used in which the driver cDNA is covalently linked to a latex bead to facilitate physical separation of hybridized target from unhybridized target cDNA [18] or mRNA [19] by centrifugation. Magnetic beads have also been used in this way [32].

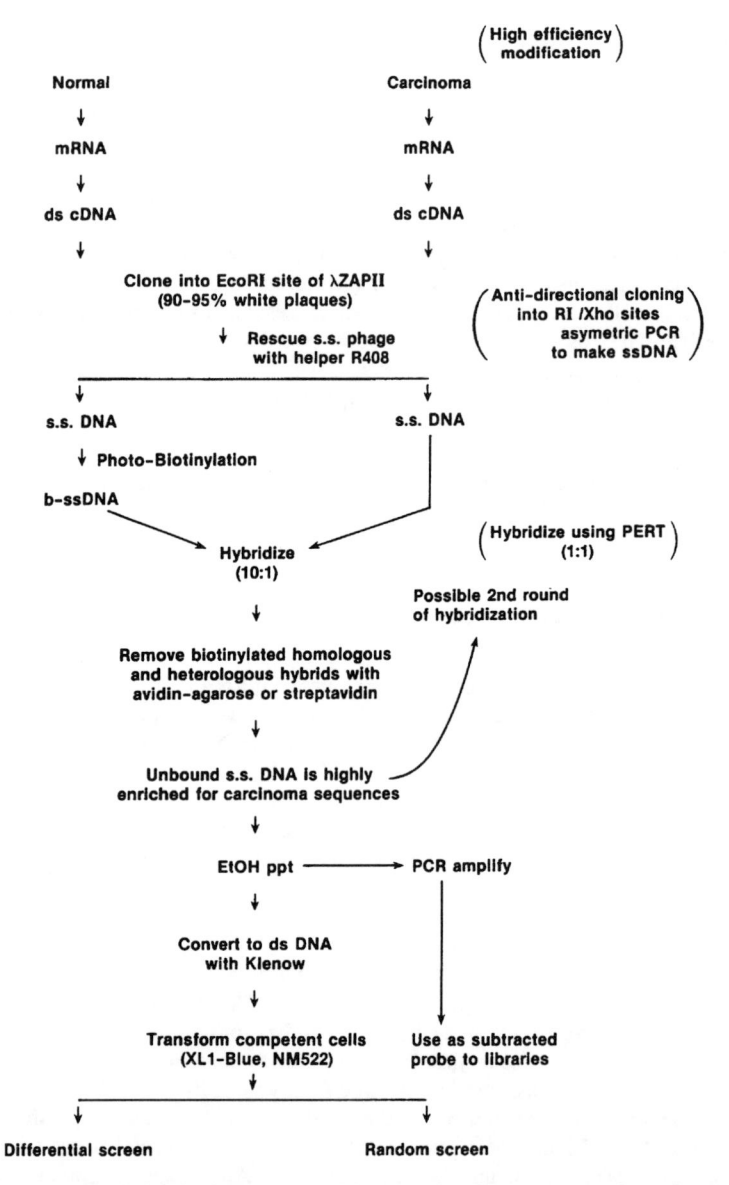

```
                                            ⎛ High efficiency  ⎞
                                            ⎝  modification    ⎠
        Normal                  Carcinoma
          ↓                        ↓
         mRNA                     mRNA
          ↓                        ↓
        ds cDNA                  ds cDNA
          ↓                        ↓
            Clone into EcoRI site of λZAPII
               (90-95% white plaques)         ⎛ Anti-directional cloning ⎞
                ↓  Rescue s.s. phage          ⎜   into RI /Xho sites     ⎟
                    with helper R408          ⎜     asymmetric PCR       ⎟
       ─────────────────────────────────      ⎝    to make ssDNA         ⎠
          ↓                        ↓
        s.s. DNA                 s.s. DNA
          ↓ Photo-Biotinylation
        b-ssDNA
                                              ⎛ Hybridize using PERT ⎞
                    Hybridize ←               ⎝        (1:1)         ⎠
                     (10:1)
                                Possible 2nd round
                       ↓         of hybridization
            Remove biotinylated homologous
             and heterologous hybrids with
             avidin-agarose or streptavidin
                       ↓
              Unbound s.s. DNA is highly ──┘
             enriched for carcinoma sequences
                       ↓
                 EtOH ppt ─────────→ PCR amplify
                       ↓
                 Convert to ds DNA
                   with Klenow
                       ↓
               Transform competent cells     Use as subtracted
                  (XL1-Blue, NM522)          probe to libraries
                       ↓
        ───────────────────────────
          ↓                        ↓
       Differential screen       Random screen
```

Fig. 2: Subtraction hybridization. cDNA libraries for the tissues to be subtracted are synthesized. Single-stranded (ss) cDNA from both libraries is rescued and one is biotinylated. The cDNAs are hybridized to each other and all biotinylated hybrids are removed (subtracted) with avidin-agarose. High-efficiency modifications using directional libraries phenol-enhanced reassociation technique (PERT) for more complete hybridization, and multiple rounds of hybridization/subtraction are indicated. In this example enrichment for cDNA expressed in carcinoma is shown. ds, double stranded; PCR, polymerase chain reaction; EtOH, ethanol

Polymerase Chain Reaction, or Cloning Without Libraries

Perhaps no technique has revolutionized molecular biology more than the polymerase chain reaction (PCR) [34]. PCR amplifies a segment of DNA exponentially, producing more than a million-fold increase in the amount of a DNA fragment (see Fig. 3). Therefore, for certain applications, PCR eliminates the need to generate cDNA libraries and genomic DNA libraries:

1. When part of the nucleotide sequence of a gene is known, it is possible to amplify and clone that DNA directly from a cellular source (genomic DNA or mRNA that is first reverse transcribed into cDNA utilizing primers derived from the known sequence). The 5' ends of the primers can be designed with restriction endonuclease sites to facilitate subsequent cloning.

2. PCR is also useful for amplifying cDNA when only very limited amounts of mRNA are available [3, 42]

3. Since it is not uncommon for cDNA clones to be incomplete, PCR can be used to clone out the remaining portion of the cDNA (typically the 5' end) by a procedure known as rapid amplification of cDNA ends or RACE [15].

4. PCR has also been applied to subtractive hybridization (see Fig. 2 and reviewed in Schweinfest and Papas, [35]) primarily to amplify the small quantities of cDNA that remain following subtraction. This amplified subtracted cDNA can then be used as a sensitive probe for differentially expressed cDNA or can be used for repeated rounds of subtraction.

Primer design should take into account the following criteria: (a) the primer pair should closely matched for length (20-30 nt) and G+C content (30%-70%); (b) regions of complementarity between the primers should be avoided; and (c) the ends of the primers should not contain long A+T stretches.

One of the most elegant uses of PCR for cloning is the technique known as differential display of mRNA [22]. In this method, PCR fragments are generated from reverse transcribed mRNA (cDNA) using primers and conditions that amplify a subset of the mRNA population rather than a single sequence of mRNA. When compared to a similarly selected subset from the mRNA population of another cell type (e.g., cancer versus normal cells; activated T cells versus resting T cells) by display of the PCR products on a sequencing gel, differences among the products become apparent. These different products are then recovered directly from the gel matrix and reamplified for cloning. In this way, gene expression differences can be cloned without making cDNA libraries. Differential display has been successfully employed to isolate differentially expressed cDNA in breast cancer compared to normal breast epithelial cells [23, 33]. The original differential display technique is biased toward the 3' untranslated region of the mRNA and rarely results in a full-length cDNA. However, a recent modification of the technique has been described in which longer cDNA biased toward the coding region are amplified [38]. Also, another thermal-stable DNA polymerase, *Tth pol*, from the bacteria *Thermus thermophilia* has been found to possess reverse transcriptase activity. This allows for both reverse transcription and PCR (RT-PCR) to be performed in the same reaction [26].

Target DNA

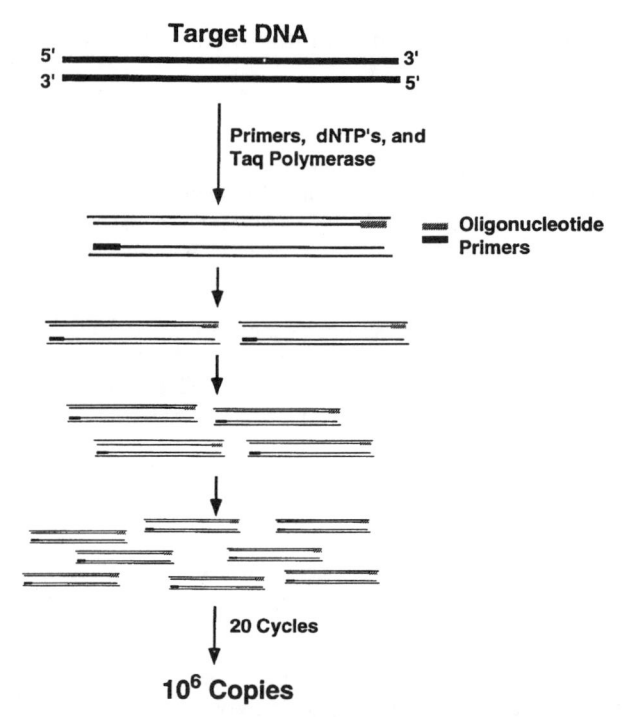

Fig. 3: Amplification of DNA by the polymerase chain reaction (PCR). Excess primers for DNA synthesis by Taq polymerase are allowed to anneal and prime DNA synthesis and are released by melting at high temperature for 20-30 cycles. NTP, nucleoside triphosphate

Genomic Cloning

In order to study the structure of genes and to understand the genetic elements controlling their expression, it is necessary to clone the genomic DNA. The ideal genomic library should contain a set of overlapping DNA fragments with sufficient redundancy to assure a high probability (>99%) that any given DNA sequence in the genome is represented in the library. The overlapping nature of the fragments allows one to "walk" from one clone to another, generating an array of clones representing DNA that is contiguous on the chromosome. Such a library of cloned DNA needs to contain n members where $n=\ln(1-p)/\ln(1-L/M)$, where p is probabilty (usually set at 99%), L is average clone size (in kilobase pairs), and M is haploid genome size (in kilobase pairs) [9]. Clearly, the larger the clone size, the fewer members are required for a complete library. We will briefly discuss the features of several genomic libraries (see also Table 2).

Lambda Replacement Vectors

As with the lambda insertion vectors described for cDNA cloning, these vector systems utilize a bacteriophage and are propagated in *E. coli*. However, unlike insertion vectors, replacement vectors *require* insert DNA (which replaces a nonessential lambda fragment called a stuffer) in order to be of the appropriate size for packaging into viable phage particles.

Table 2: Genomic cloning systems

Vector	Insert size (kbp)	Library size for complete human genome ($p=99\%$)	Host	References (commercial sources)
Lambda replacement vectors ☐ EMBL3 ☐ EMBL4 ☐ λFIX ☐ λDASH ☐ λGEM11 ☐ λGEM12	9-23	10^6	E. coli	Frischauf et al. [14] (Stratagene, Promega) Stratagene Cloning Systems Promega
Cosmids	32-45	3.5×10^5	E. coli	Collins and Hohn [11] Wahl et al. [41] (Stratagene, Gibco BRL)
P1 Phage	75-100	1.7×10^5	E. coli	Sternberg [39]
YAC	300	5×10^4	Yeast	Burke et al. [6] (Gibco BRL)

YAC, yeast artificial chromosomes.

Several lambda replacement vectors are commonly used (see Table 2) which share a few key features: (a) they accept DNA fragments 9-23 kbp in size, (b) they utilize a genetic selection system (*spi* selection) to permit growth of recombinant phage only, and (c) both single-site and directional cloning is possible. Due to their ease of handling, storage, and screening, these are the most commonly used forms of genomic libraries. High quality libraries typically yield 5×10^6 to 5×10^7 pfu/μg insert genomic DNA. Libraries for a wide variety of organisms are commercially available.

Cosmids

Cosmids are similar to lambda replacement vectors in that they can be packaged in vitro as viral phage particles due to the presence of specific DNA sequences derived from λ-phage called *cos* sites. However, cosmids are also like plasmids in that they are relatively small (<9 kbp), double-stranded circular DNA. As a result, cosmids have a larger insert capacity (32-45 kbp) than lambda replacement vectors. Cosmid library yields are similar to those of lambda replacement vectors. Cosmids do not generally provide an advantage over lambda replacement vectors unless it is truly necessary to have large contiguous segments of cloned DNA.

P1 Vectors

Bacteriophage P1 can accomodate up to 100 kbp DNA. The insert DNA is cloned between two *loxP* sites. A 162-bp *pac* site on the vector is required for packaging the DNA.

Concatenated vector plus insert DNA molecules are packaged in vitro into phage heads after which the phage tails are added. This viable phage particle is then infected into an *E. coli* host carrying a P1 gene that constitutively produces the *cre* recombinase. This allows the injected DNA to be circularized by recombination between the *loxP* sites (the same mechanism used by the *cre-lox* cDNA vectors above). A P1 plasmid replicon on the vector allows the DNA to be maintained at one copy per cell, but an inducible P1 lytic replicon permits the copy number to increase to about 20 copies per cell. Up to 10^5 clones can be obtained from 1-2 µg insert genomic DNA.

Yeast Artificial Chromosomes (YACs)

These have the largest capacity of all genomic cloning vectors, i.e., 300 kbp. YACs are linear molecules that replicate autonomously in *Saccharomyces cerevisiae*. They key features of a YAC vector include an autonomous replication sequence (ARS), centromeric DNA, telomeric DNA, selectable markers (TRP1, URA3), and a cloning site located within a phenotypically observable gene (to permit identification of recombinants). High molecular weight genomic DNA is isolated from tissues or cells embedded in agarose after partial digestion with a restriction endonuclease, size-fractionated by pulsed field gel electrophoresis, cloned into the YAC vector, and transformed into the yeast host. YAC libraries typically yield 2×10^2 to 2×10^3 colonies per µg insert genomic DNA. The library is best maintained as individually picked colonies in microtiter wells, although replica plating and colony pooling is faster.

References

1. *Alting-Mees M, Hoener P, Ardourel D, Sorge JA, Short JM (1992) New lambda and phagemid vectors for prokaryotic and eukaryotic expression. Strategies 5: 58-61*
2. *Aviv H, Leder P (1972) Purification of biologically active globin messenger RNA by chromatography on oligothymidylic acid cellulose. Proc Natl Acad Sci USA 69: 1408-12*
3. *Belyavsky A, Vinogradova T, Rajewsky K (1989) PCR-based cDNA library construction: general cDNA libraries at the level of a few cells. Nucleic Acids Res 17: 2919-2932*
4. *Berger SL (1987) Isolation of cytoplasmic RNA: ribonucleoside-vanadyl complexes. Methods Enzymol 152: 227-234*
5. *Blaese RM, Colver KW, Chang L, Anderson WF, Mullen C, Nienhuis A, Carter C, Dunbar C, Leitman S, Berger M et al. (1993) Treatment of severe combined immunodeficiency disease (SCID) due to adenosine deaminase deficiency with CD34+ selected autologous peripheral blood cells transduced with human ADA gene. Hum Gene Ther 4: 521-527*
6. *Burke DT, Carle GF, Olson MV (1987) Cloning of large segments of exogenous DNA into yeast by means of artificial chromosome vectors. Science 236: 806-812*
7. *Chirgwin JM, Przybyla AE, MacDonald RJ, Rutter WJ (1979) Isolation of biologically active ribonucleic acid from sources enriched in ribonuclease. Biochemistry 18: 5294-99*
8. *Chomczynski P, Sacchi N (1987) Single-step method of RNA isolation by acid guanidinium thiocyanate-phenol-chloroform extraction. Anal Biochem 162: 156-159*
9. *Clarke L, Carbon J (1976) A colony bank containing ColE1 hybrid plasmids representative of the entire Escherichia coli genome. Cell 9: 91-99*
10. *Clemens MJ (1984) Purification of eukaryotic messenger RNA In: Hames BD, Higgins SJ (eds.) Transcription and Translation: a practical approach. IRL, Oxford, pp. 211-230*

11. Collins J, Hohn B (1978) Cosmids: A type of plasmid gene-cloning vector that is packageable in vitro in bacteria. Proc Natl Acad Sci USA 75: 4242-4246
12. Crameri R, Suter S (1993) Display of biologically active proteins on the surface of filamentous phages: a cDNA cloning system for selection of functional gene products linked to the genetic information responsible for their production. Gene 137: 69-75
13. D'Alessio JM, Bebee R, Hartley JL, Noon MC, Polayes D (1992) Lambda Ziplox: automatic subcloning of cDNA. Focus 14: 76-79
14. Frischauf A-M, Lehrach H, Poustka A, Murray N (1983) Lambda replacement vectors carrying polylinker sequences. J Mol Biol 170: 827-842
15. Frohman MA, Dush MK, Martin GR (1988) Rapid production of full-length cDNAs from rare transcripts: amplification using a single gene-specific oligonucleotide primer. Proc Natl Acad Sci USA 85: 8998-9002
16. Gubler U, Hoffman BJ (1983) A simple and very efficient method for generating cDNA libraries. Gene 25: 263-269
17. Han JH, Rutter WJ (1987) Lambda gt22 an improved lambda vector for the directional cloning of full-length cDNA. Nucleic Acids Res 15: 6304
18. Hara E, Campisi J (1994) cDNA synthesis and asymmetric PCR on oligotex^{TM} for subtractive cDNA cloning. J NIH Res 6: 77
19. Hara E, Kato T, Nakada S, Sekiya S, Oda K (1991) Subtractive cDNA cloning using oligo(dT)30-latex and PCR: isolation of cDNA clones specific to undifferentiated human embryonal carcinoma cells. Nucleic Acids Res 19: 7097-7104
20. Hornes E, Korsnes L (1990) Magnetic DNA hybridization properties of oligonucleotide probes attracted to supermagnetic beads and their use in the isolation of poly(A) mRNA from eukaryotic cells. Gene Anal Tech Appl 7: 145-150
21. Huynh TV, Young RA, Davis RW (1985) Constructing and screening cDNA libraries in λgt10 and λgt11. In: Glover DM (ed.) DNA cloning: a practical approach, vol 1. IRL, Oxford, pp. 49-78
22. Liang P, Pardee AB (1992) Differential display of eukaryotic messenger RNA by means of the polymerase chain reaction. Science 257: 967-971
23. Liang P, Averboukh L, Keyomarsi K, Sager R, Pardee AB (1992) Differential display and cloning of messenger RNAs from human breast cancer versus mammary epithelial cells. Cancer Res 52: 6966-6968
24. Mechler B (1987) Isolation of messenger RNA from membrane-bound polysomes. Methods Enzymol 152: 241-248
25. Miki T, Fleming TP, Crescenzi M, Molloy CJ, Blam SB, Reynolds SH, Aaronson SA (1991) Development of a highly efficient expression cDNA cloning system: application to oncogene isolation. Proc Natl Acad Sci USA 88: 5167-5171
26. Myers TW, Sigua CL, Gelfand DH (1994) High temperature reverse transcription and PCR with Thermus thermophilus DNA polymerase. In: Whelan WJ, Ahmad F, Baumbach L, Bialy H, Black S, Davies K, Hodgson J, Howell RR, Huijing F, Scott WA (eds.) Advances in gene technology: molecular biology and human disease. Proceedings of the 1994 Miami bio/technology winter symposium, vol 4, p 87
27. Nabel GJ, Nabel EG, Yang Z-Y, Fox BA, Plautz GE, Gao X, Huang L, Shu S, Gordon D, Chang A (1993) Direct gene transfer with DNA-liposome complexes in melanoma: expression biologic activity and lack of toxicity in humans. Proc Natl Acad Sci USA 90: 11307-11311
28. Nelson PS, Papas TS, Schweinfest CW (1993) Restriction endonuclease cleavage of 5-methyl-deoxycytosine hemimethylated DNA at high enzyme-to-substrate ratios. Nucleic Acids Res 21: 681-686

29. Nevins JR, (1987) Isolation and analysis of nuclear RNA. Methods Enzymol 152: 234-241
30. Okayama H, Berg P (1983) A cDNA cloning vector that permits expression of cDNA inserts in mammalian cells. Mol Cell Biol 3: 280-289
31. Palazzolo MJ, Hamilton BA, Ding D, Martin CH, Mead DA, Mierendorf RC, Raghran KV, Meyerowitz EM, Lipshitz HD (1990) Phage lambda cDNA cloning vectors for subtractive hybridization fusion-protein synthesis and cre-loxP automatic plasmid subcloning. Gene 88: 25-36
32. Rodriguez IR, Chader GJ (1992) A novel method for the isolation of tissue-specific genes. Nucleic Acids Res 20: 3528
33. Sager R, Anisowicz A, Neveu M, Liang P, Sotiropoulou G (1993) Identification by differential display of alpha 6 integrin as a candidate tumor suppressor gene. FASEB J 7: 964-970
34. Saiki RK, Gelfand DH, Stoffel S, Scharf SJ, Higuchi R, Horn GT, Mullis KB, Erlich HA (1988) Primer-directed enzymatic amplification of DNA with a thermostable DNA polymerase. Science 239: 487-91
35. Schweinfest CW, Papas TS (1992) Isolation of genes differentially expressed in cancer and other biological systems (Review). Int J Oncol 1: 499-506
36. Schweinfest CW, Kwiatkowski RW, Dottin RP (1982) Molecular cloning of a DNA sequence complementary to creatine kinase M mRNA from chickens. Proc Natl Acad Sci USA 79: 4997-5000
37. Short JM, Fernandez JM, Sorge JA, Huse WD (1988) Lambda ZAP: a bacteriophage lambda expression vector with in vivo excision properties. Nucleic Acids Res 16: 7583-7600
38. Sokolov BP, Prockop DJ (1994) A rapid reverse transcription-PCR procedure for identification of tissue-specifically and differentially expressed mRNAs In: Whelan WJ, Ahmad F, Baumbach L, Bialy H, Black S, Davies K, Hodgson J, Howell RR, Huijing F, Scott WA (eds.) Advances in gene technology: molecular biology and human disease. Proceedings of the 1994 Miami bio/technology winter symposium, vol 4, p 68
39. Sternberg NL (1990) Bacteriophage P1 cloning system for the isolation, amplification, and recovery of DNA fragments as large as 100 kilobase pairs. Proc Natl Acad Sci USA 87: 103-107
40. Sykes DE, Weiser MM (1992) Identification of genes specifically expressed in epithelial cells of the rat intestinal crypts. Differentiation 50: 41-46
41. Wahl GM, Lewis KA, Ruiz JC, Rothenberg B, Zhao J, Evans GA (1987) Cosmid vectors for rapid genomic walking restriction, mapping, and gene transfer. Proc Natl Acad Sci USA 84: 2160-2164
42. Welsh J, Liu J-P, Efstratiadis A (1990) Cloning of PCR-amplified total cDNA: construction of a mouse oocyte cDNA library. Gene Anal Tech Appl 7: 5-17

Gene Cloning II: Screening and Sequencing of Genes

*D.K. Watson, P.G. Vanek, X.-K. Zhang, M.W. Graber,
C.W. Schweinfest*

Introduction

The identification of the genes or gene products that have a role in various cellular processes is fundamental to our understanding of the networks in place that allow response to environmental signals. All levels of the various signal transduction pathways can be molecularly analyzed by currently available methodologies. One important long range goal is to understand human disease and disease progression at the molecular level. The molecular nature of the deficiencies that result in several human diseases such as myotonic and muscular dystrophy, retinoblastoma, cystic fibrosis, neurofibrosarcoma and Ewing sarcoma, have been characterized, already allowing early detection and some prediction of appropriate therapeutic modalities [39]. Indeed, by understanding the normal function of genes, new therapies may be discovered that increase the probability of a successful outcome.

Once a key question for particular field of investigation is adequately defined, the appropriate experimental approaches can be selected. For those questions that require new information at the gene or gene product level, the investigator must immediately address three key issues prior to initiating molecular cloning. First, the nature of the hypothesis will determine the source of DNA: genomic DNA or a DNA copy of mRNA (cDNA, complementary DNA). If the goal is to understand the gene structure (Exon and Intron organization) and gene regulation (5' promoter elements and regulatory elements present throughout the gene), the identification of genomic clones spanning the gene of investigation is important. On the other hand, if one is interested primarily in the gene product(s), isolation of cDNA clones is more appropriate. Second, the investigator must decide on the choice of vector and material for construction of the necessary library (if one is not already available). Third, the reagents available will define the method to be used for clone identification (screening). The preceding chapter ("Gene Cloning I: Preparation of DNA Libraries") provides a discussion of the first two issues while the present chapter provides a brief overview of the methodologies currently available for library screening and sequence analysis.

Screening: Identification of Gene Segments

To test a large number of clones, a bacteriophage library is plated onto a series of bacteriological agar plates. Typically, up to 10^6 clones plated at a high density are handled in one screening experiment. After transfer onto nitrocellulose filter paper [4], an appropriate assay is devised that allows identification of the desired clone. The identification of a particular clone that contains DNA of interest is dependent upon detection of either the nucleic acid or the protein that is being produced by that defined clone present in the library being screened (Fig. 1). Once a desired clone is identified, the same assay is utilized to purify the clone by successive screening at lower densities of the identified pool of clones. The detection of nucleic acid in a clone is carried out by hybridization analysis of the library. Hybridization stringency is dependent on both the size and relatedness (nucleotide homology) of the nucleic acid probe to the target DNA. It is also important that the probe is free of any repeat sequences (e.g., Alu repeats) which might hybridize with many unrelated target clones or sequences that might cross-hybridize with the vector.

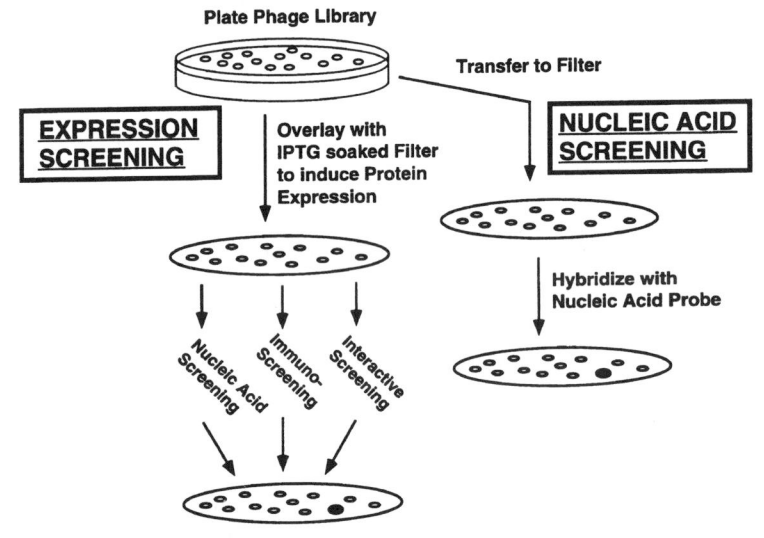

Fig. 1: Screening a bacteriophage library; methodologies used in the isolation of plaques of interest from a recombinant library (screening). IPTG, isopropylthiogalactopyranoside

DNA Probes.

Quite frequently, there might be a DNA fragment of a gene or cDNA for which additional clones must be identified. Because these fragments are longer than synthetic oligonucleotides, hybridization can be carried out under very stringent conditions; for example, 65°C in 1% bovine serum albumin (BSA), 1 mM (EDTA), 0.5 M NaHPO$_4$, pH 7.2, 7% NaDodSO$_4$ [11] for 2 h or overnight. If two regions of amino acid sequence are known, it is also possible to utilize designed oligonucleotides for polymerase chain reaction (PCR) affording amplification of a larger DNA fragment that can be utilized for screening.

Oligonucleotide Probes

The current sensitivity of automated protein sequencers is at the low picomole level and is rapidly approaching the subpicomole level. Proteins can be electroblotted onto polyvinylidene difluoride (PVDF) membranes, detected by staining with Ponceau S or Coomassie blue, released from the membrane and sequenced [34, 38]. Once some of the amino acid sequence for a protein is known, it is possible to design oligonucleotides whose precise sequence is predicted from the DNA genetic code. However, because of the redundancy of the code, several different nucleotide sequences are possible, and thus degenerate sequences are usually designated for oligonucleotide synthesis. It is preferable to design sequences that are directed towards amino acids that have single (Met and Trp) or few (Asp, Asn, Cys, Gln, Glu, His, Lys, Phe, Tyr) codons. In addition, codon preferences are sometimes quite different for different organisms [41] and must be considered when designing sequences. Oligonucleotides are usually 18 bases or longer, with no areas of self-complementarity, and if screening with multiple sequences, care should be taken such that they have similar length and G+C contents. Base pairing between the synthetic oligonucleotide and target DNA is dependent on kinetics of interaction, which is determined by concentration, temperature and salt conditions of hybridization. As a starting point, hybridization is usually carried out at 10°C-15°C below the calculated T_m, i.e., $4(G+C)+2(A+T)$ in $1\ M\ Na^+$ [30]. After overnight hybridization, filters are washed in a high salt concentration buffer (e.g., 6 x standard saline and citrate, 1x=150 mM NaCl, 15 mM sodium citrate, ph 7.0/0.05% pyrophosphate) for 5-15 min at room temperature and then for 15-30 min 45°C. Depending on the amount of background, the washing stringency can be increased by raising the buffer temperature. If multiple conditions are to be tested, it is very important that the filters are not allowed to dry prior to exposure to X-ray film.

Labeling of Probes

Oligonucleotides (5-50 pmol) can be labeled using ^{32}P-adenosine triphosphate ([^{32}P]-ATP; at least 7000 Ci/mmol) and T4 polynucleotide kinase under the conditions recommended by the supplier. DNA fragments are labeled with ^{32}P-deoxycytidine triphosphate ([^{32}P]-dCTP) using the method of random priming [17]. Probes of highly specific activity are necessary to insure that the sensitivity required for detection is achieved; at least 10^9 cpm/μg oligonucleotide or 10^8 cpm/μg DNA are required. In the last several years, many nonradioactive DNA labeling and detection kits have been developed that generate probes labeled with digoxigenin or biotin. Detection is mediated by antibodies to digoxigenin or streptavidin complexes with biotin which in turn are linked to enzymes that catalyze chemiluminescent substrates (Table 1). In addition to lack of potential health hazards and disposal problems, nonradioactive systems are more stable (over 6 months), afford rapid visualization (less than 1 h), and in some cases are more sensitive than radioactive probes. Recently, modifications have been described that have greatly reduced the previous problems with high background encountered with nonradioactive detection systems [15]. Furthermore, a novel and rapid nonradioactive PCR-based screening method has recently been described which reduces the number of cDNA clones to be analyzed [1].

Table 1. Commonly used nonradioactive detection systems

	Trade name			
	Genius	Flash	Lightsmith	Phototope
Sensitivity	1.0 µg for single copy (0.1 pg)	<2.5 µg for single copy	10 µg for single copy	<1.0pg (Target)
Detection	Dioxigenin-11-dUTP, antidigoxigenin antibodies (fluorescent dye, or enzyme linked), or chemiluminescent substrate	Biotin-conjugated (bio-11-dUTP) alkaline phosphatase conjugated probes, chemiluminescence	Direct conjugation of alkaline phosphatase, chemiluminescence	Biotinylated nucleotides, biotinylation/chemiluminescence
Reprobing	Yes	Yes	Once	Yes
Specific filters	Can use nitrocellulose	Flash membrane (neutral nylon); no charged nylon or nitrocellulose	Neutral nylon, no nitrocellulose	Neutral or slightly charged nylon, no nitrocellulose
Probe	DNA, RNA, oligonucleotides, proteins	DNA, RNA, oligonucleotides	Oligonucleotides, DNA, RNA	DNA, RNA, oligonucleotides
Source	Boehringer-Mannheim	Stratagene	Promega	New England Biolabs

dUTP, deoxyuridine triphosphate.

Functional Screening: Expression Cloning

Another approach to the identification of cDNA clones of interest is dependent upon detection of the protein being produced by specific plaques in the library being screened (Fig. 1). Protein produced by a given cDNA clone can be identified by the ability of the protein to bind labeled DNA or RNA (nucleic acid screening), antibody (immunoscreening), ligand/substrate, or defined proteins or peptides (interactive screening). Vectors, such as λgt11, allow the inserted cDNA to be expressed as fusion proteins with β-galactosidase upon induction of the *lac* promoter with IPTG (isopropylthiogalactopyranoside). Such expression is dependent upon proper codon phasing such that the cloned cDNA is expressed in frame with that of the β-galactosidase.

Expression cDNA Library Screening

Before choosing a library to screen, it is important to know that the source of the library expresses the protein of interest. Selection of a suitable library may be accomplished by incubation of protein that has been transferred onto nitrocellulose with antibody (western), labeled DNA (southwestern) or labeled protein (far western). In our laboratory, we currently use cDNA libraries in λgt11 and λZAP II vectors. For screening λgt11, libraries are plated using *Escherichia coli* strain Y1090 cells prepared by growing overnight at 32°C in LB media supplemented with MgSO$_4$ and maltose. A large number (2-3 x 10^6) of plaques gives sufficient probability that a single recombinant bacteriophage will carry a cDNA insert in the correct frame and orientation to allow for expression of the β-galactosidase fusion protein. Twenty thousand plaque-forming units (pfu) are plated per 150 mm Petri dish. Plates are incubated at 42°C (to suppress lysogeny) for 4-6 h until plaques are just visible and then are overlaid with nitrocellulose circles that have been treated with 10 mM IPTG. The plates are shifted to 37°C and incubated for 3.5 h or overnight. During this time, the plaques and the fusion proteins are transferred onto the nitrocellulose.

Nucleic Acid Screening (Southwestern Assay)

Identification of functional expression of DNA binding domains by their high affinity binding to recognition site DNA continues to be a first choice for identification and isolation of transcription factors [43]. In our laboratory, nitrocellulose filters are removed and allowed to dry for at least 15 min, and then processed using a modification of the previously described method [7]. The proteins are denatured by immersing the membranes in LBB buffer (10 mM Hepes, pH 7.8, 10 mM KCl, 3 mM MgCl$_2$, 1 μM ZnCl2, 0.5 mM dithiothreitol) containing 6 M guanidine HCl for 10 min at 4°C. Following five cycles of sequential dilution to 0.5 times the previous concentration, the filter is washed in LBB and then blocked using 5% BSA in LBB. The filter is washed twice in LBB containing 0.1% BSA, and transferred to LBB/0.1% BSA containing 10 μg/ml salmon sperm DNA, 10 μg denatured salmon sperm DNA, and 1-2 x 10^6 cpm/ml of double-stranded DNA probe containing the target sequence. The filter is incubated for 2-4 h with gentle shaking and washed three times with LBB/0.1% BSA. After blotting onto Whatman 3MM paper, the filters are exposed to Kodak XAR-5 film overnight with an intensifying screen to detect clones that produce a protein capable of interacting with the oligonucleotide probe. Positive plaques identified by the first round of screening are subject to a secondary and tertiary screen in which positive plaques are picked and replated at lower density, as described above. An alternative to denaturation - renaturation screening is accomplished by immobilizing expressed proteins on nitrocellulose and incubating directly in binding TNE buffer consisting of 10 mM TRIS-HCl (pH 7.6), 20 mM NaCl, 0.2 mM EDTA, and 0.5 mM DTT. The filters are then processed as above, but in TNE buffer containing BSA and nonspecific denatured salmon sperm DNA. The success of this alternative method requires that the protein retain its DNA-binding capability following immobilization onto nitrocellulose filters. The probe is generated by separately labeling individual strands of target oligonucleotide with [^{32}P]-ATP using T4 polynucleotide kinase according to standard protocols. Labeled complementary oligonucleotides are heated to 95°C and annealed by slow cooling. These double-stranded oligonucleotides are concatenated into longer polymers by ligating them together with T4 DNA ligase for 5 min at room temperature. The reaction is stopped by adding EDTA to a 10 mM final concentration, and heating to 65°C for 10 min. The labeled oligonucleotides are purified using Sepharose G-50. Labeling in this manner generates the very highly specific activity probe necessary for the success of the described methods.

Immunoscreening (Western Assay)

Identification of positive clones by the reaction with defined antibodies provides the investigator with a rapid method to isolate the cDNA for the protein initially utilized to raise the antibodies, as well as to identify genes that encode proteins that are related to the initial antigen [23]. Following protein transfer to nitrocellulose filters, filters can be processed by a variety of methods, including one employed in our laboratory [31]: after washing and hydration of the dried filters in buffer, e.g., TBST (50 mM TRIS, 150 mM NaCl, 0.5% Tween-20), nonspecific protein-binding sites are blocked by incubation with 1% BSA/TBST for 15-30 min. Alternatively, blocking can also be carried out using BLOTTO (5% carnation nonfat milk powder, 50 mM TRIS, pH 7.5, 50 mM NaCl, 1 mM EDTA, and 1 mM DTT; [25], calf serum, gelatin, casein, etc. Filters can then be incubated with the primary antibody (1:200 to 1:1000 dilution; 0.5-10µg/ml in TBST) for 30 min to 24 h at 4°C, followed by several washings with cold TBST buffer. Plaques producing protein that reacts with the primary antibody can be identified by subsequent incubation with ^{125}I-labeled secondary antibody or protein A (about 0.5 x 10^6 cpm/ml) for 2-16 h at 4°C, washing, and exposure to X-ray film. Use of the secondary antibody reduces background signal. Alternative methodologies exist that do not use radioisotopic detection and which are quite sensitive. One method is to use alkaline phosphatase linked to either streptavidin or to the secondary antibody, followed by detection using a colorometric enzymatic assay (BCIP/NBT, Promega).

Interactive Screening (Far Western Assay)

The ability of λgt11 expression libraries to produce expressed fusion proteins that maintain biological activity has been exploited for the identification of calmodulin ligand-binding protein [42] and opioid receptors [26]. These studies utilized labeled ligands to identify and purify plaques of interest. Protein kinase C (PKC) substrates have been recently identified and cloned by a PKC overlay assay using partially purified enzyme to bind to fusion proteins present on the nitrocellulose. After cross-linking the bound PKC with 0.5% formaldehyde, positive plaques were identified by antibody to PKC, visualized by alkaline phosphatase-conjugated second antibody and color development [8]. The interaction between proteins is often of sufficient strength to allow identification of clones expressing a protein by screening with a labeled protein. In order to screen a library, plaques capable of producing a protein or peptide are identified by incubation with a labeled protein. Several interesting genes have been identified by interactive cloning carried out by many investigators who have screened using proteins labeled with ^{125}I [5], ^{32}P [6] or biotin [12]. Presumptive protein-protein interactions may be initially identified by Far-Western blotting [29], coimmunoprecipitation, cross-linking, or protein-mediated pulldown of in vitro or in vivo labeled proteins. These initial experiments allow the investigator not only to have positive indications that protein-protein interactions exist, but also serve to define the conditions most suitable for screening of the expressed library:

1) Far Western analysis: Briefly, 25-50 mg protein is separated by sodium dodecyl sulfate polyacrylamide gel electrophoresis (SDS-PAGE). The resolved proteins are electroblotted onto either nitrocellulose or nylon membranes, followed by LBB renaturation as described above ("Nucleic Acid Screening"). After blocking with 1% BSA, filters are incubated with ^{35}S-methionine in vitro-transcribed/translated protein.
2) Co-immunoprecipitation of cellular proteins prepared with nondenaturating conditions.
3) Crosslinking (with reversible reagents, Pierce) of labeled cellular proteins after mixing with purified protein.
4) Binding of labeled proteins to bacterially expressed proteins linked to agarose beads: Protein is expressed as a fusion protein containing a biotinylated tag and is purified by binging to avidin resin. After washing (conditions identical to those recommended for protein purification), ^{35}S-labeled protein is incubated with the resin at room temperature

for 60 min, followed by repeated washes, and bound proteins are released by boiling in SDS-PAGE sample buffer. Incubation and washing buffer (initially 20 mM Hepes-NaOH, pH 7.9, 25 mM NaCl, 2.5 mM MgCl$_2$, 0.1 mM EDTA, 0.05% NP40, and 1% Triton X-100) can be modified as needed, and appropriate controls (PinPoint System vector alone, preincubation of column with BSA) can be included. Once the interactive conditions are established, labeled protein is applied to nitrocellulose filters bearing the expressed proteins.

Processing and Characterization of Positive Clones

To analyze β-galactosidase recombinant proteins by western and southwestern analysis, preparative amounts of the protein can be obtained by preparing Y1089 lysogens of λgt11 clones. Positive clones are made into phage lysogens by incubating 50 ml of a high-titre stock (over 10^{10} pfu/ml) of the clone with 10 ml of plating *E. coli* Y1089 cells(strain Y1089 lacks a *supF* gene which would enable the phage to lyse its host). Cells are plated at low density onto LB-agar (10 g bactotryptone, 5 g bactoyeast extract, 10 g NaCl, and 15 g agar per l H$_2$O). The plates are incubated at 32°C until individual colonies can be visualized. The plates are replica plated onto second, fresh LB-agar plates, and the new plates are incubated at 42°C for 3-5 h, while the original plates are returned to 32°C for the same period. Lysogens are scored for loss of colony growth at 42°C (the repressor gene of λgt11 is temperature sensitive) and are replated and grown at 32°C. Protein expression from lysogens is driven by the *lac* promoter within the λ-phage and therefore can be induced with 1-5 mM IPTG. Since expression of proteins in the λgt11 system is as a fusion product with β-galactosidase, relative efficiency of expression may be determined using anti-β-galactosidase antibodies, which may be detected using colorimetric assays with alkaline phosphatase or horseradish peroxidase conjugated secondary antibodies.

Alternative Approaches

Lysogen Screening

To increase to sensitivity of expression screening, it is possible to prepare a λ-lysogen library and screen for proteins that are produced by the bacteria containing the prophage. One study has estimated that at least ten times more protein is expressed in a colony than contains a prophage compared to that produced by a single plaque [35]. Using such a prophage library, this study was successful in isolating clones for calmodulin-binding protein by screening with labeled calmodulin; initial attempts to screen the corresponding phage library had proved unsuccessful [35].

Surface Display Libraries/Panning

Another method for functional screening is based upon the display of proteins on the surface of filamentous phage [3]. The key feature of this system is that libraries are cloned such that proteins are expressed as fusions with coat proteins. The pCBComb3 and pComb3 vectors are derivatives of pBC and pBluescript (Stratagene) that have been engineered for cloning combinatorial antibody libraries such that encoded Fab fragments will be expressed as fusions with the gene VIII product coat protein VIII. Phagemids are transformed into *E. coli* strain XL1-Blue cells (Stratagene) and cultures are infected with VCS M13 helper phage for phage rescue. To identify phage, 10^{11} cfu (colony forming units) in 50 µl are incubated in a well of a microtiter plate (Costar 3690) that has been coated with antigen (Fig. 2). Following incubation and washing, phages retained by antigen-antibody complexes are eluted and used to infect bacteria. In this study, protein expression from clones in each round of screening were induced by 5 mM IPTG and colonies were made to react with antigen-labeled alkaline phosphatase. In addition, constructs that contained Fabs of known specificity and affinity were used to demonstrate that enrichments between 10^4 and 10^5 were possible in single-pass experiments. Recently, the pComb3 vector has been modified to create the pJuFo vector system [13, 14]. This system is also based on the expression of cDNA as a fusion protein with the viral coat protein pIII. It is unique in its use of the high-affinity interaction of fos and jun leucine zippers to link pIII-jun to fos-cDNA. It also allows for the dissociation of the cDNA from the phage coat protein by mild treatment with reducing agents. The pJuFo system has been used to identify antigens in a cDNA library by panning with antibody and has afforded an enrichment of 10^7-fold after four rounds of panning. Clearly, phages bearing the expressed cDNA product on their surface can be selected by a variety of panning methods by changing the substrate (antigen, antibody, protein, or nucleic acid) in the microtiter well.

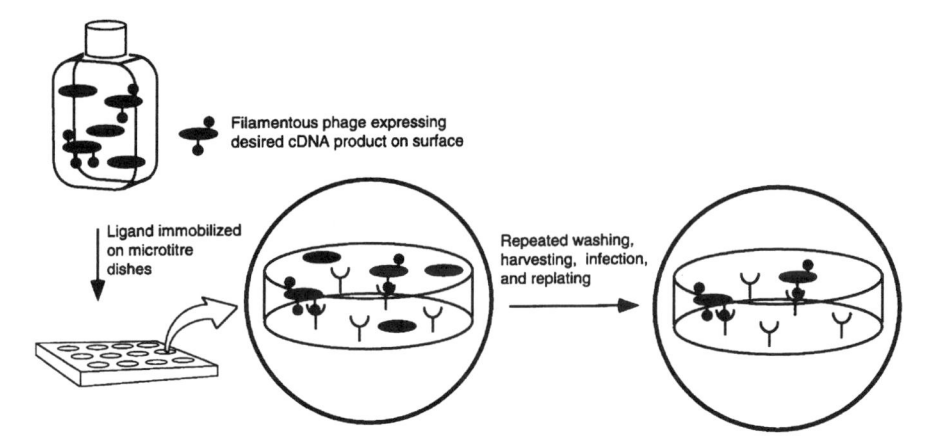

Fig. 2: Procedure for screening surface display libraries. This screening (panning) is dependent upon choice of ligand (antibody, antigen, DNA, or protein immobilized microtiter wells)

Screening other Library Systems

The above discussion has focused on the screening of bacteriophage λ-based libraries utilizing methods that employ nucleic acid hybridization, DNA-protein interaction, and protein-protein interaction. The latter two categories apply strictly to cDNA libraries, while nucleic acid hybridization applies to both cDNA and genomic libraries. More recently, investigators have been building genomic DNA libraries in vector systems other than lambda. One of the motivations for building such libraries has been the Human Genome Project's goal of mapping and sequencing the entire human genome (3×10^9 bp). Libraries with large inserts greatly facilitate the mapping and ordering of genes; several systems for cloning large segments of DNA have been described in the preceeding chapter. Here we will consider some approaches to screening such libraries.

Cosmids. Cosmids are hybrids of λ-phages and plasmids: the phage-derived *cos* sites allow the vector to be packaged as a phage particle [24], while the origin of replication and the selectable marker gene (amp^R) are plasmid-derived. Cosmids do not form plaques and, therefore, they are screened as bacterial colonies [22]. Colonies are plated at high density (10^5 colonies per 82 mm-diameter filter) onto a nitrocellulose filter by slow suction filtration. The colonies are allowed to grow overnight at 37°C or until small colonies appear (1 mm) by transferring the filter to an LB plate containing ampicillin. The colonies are replicated onto another filter and allowed to grow overnight, after which the cosmids are amplified by transferring the filter to an LB plate containing 50 μg chloramphenicol/ml and by incubating at 37°C for several hours. The bacteria are then lysed and the DNA is made accessible for hybridization to probe DNA by standard protocols [21]. Regions with positive hybridization signals are picked from the original nitrocellulose filter (the master filter) and replated at lower density for 1-2 susequent rounds of screening as described above. Some DNA sequences are unstable in cosmids, however, and alternative vectors called fosmids [27] or alternative methods [33] have been described to facilitate the handling of these clones.

P1 Phage. P1 vectors containing up to 100 kbp of DNA are packaged in vitro and injected in vivo into host *E. coli*. Once injected into the *cre*-containing host, DNA with two *loxP* sites will be circularized forming a large plasmid. Upon IPTG induction of the lytic replicon under *lacZ* control, the amount of plasmid DNA increases about 25-fold [44]. Recombinants can be selected for by cloning into the *Bacillus amyloliquifaciens sacB* gene in the vector. Interruption of this gene permits growth on sucrose-containing media [36]. Recombinants are screened as bacterial colonies by the same method described above for cosmids or as pools of clones [37]. Several hundred to a few thousand clones are assembled into primary pools, ten primary pools are combined to form a secondary pool, and five secondary pools are combined to form a tertiary pool. Pools are then screened using PCR, starting with the tertiary pools. Due to the high sensitivity of PCR, target DNA from as little as 4 μl frozen glycerol stock is used. Furthermore, prefrozen pools eliminate the need to grow cells from each level of pool every time a library is screened. Once the primary pool containing the DNA of interest is identified, the individual clone is identified by one to two rounds of colony hybridization.

Yeast Artificial Chromosomes (YAC). Screening DNA cloned into YAC vectors is best accomplished using a heirarchy of pooled clones and the PCR [20]. The YAC library is first arrayed in 96-well microtiter trays. Clones from four such trays are inoculated and grown on a nylon membrane filter, generating a primary pool of 384 clones. Five such filters are combined to generate a secondary pool of 1920 clones. From these secondary pools, DNA is isolated to be used as target DNA for PCR with primers that will amplify the DNA of interest. Once the original nylon filter is identified, clones are screened by hybridization using the PCR product as the probe.

Two Hybrid Systems.

Interactions between proteins can be identified and cloned using the yeast two-hybrid selection system [10], now commercially available (Matchmaker, Clontech, Palo Alto, CA). This method is based on functional reconstitution of the transcriptional activator GAL4. Two separate plasmids are employed, one containing the DNA-binding domain of GAL4 linked to protein X and another containing the GAL4 activation domain linked to protein Y. After introduction into yeast cells, in vivo interaction between protein X and protein Y results in functional GAL4 protein. Because the yeast cells also contain a reporter plasmid *GAL1-lacZ*, which contains a binding site for GAL4 to promote expression of the *lacZ* gene, functional GAL4 can be detected by β-galactosidase activity. In practice, DNA encoding a known protein or region of a protein is cloned to either of the plasmids (in place of X or Y), and a cDNA library is cloned to the other plasmid (in place of Y or X). For this system to be successful, the protein encoded by the gene linked to the GAL4 DNA-binding domain must not have any transcription activation sequences. A recent modification has expanded the utility of this system such that protein-peptide interactions can now be detected [47]. This modification also described cloning a mixture of random oligonucleotides that would encode 16 residue peptides into the activation domain vector. With a complexity of 10^6 different peptides, all possible pentimers and 10% of all possible hexamer peptides are present in the library.

The most important concerns are whether all necessary coponents are present in yeast cells and whether proteins produced in yeast have proper solubility, stability, and post-translational modifications. To circumvent possible limitations to the yeast two-hybrid system, mammalian two-hybrid systems have also been designed. The CRA (contingent replication assay) transfects mammalian cells with three different plasmids [45]. Plasmid G5ET directs the synthesis of SV40 T antigen under GAL4 control. The two fusion vectors (pSG424 and AASVVP16) direct the synthesis of GAL4 DNA-binding domain X and VP16 transactivation domain Y. In this system, protein-protein interaction not only allows functional reconstitution of a transcription activator, but this hybrid activator binds to the G5ET GAL4 DNA-binding site, activating the synthesis of the T antigen that is required for the replication of the AASVVP16-Y vector. Replication of this vector in mammalian cells results in unmethylated copies of AASVVP16-Y, which makes them resistant to *Dpn*I digestion, allowing for further enrichment of replicated plasmids by digestion and transformation into bacteria. The original work demonstrated an enrichment of over 200-fold. The KISS (karyoplasmic interaction selection strategy) also utilizes protein-protein interaction to result in functional reconstitution of the GAL4 activator, but uses some interesting reporter systems (e.g., CD4 and hygromycin B resistance) that may be quite useful when further developed [16]. Both CRA and KISS systems have been evaluated using model hybrids, but have not yet been developed for library screening.

Sequencing of Genes

Once a clone is isolated, it is essential that the DNA sequence of the insert be determined. The two different methods used for sequencing are the chemical cleavage method [32] and the enzymatic chain termination/dideoxy method [40]. The chemical cleavage method is based upon modification of specific bases which are subsequently cleaved by piperidine. This method requires that the radioactive label is present on only one site on the DNA, employs several toxic chemicals and requires more processing time than dideoxy sequencing. The dideoxy sequencing method uses DNA polymerase (e.g, Sequenase, USB Biochemicals) to synthesize a complementary strand from a DNA template previously annealed with a specific oligonucleotide primer (17 bases or longer). Synthesis proceeds until a dideoxynucleotide is incorporated, which blocks further elongation. In practice, each template-primer is incubated with four different mixes, each containing one of the four dideoxynucleotides.

Each sequencing technique generates a collection of oligonucleotides that have been modified/cleaved or terminated with a dideoxynucleotide in a base-specific reaction. Because the oligonucleotides have a fixed end (5'- or 3'-labeled end with chemical cleavage; 5' primer-binding site with dideoxy method) and the other end defined by a specific base, the products for each reaction as a ladder of bands after resolution on a denaturing polyacrylamide gel (5%-6% in 7M urea). Each DNA set is loaded on adjacent lanes, allowing the DNA sequence to be read off an X-ray film from the gel (Fig. 3). To sequence clones that have large inserts (over 400-500 bases), new clone-specific primers based on the sequence obtained are synthesized and sequencing is repeated until the sequence for both strands of the DNA fragment is determined. Two recent studies have described the use of multiple modular primers to speed up large-scale sequencing by "primer walking" [2, 28]. Alternatively, a series of nested deletions throughout the original insert can be constructed (e.g., ExoIII/mung bean system, Stratagene) and sequenced with a limited number of oligonucleotide primers. The creation of ordered deletions has also been improved through the use of PCR [46].

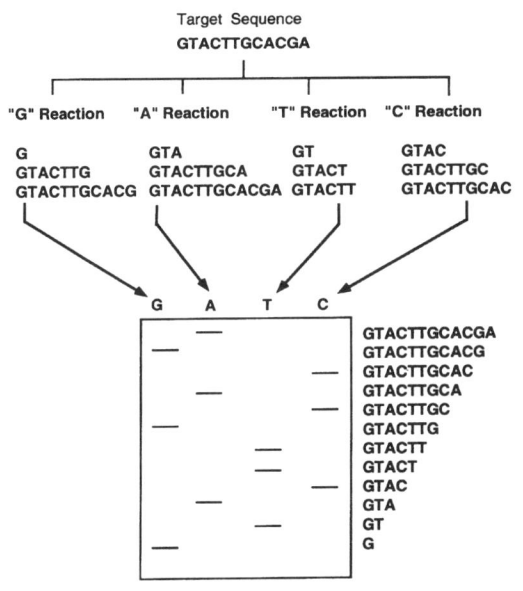

Fig. 3: General strategy for DNA sequencing. To sequence target DNA separate base-specific reactions (chemical modification reactions: G, A+G, A>C, T+C, C; dideoxy: G, A, T, C, as illustrated in diagram, are carried out. The products of these reactions have one fixed end and one end that is defined by sequential termination at each base. Oligonucleotides are separated by electrophoresis on a denaturing polyacrylamide gel, and a set of lanes are "read" off of an autoradiographic image of the gel.

Multiplex sequencing [9] is a modification of enzymatic sequencing that uses an uniquely tagged primer (37-base primer, 17 of which are used to prime DNA synthesis and a unique 20-base segment for later identification by hybridization) for each reaction. The four reactions can be pooled and electrophoretically resolved on the same gel lane. After electrophoretic separation of the oligonucleotides, the gel is transferred to a nylon membrane that is hybridized to oligonucleotide probes specific for each of the four reactions.

Many data entry computer programs have been written that reduce the time required for gel reading. A variety of film readers and automated DNA sequencers are also commercially available and have been compared [18]. Automated DNA sequencers (e.g., ABI 373) are useful for large-scale sequencing projects or are often available through core facilities to validate the large initial investment. Fluorophores specific for each terminator base now allow for single lane analysis. The overall throughput is quite good, able to sequence 36 templates per run at 450 bases each with high accuracy and automated base calling.

Sequence data can be checked against sequences in GenBank and EMBL using the UWGCG (University of Wisconsin Genetics Computer Group) [19] programs to ascertain the uniqueness of the clone identified and to identify any close DNA sequence or protein sequence motifs. The sequence information is also required prior to subcloning into prokaryotic expression vectors, e.g., pET (Novagen), PinPoint (Promega), that afford rapid protein purification. If protein modification is required, clones can be expressed in one of the available eukaryotic expression systems, e.g., Baculovirus/SF-9, pBlueBacHis or yeast, pYesHis (both from Invitrogen). The cDNA clone can also be used to obtain genomic clones to determine complexity and chromosomal position by fluorescence in situ hybridization (FISH).

References

1. Amaravadi L, King MW (1994) A rapid and efficient nonradioactive method for screening recombinant DNA libraries. Biotechniques 16: 98-101
2. Azhikina T, Veselovskaya S, Myasnikov V, Potapov V, Ermolayeva O, Sverdlov E (1993) Strings of contiguous modified pentanucleotides with increased DNA-binding affinity can be used for DNA sequencing by primer walking. Proc Nat Acad Sci USA 90: 11460-11462
3. Barbas CF III, Kang AS, Lerner RA, Benkovic SJ (1991) Assembly of combinatorial antibody libraries on phage surfaces: the gene III site. Proc Natl Acad Sci USA 88: 7978-7982
4. Benton WD, Davis RW (1977) Screening λgt recombinant clones by hybridization to single plaques in situ. Science 196; 180-182
5. Blackwood EM, Eisenman RN (1991) Max: a helix-loop-helix zipper protein that forms a sequence-specific DNA-binding complex with myc. Science 251: 1211-1217
6. Blanar MA, Rutter WJ (1992) Interaction cloning: identification of a helix-loop-helix zipper protein that interacts with c-fos. Science 256: 1014-1018
7. Bowden B, Steinberg J, Laemmli UK, Weintraub H (1980) The detection of DNA-binding proteins by protein blotting. Nucleic Acids Res 8: 1-20
8. Chapline C, Ramsay K, Klauck T, Jaken S (1993) Interaction cloning of protein kinase C substrates. J Biol Chem 10: 6858-6861
9. Chee M (1991) Enzymatic multiplex DNA sequencing. Nucleic Acids Res 19: 3301-3305
10. Chien C-T, Bartel PL, Sternglanz R, Fields S (1991) The two-hybrid system: a method to identify and clone genes for proteins that interact with a protein of interest. Proc Natl Acad Sci USA 88: 9578-9582
11. Church GM, Gilbert W (1984) Genomic sequencing. Proc Natl Acad Sci USA 81: 1991-1995
12. Cicchetti P, Mayer BJ, Thiel G, Baltimore D (1992) Identification of a protein that binds to the SH3 region of Abl and is similar to Bcr and GAP-rho. Science 257: 803-805
13. Crameri R, Suter M (1993) Display of biologically active proteins on the surface of filamentous phages: a cDNA cloning system for selection of functional gene products linked to the genetic information responsible for their production. Gene 137: 69-75
14. Crameri R, Moser M, Dudler T, Menz G, Blaser K (1994) A new cDNA expression system for cloning and selective isolation of functional gene products linked to the genetic information required for their production In: Whelan WJ, Ahmad F, Baumbach L, Bialy H, Black S, Davies K, Hodgson J, Howell RR, Huijing F, Scott WA (eds.) Advances in gene technology: molecular biology and human disease, vol 4. IRL, Oxford, p. 28

15. Engler-Blum G, Meier M, Frank J, Muller GA (1993) Reduction of background problems in nonradioactive northern and southern blot analyses enables higher sensitivity than ^{32}P-based hybridizations. Anal Biochem 210: 235-244
16. Fearon ER, Finkel T, Gillison ML, Kennedy SP, Casella JF, Tomaselli GF, Morrow JS, Dang CV (1992) Karyoplasmic interaction selection strategy: a general strategy to detect protein-protein interactions in mammalian cells. Proc Natl Acad Sci USA 89: 7958-7962
17. Feinberg AP, Vogelstein B (1984) A technique for radiolabeling DNA restriction endonuclease fragments to high specific activity. Anal Biochem 137: 266-267
18. Fox S (1991) Applications for synthesizing and sequencing DNA beyond the genome project. Gene Eng News 11: 6-8
19. Genetics Computer Group (1991) Program manual for the GCG package, version 7
20. Green ED, Olson MV (1990) Systematic screening of yeast artificial-chromosome libraries by use of the polymerase chain reaction. Proc Natl Acad Sci USA 87: 1213-1217
21. Grunstein M, Hogness DS (1975) Colony hybridization: a method for the isolation of cloned DNAs that contain a specific gene. Proc Natl Acad Sci USA 72: 3961-3965
22. Hanahan D, Meselson M (1983) Plasmid screening at high density. Methods Enzymol 100: 333-342
23. Helfman DM, Feramisco JR, Fiddes JC, Thomas GP, Hughes SH (1983) Identification of clones that encode chicken tropomyosin by direct immunological screening of a cDNA expression library. Proc Natl Acad Sci USA 80: 31-35
24. Ish-Horowitz D, Burke JF (1981) Rapid and efficient cosmid cloning. Nuc Acids Res 9: 2989-2998
25. Johnson DA, Gautsch JW, Sportsman JR, Elder JH (1984) Improved technique utilizing nonfat dry milk for analysis of proteins and nucleic acids transferred to nitrocellulose. Gene Anal Tech 1: 3-8
26. Kieffer BL, Befort K, Gaveriaux-Ruff C, Hirth CG (1992) The δ-opioid receptor: Isolation of cDNA by expression cloning and pharmacological characterization. Proc Natl Acad Sci USA 89: 12048-12052
27. Kim UJ, Shizuya H, de Jong PJ, Birren B, Simon MI (1992) Stable propagation of cosmid sized human DNA inserts in F factor based vector. Nucleic Acids Res 20: 1083-1085
28. Kotler LE, Zevin-Sonkin D, Sobolev IA, Beskin AD, Ulanovsky LE (1993) DNA sequencing: Modular primers assembled from a library of hexamers or pentamers. Proc Natl Acad Sci USA 90: 4241-4245
29. Liu X, Miller CW, Koeffler PH, Berk AJ (1993) The p53 activation domain binds the TATA box-binding polypeptide in holo-TFIID, and a neighboring p53 domain inhibits transcription. Mol Cell Biol 13: 3291-3300
30. Mason PJ, Williams JG (1985) Hybridization in the analysis of recombinant DNA In: Hames BD, Higgins SJ (eds.) Nucleic acid hybridisation: a practical approach. IRL, Oxford, pp. 113-137
31. Mavrothalassitis G, Fisher RJ, Smyth F, Watson DK, Papas TS (1994) Structural inferences of the ETSI DNA-binding domain determined by mutational analysis. Oncogene 9: 425-435
32. Maxam AM, Gilbert W (1977) A new method for sequencing DNA. Proc Natl Acad Sci USA 74: 560-564
33. Millar SJ, Dempsey D, Dickinson DP (1992) High yield recovery of recombinant DNA from poorly growing cosmid and lambda genomic clones. Biotechniques 13: 554-556
34. Mozdzanowski J, Speicher DW (1992) Microsequence analysis of electroblotted proteins. I. Comparison of electroblotting recoveries using different types of PVDF membranes. Anal Biochem 207: 11-18

35. Mutzel R, Baeuerle A, Jung S, Dammann H (1990) Prophage lambda libraries for isolating cDNA clones by functional screening. Gene 96: 205-211
36. Pierce JC, Sauer B, Sternberg N (1992a) A positive selection vector for cloning high molecular weight DNA by the bacteriophage P1 system: improved cloning efficacy. Proc Natl Acad Sci USA 89: 2056-2060
37. Pierce JC, Sternberg N, Sauer B (1992b) A mouse genomic library in the bacteriophage P1 cloning system: organization and characterization. Mammalian Genome 3: 550-558
38. Reim DF, Speicher DW (1992) Microsequence analysis of electroblotted proteins. II. Comparison of sequence performance on different types of PVDF membranes. Anal Biochem 207: 19-23
39. Rowley JD, Aster JC, Sklar J (1993) The clinical applications of new DNA diagnostic technology on the management of cancer patients. JAMA 270: 2331-2337
40. Sanger F, Nicklen FS, Coulson AR (1977) DNA sequencing with chain-terminating inhibitors. Proc Natl Acad Sci USA 74: 5463-5467
41. Sharp PM, Cowe E, Higgins DG, Shields DC, Wolfe KH, Wright F (1988) Codon usage patterns in Escherichia coli, Bacillus subtilis, Saccharomyces cerevisiae, Schizosaccharomyces pombe, Drosophila melanogaster and Homo sapiens; a review of the considerable within-species diversity. Nucleic Acids Res 16: 8207-8211
42. Sikela JM, Hahn WE (1987) Screening an expression library with a ligand probe: Isolation and sequence of a cDNA corresponding to a brain calmodulin-binding protein. Proc Natl Acad Sci USA 84: 3038-3042
43. Singh H, LeBowitz JH, Baldwin AS Jr, Sharp PA (1988) Molecular cloning of an enhancer binding protein: isolation by screening of an expression library with a recognition site DNA Cell 52: 415-423
44. Sternberg N (1990) Bacteriophage P1 cloning system for the isolation amplification and recovery of DNA fragments as large as 100 kilobase pairs. Proc Natl Acad Sci USA 87: 103-107
45. Vasavada HA, Ganguly S, Germino FJ, Wang ZX, Weissman SM (1991) A contingent replication assay for the detection of protein-protein interactions in animal cells. Proc Natl Acad Sci USA 88: 10686-10690
46. Whitcomb JM, Rashtchian A, Hughes SH (1993) A new PCR based method for generation of nested deletions. Nucleic Acids Res 17: 4143-4146
47. Yang M, Fields S (1994) Use of the two-hybrid system to detect protein-peptide interactions In: Whelan WJ, Ahmad F, Baumbach L, Bialy H, Black S, Davies K, Hodgson J, Howell RR, Huijing F, Scott WA (eds.) Advances in gene technology: molecular biology and human disease, vol 4. IRL, Oxford, p. 40

Section 4:

*Regulation and Dysregulation of the
Systemic Mediator Response in Injury and Sepsis*

Alphabet Soup: An Analysis of Mediators of Sepsis

J.W. Holaday, C.A., Nacy, E.A. Neugebauer

Introduction

As with any disease, clinical strategies to improve outcome in patients with septic shock evolve from investigations into the underlying mediators and mechanisms. The complexity of bacterially induced septic shock involves a cascade of events that occur over time, beginning with the proliferation of offending organisms, followed by the release of toxic mediators from the bacteria, that, in turn, activate a series of host responses that further exacerbate the problem. Ultimately, decreased tissue perfusion and further metabolic derangements lead to respiratory dysfunction, multiple organ failure and death (Fig. 1).

Over the past century, hundreds of mediators have been proposed to serve as pathophysiological substances that contribute to the sequelae of septic shock. An "alphabet soup" of abbreviations are used to describe these septic shock mediators that include toxins (e.g., LPS), cytokines (e.g, TNF, IL-1), eicosanoids (e.g., PAF, PGE, TXA_2), biogenic amines (e.g., H2, NE, DA), kinins (e.g., BK), peptides (e.g., Enk, VIP), ions (e.g., Ca^{2+}), and hormones (e.g., ACTH, BEP). Without doubt, many of these "alphabet" mediators contribute to the cascade of septic shock pathophysiology [1]; however, to focus solely on their adverse effects implies that they lack a role in maintaining healthy homeostasis.

Many "mediators of septic shock" subserve both *beneficial and adverse* effects, depending upon the amount and timing of their activation. Thus, as with any drug, too much may be as bad as too little. Their release in *supra*homeostatic amounts may be deleterious and prompt their consideration as "mediators of septic shock" (e.g., endorphins), whereas when their release is inhibited by septic shock the body may be deprived of essential homeostatic regulators. In the latter case, the absence of "mediators" may even exacerbate shock (e.g., glucocorticoids), and rational therapeutic strategies may require their replacement. This conundrum is further complicated by timing; although the amounts of mediators released may be within homeostatic ranges, when considered in concert with the emerging pathophysiology of septic shock, changes in mediator levels may be too early or too late, and thus either help or hinder recovery.

Recent advances in septic shock research have brought into focus many new putative mediators and mechanisms, and physiological events that were once medical mysteries now can be attributed to the specific effects of these individual biological substances. Despite such revelations, an evaluation of the literature on septic shock leaves the investigator with a sense

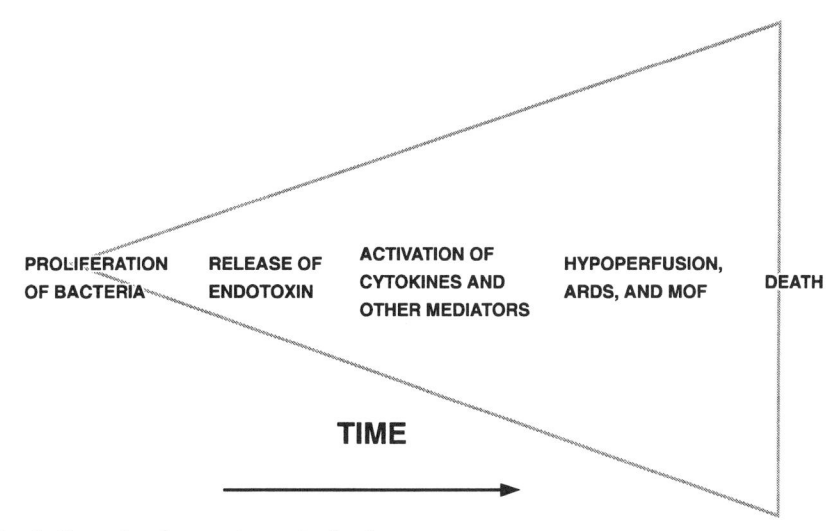

Fig. 1: Cascade of events in septic shock

PROLIFERATION OF BACTERIA → RELEASE OF ENDOTOXIN → ACTIVATION OF CYTOKINES AND OTHER MEDIATORS → HYPOPERFUSION, ARDS, AND MOF → DEATH

TIME →

that, although many pieces of the septic shock puzzle have been presented, no clue was provided to indicate how these pieces fit together. Furthermore, despite this wealth of accumulating knowledge, application of these emerging technologies to the clinic has yet to alter significantly the morbidity and mortality of septic shock.

This chapter will provide a brief overview of the mediators of septic shock, with emphasis on the application of Koch-Dale criteria and meta-analysis as useful, objective tools by which to integrate the existing literature for individual mediators [1]. These tools were employed to assess the "state-of-the art" research in septic shock by analyzing the sufficiency of published data in ascribing casual roles for over 24 single mediators (e.g., histamine) or categories of mediators (e.g., interleukins).

What Initiates Septic Shock?

One focus of shock research has been to investigate the cascade of events that result from the release of bacterial toxins. Endotoxins (e.g., lipopolysaccharides) for gram-negative bacteria initiate septic shock by precipitating a systemic inflammatory response syndrome (SIRS) through activation of a broad spectrum of host-derived mediators [2]. The mechanisms by which gram-positive endotoxins contribute to septic shock are less well defined, with some evidence to indicate that their pathological effects are due to the formation of pores in biologic membranes [3]. However important these toxins are to pathophysiological events that follow their release, it may be even more important to first address their source, namely proliferating bacteria in the bloodstream (Fig. 1).

Although the advent and refinement of antibiotic drugs has revolutionized medicine, their use has not significantly altered the mortality of septic shock once it is underway. In fact, many bacteria release their toxins after they are killed by antibiotics, thus initiating the septic shock cascade. Furthermore, over time, the use of antibiotics has resulted in the evolution of resistant strains of bacteria that no longer respond to these drugs. The likelihood of bacteremia progressing to sepsis and septic shock is increasing, and efforts to find new ways to prevent and to treat this lethal disease may require new strategies for killing bacteria.

Cascade of Mediators

In an attempt to assess objectively the causal role of individual mediators in septic shock, Neugebauer and Holaday [1] recently completed a collective meta-analysis of 24 mediators that were individually reviewed and subjected to Koch-Dale analysis of causality by distinguished authorities in the field. Done correctly, this effort requires an impartial review of all available literature to assess whether studies were appropriately performed before allowing their inclusion of the data-base. Once this hurdle is completed, those studies judged to be suitable for further analysis are subjected to a structured evaluation to establish evidence for causality.

Because of limitations in available data and/or the different strategies in evaluating mediators employed by individual authors, it was impossible to organize each chapter according to the rigid analytical criteria required for causality assessment. Six different "categories" of mediators were presented, including toxins, biogenic amines, oligo- and polypeptides, proteins, fatty acid derivatives, and varia (miscellaneous). Most authors did attempt to subject their "mediators" to the rigors of Koch-Dale analysis, a process that asks four questions: (1) is the mediator present in disease, or... (2) absent in health? (3) can one elicit the disease by administration of the mediator? (4) can one block or prevent disease by using mediator antagonists? As reviewed above, this approach is based upon the definition of "mediators of sepsis" as "bad guys," and does not consider that the absence of a beneficial mediator may be as detrimental as the presence of a detrimental mediator.

As with any attempt to provide a consensus, the ultimate evaluation involves a degree of subjectivity. Despite the attempt to overcome subjectivity through the use of a structured analysis of individual mediators by Koch-Dale and meta-analysis, a subjective assessment was necessarily involved in generalizing on the state-of-the-art knowledge on mediators of septic shock (Fig. 2). The concluding chapter of the book by Neugebauer and Holaday [1] provided an attempt to assess collectively individual chapters about mediators, with the caveat that the groupings of related mediators within prescribed categories may have further obscured an evaluation of the roles of individual mediators [4].

Among the toxins, strong evidence was available to support a role of endotoxin in the pathogenesis of septic shock, whereas weak evidence was available for exotoxins. Within the biogenic amines, histamine and the catecholamines were supported by moderate evidence, whereas the role of serotonin as a mediator of sepsis was less well established or nonexistent. Among the oligopeptides and polypeptides, strongest evidence was available to support a role of endorphins, complement (C3a, C5a), interleukins-1, -2, and -6, and tumor necrosis factor (TNF). Vasoactive intestinal peptide (VIP), kallikrein, vasopressin, renin-angiotensin, and neuropeptide Y were less well supported by evidence for their roles in septic shock pathogenesis. A role for the protein mediators in septic shock, represented by fibronectin, PMN elastase, cathepsin B, EDRF/nitric oxide, and endothelin, was only weakly or moderately supported by available experimental evidence. Fatty acid derivatives, including cyclooxygenase metabolites, peptidoleukotrienes, and platelet-activating factor, were all supported by strong evidence as mediators of sepsis. The final category of mediators, varia, included strong evidence for an involvement of Ca^{2+} and moderate evidence for an involvement of oxygen free radicals and cortisol.

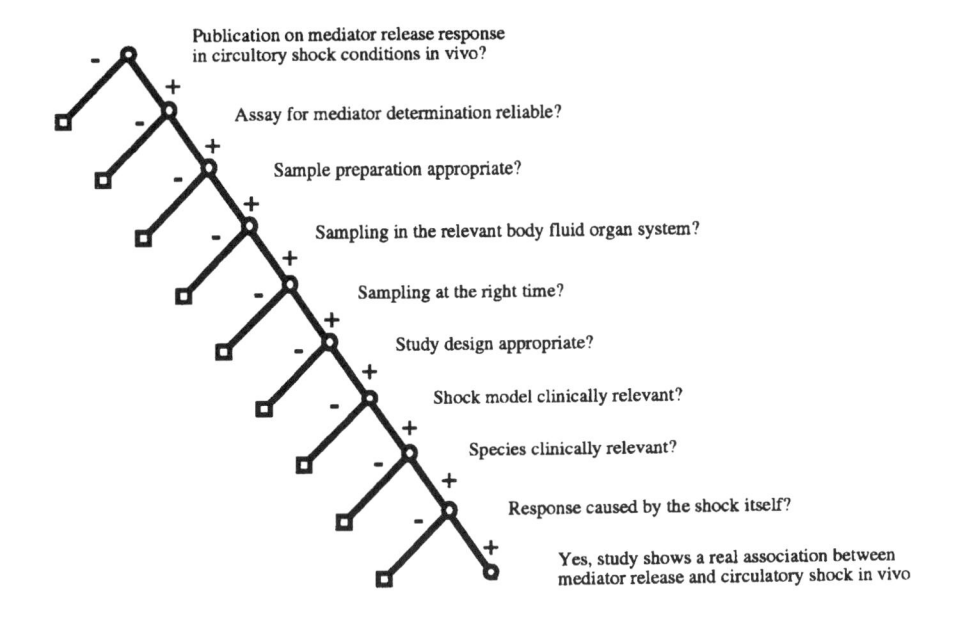

Fig. 2: An example of a decision tree for evaluating the potential relationship between a deleterious mediator and its involvement in septic shock

References

1. Neugebauer EA, Holaday JW (eds.) (1993) Handbook of mediators of septic shock. CRC, Boca Raton
2. Cody CS, Dunn DL (1993) Endotoxins in septic shock. In: Neugebauer EA, Holaday JW (eds.) (1993) Handbook of mediators of septic shock. CRC, Boca Raton, pp. 1-38
3. Bhakdi S (1993) Possible relevance of bacterial endotoxins in the pathogenesis of septic shock. In: Neugebauer EA, Holaday JW (eds.) (1993) Handbook of mediators of septic shock. CRC, Boca Raton, pp. 39-48
4. Holaday JW, Neugebauer EA, Carr DB (1993) M^2 - an analysis of meta-analysis of mediators of septic shock. In: Neugebauer EA, Holaday JW (eds.) (1993) Handbook of mediators of septic shock. CRC, Boca Raton, pp. 523-534

Humoral Manifestations of Regulation and Dysregulation of the Systemic Mediator Response in Injury and Sepsis

B.A. Pruitt, Jr., D.G. Burleson, A.C. Drost, W.G. Cioffi, A.D. Mason, Jr.

The mediators liberated by an injury orchestrate and integrate the responses of cells, tissues, and organs to increase blood flow and oxygen delivery to injured tissues, mobilize and direct nutrients to effect cell repair and wound healing, and enhance immune function to prevent and control infection. These initial inflammatory changes activate platelets and macrophages or monocytes which release a variety of mediators that induce what is termed the acute-phase response. The mediators include the "early" or "alarm" cytokines, interleukin-1 (IL-1) [18], and tumor necrosis factor (TNF) [19], which induce cells in the area of injury to release other "secondary" cytokines, such as IL-8 and other interleukins, and monocyte chemoattractant protein (MCP) [27]. Those secondary mediators amplify the initial signals and elicit changes in leukocyte density and metabolite production that orchestrate the acute-phase response. Chemotactic agents produced locally control cell migration into the injured tissue [30]. Neutrophils and other granulocytic cells are activated as are the endothelial cells with expression of the selectin, integrin, and pecam surface molecules on the former and the counterreceptor intercellular adhesion molecules on the latter [9, 10, 33, 39].

Microvascular alterations resulting in edema and erythema in the area of tissue damage have been attributed to excited oxygen radicals, nitric oxide, and arachidonic acid metabolites [2, 5, 7]. The balance between thromboxane, the prostaglandins, and the leukotrienes, determines the state of constriction or dilatation of the vessels in the area of tissue injury. Histamine, serotonin, and platelet-activating factor (PAF) which are also liberated by injury can alter microvascular permeability in that area and promote platelet aggregation, which further alters blood flow [12, 13, 26, 45].

These cytokines typically exert systemic as well as local inflammatory effects. IL-1 and TNF, as well as IL-6, interferon-alpha (IFN-α), and macrophage inflammatory protein-1, which are all "endogenous pyrogens," induce and regulate the febrile response apparently by increasing prostaglandin E_2 production [20]. Central thermoregulatory mechanisms are reset and other hypothalamic functions are altered [44]. This results in disruption of the normal pituitary-adrenal relationship, a blunted growth hormone response to arginine stimulation, altered responsiveness to the administration of narcotics, altered anti-diuretic hormone secretion, decreased thyroid-stimulating hormone responsiveness, central hypogonadism, and altered pineal melatonin content [43]. These functional alterations are associated with emergence of a new population of neurons on the surface of the floor of the third ventricle [41].

Function of the liver is also profoundly influenced by systemic inflammatory mediators. In response to those mediators, marked changes in hepatic metabolic activity occur, associated with increased production of the acute-phase plasma proteins. The inflammatory mediators that influence hepatic metabolism include the IL-1-type cytokines, the IL-6-type cytokines, glucocorticoids, and several growth factors. The IL-1-type cytokines include the α and β forms of both IL-1 and TNF; the IL-6-type cytokines include IL-6, IL-11, leukemia inhibitory factor (ILF), oncostatin M (OSM), and ciliary neurotrophic factor (CNTF). The involved growth factors include insulin, hepatocyte growth factor (HGF), transforming growth factor-β (TGF-β), and fibroblast growth factor (FGF). The principal activity of the cytokines is to stimulate gene expression for the acute-phase plasma proteins, and the growth factors and glucocorticoids either amplify or dampen these actions.

The IL-1-type cytokines regulate acute-phase protein genes which increase expression of C-reactive protein, serum amyloid A, α_1-acid glycoprotein, complement component C3, and haptoglobin. The IL-6-type cytokines enhance the production of other acute-phase plasma proteins including fibrinogen, α_1-antichymotrypsin, α_1-antitrypsin, thiostatin, α_2-macroglobulin, and haptoglobin [7]. The increased production of acute-phase plasma proteins, resulting from a reprogramming of protein synthesis priorities, may be associated with a decrease in hepatic albumin synthesis. In hypermetabolic burn patients hepatic albumin synthesis is elevated unless infection occurs, in which case albumin production is decreased [14].

The circulating mediators elicit a broad range of systemic effects which are common to both injury and sepsis, i.e., tachycardia, tachypnea, and leukocytosis or leukopenia in addition to fever and hypermetabolism. The inflammatory cytokines also evoke alterations in organ function that are common to both injury and sepsis. The cardiovascular changes are manifest in the hyperdynamic circulation as well as altered renal function, which is characterized by variable degrees of oliguria and azotemia or, alternatively, inappropriate diuresis. Altered pulmonary function is indexed by an increase in minute ventilation and altered gastrointestinal function by ileus and increased permeability. The effects of inflammatory mediators on the central nervous system, which can be modified by altered function of other organ systems, include varying degrees of agitation, disorientation, and obtundation. Many of the changes in immune cell populations and function also characterize the response to both injury and sepsis [37].

The initial organ dysfunction following injury is typically short lived and lasts only 48-72 h with progressive restoration of organ function if the injury is promptly and definitively repaired and effective organ support is provided. However, the acute inflammatory response may convert to a state of chronic, progressively severe inflammation, a condition which has been termed the "systemic inflammatory response syndrome" [6, 8]. This syndrome occurs if the acute-phase response is prolonged because of the continued presence of necrotic tissue, persistent stimulation by undiagnosed infection, or disruption of the mechanisms controlling the production of inflammatory mediators as may occur when the wound is not closed in a timely fashion. A secondary stress such as an episode of physiologically significant hypovolemia, the development of a complicating infection, or recurrent injury causing further tissue damage, such as another operative procedure or a complication such as acute pancreatitis associated with tissue destruction, can also evoke the syndrome [35].

If the systemic inflammatory response syndrome does develop, what has been termed secondary organ dysfunction occurs with persistence or recrudescence of the previously described organ dysfunctions and may relentlessly progress to sequential failure of multiple organs. In this situation, it becomes even more important to differentiate the response to injury from that to sepsis in order to institute effective support measures before irreversible organ failure occurs or unnecessary broad-spectrum antibiotic therapy is instituted. Measurement of various nutrients and other products of cell metabolism, although attractive as a diagnostic approach, is incapable of making the necessary differentiation because changes in those variables parallel one another in the response to injury and in the early stages of sepsis [37]. Hyperglycemia as well as elevated circulating levels of complement activation products, arachidonic acid metabolites, and various cytokines occur both in patients following injury and in patients with sepsis. Similarly, a decrease in circulating levels of fibronectin and of the coagulation factors is seen in both conditions. Alterations in hormone production are also similar in patients soon after injury and those with early sepsis. The production of catecholamines, corticosteroids, and glucagon is increased and the production of insulin, thyroid hormone sex hormones, melatonin, and growth hormone is decreased [43]. In short, the common features of responses to injury and sepsis make the differentiation of the two conditions difficult by either standard measurements of organ function or commonly employed biochemical assays.

Numerous humoral substances and mediators including endotoxin per se, tumor necrosis factor, the interleukins, platelet-activating factor, and neopterin have been evaluated as monitors of the response to injury and indices of systemic inflammation as well as for their ability to differentiate the two. Tests for endotoxin, such as the limulus lysate assay, have been used to evaluate the association of endotoxemia and bacteremia in critically ill burn patients [32]. Blood cultures and endotoxin assays were performed simultaneously in 25 consecutively admitted burn patients during the intensive phase of their care. Endotoxemia and positive blood cultures were found to be randomly associated. That random association was maintained even between the presence of endotoxemia and the occurrence of a positive blood culture during the subsequent 48 h. Additional studies indicated that 78% of patients dying with severe burns had measurable levels of endotoxin in the liver, a finding consistent with the notion that endotoxemia was a major factor in fatal sepsis [29]. In 65 patients who died with burns, 61 had endotoxin present in the liver but only 54 (or 89%) of those patients had a positive blood culture during life and 7 (or slightly more than 1 in 10) never had a positive blood culture. The uncertain specificity of the endotoxin assay results and the lack of assay correlation with clinical status severely limit the usefulness of such tests.

A variety of blood-borne metabolic products of inflammatory cells have also been evaluated to determine their usefulness in differentiating the response to injury from that to infection early in the course of the septic process when therapeutic intervention can be effective. Plasma levels of TNF-α, IL-1β, and IL-6 were measured throughout the hospital course of 27 burn patients. IL-1β and IL-6 were highest during the first postburn week and declined thereafter in uncomplicated patients. IL-1β levels correlated with burn size but were not affected by infection [21] (Fig. 1). IL-6 and TNF-α showed little response to injury per se and were not elevated in proportion to extent of burn. TNF-α, which was undetectable in most plasma samples, was elevated in infected patients. IL-6 to the contrary, was detected in all nonsurvivors, and the levels of that cytokine were significantly higher than in survivors (Table 1). The observed correlations of IL-1β and TNF-α levels with IL-6 levels appear to reflect the induction of IL-6 by both of the "alarm" cytokines. Interestingly, IL-6 levels were increased before infection was clinically diagnosed in both surviving and nonsurviving patients, suggesting that serial measurements of IL-6 may enable one to identify an early stage of infection before clinical signs are evident [22]. Alternatively, the rise in IL-6 levels prior to the clinical diagnosis of an infection may indicate that increased IL-6 levels predispose injured patients to infection.

Table 1: Influence of infection on IL-6 and TNF levels in burn patients

	No infection	Infection	
IL-6 (ng/ml)	0.13±0.03 (n=109)	0.66±0.06**	
		Lived	Died
		0.56±0.04 (n=165)	1.62±0.45** (n=16)
TNF (pg/ml)	2.52±0.77 (n=29)	9.7±0.93***	
		Lived	Died
		9.47±0.91 (n=61)	16.7±10.17 (n=2)

**$p < 0.01$ vs. infected lived.
***$p < 0.00001$ vs. no infection.

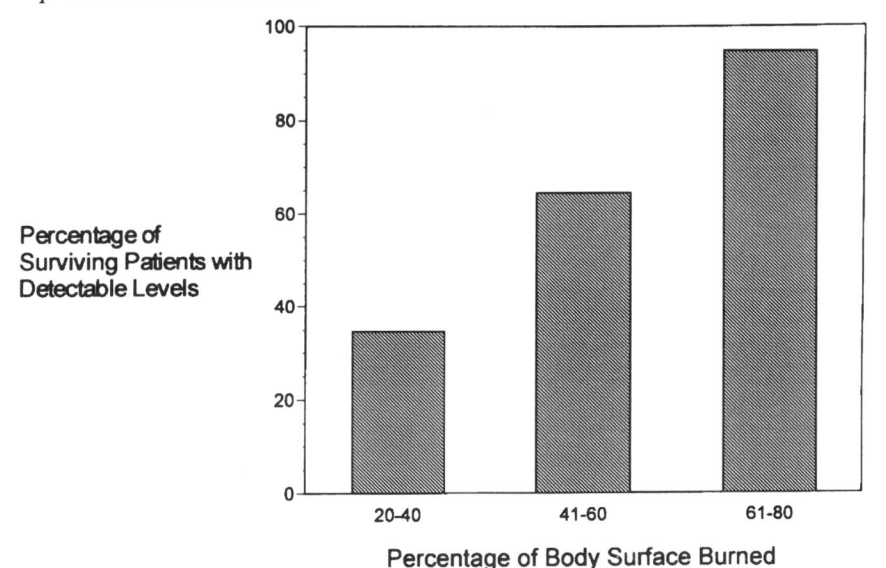

Fig. 1: *Relationship of injury severity to the presence of detectable levels of IL-1 in surviving burn patients*

Several fluorescent substances appear in the supernatants of acid-precipitated blood or plasma from burn patients and change in relationship to infection and sepsis. Initial studies in animal models revealed three humoral fluorescent materials [36], one of which, with absorbance at 398 nm, appears to consist of heme compounds such as fetal hemoglobin. A second material which fluoresces at 340 nm consists of acute-phase or stress proteins. The third material, which fluoresces at 420 nm, appears to be related to the nucleotides, principally neopterin. The latter compound was present in increased concentration in both the plasma and the kidneys of uninfected burn patients as compared with controls and in even greater concentrations in infected burn patients as compared with uninfected burn patients.

Malondialdehyde concentrations in the kidney, as an index of oxidative injury, increased in concert with increases in this fluorescent factor [28].

Neopterin, a member of the pterin family, is produced by both macrophages and B-lymphocytes. The production of neopterin is stimulated by γ-interferon and elevated in patients with intracellular infections and other diseases which affect cell-mediated immunity. In early studies in burn patients, a correlation was identified between the concentration of neopterin, as determined by high-pressure liquid chromatography, and the presence of bacteremia, suggesting that neopterin was a potentially useful indicator of infection in such patients [15]. Subsequent studies have identified a progressive rise in both urine and serum neopterin levels during the first 5 weeks following burn injury, with no correlation between neopterin levels and burn size [4].

Serum neopterin levels appear to be sensitive to renal insufficiency, with a marked elevation in serum levels when creatinine clearance is below 50 ml/min. When serum samples were screened to exclude those from patients with renal insufficiency, serum levels of neopterin in patients with systemic infection were not different from those in uninfected patients. However, depressed urine levels of neopterin characterized the preinfection state of those patients who ultimately developed an infection. In the infected patients, those depressed levels had risen to the levels measured in uninfected patients by the time the infection was diagnosed and declined thereafter (Fig. 2). The lower levels of neopterin present in the urine of patients prior to infection may indicate decreased immune activation and reflect a predisposition of those patients to infection. Conversely, rising levels in the absence of renal dysfunction appear to be indicative of developing infection and markedly increased levels have been correlated with an undrained abscess [42].

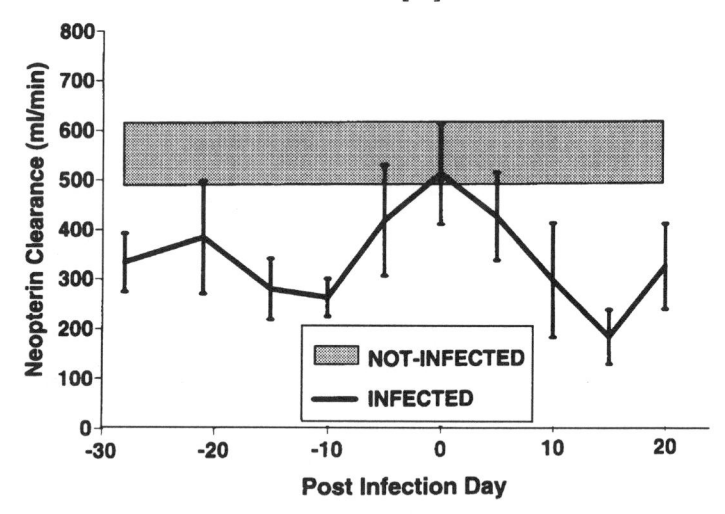

Fig. 2: Relationship of neopterin clearance to the occurrence of infection in burn patients

The limitations of even novel biochemical assays dictate that in diagnosing systemic inflammation reliance be placed upon clinical signs of progressive organ impairment that are inconsistent in terms of magnitude and duration with the status of the patient's injury. The acute-phase reaction typically subsides over a 24- to 48-h period following successful resuscitation. This resolution is promoted by both naturally occurring antagonists such as IL-1 receptor antagonists and soluble TNF receptor as well as the counterregulatory effects of IL-4 and IL-10, which down-regulate the production of cytokines and other inflammatory mediators [7, 16, 23, 40]. IL-4 down-regulates IL-1 and TNF gene expression in monocytes and reciprocally up-regulates IL-1 receptor antagonist expression [24]. IL-4 also inhibits monocyte superoxide production and further reduces inflammatory cytokine production by enhancing apoptosis in stimulated monocytes [1, 31]. Resolution of the acute-phase reaction is also promoted by IL-10 which inhibits monocyte production of IL-1α and IL-1β, IL-6, IL-8, TNF-α, granulocyte macrophage colony-stimulating factor and granulocyte colony-stimulating factors [17]. This cytokine also acts synergistically with IL-4 and TGF-β to inhibit macrophage cytotoxic activity and decrease production of reactive nitrogen oxides [11, 34]. Additionally, IL-10 up-regulates IL-1 receptor antagonist.

Corticosteroids also promote resolution of the acute-phase reaction by inhibiting monocyte cytokine production [3]. Failure of the acute-phase reaction to resolve within the customary time frame or progressive exaggeration and systemic expression of the inflammatory response should prompt a thorough search for the persistent inflammatory stimulus [38]. If the cause, usually a focus of infection or necrosis, remains unidentified and unresolved, generalized dysregulation of organ function and metabolic processes will occur, resulting in progressive sequential organ failure and a fatal outcome [25].

Certain measurable humoral indicators such as IL-1 appear to reflect injury severity but are little affected by sepsis, while TNF-α and IL-6 respond to infection but show relatively little response to the magnitude of the initial injury. Isolated measurements of those cytokines are difficult to interpret but serial measurements may enable one to diagnose an infection prior to the time when it is clinically evident. In similar fashion serial assays of neopterin clearance may be useful in identifying patients at risk to infection (low values) as well as those in whom an infection is developing (rising values). The refinement of currently available assays and the development of new diagnostic techniques that are both sensitive and specific in distinguishing between the responses to injury and sepsis and in identifying early signs of organ dysfunction will permit timely therapeutic intervention to prevent the occurrence of mediator dysregulation. The early diagnosis of systemic inflammation, effective support of organ function, and targeted therapeutic intervention to counteract the systemic inflammatory mediators will reduce postinjury complications, hasten convalescence, and increase survival of surgical patients.

References

1. Abramson SL, Gallin JI (1990) IL-4 inhibits superoxide production by human mononuclear phagocytes. J Immunol 144: 625-630
2. Alexander F, Mathieson M, Teoh KHT, Huval WV, Lelcuk S, Valeri CR, Shepro D, Hechtman HB (1984) Arachidonic acid metabolites mediate early burn edema. J Trauma 24: 709-712
3. Arzt E, Saver J, Pollmacher T, Lauber M, Holsboer F, Reul JMHM, Stalla GK (1994) Glucocorticoids suppress interleukin-1 receptor antagonist synthesis following induction by endotoxin. Endocrinology 134: 672-677
4. Balogh D, Lammer H, Kornberger E, Stuffer M, Schonitzer D (1992) Neopterin plasma levels in burn patients. Burns 18: 185-188
5. Baudry N, Vicaut E (1993) Role of nitric oxide in effects of tumor necrosis factor-alpha on microcirculation in rat. J Appl Physiol 75: 2392-2399
6. Baue AE (1992) The horror autotoxicus and multiple-organ failure. Arch Surg 127: 1451-1462

7. Baumann H, Gauldie J (1994) The acute phase response. Immunol Today 15: 74-80
8. Beal AL, Cerra FB (1994) Multiple organ failure syndrome in the 1990s: systemic inflammatory response and organ dysfunction. JAMA 271: 226-233
9. Benton LD, Khan M, Greco RS (1993) Integrins, adhesion molecules and surgical research. Surg Gynecol Obstet 177: 311-327
10. Bevilaqua MP, Nelson RM (1993) Selectins. J Clin Invest 91: 379-387
11. Bogdan C, Vodovotz Y, Nathan C (1991) Macrophage deactivation by interleukin 10. J Exp Med 174: 1549-1555
12. Boykin JV Jr, Eriksson E, Sholley MM, Pittman RM (1980) Histamine-mediated delayed permeability response after scald burn inhibited by cimetidine or cold-water treatment. Science 209: 815-817
13. Braquet P, Hosford D, Braquet M, Burgain R, Bussolino F (1989) Role of cytokines and platelet-activating factor in microvascular immune injury. Int Arch Allergy Appl Immunol 88: 88-100
14. Brown WL, Bowler EG, Mason AD Jr, Pruitt BA Jr (1976) Protein metabolism in burned rats. Am J Physiol 231: 476-482
15. Burleson DG, Johnson A, Salin M, Mason AD Jr, Pruitt BA Jr (1992) Identification of neopterin as a potential inhibitor of infection in burned patients. Proc Soc Exp Biol Med 199: 305-310
16. Damtew B, Rzewnicki D, Lozanski G, Kushner I (1993) IL-1 receptor antagonist affects the plasma protein response of Hep 3B cells to conditioned medium from lipopolysaccharide-stimulated monocytes. J Immunol 150: 4001-4007
17. De Waal Malefyt R, Abrams J, Bennett B, Figdor CG, de Vries JE (1991) Interleukin 10 (IL-10) inhibits cytokine synthesis by human monocytes: an autoregulatory role of IL-10 produced by monocytes. J Exp Med 174: 1209-1220
18. Dinarello CA (1984) Interleukin-1. Rev Infect Dis 6: 51-95
19. Dinarello CA, Cannon JG, Wolff SM, Bernheim HA, Beutler B, Cerami A, Figari IS, Palladino MA Jr, O'Common JV (1986) Tumor necrosis factor (cachectin) is an endogenous pyrogen and induces production of interleukin 1. J Exp Med 163: 1433-1450
20. Dinarello CS, Cannon JG, Mancilla J, Bishai I, Lees J, Coceani F (1991) Interleukin-6 as an endogenous pyrogen: induction of prostaglandin E_2 in brain but not in peripheral blood mononuclear cells. Brain Res 562: 199-206
21. Drost AC, Burleson DG, Cioffi WG Jr, Jordan BS, Mason AD Jr, Pruitt BA Jr (1993) Plasma cytokines following thermal injury and their relationship with patient mortality, burn size, and time postburn. J Trauma 35: 335-339
22. Drost AC, Burleson DG, Cioffi WG Jr, Mason AD Jr, Pruitt BA Jr (1993) Plasma cytokines after thermal injury and their relationship to infection. Ann Surg 218: 74-78
23. Essner R, Rhodes K, McBride WH, Morton DL, Economou JS (1989) IL-4 down-regulates IL-1 and TNF gene expression in human monocytes. J Immunol 142: 3857-3861
24. Fenton MJ, Buras JA, Donnelly RP (1992) IL-4 reciprocally regulates IL-1 and IL-1 receptor antagonist expression in human monocytes. J Immunol 149: 1283-1288
25. Fry DE, Pearlstein L, Fulton RL, Polk HC Jr (1980) Multiple system organ failure: the role of uncontrolled infection. Arch Surg 115: 136-140
26. Lefer AM (1989) Significance of lipid mediators in shock states. Circ Shock 27: 3-12
27. Liebler JM, Kunkel SL, Burdick MD, Standiford TJ, Rolfe MW, Strieter RM (1994) Production of IL-8 and monocyte chemotactic peptide-1 by peripheral blood monocytes. J Immunol 152: 241-249
28. Lin KD, Burleson DG, Powanda MC (1984) Alteration of host resistance in burned soldiers: characterization of biochemical indicators of infection in the thermally injured. US Army Institute of Surgical Research, Brooke Army Medical Center, Fort Sam Houston, pp. 200-207 (Annual research progress report)

29. Lindberg RB, English VC, Mason AD Jr, Pruitt BA Jr (1976) Detection of endotoxin in burned soldiers with sepsis. US Army Institute of Surgical Research, Brooke Army Medical Center, Fort Sam Houston, pp. 54-61 (Annual research progress report)
30. Locati M, Zhou D, Luini W, Evangelista V, Mantovani A, Sozzani S (1994) Rapid induction of arachidonic acid release by monocyte chemotactic protein-1 and related chemokines. J Biol Chem 269: 4746-4753
31. Mangan DF, Robertson B, Wahl SM (1992) IL-4 enhances programmed cell death (apoptosis) in stimulated human monocytes. J Immunol 148: 1812-1816
32. McManus AT, Lindberg RB, Pruitt BA Jr, Mason AD Jr (1979) Association of endotoxemia and bacteremia in burn patients: a prospective study. In: Cohen E (ed.) Biomedical applications of the horseshoe crab (Limulidae). Liss, New York, pp. 275-278
33. Muller WA, Weigl SA, Deng X, Phillips DM (1993) PECAM-1 is required for transendothelial migration of leukocytes. J Exp Med 178: 449-460
34. Oswald IP, Gazzinelli RT, Sher A, James SL (1992) IL-10 synergizes with IL-4 and transforming growth factor-beta to inhibit macrophage cytotoxic activity. J Immunol 148: 3578-3582
35. Parrillo JE (1993) Pathogenetic mechanisms of septic shock. N Engl J Med 328: 1471-1477
36. Powanda MC, Dubois J, Villarreal Y, Walker HL, Pruitt BA Jr (1981) Detection of potential biochemical indicators of infection in the burned rat. J Lab Clin Med 97: 672-679
37. Pruitt BA Jr (1987) Infection: cause or effect of pathophysiologic change in burn and trauma patients. In: Paubert-Braquet M, Braquet P, Demling R, Fletcher R, Foegh M (eds.) Lipid mediators in the immunology of shock. Plenum, New York, pp. 31-42
38. Pruitt BA Jr, Goodwin CW Jr, Vaughan GM, Aulick LH, Newman JJ, Strome DR, Mason AD Jr (1985) The metabolic problems of the burn patient. Acta Chir Scand Suppl 522: 119-139
39. Ruoslahti E (1991) Integrins. J Clin Invest 87: 1-5
40. Scannell G, Waxman K, Kaml GJ, Ioli G, Gatanaga T, Yamamoto R, Granger GA (1993) Hypoxia induces a human macrophage cell line to release tumor necrosis factor-alpha and its soluble receptors in vitro. J Surg Res 54: 281-285
41. Scott DE, Vaughan GM, Pruitt BA Jr (1986) Hypothalamic neuroendocrine correlates of cutaneous burn injury in the rat. I. Scanning electron microscopy. Brain Res Bull 17: 367-378
42. Strohmaier W, Mauritz W, Gaudernak T, Grunwald C, Schuller W, Schlag G (1992) Septic focus localized by determination of arterio-venous difference in neopterin blood levels. Circ Shock 38: 219-221
43. Vaughan GM (1990) Neuroendocrine and sympathoadrenal response to thermal trauma. In: Dolacek R, Brizio-Molteni L, Molteni A, Traber D (eds.) Endocrinology of thermal trauma. Pathophysiologic mechanisms and clinical interpretation. Lea and Febiger, Philadelphia, pp. 267-306
44. Wilmore DW, Orcutt TW, Mason AD Jr, Pruitt BA Jr (1975) Alterations in hypothalamic function following thermal injury. J Trauma 15: 697-703
45. Yurt RW, Pruitt BA Jr (1986) Base-line and postthermal injury plasma histamine in rats. J Appl Physiol 60: 1782-1788

Humoral Mediators in Surgical Stress and Multiple Organ Failure

M. Miyashita, M. Onda, K. Sasajima, T. Matsutani, Y. Akiya, K. Okawa, H. Maruyama, T. Nakamura, K. Furukawa, K. Yamashita

Introduction

Systemic inflammatory response syndrome (SIRS) is often encountered in patients who undergo major surgery [8]. An associated impaired host defense dysfunction with altered immune reactions is related to serious postoperative complications. Postoperative SIRS is frequently associated with multiple organ failure (MOF) including respiratory distress and/or disseminated intravascular coagulation (DIC). Recently, it has been suggested that systemic interleukin-1β (IL-1β) and interleukin-6 (IL-6) response to surgical trauma increases with the severity of the surgical insult and that an early exaggerated IL-6 response is associated with the clinical development of major complications [1]. Activation of polymorphonuclear leukocyte (PMN) is considered to be one of the most important mechanisms of tissue injury. Granulocyte colony-stimulating factor (GCSF) induces differentiation of PMN, and interleukin-8 (IL-8) is related to chemotaxis. IL-6 is a pleiotropic cytokine which serves to regulate several components of hepatic acute-phase response as well as to promote B-cell differentiation and costimulation of T cell in the presence of prior activation of tumor necrosis factor and/or IL-1 [6]. IL-6 also stimulates multilineage hematopoiesis including leukocyte and thrombocyte [11]. Oxy-radicals generated from respiratory bursts of PMN cause endothelial cell damage [13], and alteration of thiol-Ca^{2+} homeostasis is proposed in the mechanisms of oxidant-induced cell damage [9]. Further, PMN protease causes increased vascular permeability in ischemic injury [10]. An important source of nitrate is the conversion of L-arginine into L-citrulline and nitric oxide (NO) [3], and increased production of NO by endotoxin or cytokines causes hypotension by inducing vasodilation [14]. Coexistence of NO and O_2- forms peroxynitrite, which is extremely reactive. Thus, it is proposed that tissue damage found in the sequential process of augmented cytokine responses and PMN activation finally leads to organ dysfunctions in surgical stress.

Glucocorticoid is supposed to protect organs in endotoxin shock partly because of the attenuating lipid peroxidation reaction caused by leukocyte-derived oxy-radicals [7]. Recently, there has been an accumulation of reports in which glucocorticoid inhibits production of cytokines; IL-6 in human blood monocytes [2], IL-6 in human dermal microvascular endothelial cells [4], IL-6, IL-8, and GCSF in human bronchial epithelial cells [5], with inflammatory bowel disease [12]. We describe the clinical basis of cytokine responses and related biochemical evidence following a major operation. Furthermore, the effect of glucocorticoid on modulation of cytokine responses to reduce surgical risk is discussed.

Patient Characteristics

Nineteen patients with squamous cell carcinoma of the esophagus who underwent esophagectomy through laparotomy and thoracotomy followed by reconstruction with gastric tube or colon were studied. For evaluation of cytokine responses, 30 mg and 15 mg methylprednisolone/kg body weight were administered i.v. before and after the operation, respectively, in seven randomly selected patients. The patients were divided into two groups: six patients with MOF who had postoperative respiratory distress, DIC, liver dysfunction, and/or renal failure, and 13 patients with no MOF who had no serious organ dysfunction. Two out of the seven patients with methylprednisolone infusion developed DIC, respiratory distress, and renal failure. Age, duration, and bleeding volume in each group were 67 ± 7 (mean $\pm$ SD) years, 513 ± 206 min, and 1448 ± 504 ml in patients with MOF and 64 ± 9 years, 417 ± 63 min, and 668 ± 458 ml in patients with no MOF, respectively. Statistical analysis revealed a significant difference ($p < 0.01$) in bleeding volume between patients with and without MOF.

Peripheral Blood Platelet and Lymphocyte Counts

Platelet count in the peripheral blood decreased until the third postoperative day (POD) to approximately one-third of that before the operation and returned to its normal level on the seventh POD. There were no significant differences between patients with and without MOF. An effect of glucocorticoid on platelet count was also not found. Peripheral blood lymphocyte count was similar to the platelet count, and there was also no significant effect of glucocorticoid on lymphocyte count.

Responses of Cytokines

Plasma IL-6 and GCSF were chosen for surgically induced cytokines and were assayed by ELISA. IL-6 transiently increased immediately after the operation in patients with no MOF. Furthermore, patients with MOF had increased levels of IL-6 twice those of patients with no MOF ($p<0.05$). In patients with no MOF, the IL-6 level on the first POD in patients with glucocorticoid infusion was significantly lower than in patients without the infusion ($p<0.05$) (Fig. 1). GCSF in patients with no MOF also increased after the operation ($p<0.01$) and decreased immediately, returning to its normal level on the third POD. In contrast, GCSF in patients with MOF showed a small increase on the first POD ($p<0.01$) and tended to rise again on the fifth and seventh PODs with evidence of complications. It appeared that glucocorticoid infusion reduced the increase in GCSF after the operation in patients with no MOF (Fig. 2). However, these changes were not statistically significant because of the interindividual variation in GCSF response. Despite the remarkable increase in GCSF, the peripheral blood leukocyte count remained slightly increased until the fifth POD in patients both with and without MOF. The leukocyte count increased more in patients with MOF on the fifth POD when the infection became manifest.

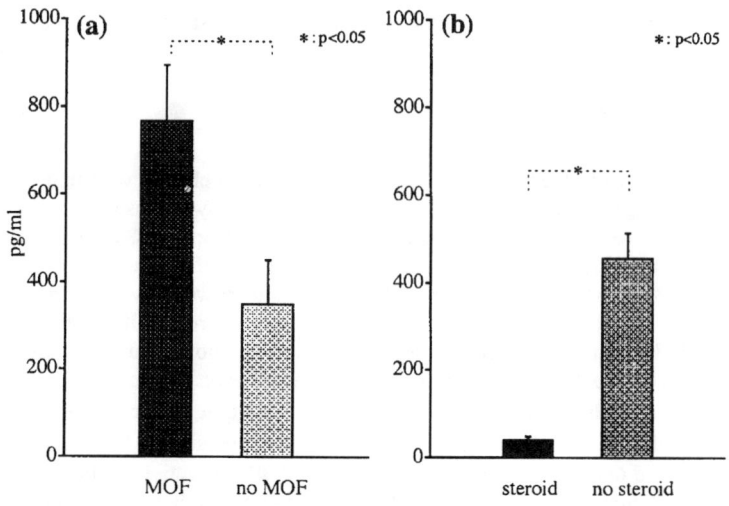

Fig. 1: Plasma IL-6 level after the operation in patients who developed MOF was significantly higher than that in patients with no MOF. Glucocorticoid infusion significantly reduced the IL-6 level at first POD in patients with no MOF

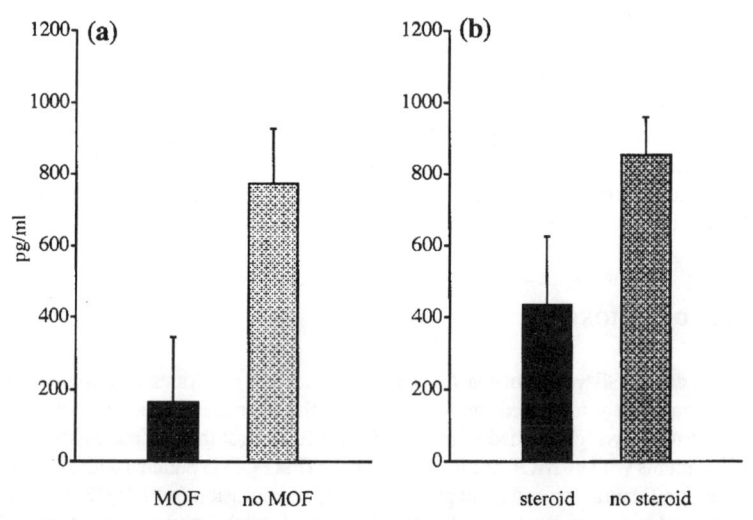

Fig. 2: Patients with MOF tended to have a lower plasma GCSF level after the operation than those with no MOF. It seems that the GCSF level after the operation might have been reduced by glucocorticoid infusion in patients with no MOF. However, no statistically significant differences were found in this study

C-Reactive Protein

Measurements were taken of C-reactive protein (CRP) as one of the acute-phase proteins which were induced in the liver by the stimulus of IL-6. CRP had a maximal increase on the third POD in patients with no MOF. However, patients with MOF showed a greater increase, with no return to normal until the seventh POD ($p<0.05$). When they were infused with glucocorticoid, the rise in CRP became less pronounced (p<0.05) (Fig. 3). These results were compatible with the changes of IL-6.

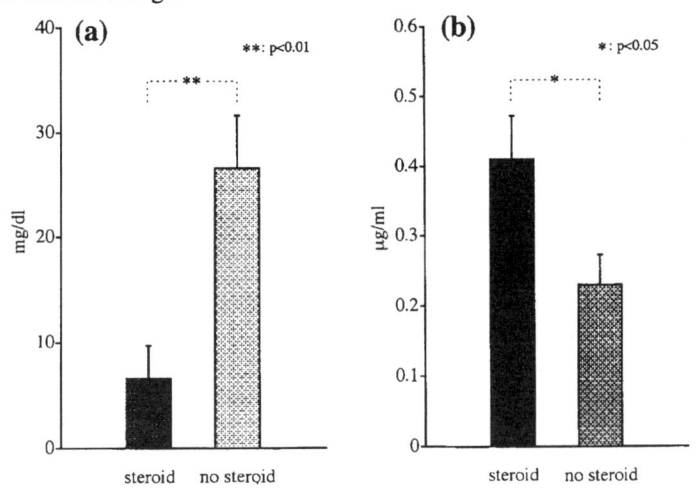

Fig. 3: In patients with no MOF, glucocorticoid infusion significantly reduced serum CRP level (a) and minimized the decrease in coenzyme Q_{10} (b)

Oxy-Radicals, Antioxidants, and Nitric Oxide

As a function of activated PMN, superoxide anion (O_2^-) production of PMN stimulated by phorbol myristate acetate was measured by cytochrome C assay. There was a decreased O_2^- production/10^6 PMNs on the third POD in patients without MOF ($p<0.05$), while there were no significant changes in patients with MOF until the fifth POD before the infection became manifest. However, because there was an increase in the peripheral blood PMN count, the total O_2^- production from circulating PMN tended to increase after the operation. Antioxidants are the host defense against oxidative stress and include enzymes (i.e., superoxide dismutase, catalase) and vitamins (i.e., α-tocopherol, β-carotene, ascorbic acid). In this study, α-tocopherol, β-carotene, and coenzyme Q_{10} were measured. Levels of coenzyme Q_{10} decreased on the first POD ($p<0.05$) and did not return until the seventh POD. There was no significant difference in coenzyme Q_{10} changes between patients with and without MOF. In those who had no MOF, no reduction in coenzyme Q_{10} was found when they were infused with glucocorticoid, while patients without glucocorticoid showed a reduction of coenzyme Q_{10} ($p<0.05$) (Fig. 3). However, there were no significant changes in either α-tocopherol or β-carotene because of the interindividual variation in their background levels. NO_x (NO_2 and

NO_3), which are stable end products of NO, were measured by the reaction with $NaNO_2$ and $NaNO_3$ as standard. A reduction in urinary NO_3, a predominant form of NO_x in the preoperative urine samples, was found on the operative day ($p<0.05$). It was then followed by an induction of endogenous NO synthesis and NO_x returned to the preoperative level on the first POD ($p<0.05$) in patients with no MOF. However, an increase in urinary NO_x was found in the presence of sepsis.

Discussion

Augmented responses of IL-6 and an abnormal pattern of GCSF were caused by surgical stress including massive bleeding during the major operation and were associated with development of MOF. Following the operation, circulating platelet and lymphocyte counts decreased. These were glucocorticoid-independent phenomena, and the precise mechanisms of postoperative platelet aggregation and immunosuppression remain unclear. The proposed surgical stress mechanism relevant to IL-6 and GCSF in the complex cytokine interrelationships is shown in Fig. 4. We found major surgical stress-activated cytokine-producing cells such as mononuclear cells, an augmented IL-6 response, and abnormal patterns of GCSF response to finally cause tissue damage and organ dysfunction through PMN activation and altered endothelial NO production. Glucocorticoid infusion might have exerted suppression on cytokine-producing cells and might have been effective in reducing IL-6 and probably GCSF. The results of our clinical study were supported by those of several in vitro studies in which corticosteroids were said to inhibit the secretion of IL-6 [2, 4, 5], the accumulation of the IL-6 messenger RNA [5], and GCSF secretion [12]. Consequently, glucocorticoid infusion inhibited hepatic synthesis of acute-phase protein and minimized the decrease in antioxidant. These results suggested that glucocorticoid infusion might reduce surgical stress by suppressing functions of cytokine-producing cells and might prevent deteriorated host defense responses in the cytokine network.

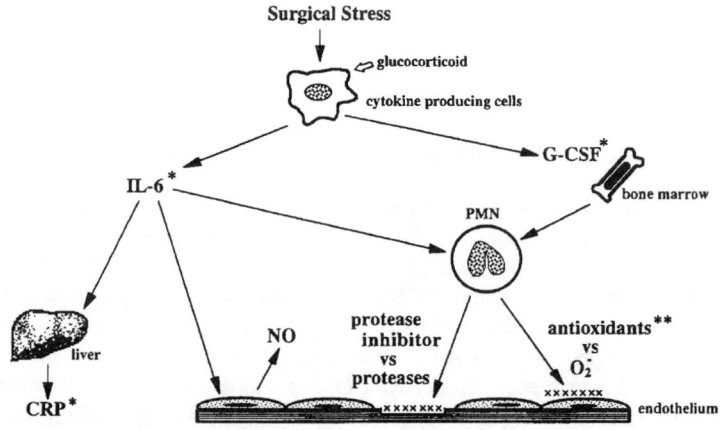

Fig. 4: Molecular scheme of surgical stress proposed on the basis of the present clinical evidence. The network of IL-6 and GCSF with acute-phase protein induction, NO production, and PMN activation was specifically studied in complex cytokine interrelationships. Effects of glucocorticoid infusion on suppression of surgically induced IL-6, GCSF, and CRP (*) and minimizing decreased antioxidants (**) are shown

References

1. Baigrie RJ, Lamont PM, Kwiatkowski D, Dallman MJ, Morris PJ (1992) Systemic cytokine response after major surgery. Br J Surg 79: 757-760
2. Breuninger LM, Dempsey WL, Uhl J, Murasko DM (1993) Hydrocortisone regulation of interleukin-6 protein production by a purified population of human peripheral blood monocytes. Clin Immunol Immunopathol 69: 205-214
3. Green LC, Luzuriaga KR, Wagner DA, Rand W, Istfan N, Young VR, Tannenbaum SR (1981) Nitrate biosynthesis in man. Proc Natl Acad Sci USA 78: 7764-7768
4. Hettmannsperger U, Detmar M, Owsianowski M, Tenorio S, Kammler H, Orfanos CE (1992) Cytokine-stimulated human dermal microvascular endothelial cells produce interleukin 6-inhibition by hydrocortisone, dexamethasone, and calcitriol. J Invest Dermatol 99: 531-536
5. Levine SJ, Larivee P, Logun C, Agnus CW, Shelhamer JH (1993) Corticosteroids differentially regulate secretion of IL-6, IL-8, and G-CSF by a human bronchial epithelial cell line. Am J Physiol 265: L-360-L368
6. Lowry SF (1993) Cytokine mediators of immunity and inflammation. Arch Surg 128: 123501241
7. Matsuda T, Miyashita M, Kojima N, Egami K, Adachi K, Yamashita K, Onda M, Kawanami O (1985) Endotoxin-induced lung injury: role of oxidant and efficacy of steroid. Circ Shock 16: 66
8. Members of the American College of Chest Physicians/Society of Critical Care Medicine Consensus Conference Committee (1992) Definitions for sepsis and organ failure and guidelines for the use of innovative therapies in sepsis. Chest 101: 1644-1655
9. Orrenius S, McConkey DJ, Nicotera P (1988) Mechanisms of oxidant-induced cell damage. In: Cerutti PA, Fridovich I, McCord JM (eds.) Oxy-radicals in molecular biology and pathology. Liss, New York, pp. 327-339
10. Parks DA, Granger DN, Bulkley GB, Shah AK (1985) Soy bean trypsin inhibitor attenuates ischemic injury to the feline small intestine. Gastroenterology 89: 6-12
11. Patchen ML, MacVittie TJ, Williams JL, Schwartz GN, Souza LM (1991) Administration of interleukin-6 stimulates multilineage hematopoiesis and accelerates recovery from radiation-induced hematopoietic depression. Blood 77: 472-480
12. Pullman WE, Elsbury S, Kobayashi M, Hapel AJ, Doe WF (1992) Enhanced mucosal cytokine production in inflammatory bowel disease. Gastroenterology 102: 529-537
13. Sacks T, Moldow CF, Craddock PR, Bowers TK, Jacob HS (1978) Oxygen radical mediated endothelial cell damage by complement-stimulated granulocytes. An in vitro model of immune vascular damage. J Clin Invest 61: 1161-1167
14. Vane JR, Anggard EE, Botting RM (1990) Regulatory function of the vascular endothelium. N Engl J Med 323: 27-36

Neurohormone and Neuropeptide Regulation of the Posttraumatic Immune Response

J. Shelby, W.W. Ku, H. C. Nielson

Introduction

Alterations in immune response following traumatic injury, including dysregulation of immune cell cytokine secretion, are a result of a dynamic neuroendocrine process reflecting the attempted adaptive response of the injured host. The most widely investigated component of this process of adaptation to a stressful challenge is the hypothalamic-pituitary-adrenal (HPA) axis, the activation of which results in the well known elevation of glucocorticoid levels in trauma patients [1]. There is considerable evidence for the suppressive effects of glucocorticoid on immune function [2], which may play a role in trauma associated immune suppression.

Recent work has revealed that other neural products associated with the stress response also have immune regulating activity, suggesting that both the nervous and immune systems use these signal molecules in adaptive responses [3-5]. Neuropeptides influence immune reactivity by direct and indirect pathways, including tissue distribution, proliferative and synthetic responses, and cytotoxic activities of lymphocytes. Evidence for direct effects on immune response is strengthened by the discovery that immune cells possess receptors for these natural derived molecules [6] (Table 1) These neural/immune system interactions may occur in a hormonal (via circulation), paracrine (released from nerves), or autocrine (produced by immune cells themselves) fashion.

The nerve mapping studies by the Feltons and others [7] have revealed innervation of lymphoid organs, including the thymus, spleen, lymph nodes and bone marrow, with evidence for secretion of neurotransmitters in the immediate lymphoid microenvironment. Additionally, there is evidence that T cells produce ACTH, β-endorphin, and corticotropin-releasing hormone molecules that are identical to the neural product [8, 9], thereby setting the stage for paracrine and autocrine delivery to immune cells of these regulatory mechanisms.

Discoveries in neuroimmunologic research have also revealed that immune cell cytokine secretion is under neuroendocrine control [10-12] (Table 2). However, understanding of the mechanisms responsible for CNS regulation of immune response and cytokine production is incomplete, and very little is known about the role of this process in regulation of host immune response following trauma.

Table 1: Some regulatory molecules and receptors common to the nervous and immune system

Agent	Synthesized immune cells	Immune cell receptor	Action on immune cell function
ACTH	+	+	Inhibits T and B cells
Substance P	?	+	Enhances T cells
Somatomedin	?	+	Inhibits T cells
VIP	?	+	Alters lymphocyte homing and inhibits T cells
CRH	?	+	Inhibits T and B cells
NGF	?	+	Enhances mitogenesis/ IL-2R
Opiates	?	+	Inhibits T cells
Norepinephrine	?	+	Inhibits T cells; enhances B cells
β-Endorphin	+	+	Inhibits B cells
Melatonin	?	+	Enhances T and B cells
Serotonin	?	+	Enhances NK cells

IL-2R, interleukin-2 receptor; NK, natural killer; VIP, vasoactive intestinal peptide; CRH, corticotropin releasing hormone; NGF, nerve growth factor.

Table 2: Regulatory molecules of the nervous system: cytokine modulation

Agent	Cytokine / effect	Target cell
Substance P	IL-1, 2, 6, TNFα, IFN-γ / increase	Multiple / monocytes
VIP	IL-2, 6 / increase	T cell / monocytes
Melatonin	IL-2 / increase IL-6, IFN-γ / decrease	T cell / serum
Serotonin	IFN-γ / increase	NK cells
Somatostatin	IL-2 / increase	T cell

VIP, vasoactive intestinal peptide; IL, interleukin; TNF, tumor necrosis factor; IFN, interferon; NK, natural killer

Of interest to us is the neurohormone melatonin, which appears to have immunostimulatory effects in models of stress [13, 14]. Recently it has been observed that disruption of light/dark cycles induces significant changes in the CNS, with subsequent alterations in several physiologic functions, including immune response [15, 16]. Mediation of these changes appears to be linked to the pineal gland and its best known and most widely investigated product, the indole melatonin [17, 18]. Melatonin is known to act at the hypothalamic level [19], affecting thermoregulation and pituitary release of certain hormones [19, 20]. The pineal gland and melatonin have been reported to exert an oncostatic effect on carcinogenesis and tumor growth [21], and neoplastic diseases have been associated with immune depression and altered plasma melatonin levels [22, 24]. Administration of exogenous melatonin has been shown to enhance several immune parameters in normal and restraint stressed mice [25]. There have also been reports of melatonin mediated up-regulation of T cell interleukin-2 (IL-2) production in mice which were immunodeficient because of extremes of age or cyclophosphamide therapy [10]. Similarly, pinealectomy was shown to inhibit IL-2 production and natural killer (NK) cell activity in mice, while administration of exogenous melatonin in pinealectomized mice restored IL-2 production and NK activity [11]. Thus, melatonin appears to exert immunoenhancing effects in several models of immunodeficiency. Additionally, peak plasma melatonin levels have been shown to be significantly depressed in burn patients [26], suggesting a decreased availability of endogenous melatonin following severe injury. The possible role for melatonin in immune function alterations following thermal injury has not been previously evaluated.

Cytokine secretion alterations have been noted following injury, including decreases in IL-2 and excessive production of IL-6 and interferon-γ (IFN-γ) [27]. To investigate the possible immunoregulatory role of melatonin following traumatic injury, we have examined the effect of in vivo administration of exogenous melatonin on splenocyte cytokine production and contact sensitivity response in a murine model of thermal injury. The data presented indicate that melatonin has significant in vivo cytokine regulatory activity and influences cellular immune response in thermally injured mice.

Mouse Thermal Injury Model

Male Balb/c strain mice were obtained from the National Cancer Institute and housed in the pathogen free University of Utah vivarium rodent facility. The mice were rested for 2 weeks following shipment to the rodent facility before initiation of experiments. Age matched mice housed together in groups of four to six mice, ranging in age from 8-10 weeks, were used in any single experiment. Separate groups of mice were assessed for contact sensitivity response and cytokine secretion. Scald burns (20%-25% total body surface area) were given in a standardized manner. Full-thickness injury using this protocol has been documented by histologic examination. Burn injured mice were given intraperitoneal injections for fluid resuscitation of normal sterile saline: 2 ml in the first 24 h, followed by 1 ml on days 1 and 2. All animals were maintained in a controlled environment, with a standard 12 h/light/dark cycle (6 a.m. to 6 p.m. light on, 6 p.m. to 6 a.m. dark). Sham stressed mice received identical treatment as described for injured mice, including depilation, saline and vehicle injections and anesthesia, but they were not injured. Intact controls were not handled until spleen harvest (cytokine analysis group). Intact controls for the contact sensitivity response group were sensitized and challenged as described.

Materials and Methods

Reagents and Culture Conditions

Melatonin (N-acetyl-5-methoxytryptamine) (Sigma Chemical Co., St. Louis, MO) was dissolved in a minimal volume of ethanol and diluted with sterile phosphate buffer saline (PBS) to a final 0.2% ethanol PBS solution. The same ethanol-PBS solution was used as a vehicle in sham stressed mice. The melatonin was diluted to the appropriate concentration in PBS just before subcutaneous injection of 0.1 ml into the mice. It was injected at 4:00 p.m. daily.

Monoclonal antibodies and reference standards used in this study were a gift from Dr. Barbara Araneo, University of Utah. The monoclonal antibodies were prepared from culture supernatants of appropriate B cell hybridomas grown in serum-free conditions. The antibodies were from the following hybridoma clones: S4B6, rat anti murine IL-2; XMG1.2, rat anti

IFN-γ; 1452C-11.2, hamster anti murine CD3e; 11B11, rat anti-murine IL-4; MP5-20F3, rat anti murine IL-6. Murine recombinant IFN-γ, IL-2, and IL-4 and human recombinant IL-6 were used as reference standards in the bioassays and ELISAs.

Single cell suspensions of splenocytes harvested at day 5 postburn injury were prepared from spleens of control and experimental mice, washed twice in sterile balanced salt solution and placed in culture in RPMI 1640 supplemented with 1% Nutridoma-NS (serum-free) (Boehringer-Mannheim), antibiotics, 200 mM L-glutamine and 5×10^5 M^{2-}mercaptoethanol, at a density of 1×10^7 cells/ml per well. Cells were cultured with and without 1.5 mg of the T cell-specific mitogen anti CD3e, in a 24-well cluster culture plate for 24 h to induce cytokine release. Cell-free supernatants were collected and stored at 4°C for quantitation of cytokine content. The culture conditions have previously been assessed as providing optimal conditions for evaluation of splenocyte cytokine secretion [28].

Cytokine Assessment and Contact Sensitivity Assay

Both IL-2 and IL-4 production were assessed using a standard bioassay, as previously described [29]. HT-2 cells were the indicator cell line, and IL-2 was distinguished from IL-4 by using either monoclonal anti-IL-2 or anti-IL-4 antibodies in the culture media, which was supplemented with Nutridoma-NS(serum-free). A modified 3-{4,5-Dimethylthiazole-2-yl}-2,5 diphenyl tetrazolium bromide (MTT)-based colorimetric assay was performed with spectrophotometric readings for each titration analyzed by least squares regression using a second-degree polynomial curve-fitting program to obtain a unit value to the interleukin under evaluation, with the mean and standard deviation reported.

The levels of the cytokines IL-6 and IFN-γ were quantitated by a capture ELISA [29]. The appropriate capture antibody was absorbed to the wells of a 96-well microtest plate. Test supernatants were diluted (1:10) and twofold serial dilutions of the appropriate reference cytokine were added to the wells, followed by biotinylated detection antibody. The ELISA was developed using an avidin-horseradish peroxidase conjugate and appropriate substrate. Optical density readings were taken at 405 nmol/l using a 96-well microtest plate spectrophotometer. The lower limit of detection for most of these cytokines are levels which are less than 50 pg/ml.

Mice were sensitized on 2 consecutive days (postburn days 1 and 2) with the contact sensitizing antigen dinitrofluorobenzene (DNFB). A solution of 0.25% DNFB (Sigma Chemical Co., St. Louis, MO) was prepared in a 4:1 acetone-olive oil mixture, and 25 ml was applied to the shaved ventral surface. On postburn day 5 the contact sensitivity (CS) response was elicited by applying 10 μl of a challenge dose of the DNFB solution to the right hind footpads. The extent of swelling in all challenged mice, measured with an engineer's micrometer in 10^{-3} inches, is expressed as the difference in thickness between the challenged right hind footpad and unchallenged left hind footpad 24 h after challenge (postburn day 6).

Results

Contact Sensitivity

The CS response was inhibited in untreated sham stress and burn injured mice as compared to intact controls (Fig. 1), an observation which has previously been reported [29]. Melatonin (40 mg/kg) was administered at 4:00 p.m. daily starting the day of burn injury, until postburn day 6, when the footpads were measured. Sham stressed and injured mice receiving daily evening

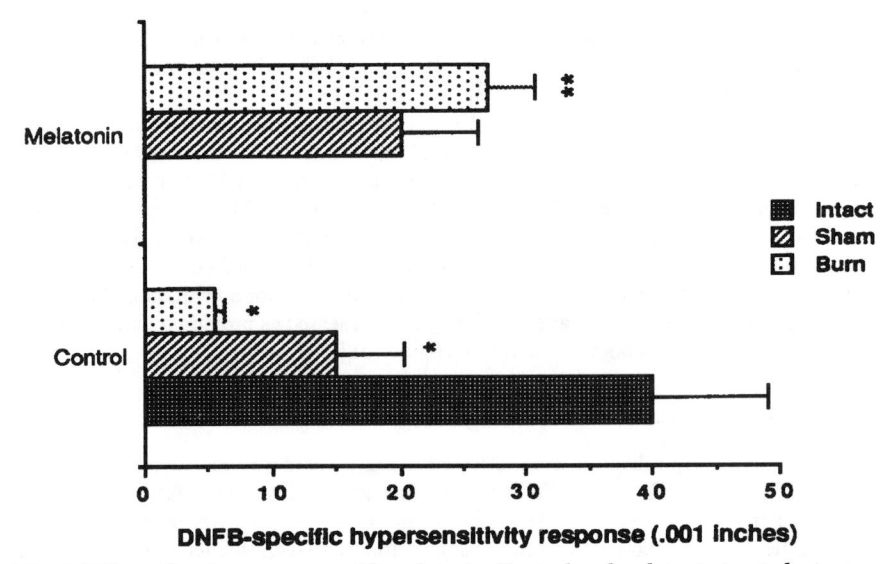

*Fig. 1: Effect of in vivo treatment with melatonin. Control and melatonin treated mice were assessed for contact sensitivity response. Bars indicate mean difference between challenge and unchallenged footpad measurements, and standard error. *$p<0.05$ compared with intact control mice; **$p<0.01$ compared with burn control group*

melatonin showed a significantly greater magnitude of contact hypersensitivity response, as compared to intact controls ($p<0.05$). These data indicate that melatonin administration influenced the development of a cell mediated immune response to the contact antigen DNFB, resulting in enhanced reactivity in sham stressed and burn injured mice.

Splenocyte Cytokine Secretion

Anti-CD3e stimulated splenocyte IL-2 secretion was reduced in sham stressed and thermally injured mice compared to controls ($p<0.05$), while IL-4 levels were increased (Fig. 2A, B). Melatonin (20 mg or 40 mg/kg) was given daily, starting on the day of injury through postburn day 4, with splenocyte harvest on postburn day 5. Thermally injured mice receiving evening melatonin at the concentration of 40 mg/kg showed increased splenocyte secretion of IL-2 (Fig. 2A), with no change observed in IL-4 levels (Fig. 2B). This would indicate that in vivo exogenous melatonin therapy increased the potential for IL-2 secretion by stimulated splenocytes from sham stressed and burn injured mice, while having little or no effect on IL-4 secretion in this population of cells.

In contrast to depressed IL-2 secretion observed in supernatants from stimulated splenocytes from burn injured Balb/c mice, spontaneous secretion of IL-6 and IFN-γ by unstimulated splenocytes from these mice was increased at postburn day 5, in comparison with spontaneous splenocyte secretion of these cytokines from sham stressed and intact control mice. ($p<0.001$) (Fig. 2C, D). Secretion of IFN-γ was reduced in thermally injured mice receiving 40 mg/kg evening melatonin ($p<0.05$) (Fig. 2C). Similarly, splenocyte production of IL-6 was significantly reduced in thermally injured mice receiving 20 mg/kg and 40 mg/kg evening melatonin ($p<0.001$) (Fig. 2D).

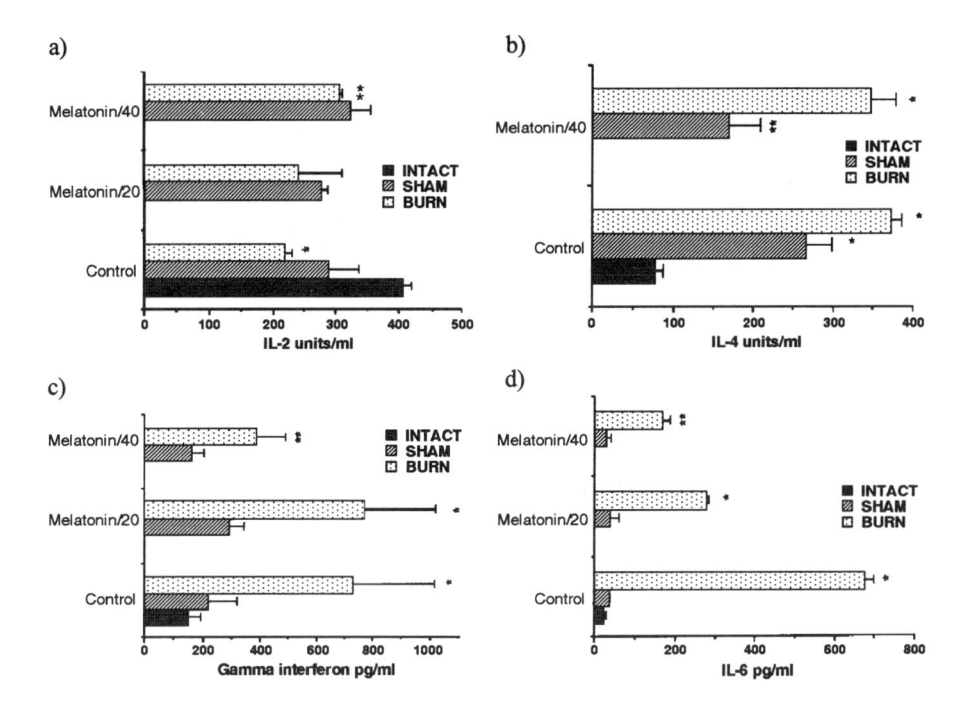

Fig. 2: a) Effect of in vivo treatment with melatonin on splenocyte interleukin (IL)-2 secretion. Spleen cells from control and melatonin treated mice were activated and culture supernatants were evaluated for IL-2 levels. Bars indicate the mean unit levels and standard errors for each group. *p<0.01 compared with intact control; **p<0.01 compared with burn control. b) Effect of in vivo treatment with melatonin on splenocyte IL-4 secretion. Spleen cells from control and melatonin treated mice were activated and culture supernatants were evaluated for IL-4 levels. Bars indicate the mean unit levels and standard errors for each group. *p<0.001 compared with intact control; **p<0.05 compared with intact control. c) Effect of in vivo treatment with melatonin on splenocyte interferon (IFN)-γ secretion. Spleen cells from control, melatonin (20 mg/kg), and melatonin (40 mg/kg) treated mice were placed in culture without further activation, and the supernatants were evaluated for IFN-γ levels. Bars indicate the mean pg/ml and standard error for each group. *p<0.05 compared with intact control; **p<0.05 compared with burn control. d) Effect of in vivo treatment with melatonin on splenocyte IL-6 secretion. Spleen cells from control, melatonin (20 mg/kg) and melatonin (40 mg/kg) treated mice were placed in culture without further activation, and the supernatants were evaluated for IL-6 levels. Bars indicate the mean pg/ml and standard error for each group. *p<0.001 compared with sham and intact controls; **p<0.001 compared with burn control

These results suggest that exogenous melatonin has cytokine secretion regulatory activity in thermally injured animals, as manifest by the enhancement of IL-2 production and the concurrent reduction in high levels of IFN-γ and IL-6.

Discussion

Recent work has indicated that the circadian synthesis and release of melatonin modulates several immune parameters including antibody response [17], IL-2 production (10, 11), and cellular response [30]. Melatonin appears to antagonize the immunosuppressive effects of corticosterone [17], cyclophosphamide [10] and restraint stress [25], in studies in which exogenous melatonin was administered. Only evening administered melatonin was effective in up-regulating immune response in these studies, a reminder of the circadian dependence of melatonin mediated effects.

Our findings further confirm the role for melatonin as an anti-stress immunoregulatory neurohormone. Cell mediated CS response was up-regulated by exogenous melatonin treatment of burn injured mice, in association with an enhancement of splenic IL-2 secretion. In contrast, IL-4 secretion, which is increased in injured mice, was not affected by melatonin treatment. Antibody production following thermal injury has been characterized as being initially reduced (both IgM and IgG), followed by a return to supernormal production levels, which is associated with increased production of IL-6, a cytokine with varied bioactivity, including B cell growth and differentiation stimulus [31]. Similarly, IL-4 and IFN-γ are known to promote B cell differentiation and immunoglobulin isotype switching [32].

Excessive systemic and local levels of some cytokines are associated with pathogenic processes following burn injury and various inflammatory and autoimmune states [33-35]. In our study we observed increased levels of IL-6 and IFN-γ in untreated burn injured Balb/c mice, with significant reductions of these two cytokines in burn injured mice treated with melatonin. Whether or not melatonin treatment will have beneficial effects on cytokine related pathology following injury is not known.

Plasma melatonin levels peak at night in higher mammals, including humans [18]. There are situations in which derangements of circadian melatonin rhythm are associated with morbidity and altered immune function, including in cancer patients and the aged [18, 24, 36]. The inbred murine strain in this study, Balb/c, is characterized as having exaggerated glucocorticoid responses to stressful stimuli and increased susceptibility to cellular infections and autoimmunity [37]. The Balb/c strain was also defined as having the lowest melatonin nocturnal peak plasma levels out of three strains tested [18]. Possibly the predisposition of Balb/c mice to immune dysregulation is the result of an imbalance between circadian glucocorticoid and melatonin levels, with the glucocorticoids predominating. In our model of thermal injury and stress, melatonin appeared to bring back into balance immune parameters in treated burn injured Balb/c mice.

In models of endogenous melatonin elevation or inhibition, by pharmacologic, environmental (constant light or dark), or surgical (pinealectomy) means, several changes in immune reactivity have been observed. In a murine model of autoimmune type II collagen with subsequent development of collagen-induced arthritis, constant darkness enhanced the magnitude of autoimmunity and exaggerated the development of arthritis [38]. In another study, pinealectomy of young mice resulted in decreased IL-2 secretion and NK activity [11]. Additionally, pharmacologic inhibition of melatonin was associated with depressed primary antibody response [8]. Endogenous melatonin secretion appears to be lower following traumatic injury, with evidence for depressed peak plasma levels [26]. Our findings of immune modulation by melatonin in burn injured mice, along with evidence for deficient endogenous levels of melatonin following severe injury, suggest a possible role for melatonin in adaptive immune response.

The precise mechanism by which melatonin exerts its effects on immune cells in uncertain. However, there is evidence that melatonin stimulates T cell production of opioids which then mediated melatonin-induced immune enhancement in a model of restraint stress [39]. Other investigators have suggested that melatonin affects the affinity and density of thymus steroid receptors in rats undergoing challenge with T-dependent antigens [40]. These approaches suggest than melatonin has an indirect influence on immune cell function, but there is also evidence that spleen cells possess receptors for melatonin, leaving open the possibility of direct effects [41].

The mechanisms by which melatonin increased IL-2 secretion and CS response, and modulated spontaneous IFN-γ and IL-6 levels in thermally injured mice is unclear. Further studies of melatonin therapy following stress and injury will delineate the mediating pathways and show whether or not these changes in immune function and cytokine profiles will result in enhanced infectious resistance and reduced immune/cytokine mediated pathogenic processes.

Additionally, there is a wealth of work waiting to be done: (1) to focus on all neural products produced during an adaptive stress response following severe injury, (2) to learn more about the possible influence these molecules may have on immune function, and (3) to design novel therapeutic interventions.

References

1. Vaughan VM, Becker RA, Allen JP, Goodwin CV, Pruitt BA, Mason DA (1982) Cortisol and corticotropin in burned patients. J Trauma 22: 263-273
2. Cupps TR, Fauci AC (1982) Corticosteroid-mediated immunoregulation in man. Immunol Rev 65: 134-155
3. Dunn AJ (1990) recent advances in psychoneuroimmunology. Cur Opin Psychiatr 3: 103-107
4. Dantzer R, Kelley KW (1989) Stress and immunity: an integrated view of relationships between the brain and immune system. Life Sci 44: 1995-2008
5. Roszman TL, Carlson SL (1981) Neurotransmitters and molecular signalling in the immune response. In: Ader R, Felten DL, Cohen N (eds.) Psychoneuroimmunology, Academic, New York, pp. 311-335
6. Carr DJJ, Blalock JE (1991) Neuropeptide hormones and receptors common to the immune and neuroendocrine systems: bidirectional pathway of intersystem communication. In: Ader R, Felten DL, Cohen N (eds.) Psychoneuroimmunology, Academic, New York, pp. 573-588
7. Felten SY, Felten DL (1991) Innervation of lymphoid tissue. In: Ader R, Felten DL, Cohen N (eds.) Psychoneuroimmunology, Academic, New York, pp. 27-69
8. Goetzl EJ, Turck CW, Sreedharan SP (1991) Production and recognition of neuropeptides by cells of the immune system. In: Ader R, Felten DL, Cohen N (eds.) Psychoneuroimmunology, Academic, New York, pp. 263-282
9. Besedovsky HO, Del Rey A (1991) Physiological implications of the immune-neuro-endocrine network. In: Ader R, Felten DL, Cohen N (eds.) Psychoneuroimmunology, Academic, New York, p. 589-608
10. Caroleo MC, Frasca D, Giuseppe N, Doria G (1992) Melatonin as immunomodulator in immunodeficient mice. Immunopharmacology 23: 81-89
11. Gobbo VD, Libri V, Villani N, Calio R, Nistico G (1984) Pinealectomy inhibits interleukin-2 production and natural killer cell activity in mice. Int J Immunopharmacol 11: 567-573

12. Spector NH, Korneva EA (1981) Neurophysiology, immunophysiology, and neuroimmunomodulation. In: Ader R, Felten DL, Cohen N (eds.) Psychoneuroimmunology, Academic, New York
13. Maestroni GJ, Conti A, Pierpaoli W (1988) Role of the pineal gland in immunity III. Melantonin antagonizes the immunosuppressive effect of acute stress via an opiatergic mechanism. Immunology 63: 465-469
14. Maestroni GJ, Conti A, Pierpaoli W (1987) Role of the pineal gland in immunity II. Melantonin enhances the antibody response via an opiatergic mechanism. Clin Exp Immunol 68: 384-391
15.. Radosevic-Stasic B, Jonjic S, Rukavina D (1983) Immune response of rats after pharmacologic pinealectomy. Period Biol 5: 282-297
16. Wurtman R (1986) Melatonin in humans. J Neural Trans Suppl 21: 1-8
17. Maestroni GJM, Conti A, Pierpaoli W (1986) Role of the pineal gland in immunity; circadian synthesis and release of melatonin modulates the antibody response and antagonizes the immunosuppressive effect of corticosterone. J Neuroimmunol 13: 19-30
18. Maestroni GJM, Conti A (1991) Role of the pineal neurohormone melatonin in the psycho-neuroendocrine-immune network. In: Ader R, Felten DL, Cohen N (eds.) Psychoneuroimmunology, 2nd edn. Academic, New York, pp. 495-513
19. Pierpaoli W, Changxian Y (1990) The involvement of pineal gland and melatonin in immunity and aging. I. Thymus-mediated, immunoreconstituting and antiviral activity of thyrotropin-releasing hormone. J Neuroimmunol 27: 99-109
20. Beck-Friis J, Kjellman BF, Ljunggren J-G, Wetterberg L (1985) The pineal gland in affective disorders. In: Brown GM, Wainwright SD (eds.) The pineal gland: endocrine aspects, Pergamon, New York, pp. 313-325
21. Regelson W, Pierpaoli W (1987) Melatonin: a rediscovered antitumor hormone? Its relation to surface receptors, sex steroid metabolism, immunologic response, and chronobiologic factors in tumor growth and therapy. Cancer Invest 5: 379-385
22. Lissoni P, Barni S, Archili C, Cattaneo G, Rovelli F, Conti A, Maestroni GJM, Tancini G (1990) Endocrine effects of a 24 hour intravenous infusion of interleukin-2 in the immunotherapy of cancer. Anticancer Res 10: 753-758
23. Lissoni P, Barni S, Crispino S, Tancini G, Fraschini F (1989) Endocrine and immune effects of melatonin therapy in metastatic cancer patients. Eur J Cancer 25: 789-795
24. Lissoni P, Tancini G, Barni S, Viviani S, Archili C, Cattaneo G, Fiorelli G (1990) Alterations of pineal gland and of T lymphocyte subsets in metastatic cancer patients: preliminary results. J Biol Regul Homeost Agents 3: 181-183
25. Maestroni GJM, Conti A, Pierpaoli W (1988) Pineal melatonin, its fundamental immunoregulatory role in aging and cancer. Ann NY Acad Sci 521: 141-149
26. Vaughn G, Taylor TJ, Pruitt BA, Mason AD (1985) Pineal function in burns: melatonin is not a marker for general sympathetic activity. J Pineal Res 2: 1-12
27. Moss NM, Gough DB, Jordan AL et al. (1988) Temporal correlation of impaired immune response after thermal injury with susceptibility to infection in a murine model. Surgery 104: 882-887
28. Daynes RA, Araneo BA, Dowell TA, Huang K, Dudley D (1990) Regulation of murine lymphokine production in vivo. III. The lymphoid microenvironment exerts regulatory influences over T helper function. J Exp Med 171: 979-996
29. Araneo BA, Shelby J, Gang-Zhou L, Ku WW, Daynes R (1993) Administration of dehydroepiandrosterone to burned mice preserves normal immunologic competence. Arch Surg 128: 318-325
30. Shelby J, Ku WW, Nelson EW (1993) Immunomodulatory role for melatonin in allograft rejection. In: Abstract book, Tolerance Induction Symposium, Breckenridge, Colorado, 1993

31. Isakson P (1992) Interleukin 4. Adv Neuroimmunol 2: 55-65
32. Finkelman FD, Katona I, Mosmann TR, Coffman RL (1988) Interferon-γ regulates the isotypes of immunoglobulin secreted during in vivo humoral responses. J Immunol 140: 1022-1027
33. Schluter B, Konig B, Bergmann U, Muller FE, Konig W (1991) Interleukin-6 - a potential mediator of lethal sepsis after major thermal trauma: evidence for increased IL-6 production by peripheral blood mononuclear cells. J Trauma 31: 1663-1670
34. Gijbels K, Billiau A (1992) Interleukin 6: general biological properties and possible role in the neural and endocrine systems. Adv Neuroimmunol 2: 83-97
35. Vankelecom H, Billiau A (1992) Interferon-γ in neuroimmunology and endocrinology. Adv Neuroimmunol 2: 139-161
36. Armstrong SM, Redman JR (1991) Melatonin. A chronobiotic with anti-aging properties? Med Hypotheses 34: 300-309
37. Mason D (1991) Genetic variation in the stress response: susceptibility to experimental allergic encephalomyelitis and implications for human inflammatory disease. Immunol Today 12: 57-60
38. Hansson I, Holmdahl R, Mattsson R (1990) Constant darkness enhances autoimmunity to type II collagen and exaggerates development of collagen-induced arthritis. J Neuroimmunol 27: 79-84
39. Maestroni GJM, Conti A (1989) Beta-endorphin and dynorphin mimic the circadian immunoenhancing and anti-stress effects of melatonin. Int J Immunopharmac 11: 333-340
40. Persengiev S, Patchev V, Velev B (1991) Melatonin effects on thymus steroid receptors in the course of primary antibody responses: significance of circulating glucocorticoid levels. Int J Biochem 23: 1487-1489
41. Yu ZH, Yuan H, Lu Y, Pang SF (1991) (^{125}I)Iodomelatonin binding sites in spleens of birds and mammals. Neurosci Let 125: 175-178

Endocrine Responses to Mesenteric Traction During Major Abdominal Surgery

Ch.-F. Wolf, A. Brinkmann, D. Berger, E. Kneitinger, H. Wiedeck, R. Wennauer, M.Büchler, M. Georgieff, A. Grünert, W.D. Seeling

Introduction

Mesenteric traction during abdominal surgery results in lowered blood pressure for 20 - 40 min and eventually in a facial flush [7, 8]. These symptoms are accompanied by a dramatic release of prostacyclin (PGI_2) following the manipulation of the mesentery. Blood pressure returns to pretraction values after 20 - 40 min while the plasma concentration of 6-keto-$PGF_1\alpha$, which is a detectable degradation product of PGI_2, is still enhanced [7, 8]. Apart from the clinical complication as indicated by the hemodynamic disturbances, the pathomechanisms of the syndrome have been the focus of several studies [2, 4, 9, 10]. Cyclooxygenase inhibition protects against hemodynamic instability following exploration of the abdominal contents [2, 4, 10]. Further insights into counteraction of profound endogenous prostacyclin liberation during abdominal surgery have not so far been definitively described. An approach to the investigation of the physiological endocrine response, which plays a role in the maintenance of blood pressure, is presented in this study.

Methods

Fifty patients (28 male, 22 female) undergoing major abdominal surgery (including surgery of the infrarenal aorta and pancreas) were studied in a prospective randomized, double-blinded protocol, which had been approved by the local ethics committee. Ages ranged between 37 and 78 years (ASA II-IV). Mesenteric traction was performed in a uniform fashion by the surgeon at time point 0 in the opened abdominal cavity. A combined technique was used on patients with general anesthesia plus continuous supplemental thoraco-epidural anesthesia providing a sensory blockade from T4 to L1. Either 400 mg ibuprofen i.v. ($n = 25$) or a placebo aliquot ($n = 25$) was administered to patients 15 min before induction of anesthesia. At time points 0, 5, 15, 30, 45, and 90 min (6 h) before and after mesenteric traction (baseline) we determined the plasma concentrations of 6-keto-PGF$_{1\alpha}$, epinephrine, norepinephrine, dopamine, renin, aldosterone, vasopressin and cortisol. Hemodynamic measurements were continuously made over the observation period. For determination of plasma catecholamine levels we performed reversed-phase high-performance liquid chromatography (Waters) with aluminum extraction and electrochemical detection. Plasma aldosterone concentrations were detected with a Coat-A-Count radioimmunoassay (RIA) from Hermann Biermann Diagnostica (Bad Nauheim). Cortisol plasma concentration (PC) was measured with a Coat-A-Count cortisol RIA from Hermann Biermann Diagnostica (Bad Nauheim). Determination of active renin PC was performed with an RIA [active renin immunoradiometric assay (IRMA) Nichols]. Vasopressin concentrations were measured by RIA (vasopressin direct RIA, Bühlmann Laboratories). All plasma samples (renin, aldosterone, vasopressin, 6-keto-PGF$_{1\alpha}$, cortisol and catecholamines) were analyzed in duplicate.

Data are presented as means ± SEM. Statistical analysis was performed using the Mann-Whitney test to analyze for the effects of Ibuprofen on vasopressor hormone levels. Differences between pre- and post-traction values were tested with a Wilcoxon signed-rank test for paired data. An α-value of $p < 0.05$ was considered significant, applying a Bonferroni correction for multiple test procedures.

Results

Hemodynamic instability occurred as expected in the placebo group (data not shown). Blood pressure returned to pretraction values after 30-40 min. We were unable to detect any difference between the two groups at the baseline time point. The PC of 6-keto-PGF$_{1\alpha}$ peaked 5 min after mesenteric traction (2274±284 ng/l; ibuprofen-pretreated group, 102±12 ng/l; baseline, 60±1 ng/l; Fig. 1), remained elevated for 90 min by a statistically significant amount compared with the ibuprofen-pretreated group, and decreased steadily over 6 h (203±42 ng/l; ibuprofen-pretreated group, 84±12 ng/l; reference values $p < 60$ ng/ml). The PC of catecholamine barely exceeded the upper limit of the reference range during the observation period (Fig. 2; reference values: epinephrine, 10-120 ng/l; norepinephrine, 100-600 ng/l). The PC of epinephrine showed a detectable reaction to traction on the mesenteric root, whereas the PC of norepinephrine showed no such reaction. The PC of ADH peaked 5 min after mesenteric traction (71±7 pg/l; ibuprofen-pretreated group, 20±6 pg/l; baseline, 5±1 pg/l; Fig. 1; expected "normal" values, 0-6.7 pg/ml) and showed, analogously to the PC of 6-ketp-PGF$_{1\alpha}$, a steady decrease over the observation period.

The PC of renin peaked after 45 min (66±23 µU/ml; ibuprofen-pretreated group, 18±3 µU/ml; baseline, 16±2 µU/ml: reference values: 10-22 µU/ml with the patient in the supine position). Aldosterone also showed a maximum after 45 min compared with the ibuprofen-pretreated group (110±12 pg/ml; ibuprofen-pretreated group, 66±16 pg/ml; baseline, 56±7 pg/ml; reference values, 35-100 pg/ml with the patient in the supine position; Fig. 3) whereas cortisol demonstrated plasma values within the reference ranges in respect to the circadian rhythms with a reasonable (end of anesthesia) maximum 6h after mesenteric traction (26±1 µg/l; ibuprofen-tretreated group, 24±3 µg/l; baseline, 10±1 µg/l; reference values, 2-46 µg/l (morning), 2-27 µg/l (afternoon); Fig. 2).

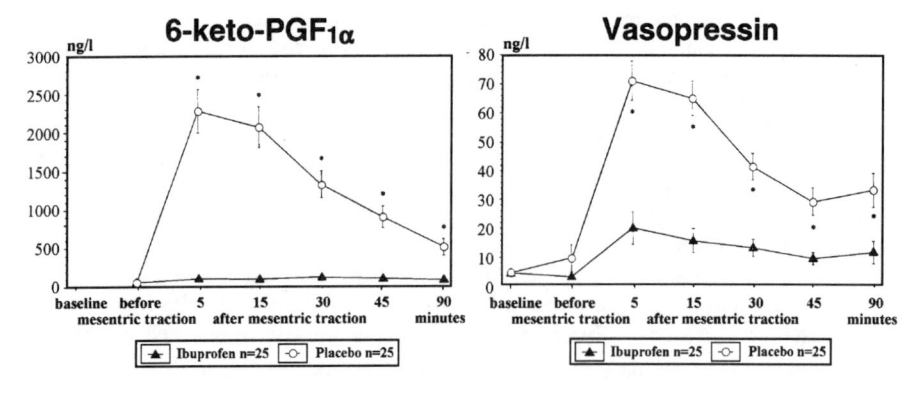

*Fig. 1: Plasma concentrations of 6-keto-PGF$_{1\alpha}$ and vasopressin during the observation period. Statistical analysis comparing ibuprofen-treated patients with the placebo group. *$p<0.05$*

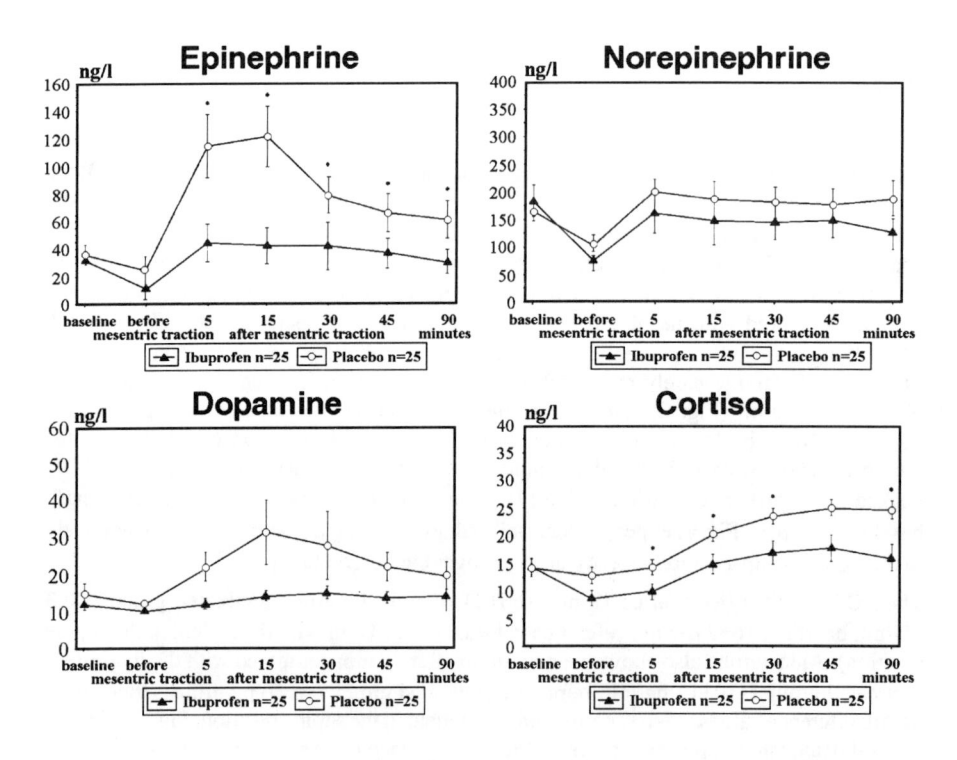

*Fig. 2: Plasma concentrations of epinephrine norepinephrine dopamine and cortisol during the observation period. Statistical analysis comparing ibuprofen-treated patients with the placebo group. *$p<0.05$*

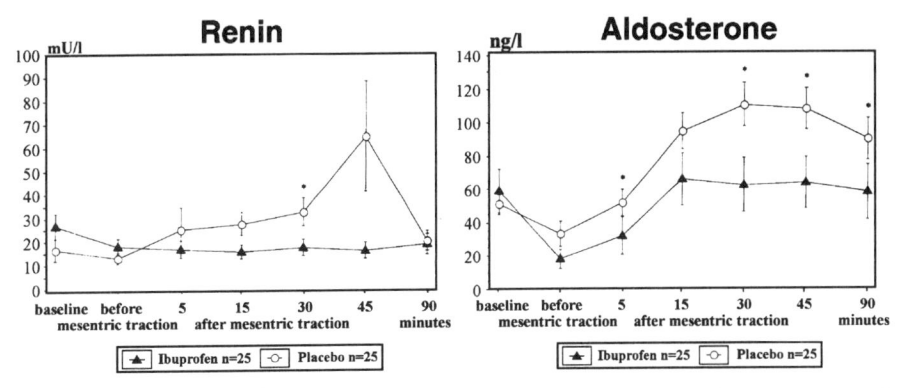

Fig. 3: *Plasma concentrations of renin and aldosterone during the observation period. Statistical analysis comparing ibuprofen- treated patients with the placebo group.* $*p<0.05$

Discussion

As predicted, significant hypotension, tachycardia, decreased systemic vascular resistance (SVR) and a considerable release of PGI_2 follow mesenteric traction. Declining but substantially enhanced plasma concentrations of 6-keto-$PGF_{1\alpha}$ are recorded over 90 min. Since the plasma half-life of both, PGI_2 and 6-keto-$PGF_{1\alpha}$ is reported to be less than 90 min [5], a continuing PGI_2 liberation following the initial prostacyclin release has been recorded. Our data clearly signify the importance of vasopressin and the renin-angiotensin-aldosterone system (RAAS) in maintaining stable hemodynamic circulation after an acute, endogenous prostacyclin release.

In contrast to vasopressin and to the RAAS, epinephrine plasma levels barely exceeded the upper reference limit in their reaction to systemic vasodilation. The blockade of the efferent sympathetic drive, as associated with epidural anesthesia, partially explains this reduced sympathoadrenergic response. However, as observed in a pilot study [1], epidural blockade reduces sympathoadrenergic response to mesenteric traction to a lower level, but even without spinal blockade no sufficient catecholamine release can be recorded following initial PGI_2 liberation. The PC of epinephrine, which increases only within its "normal" range after mesenteric traction, and the unchanged PC of norepinephrine reflect both the inadequate catecholamine response to prostacyclin release and the adequate spinal blockade, respectively.

The advantage of our design regarding an epidural blockade is its exclusion of interfering neuronal reflex arcs. We therefore focused our attention on the endocrine reaction to prostacyclin liberation. We identified ADH as the first vasopressor hormone that increases counteractively to mesenteric traction. This vasopressin PC corresponded perfectly to the PC of 6-keto-$PGF_{1\alpha}$ as demonstrated in Fig. 1. Data from patients and from animal models indicate that the non-osmotic release of ADH is virtually always accompanied by a simultaneous activation of the RAAS and the sympathetic nervous system [6]. In our experimental design we observed the main activation of the RAAS about 30-45 min after mesenteric traction. Although one stimulus for renin release, i.e., the adrenergic system, had been inhibited by epidural blockade, other stimuli such as baroreceptor, macula densa and prostacyclin itself may have activated the RAAS [3]. The coincidence of restored blood pressure, restored systemic vascular resistence and restored hear-trate, on one hand, with the main activation of the RAAS and vasopressin, on the other hand make major vasoconstrictive action of these hormones very likely. However, additional interference of further vasoconstricting agents, e.g., endothelin or neurotensin, etc., cannot be excluded.

The PC of cortisol, which is an indicator of surgical stress or trauma, demonstrated slightly increasing plasma values in our placebo group compared with the ibuprofen-pretreated group. As observed for a second indicator of stress, i.e., epinephrine, cortisol plasma concentrations did not exceed the reference values. Such "normal" plasma concentrations of epinephrine and cortisol indicate that the endocrine response documented in this study is not a general response to something like "stress," but an explicit reaction to vasodilation mediated by prostacyclin.

We therefore summarize that the earliest detected counteraction to PGI_2 release and consecutive vasodilation is mediated via ADH secretion. The second regulatory factor is the renin-angiotensin-aldosterone system (RAAS); its activation is found 30-45 min after mesenteric traction. A substantial regulatory release of catecholamines could not be documented. The activation of ADH and RAAS after mesenteric traction is not a hormonal response primarily related to surgical trauma and/or stress but a counteraction to systemic vasodilation induced by prostacyclin.

References

1. Brinkmann A, Wolf C-F, Walther F-G, Junger S, Duntas L, Oettinger W, Seeling W (1991) Mesenteric traction syndrome - aspects of pathophysiology and treatment. In: Eyrich K, Dennhardt R, Voigt KH, Egerer K, Gramm H-J (eds.) Endocrinology in anesthesia and critical care medicine. Berlin, p 27
2. Brinkmann A, Wolf C-F, Walther F-G, Junger S, Duntas L, Oettinger W, Rosenthal J, Seeling W, Ahnefeld FW (1993) Mesenteric traction syndrome during major abdominal surgery: part I Relevance of cyclooxygenase inhibition by intravenous ibuprofen. Clin Physiol Biochem 10: 8-85
3. Dunn MJ (1989) Prostaglandin I_2 and the kidney Arch Mal Coeur 82(4): 27-31
4. Hudson JC, Wurm WH, O'Donnel TF Jr, Kane FR, Mackey WC, Su YF, Watkins WD (1990) Ibuprofen pretreatment inhibits prostacyclin release during abdominal exploration in aortic surgery. Anesthesiology 72: 443-449
5. Patrono C, Pugliese F, Ciabattoni G, Patrignani P, Maseri A, Chierchia S, Peskar BA, Cinotti GA, Simonetti BM, Pierucci A (1982) Evidence for a direct stimulatory effect of prostacyclin on renin release in man. J Clin Invest 69: 231-239
6. Schrier RW (1988) Pathogenesis of sodium and water retention in high-output and low-output cardiac failure nephrotic syndrome cirrhosis and pregnancy (1). N Engl J Med 319: 1065-1072
7. Seeling W, Heinrich H, Oettinger W: Das Eventerationssyndrom: Prostacyclinfreisetzung und akuter paO_2-Abfall durch Duenndarmeventeration. (The eventration syndrome: prostacyclin liberation and acute hypoxemia due to eventration of the small intestine). Anaesthesist 35: 738-743
8. Seltzer JL, Ritter DE, Starsnic MA, Marr AT (1985) The hemodynamic response to traction on the abdominal mesentery. Anesthesiology 63: 96-99
9. Seltzer JL, Goldberg ME, Larijani GE, Ritter DE, Starsnic MA, Stahl GL, Lefer AM (1988) Prostacyclin mediation of vasodilation following mesenteric traction. Anesthesiology 68:514-518 1988
10. Wolf C-F, Brinkmann A, Duntas L, Oettinger W, Walther F-G, Junger S, Rosenthal J, Keck FS, Seeling WD (1991) Interaktion von Prostaglandinen Renin und ANP bei der Beeinflußung des intraoperativen Blutdruckes. Nieren- und Hochdr 10:580-581 1991

Histamine in Septic/Endotoxic Shock

S. Dimmeler, E. Neugebauer, A. Lechleuthner

Introduction

The biogenic amine histamine, discovered as a shock mediator in 1920 by Sir Henry Dale [1], was one of the most well studied mediators 20 years ago. During the past 15 years, however, various other, diverse mediators have been discovered. As there newly discovered mediators, such as cytokines, arachidonate acid metabolites, oxygen radicals or nitric oxide receive increasing attention, histamine seems to have become "out of date" mediator, no longer challenging pharmacologists and physiologists in shock research. Nonetheless, the important role of histamine in anaphylactic shock [2] and more recent results in septic/endotoxic shock research have led us to assume that histamine plays a role in pathophysiology of septic/endotoxic shock. Thus, its part in the mediator network has still not been elucidated. To establish a cause/effect relationship between a mediator and a specific disease, i.e., septic/endotoxic shock, the four Koch-Dale criteria should be met. These are:
1. The presence of the mediator in the disease
2. The absence of the mediator in health
3. Elicitation of the disease by exogenous administration or endogenous formation/release of the mediator
4. The blockade of the mediator's effect(s) by inhibition of synthesis/release, by specific antagonists, or preventing or ameliorating the disease

To evaluate the evidence that the single mediator histamine is a causal chemical factor in clinical and experimental septic/endotoxic shock, a meta-analysis in combination with a decision tree was performed. An excerpt of the results is presented here; for further details see the publications of Neugebauer and coworkers [3, 4].

Increased Histamine Levels in Septic/Endotoxic Shock

Until December 1990 29 studies in seven species had been published on the topic of histamine release in septic/endotoxic shock conditions in vivo. The majority of the studies in animals demonstrated histamine release under endotoxic/septic conditions. However, three out of seven studies in man did not report any increase in blood histamine concentration.

The reliabiliy of histamine assays, the rapid release of histamine by other interventions (incorrect blood sampling, application of histamine-releasing drugs), the instability of histamine, the need for correctly timed blood sampling, and the choice of a control group are critical factors which have to be well considered in studies with critically ill patients. In order to answer the question whether or not histamine is released in septic shock, a cross-sectional study was designed comparing daily plasma histamine levels in 20 patients in septic shock (inclusion criteria according to the VA study [10]) with a control group consisting of 20 patients with peripheral trauma who did not show any signs of local of systemic infection after surgery. Up to the fourth day after inclusion into the study, plasma histamine concentrations in septic patients were significantly elevated ($p<0.05$). Furthermore, plasma histamine concentrations were higher in nonsurvivors than in survivors. In the group of nonsurvivors (nine patients) eight patients had plasma levels higher than the designated "cut-off point" (1 ng/ml) at the day of enrollment into the study. Only one patient survived with a histamine concentration over 1 ng/ml. Although the absolute number of patients is small, these results indicate that histamine is released or formed in septic/endotoxic shock.

Elicitation of Septic/Endotoxic Shock by Exogenous Administration, Endogenous Release, or Formation of Histamine

As histamine is only one of the mediators involved in the pathogenesis of endotoxic shock, it is unrealistic to expect that all pathophysiological reactions observed in the complex setting of septic/endotoxic shock can be mimicked only by histamine itself. However, if the hypothesis is correct, that histamine is a harmful mediator in septic/endotoxic shock, it should be possible to experimentally induce hemodynamic, respiratory, biochemical and/or morphological alterations resembling those in septic shock by exogenous administration of histamine or by endogenously released/formed histamine. The problem is that the influence of histamine can only be evaluated with regard to the diverse actions of histamine on its receptors (H_1-, H_2- or H_3-receptors). Table 1 illustrates the effects of histamine via H_1- and H_2-receptor stimulation, as described in the literature. Overall, stimulation of H_1-receptors seems to be associated with negative effects such as bronchial constriction or increased vascular permeability, whereas H_2-activation has anti-inflammatory and positive inotropic effects and may therefore ameliorate septic/endotoxic shock.

This hypothesis is supported by a reduction of mortality in rat endotoxic shock by H_2-agonism [11]. Endotoxic shock in rats ($n = 40$ per group) was induced by administration of 45 mg endotoxin/kg body weight intraperitoneally, followed by a continuous subcutaneous infusion of saline (control group) or the arpromidine-related H_2-agonist BU-E-75 (treatment group). After 96 h, 80% (32 out of 40) died in the control group, whereas the group treated with BU-E-75 (100 µg/kg body weight per hour) showed a significantly lower mortality rate (50%; $p = 0.009$).

Blockade of Histamine Effects with Antagonists and Prevention or Amelioration of Septic/Endotoxic Shock

The treatment of septic/endotoxic shock with histamine-antagonists was possible after the discovery of specific H_2-receptor antagonists by Black and coworkers [5] and H_1-antagonists by Ash and Schild [6]. The novel class of H_3-receptor antagonists, involved in neuronal transmission, and the intracellular receptor antagonists (Hic) have yet not been used in the treatment of septic/endotoxic shock.

Treatment with H_1-antagonists reduced the mortality of septic/endotoxic shock in rats [7,8,11] and mice [9]. H_1-antagonists prevented the decrease in blood pressure and endotoxin-induced heart ischemia and necrosis and reduced endotoxin effects on lung vascular permeability [12]. Best results were obtained by treatment with H_1-antagonists in the early phase of septic shock [13]. A study in porcine hyperdynamic shock (six pigs/group) revealed an amelioration of cardiovascular dysfunction and improved tissue oxygenation following administration of the H_1-antagonist dimethindene (2 mg/kg), as summarized in Table 2.

H_2-antagonists seemed to be less effective than H_1-antagonists. Seven animal studies (endotoxic shock in cats, mice and rats) did not show increased survival, rather in some studies H_2-antagonists had harmful effects [4].

In summary, meta-analysis of the four Koch-Dale criteria and of our own results showed a significant association of histamine with septic/endotoxic shock. Its influence is time-dependent and receptor-related. Early blockade of the H_1-receptors and stimulation of H_2-receptors may be appropriate therapeutic approaches. The interaction of histamine with other mediators, such as cytokines or nitric oxide, on the cellular and systemic level needs further investigation.

Table 1: Shock-related biological effects of histamine in humans via H1- and H2-receptors

H1-receptors	H2-receptors
Cardiovascular effects	
☐ Decrease in atrioventricular node conductance ☐ Coronary artery constriction ☐ Vasoconstriction (blood vessels > 80 %m) ☐ Vasodilation (blood vessels < 80 %m) ☐ Increased vascular permeability	☐ Increase in heart rate and myocardial contractility ☐ Reduction of cardiac preload ☐ Reduction of cardiac afterload ☐ Coronary vasodilatation ☐ Vasodilation (blood vessels <80 %m)
Pulmonary effects	
☐ Bronchial constriction	☐ Bronchial dilatation ☐ Increase in airway mucus secretion
Immunological effects	
☐ Proinflammatory	☐ Feedback inhibition of histamine release ☐ Inhibition of superoxide production ☐ Inhibition of cytokine production (TNF, IL-1, IL-2, IFN-γ) ☐ Immunosuppressive effect of T cells

For further details, see [14].
TNF, tumor necrosis factor; IL, interleukin; IFN, interferon

Table 2: Effect of the H_1-antagonist dimethindene in hyperdynamic porcine shock

		NaCl+endotoxin[a]	Dimethindene+endotoxin[a]
Cardiovascular system	MAP	↓↓	↓
	SVR*	↓↓	-
Pulmonary system	PVR	↑↑	↑
	MPAP	↑↑	↑
	PaO_2/FiO_2*	↓↓	↓
Metabolic function	BE*	↓↓	↓
	Lactate*	↑↑	↑
Inflamation	TNF	↑	↑

The H1-agonist dimethindene (2 mg/kg) or NaCl was administered 15 min before induction of endotoxic shock by continuous infusion of 5 µg/kg body weight per hour endotoxin. Cardiovascular, pulmonary and metabolic function was monitored for 5 h.
MAP, mean arterial pressure; SVR, systemic vascular resistance; MPAP, mean pulmonary arterial pressure; PVR, pulmonary vascular resistance: BE, base excess; TNF, tumor necrosis factor; * significant difference ($p<0.05$) between the NaCl- and dimethindene-treated groups.
[a]Changes compared to steady state values before endotoxin infusion.

References

1. Dale HH (1920) Conditions which are conductive to the production of shock by histamine. Br J Exp Pathol 1: 103
2. Lorenz W, Duda D, Dick W, Sitter H, Doenicke A, Black A, Weber D, Menke H, Stinner B, Junginger T, Rothmund M, Ohmann C, Healy MJR and the trial group Mainz/Marburg (1994) Incidence and clinical importance of perioperative histamine release: randomized study of volume loading and antihistamines after indution of anaesthesia. Lancet 343: 933
3. Neugebauer E, Rixen D, Lorenz W (1993) Histamine in septic/endotoxic shock. In: Neugebauer E, Holaday JW (eds.) Handbook of mediators in septic shock. pp 51 ff
4. Neugebauer E, Lorenz W, Maroske D, Barthlen W, Ennis M (1987) The role of mediators in septic/endotoxic shock - a meta-analysis evaluating the current status of histamine. Theor Surg 2 :1
5. Black JW, Duncan WAM, Durant CJ, Ganellin CR, Parsons EM (1972) Definition and antagonism of histamine H_2-receptors. Nature 236: 385
6. Ash ASF, Schild HO (1966) Receptors mediating some actions of histamine. Br J Pharmacol Chemother 27: 427
7. Brackett DJ, Schaefer CF, Wilson MF (1985) The effects of H_1 and H_2-receptors antagonists on the development of endotoxemia in the conscious, unrestrained rat. Circ Shock 16: 141
8. Neugebauer E, Lorenz W, Beckurts T, Maroske D, Merte H (1987) Significance of histamine formation and release in the development of endotoxic shock: proof of current concepts by randomized controlled studies in rats. Rev Infect Dis 9: 585
9. Wittig H, Cook TJ, Rittmanic T. (1978) Protection against fatal endotoxin shock in mice by antihistamines. Allergol Immunopathol VI: 409

10. Veteran Administration Systemic Sepsis Cooperative Study Group (1987) Effects of high-dose glucocorticoid therapy on mortality in patients with clinical signes of sepsis. N Engl J Med 317: 659
11. Rixen D, Neugebauer E, Lechleuthner A, Buschauer A, Nagelschmidt M, Thoma S, Rink A (1994) Beneficial effects of H_2-agonism and H_1-antagonism in rat endotoxic shock. Shock 2: 47-52
12. Brigham KL, Padove SJ, Bryant D, McKeem CR, Bowers RE (1980) Diphenhydramine reduces endotoxin effects on lung vascular permeability in sheep. Am J Physiol 40: 516
13. Dimmeler S, Lechleuthner A, Auweiler M, Troost C, Nagelschmidt M, Neugebauer E. (1995) H1-Antagonism has beneficial effects on cardiovascular and pulmonary function in porcine hyperdynamic shock. Shock 3: 416-421
14. Uvnäs B (ed.) Histamine and histamine antagonists. Springer, Berlin, Heidelberg, New York (Handbook of experimental pharmacology, vol 97)

Immune Complexes: Mediators of Sepsis and Immune Dysfunction

J.K. Horn, G.A. Hamon, R.H. Mulloy, C. Birkenmaier

Clinical Incidence of Immune Complex Formation

Circulating immune complexes have been detected in a wide range of diseases and are etiologic for certain forms of renal disease and arthritis. Aside from immune complex-mediated diseases, there is evidence that these immune complexes are also found in a wide range of other inflammatory diseases such as infection and sepsis (Table 1).
Immune complexes have been demonstrated in patients with bacteriemia [10, 11, 43]. As would be expected, bacterial antigens have been recovered from the immune complexes in these patients [17]. This has been reported in patients with gram-positive [13, 18, 28, 39] and gram-negative [7, 10, 43] infections. The disappearance of immune complexes from the circulation coincides with loss of complement activity in patients with gram-negative septic shock. This was interpreted as evidence of a pathological role for immune complexes in this disease process [11]. It is of interest, however, that in septic patients the presence of immune complexes failed to correlate with the severity of disease [35].
Plasma obtained from patients with bacterial endocarditis also display evidence of immune complexes [3, 5]. The presence of the immune complexes correlates with the subacute forms of the disease and levels appear to drop in acute episodes [19]. Other specific infections that have been shown to be associated with immune complex formation include *Echinococcus* [23], dengue virus infection [33], and schistosomiasis [6].
Multiple transfusions of blood products to an individual increase the risk of interactions between preformed immunoglobulins and cellular antigens which are commonly found on leukocyte surfaces. Studies from transplantation tissue typing indicate that the incidence of sensitization to leukocyte antigens in the general population increases following prior transfusion or childbirth. Likewise, circulating immune complexes are commonly detected in the plasma of hemophiliacs, and the incidence increases with age or the number of transfusions [1]. There is also evidence obtained from patients with chronic immune complex-mediated diseases demonstrating that such complexes are cleared by erythrocytes through binding to CR1, with eventual destruction by complement, lending indirect evidence to the existence of circulating immune complexes associated with the disease. This was demonstrated by showing a decrease in circulating

Table 1: Diseases associated with circulating immune complexes

Disease	Reference
Septic syndrome	Gutierrez-Fernandez et al. [14]
Bacteremia	Mellencamp et al. [28]
Endocarditis	Schned et al. [36]
Multiple transfusions	Giacchino et al. [12]
Burn injury	Kulick et al. [22]

immune complexes following transfusion [34]. We have hypothesized that immune complex formation through coating of leukocytes with immunoglobulins would be more likely to occur in massively transfused patients due to donor-donor interactions that are not screened by the traditional donor-recipient cross-match.

The immunosuppressive effect of transfusion has been established through clinical studies demonstrating protection of cadaver transplants by transfusion [15] and by showing increased risk of metastases following transfusion at the time of primary cancer resection [40]. Studies with uremic patients receiving chronic transfusions demonstrated the presence of circulating immune complexes concomitant with depressed lymphocyte function [12].

Following general surgical procedures, circulating immune complexes have been detected in patients with inflammatory bowel disease [8, 20], and in some patients with various hepatobiliary diseases [24]. For example, immunoglobulin A-containing circulating immune complexes, immunoglobulin G-containing circulating immune complexes, and endotoxin were measured in the sera of patients with obstructive jaundice [31]. Following jejunal-ileal bypass surgery, intravascular hemolysis, thrombocytopenia, leukopenia, and circulating immune complexes have been detected [30]. In patients undergoing cardiovascular surgery complement levels and immune complexes dropped significantly immediately after surgery, followed by a late rise in non-complement-fixing immune complexes. These complexes are suspected to be the product of polyclonal immune stimulation [26]. Immune complexes have been detected in burn patients [22, 32]; however, few studies have sampled post-traumatic patients for the presence of circulating immune complexes.

Model for Study of Immune Complexes

We hypothesized that factors other than the lipopolysaccharide (LPS) portion of endotoxin are capable of mediating the events that lead to sepsis in individuals following surgery, or infection. Since immune complexes are commonly encountered in many pathological states that precede sepsis and multiple organ failure, we were interested in establishing whether immune complexes were sufficient and capable of modulating the septic response. To investigate this process we studied the effects of insoluble immune complexes upon monocytes. Our model attempts to mimic the exposure of monocytes to cells coated with IgG that would occur following massive transfusion.

These interactions serve as a model for events that likely occur in various disease states associated with high levels of circulating immune complexes. Our studies were performed with insoluble complexes of bovine serum albumin (BSA) and rabbit polyclonal anti-BSA IgG formed in antigen excess. The precipitate resolved into three bands on SDS-polyacrylamide gel electrophoresis: heavy and light chains of rabbit IgG, and BSA. Monocytes taken from normal individuals were exposed to immune complexes at concentrations between 0 and 200 µg/ml.

In Fig. 1 are displayed the results of an experiment in which neutrophils were exposed to insoluble immune complexes to which was attached a sensitive probe of hydrogen peroxide (2',7'-dichlorofluorescein). When ingested, fluorescence is released in proportion to the amount of intracellular peroxidation that occurs. The fluorescence is assayed with flow cytometry. As shown, binding of the complexes is reflected by autofluorescence of complexes that attach to cells maintained at 4°C to prevent internalization. Incubation at 37°C induces a dramatic rise in fluorescence, indicating intracellular uptake and activation of cytoplasmic oxidases. Phagocytosis of insoluble immune complexes occurs within minutes of stimulation. This uptake is mediated by immunoglobulin Fc receptors and appears to cause activation of the phagocytic cell.

In Fig. 2 are displayed results of immune complex stimulation of monocytes assayed for intracellular oxidation. Normal monocytes are preloaded with 2',7'-dichlorofluoresceindiacetate, which is trapped within the cell and becomes fluorescent in the presence of products of intracellular peroxidation. The fluorescence was then analyzed by flow cytometry [2]. Unstimulated control cells failed to significantly increase their production of oxidants over 15 min, whereas cells that were exposed to insoluble immune complexes produced intracellular oxidant products in a dose-dependent fashion.

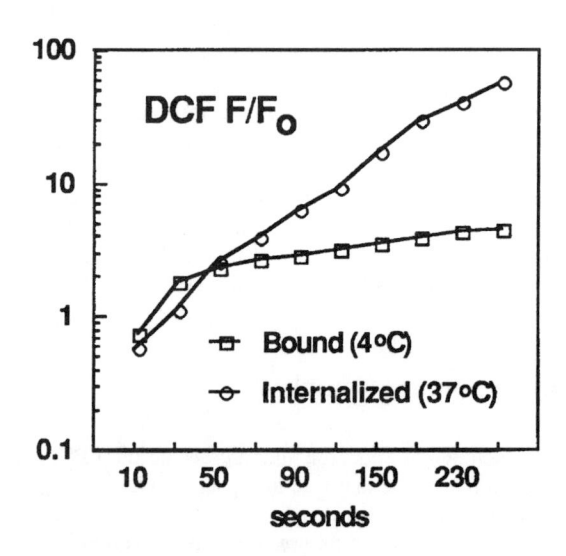

Fig. 1: Phagocytosis of insoluble immune complexes by neutrophils. Fluorescence expressed as a ratio to unstimulated controls (F/F_o) exhibited by neutrophils stimulated with insoluble immune complexes attached to a fluorescein derivative (2',7'-dichlorofluorescein, DCF). The quantity of bound (hollow squares) versus internalized (hollow circles) immune complexes is displayed

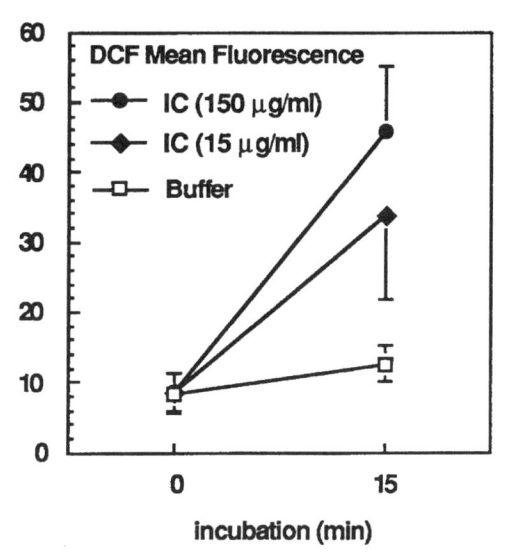

Fig. 2: Intracellular oxidation within monocytes stimulated with immune complexes (IC). Mean fluorescence (± SEM) exhibited by intracellular 2',7'-dichlorofluorescein (DCF) from normal monocytes stimulated by buffer alone (hollow squares), IC (15 µg/ml, solid rhombi), or IC (150 µg/ml, solid circles)

Alterations of Phenotype

The phenotype displayed by normal monocytes reflects the presence of several important cell surface receptors that are critical for responses of the monocyte to chemotactic stimuli; adhesion to endothelium and tissue matrix; phagocytosis; and production of cytokines. Table 2 displays a number of common receptors that can be readily assayed by direct immunofluorescent staining and flow cytometric analysis. They participate in stimulation of cytokine production (CD14), binding of complement-opsonized particles (CD35, CD11b), endothelial cell adhesion (CD11b), and uptake of immunoglobulins.

Table 2: Common monocyte receptors

Type	Name	Ligand
Lipopolysaccharide	CD14	LPS-LPS binding protein
Complement	CD11b (MAC-1, CR3) CD35(CR1)	ICAM-1, C3bi, C3b
Immunoglobulin	CD64 (FcγI) CD32 (FcγII) CD16 (FcγIII)	Monomeric IgG Polymeric IgG Polymeric IgG

Figure 3 displays alterations in the monocyte receptors following exposure of the cells to 150 μg/ml insoluble immune complexes. Over a 2-h incubation period, immune complexes alone caused downregulation of CD14, CD32, and CD64, whereas CD35 and CD16 were upregulated. CD11b failed to show significant changes during phagocytosis. Opsonization of the immune complexes with complement by incubation with serum further enhanced the downregulation of CD14 and CD32, while considerably enhancing the upregulation of CD16. These results indicate that immune complex uptake altered the monocyte phenotype, rendering the cell less responsive to immunoglobulins through the constitutively expressed Fc receptors (CD32 and CD64) and less responsive to LPS (CD14). Display of CD16 on monocytes may represent auto-activation by TGF-β1 [41]. CD35 is commonly upregulated by stimulation of monocytes by cytokines, also indicating that auto-activation can occur [25]. The enhancement of certain phenotypic alterations (downregulation of CD14/CD32 and upregulation of CD16) observed with complement opsonization most likely represent facilitation by phagocytosis (i.e., increased cell activation) through enhanced binding to complement receptors. In this case, engagement of CR3 (CD11b) by particles displaying C3bi may have caused internalization of these receptors which are normally upregulated by cell stimulation. The inability to further downregulate the high affinity Fc receptor (CD64) may reflect lack of participation in the phagocytic process, since this receptor normally recognizes soluble immune complexes (monomeric IgG).

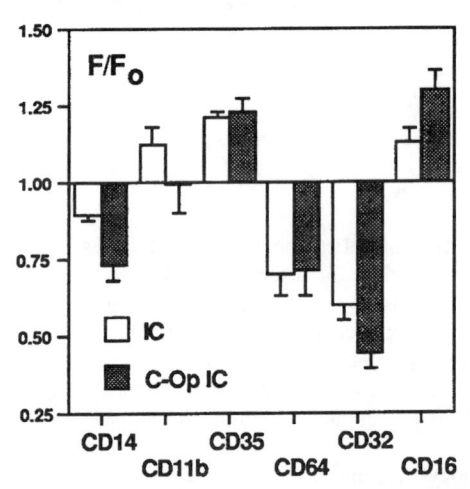

Fig. 3: Changes in phenotypic expression of common monocyte surface receptors. Fluorescence (mean±SEM) expressed as a ratio to unstimulated controls (F/F_o) exhibited by monocytes stimulated with insoluble immune complexes (IC, open bars) or insoluble immune complexes that were opsonized with complement (C-Op IC, hatched bars) for 2 h

Alteration of CD14 Expression by Immune Complexes

CD14, a 55-kDa myeloid differentiation antigen on monocytes, is capable of binding gram-negative bacteria and LPS when they become complexed with a plasma protein called lipopolysaccharide-binding protein (LBP) [37, 42]. CD14 participates in transduction of signals by bacteria and bacterial products which result in monocyte cytokine production and elimination of the bacteria. Other mechanisms also account for clearance of LPS by monocytes. Thus, the expression of CD14 by monocytes reflects their sensitivity to LPS.

As shown earlier, CD14 was considerably downregulated by phagocytosis of immune complexes. Figure 4 confirms that the depression in CD14 expression is dose and time dependent following exposure to insoluble immune complexes. This phenotypic alteration appears to be similar to that observed in septic and traumatized patients [4, 21]. It is possible that decreased expression of CD14 may render the cells less responsive to LPS and may represent a mechanism for regulation of cytokine production.

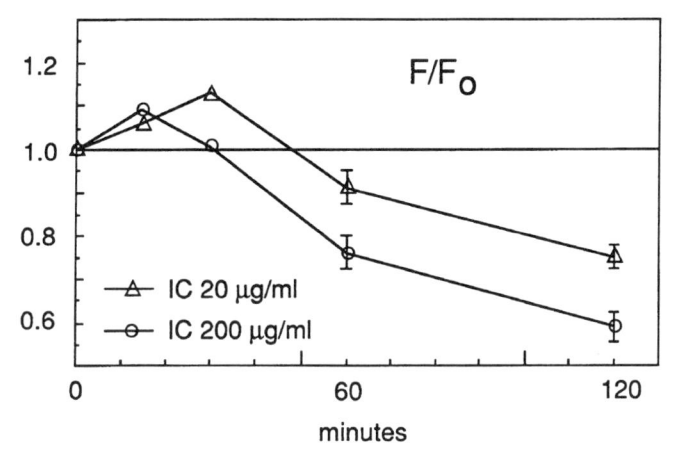

Fig. 4: Time and dose dependence observed in monocytes stimulated by insoluble immune complexes. Fluorescence (mean ± SEM) as a ratio of unstimulated controls (F/F_o) exhibited by monocytes stimulated with insoluble complexes over 2 h with concentrations of 20 µg/ml (hollow triangles) or 200 µg/ml (hollow circles) is displayed

Several investigators have shown that following stimulation of monocytes by the soluble chemoattractant N-formyl-methionyl-leucyl-phenylalanine (f-MLP), CD14 expression is decreased and soluble CD14 is found in the supernatant [16, 38]. The size of the soluble CD14 shed from the monocytes in vitro was smaller than that of either the membrane-bound form or a soluble CD14 cleaved from the cell surface by phosphatidyl inositol-specific phospholipase C, but identical to the size of one or two major soluble CD14 forms normally found in human serum.

We were interested in documenting whether CD14 was internalized or shed from the surface following immune complex stimulation. In Fig. 5 is displayed both the CD14 expression on the surface (CD14 mean fluorescence) and the quantity of soluble CD14 (sCD14) shed from the surface into the supernatant. As cells are warmed from 4°C to 37°C over 2 h, there is a dramatic increase in surface CD14 expression with some shedding of CD14 from the surface. Stimulation of the cells with insoluble immune complexes over the same period causes loss of CD14 from the surface without any appreciable shedding into the supernatant. Thus, phagocytosis of CD14 appears to be associated with internalization of CD14. As a control, phospholipase C liberated considerable amounts of soluble CD14 into the supernatant and concomitantly lowered CD14 surface expression.

To study internal levels of CD14 we treated cells with 0.4% saponin to permeabilize them to the fluorescent antibody used to assess CD14. In Fig. 6 are displayed data from a representative experiment in which baseline cells maintained at 4°C were warmed to 37°C for 2 h

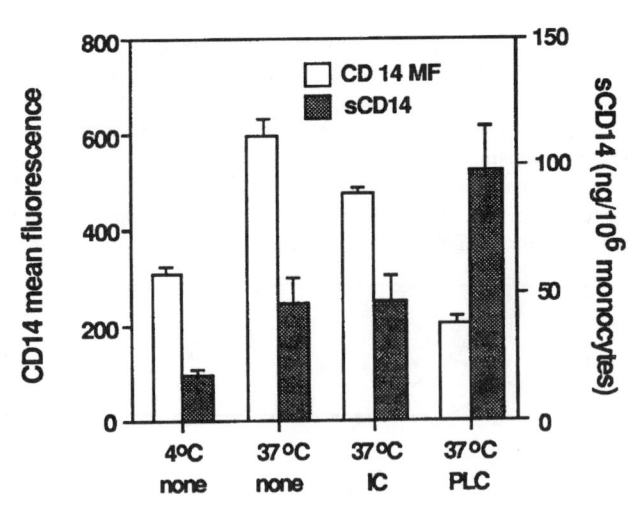

Fig. 5: *Comparison of surface CD14 expression and soluble CD14 obtained from supernatants of monocytes stimulated with insoluble immune complexes. Surface CD14 (open bars, ± SEM) was measured by direct immunofluorescent staining and flow cytometry. Concomitantly, soluble CD14 (sCD14, ± SEM) was assayed in supernatants by ELISA (hatched bars). Cells were incubated at the indicated temperatures with buffer alone (none), 150 µg/ml immune complexes (IC), or 0.01 U/ml phospholipase C (PLC)*

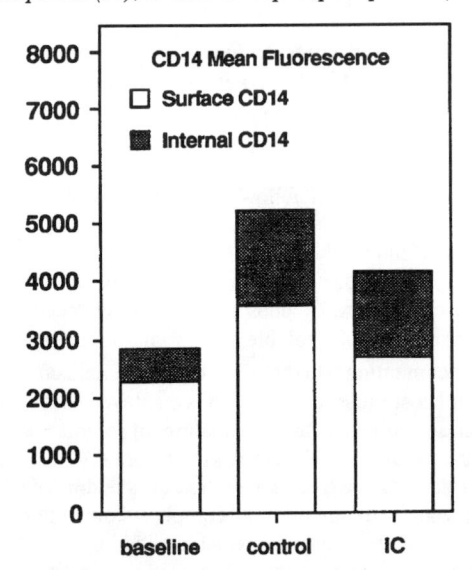

Fig. 6: *Simultaneous measurement of external and internal CD14 in monocytes following immune complex stimulation. Following stimulation with 150 µg/ml immune complexes, cells were assayed for surface expression of CD14 (external) or were permeabilized with 0.4% saponin and then assayed for total CD14 expression. Internal CD14 represents the difference between total and external levels*

and compared to cells incubated with insoluble immune complexes. The additional internal CD14 represents the total amount of fluorescence the cells displayed after treatment with saponin. Internal levels of CD14 are similar for control and immune complex-stimulated cells. Interpreted with results of soluble CD14 measurements, it appears that phagocytic internalization of CD14 leads to destruction of the material in the phagocytic vacuole, with failure by the cell to restore the internalized CD14 to the cytoplasmic pool.

Production of Mediators by Immune Complex-Stimulated Monocytes

Elevated levels of TNFα have been observed in patients with septic shock [27]. In animal studies, pro-inflammatory cytokines are thought to induce changes that mimic the events which lead to the septic syndrome in humans. In these animal models, pretreatment with antibodies directed against cytokines can prevent the lethal consequences of the cytokine actions. We were interested in determining whether the insoluble immune complexes used in our model were capable of inducing cytokine production. Table 3 displays levels of immunoreactive TNFα following stimulation with either immune complexes or with two different doses of *E. coli*-LPS in the presence or absence of plasma. The immune complexes produced significant amounts of TNFα while LPS without the binding protein (RPMI/BSA) failed to generate significant amounts of TNFα compared to buffer controls. In contrast, the LPS was competent in the presence of serum containing LBP (RPMI/serum) to produce immunoreactive TNFα at higher levels than the control.

Table 3: Effects of insoluble immune complexes on monocyte TNFα and PGE$_2$ production

	Buffer	Incubation (min)	Stimulus	Mean ± SD	p
TNFα (pg/ml)	RPMI/BSA	120	None	250 ± 142	
	RPMI/BSA	120	IC (150 μg/ml)	601 ± 189	0.0177*
	RPMI/BSA	120	LPS (1.0 ng/ml)	326 ± 259	NS
	RPMI/BSA	120	LPS (10 ng/ml)	386 ± 246	NS
	RPMI/serum	120	None	186 ± 55	
	RPMI/serum	120	LPS (1.0 ng/ml)	261 ± 74	0.0465*
	RPMI/serum	120	LPS (10 ng/ml)	325 ± 88	0.0412*
PGE$_2$ (ng/ml)	RPMI/BSA	120	None	12 ± 14	
	RPMI/BSA	120	IC (15 μg/ml)	203 ± 65	0.0165*
	RPMI/BSA	120	IC (150 μg/ml)	684 ± 108	0.0037*
	RPMI/BSA/indo.[a]	120	IC (150 μg/ml)	0.36 ± 0.34	

RPMI/BSA, RPMI 1640 + 2.5% (w/v) BSA; RPMI/serum, RPMI 1640 + 10% (v/v) autologous serum; IC, immune complexes; LPS, *E. coli* lipopolysaccharide; NS, not significant
[a]Cells pre-incubated with 1.0 μ*M* indomethacin for 15 min at 37°C.
*Vs. none, Student's *t*-test, *n*=6

Prostaglandin E_2 (PGE_2) is a well-studied immunosuppressive agent and has been demonstrated as one of the prostaglandins released by human monocytes when stimulated by LPS [9, 29]. In Table 3 we demonstrate that immune complexes at concentrations of 15 and 150 μg/ml are able to mediate a significant release of immunoreactive PGE_2 (ELISA) from normal human monocytes. The amount of PGE_2 produced was significantly higher for the 150 μg/ml concentration of immune complexes. Pre-incubation of the monocytes with indomethacin completely abrogated the effect of immune complexes. Thus, ingestion of immune complexes activates cyclooxygenase activity in monocytes, which results in production of an immunosuppressive agent.

Acknowledgement

This study was supported by a grant from the Centers for Disease Control (R49/CCR604-382).

References

1. *Andreeva TA, Fedorova ZD, Khanin TM et al. (1991) The effect of specific transfusion therapy on the level of circulating immune complexes in hemophilia patients. Ter Arkh 63(7): 50-53*
2. *Bass DA, Parce JW et al. (1983) Flow cytometric studies of oxidative product formation by neutrophils: a graded response to membrane stimulation. J Immunol 130: 1910-1917*
3. *Bayer AS, Theofilopoulos AN, Eisenberg R et al. (1976) Circulating immune complexes in infective endocarditis. N Engl J Med 295(27): 15001505*
4. *Birkenmaier CB, Hong YS, Horn JK (1992) Modulation of the endotoxin receptor (CD14) in septic patients. J Trauma 32: 473-478*
5. *Cabane J, Godeau P, Herreman G et al. (1979) Fate of circulating immune complexes in infective endocarditis. Am J Med 66(2): 277-282*
6. *Carvalho EM, Andrews BS, Martinelli R et al. (1983) Circulating immune complexes and rheumatoid factor in schistosomiasis and visceral leishmaniasis. Am J Trop Med Hyg 32(1):61-68*
7. *Danielsson D, Norberg R, Svanbom M (1975) Circulating immune complexes in a patient with prolonged gonococcal septicemia. Acta Derm Venereol (Stockh) 55(4):301-304*
8. *Fagan EA, Elkon KB, Griffin GF et al. (1982) Systemic inflammatory complications following jejuno-ileal bypass. Q J Med 51(204): 445-460*
9. *Faist E, Mewes A, Baker CC et al. (1987) Prostaglandin E_2 (PGE_2)-dependent suppression of interleukin 2 (IL-2) production in patients with major trauma. J Trauma 27:837-848*
10. *Galli M, Del GG, Fiorenza AM et al. (1982) Cryoglobulinaemia in a patient with Proteus mirabilis sepsis. Infection 10(6): 352-353*
11. *George C, Carlet J, Sobel A et al. (1980) Circulating immune complexes in patients with gram negative septic shock. Intensive Care Med 6(2): 123-127*
12. *Giacchino F, Belardi P, Coppo R et al. (1981) Effects of blood transfusion on cellular immunity. Proc Eur Dial Transplant Assoc 18: 465-468*
13. *Gurevich PS, Barsukov VS, Popov NP (1983) Vascular changes in hyperacute meningococcal sepsis as a manifestation of pathogenic action of immune complexes. Cor Vasa 25(6): 443-449*

14. Gutierrez-Fernandez J, Maroto MC, Piedrola G et al. (1989) Dysfunction of the mononuclear phagocytic system in sepsis. APMIS 97(5): 441-446
15. Hanto DW, Simmons RL (1987) Renal transplantation: clinical considerations. Radiol Clin North Am 25(2): 239-248
16. Haziot A, Chen S, Ferrero E et al. (1988) The monocyte differentiation antigen, CD14, is anchored to the cell membrane by a phosphatidylinositol linkage. J Immunol 141(2): 547-552
17. Inman RD, Redecha PB, Knechtle SJ et al. (1982) Identification of bacterial antigens in circulating immune complexes of infective endocarditis. J Clin Invest 70(2): 271-280
18. Kaplan JE, Palmer DL, Tung KS (1981) Teichoic acid antibody and circulating immune complexes in the management of Staphylococcus aureus bacteremia. Am J Med 70(4): 769-774
19. Kauffmann JE, Thompson J, Valentijn EM et al. (1981) The clinical implications and the pathogenic significance of circulating immune complexes in infective endocarditis. Am J Med 71(1):17-25
20. Kemler BJ, Alpert E (1980) Inflammatory bowel disease associated circulating immune complexes. Gut 21(3): 195-201
21. Krüger C, Schütt C, Obertacke U et al. (1991) Serum CD14 levels in polytraumatized and severely burned patients. Clin Exp Immunol 85(2): 297-301
22. Kulick MI, Wong R, Okarma TB et al. (1985) Prospective study of side effects associated with the use of silver sulfadiazine in severely burned patients. Ann Plast Surg 14(5): 407-419
23. La-Ganga V, Robecchi A, Camussi G et al. (1980) Immune complex monitoring in Echinococcus infections. Minerva Med 71(42): 3057-3061
24. Lawley TJ, James SP, Jones EA (1980) Circulating immune complexes: their detection and potential significance in some hepatobiliary and intestinal diseases. Gastroenterology 78(3):626-641
25. Limb GA, Hamblin AS, Wolstencroft RA et al. (1992) Rapid cytokine upregulation of integrins, complement receptor 1 and HLA-DR on monocytes but not on lymphocytes. Immunology 77(1): 88-94
26. Maerker AG, Dienst C, Schumacher K et al. (1985) Circulating immune complexes and complement factors in patients following cardiosurgical operations. Immun Infekt 13(2): 83-85
27. Marks JD, Marks CB, Luce JM et al. (1990) Plasma tumor necrosis factor in patients with septic shock. Am Rev Respir Dis 141: 94-97
28. Mellencamp MA, Preheim LC, McDonald TL (1987) Isolation and characterization of circulating immune complexes from patients with pneumococcal pneumonia. Infect Immun 55(8):1737-1742
29. Miller-Graziano CL, Fink M, Wu JY et al. (1988) Mechanisms of altered monocyte prostaglandin E_2 production in severely injured patients. Arch Surg 123: 293-299
30. Moake JL, Kageler WV, Cimo PL et al. (1977) Intravascular hemolysis, thrombocytopenia, leukopenia, and circulating immune complexes after jejunal-ileal bypass surgery. Ann Intern Med 86(5):576-578
31. Ohshio G, Manabe T, Tobe T et al. (1988) Circulating immune complex, endotoxin, and biliary infection in patients with biliary obstruction. Am J Surg 155(2): 343-347
32. Pashutin SB, Borisova TG, Belotskii SM (1984) Circulating immune complexes and heterophilic hemolysis in burn injury. Biull Eksp Biol Med 97(3): 324-326
33. Phan DT, Ha NT, Thuc LT et al. (1991) Some changes in immunity and blood in relation to clinical states of dengue hemorrhagic fever patients in Vietnam. Haematologia (Budap) 24(1):13-21
34. Pintera J (1981) Screening for circulating immune complexes in blood donors as an effective method of further HBsAg carriers detection. Folia Haematol (Leipz) 108(3):455-461

35. Pocidalo MA, Gilbert C, Verroust P et al. (1982) Circulating immune complexes and severe sepsis: duration of infection as the main determinant. Clin Exp Immunol 47(3):513-519
36. Schned ES, Inman RD, Parris TM et al. (1983) Serial circulating immune complexes and mononuclear phagocyte system function in infective endocarditis. J Lab Clin Med 102(6):947-959
37. Schumann RR, Leong SR, Flaggs GW et al. (1990) Structure and function of lipopolysaccharide binding protein. Science 249: 1429-1431
38. Simmons DL, Tan S, Tenen DG et al. (1989) Monocyte antigen CD14 is a phospholipid anchored membrane protein. Blood 73(1): 284-289
39. Tabbarah ZA, Wheat LJ, Kohler RB et al. (1980) Thermodissociation of staphylococcal immune complexes and detection of staphylococcal antigen in serum from patients with Staphylococcus aureus bacteremia. J Clin Microbiol 11(6): 703-709
40. Tartter PI (1988) Blood transfusion history in colorectal cancer patients and cancer-free controls. Transfusion 28(6): 593-596
41. Wong HL, Welch GR, Brandes ME et al. (1991) IL-4 antagonizes induction of Fc gamma RIII (CD16) expression by transforming growth factor-beta on human monocytes. J Immunol 147(6): 1843-1848
42. Wright SD, Tobias PS, Ulevitch RJ et al. (1989) Lipopolysaccharide (LPS) binding protein opsonizes LPS-bearing particles for recognition by a novel receptor on macrophages. J Exp Med 170: 1231-1241
43. Young LS, Stevens P, Kaijser B (1982) Gram-negative pathogens in septicaemic infections. Scand J Infect Dis Suppl 31: 78-94

Section 5:

Indicators and Crucial Functional Mechanisms for the Development of MODS/MOF and SIRS

Shock, Tissue Damage and Immune Dysfunction: Blood Flow Mediated or Persistent Inflammatory Cascade

A.E. Baue

Introduction

It has been well established that injury and operations produce immunosuppression or dysfunction. The details of these changes have been studied extensively and will be the subject of many presentations at this congress and chapters in this book. Therapeutic programs of immunomodulation have been proposed and studied in laboratory animals and patients. Many of the abnormalities of the specific immune system can be brought back to normal in patients, as shown by Markewitz et al. [1] and others. Modulation of changes in the nonspecific immune system are being evaluated but have not been proven effective clinically as yet. The question that I have been asked to address is whether the immune dysfunction that occurs after injury is because of shock, and is therefore blood flow-mediated, or due primarily to tissue injury (damage) and the inflammatory response (cascades) resulting from the injury. There is considerable evidence for both of these factors. It is also possible that shock and tissue damage are both involved in this abnormality. The teleological reason for altered immune function after injury remains elusive. The injured, operated shocked patient should have maximal host resistance but has an increased likelihood of infection. As shown in Fig. 1, shock produces altered cell and organ function and eventually cell and organ damage. This contributes to immune dysfunction. Shock, however, also produces an ischemia-reperfusion injury. There may be a no-reflow problem, and there may often be inadequate microcirculatory blood flow, even after what seems to be adequate resuscitation. These factors also occur in the traumatized patient who has in addition tissue, cell and organ damage, which contributes directly to immune dysfunction. Tissue damage from trauma also leads to mediator activation. The inflammatory cascades contribute further to immune dysfunction. This allows sepsis and/or multiple organ failure (MOF) to develop with the possibility of eventual death in many patients. Thus at the outset I will say that it is my belief that, in patients, both shock and trauma are related to the altered immune function that contributes to eventual problems. Both decreased blood flow and inflammation contribute to the problem.

Cell Alterations and Damage with Shock

Many years ago, in St. Louis, Drs. Mohammad Sayeed, Irshad Chaudry and I joined forces to explore cellular abnormalities with shock. We found a number of abnormalities in cell membrane, mitochondrial and energy metabolism. We were interested, at that time, in those processes which took time to recover after a short and finite period of shock. The principal changes that had a prolonged recovery time were cell membrane transport of sodium and potassium and decreased energy levels [2-8] (Table 1). This led to what we interpreted as an energy crisis for cells and organs after decreased blood flow. Such energy crises could occur after arterial reconstruction, with aortic cross clamping during cardiac procedures, with the preparation and preservation of organs for transplantation and with simply an inadequate

Shock → altered cell and organ function

a. ischemia/reperfusion injury
b. the no reflow problem
c. inadequate microcirculatory resuscitation and/or blood flow

→ immune dysfunction

Trauma → tissue (cell and organ) damage

mediator activation (inflammatory cascade)   sepsis and/or MOF

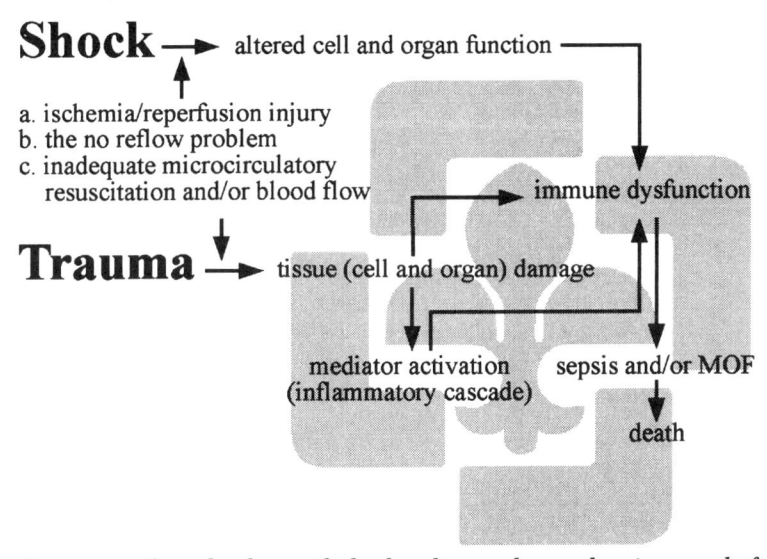

→ death

Fig. 1: The changes that take place with shock and injury that produce immune dysfunction

Table 1: Cellular alterations with hemorrhagic shock

Decreased mitochondrial capacity	Quickly reversed with treatment
Increased Na^+/K^+ ATPase activity	Quickly reversed with treatment
Mitochondrial cation changes Increased Na Decreased K Labile Mg	Quickly reversed
Cell membrane Decreased Na^+/K^+ transport	Returns slowly
Decreased ATP, ADP, AMP levels	Return slowly

circulation such as hemorrhagic shock. The abnormalities in cell membrane function produce cell swelling, as shown in Fig. 2. In Fig. 3 a small blood vessel from an animal in hemorrhagic shock is shown with endothelial swelling. In addition, we know that white blood cells are trapped in capillaries after severe hemorrhage and contribute to a no-reflow phenomenon [9]. With ischemia or shock, the question has been raised where is the impact of the energy crisis? Is it in parenchymal cells, in the microcirculation or in endothelial cells? We have provided evidence that it occurs in all of these cells. Cell damage progresses as the period of shock continues. Since those early days, much more has been learned about altered cell and membrane function with shock and injury.

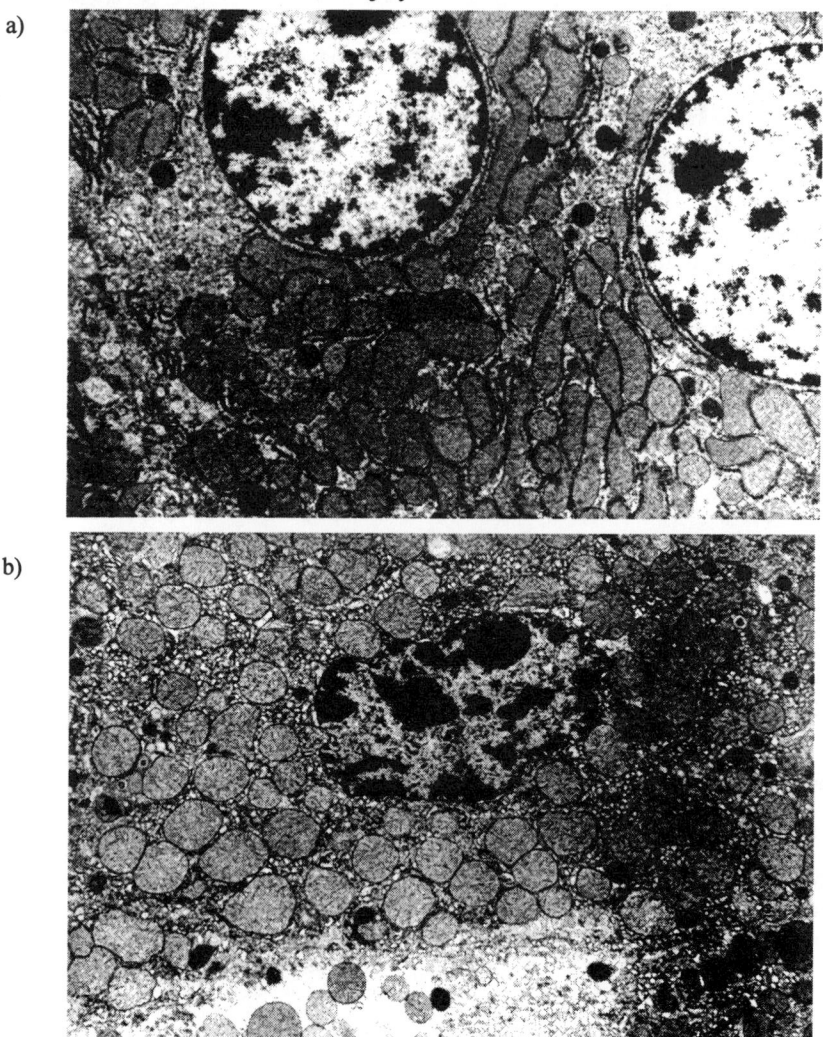

Fig. 2: a) A normal hepatocyte from an experimental animal. Note the normal ovoid mitochondria. b) A hepatocyte from an animal in shock, showing round, swollen mitochondria and a compressed nucleus

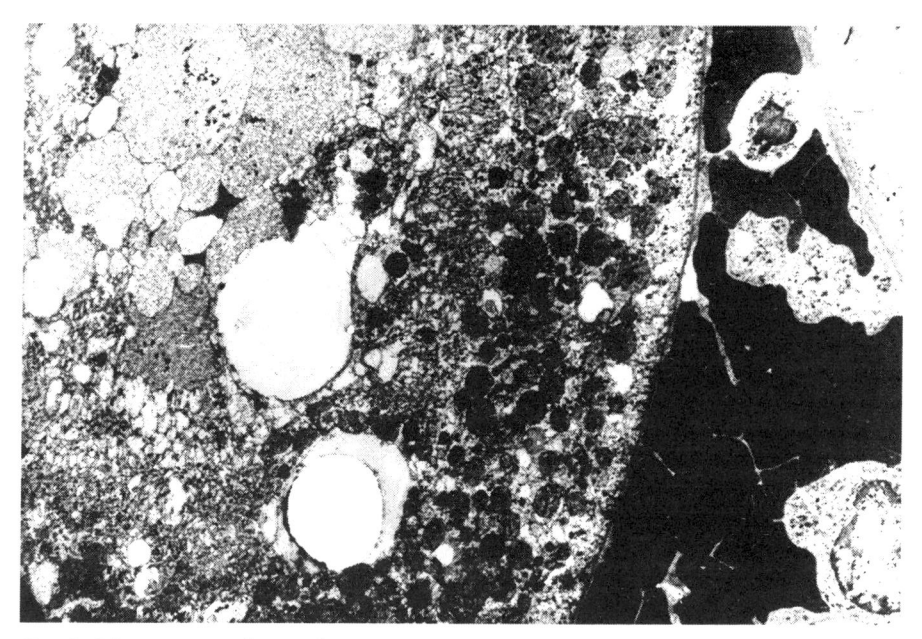

Fig. 3: The microcirculation from an animal in shock, showing swollen endothelial cells which impinge on the lumen of the vessel

Immune Alterations with Shock

Stephan, in our laboratory at Yale [10], demonstrated that hemorrhage without tissue trauma produces immunosuppression, as measured by the altered proliferative responses to mitogen stimulation and altered mixed lymphocyte reactions. Stephan also showed that a group of mice subjected to sepsis by cecal ligation and puncture 3 days after resuscitation from shock had an increased mortality as compared to those who did not have hemorrhage. Thus the altered immune response or immunosuppression with hemorrhage was a real event and seemed clinically relevant. He next demonstrated that there was decreased interleukin-2 (IL-2) production following simple hemorrhage [11]. Following this, an extensive series of studies have been carried out in Dr. Chaudry's laboratory in Michigan, with Ayala, Ertel and many other coworkers [12]. A summary of their findings and others are shown in Table 2, which is adapted from an article by Chaudry and Ayala on the mechanism of increased susceptibility to infection following hemorrhage [13]. This summarizes these extensive and detailed studies and shows the many and complex alterations that occur with shock alone. Defective antigen presentation after hemorrhage and altered receptors contribute greatly to the problem [14, 15]. From this extensive work, Chaudry and Ayala have developed an hypothesis for how hemorrhage produces immunosuppression and increases susceptibility to infection (Fig. 4). Hemorrhagic shock also increases bacterial translocation. It decreases the clearance of injected *Escherichia coli* in experimental animals, and there is increased microvascular blood flow after what seems to be adequate resuscitation.

Table 2: Alteration in immune functions produced by hemorrhagic shock (from [13])

Affected cells	Observed findings
Reticuloendothelial cells	↓ Phagocytic activity
Phagocytes	↓ Hepatic macrophage complement-receptor clearance
Pertitoneal and splenic macrophages	↓ Decreased cytotoxicity
	↓ Fc and C3b receptor expression
	↑ TGF-β productive capacityKupffer cells
Kupffer cells	↑ Capacity to release inflammatory cytokines (TNF, IL-1 and IL-6)
	↑ Cytotoxicity
Monocytes	↑ IL-1 productive capacity
Natural killer cells	↓ Cytotoxicity
Neutrophils	↑ Neutrophil adhesiveness
T cells	↓ Blastogenesis
	↓ Lymphocyte reactivity
	↓ Lymphokine release
B cells	↓ Antibody production
	↓ Frequency and number of B-cell clonal precursors specific for bacterial antigens
Accessory cells	
Monocytes, peritoneal, splenic macrophage, and Kupffer cells	↓ Antigen presentation
	↓ MHC class II expression
	↓ Number of Ia antigen positive cells
	↓ Antigen catabolism
	↑ PGE_2 release

TGF-β, transforming growth factor type beta; TNF, tumor necrosis factor; IL, interleukin; MHC, major histocompatibility complex; PGE_2, prostaglandin E_2

Reversal of the Immunosuppressive Effects of Hemorrhage

Dr. Chaudry's laboratory then set out on an extensive series of experiments to determine if there were agents that would counteract or correct the immunosuppression of hemorrhage and, particularly, to immunomodulate these various changes back to a more normal level. These agent are listed in Table 3. The question is, are there any common characteristics that these substances share which would lead to a better understanding of the mechanisms of immunosuppression? Anyone knowing Dr. Chaudry and me would recognize that adenosine triphosphate complexed with magnesium chloride (ATP-$MgCL_2$) would be at the top of the list [16-23]. These factors may exert their effects at various levels in the hypothesis presented by Chaudry and Ayala (Fig. 4).

Hemorrhage

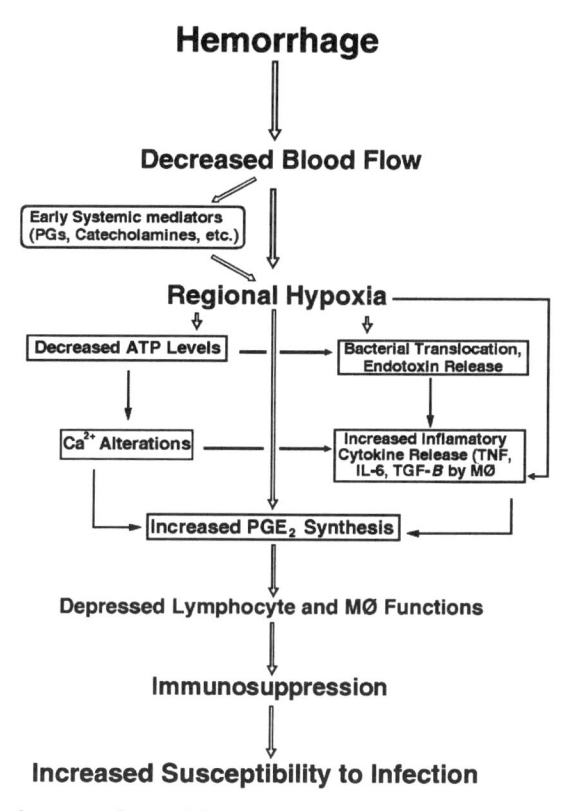

```
Hemorrhage
    ↓
Decreased Blood Flow
    ↓  ← Early Systemic mediators (PGs, Catecholamines, etc.)
Regional Hypoxia
    ↓
Decreased ATP Levels → Bacterial Translocation, Endotoxin Release
    ↓                        ↓
Ca²⁺ Alterations → Increased Inflamatory Cytokine Release (TNF, IL-6, TGF-β by MØ)
    ↓
Increased PGE₂ Synthesis
    ↓
Depressed Lymphocyte and MØ Functions
    ↓
Immunosuppression
    ↓
Increased Susceptibility to Infection
```

Fig. 4: The hypothesis put forward by Chaudry and Ayala on how hemorrhage produces immunosuppression. PG, prostaglandin; IL, interleukin; TNF, tumor necrosis factor; TGF transforming growth factor; MØ, macrophage

Table 3: Factors that block the immunosuppression after hemorrhage or restore it to normal

Cascade inhibitors	☐ ATP-MgCl₂ ☐ Ca²⁺ antagonists ☐ Cyclo-oxygenase inhibitors ☐ Chloroquine
Antibodies	☐ Lipopolysaccharide ☐ Tumor necrosis factor ☐ Interleukin-6
Growth factors	☐ Transforming growth factor-β
Additives	☐ N-3 PUFA ☐ Interferon-γ

Hemorrhagic Shock and Neutrophil Function

There have also been extensive studies of what happens experimentally with hemorrhagic shock as related to white blood cells and, particularly, polymorphonuclear neutrophils (PMNs). A no-reflow effect has been demonstrated in capillaries, resulting in their becoming plugged with activated aggregated white cells [9]. With hemorrhage, there is spontaneous activation of white blood cells [24], and the more active white cells there are, the greater the mortality. Activated PMNs produce greater endothelial adhesion and greater cytotoxicity. Related to this is the fact that an antibody to the primary human neutrophil adherence molecule (CD-18) protects against these effects of white cells [25]. Remote organ damage is also caused by white cells after hemorrhagic shock. Migratory activity of neutrophils is decreased by shock [26], and the number of nitroblue tetrazolium (NBT)-positive neutrophils correlates with irreversibility [27, 28]

Hemorrhage and the Inflammatory Response

Abraham and Chang [29] have shown that carrageenan-induced inflammation was suppressed after hemorrhage and that the degree of depression was related to the time that the animals stayed in shock. This was not a vasconstrictive phenomenon. Fink et al. [30] have also shown that sublethal hemorrhage in rats inhibits the acute peritoneal inflammatory response, but this does not affect the early removal of bacteria from the peritoneal cavity. Complement cascade receptors are also altered in shock [31].

Hemorrhage and Cytokine Production

Ayala et al. found that hemorrhage in experimental animals resulted in an increase in serum tumor necrosis factor (TNF) which was not associated with elevated levels of endotoxin [32]. In their study, IL-6 levels tended to increase later and were sustained longer. This was a trend and not a significant change. Abraham and Freitas found that interferon-γ (IFN-γ) production increased 24 and 48 h after hemorrhage in mice [33]. There were decreases in IL-2, IL-3 and IL-5 generation 2 h after blood loss. IL-1 levels have also been found to increase within 2 h of blood loss in experimental animals.

Is There an Increased Risk of Infection After Hemorrhage

I previously cited the work of Stephan from our laboratory, showing that mice had a significantly higher mortality when they were bled 3 days before cecal ligation and puncture. Many years earlier, Esrig et al. [34] showed that, following hemorrhagic shock and resuscitation, rats had increased mortality from the intraperitoneal injection of *E. coli*. They suggested that hemorrhagic shock, even when treated promptly and effectively, predisposes to infection. Esrig and Fulton also showed that dogs submitted to hemorrhagic shock and resuscitation alone had no difficulty [35]; however, if a sublethal dose of microorganisms was put in the tracheobronchial tree, it was lethal. We had previously shown that hemorrhagic shock per se does not damage the lung [36]. That is not to say, however, that it may not predispose it to insults later on. Impaired bacterial clearance of *E. coli* has been shown with hemorrhage [37].

Hemorrhagic Shock in Humans

Hemorrhagic shock alone is unusual in humans. It may occur with gastrointestinal bleeding in patients or with isolated vascular or peripheral extremity injuries. By and large, in patients there are no major problems, if bleeding is controlled and the circulation restored. Hemorrhagic shock in itself does not frequently lead to remote organ damage. In animal experiments and clinical experiences in Korea and Vietnam, shock per se was not associated with lung damage, renal failure or the adult respiratory distress syndrome (ARDS) [38]. The same has been true of gastrointestinal bleeding. However, when shock is due to trauma or associated with tissue injury, then organ malfunction and damage is frequent. Shock is believed to increase the frequency of infection, and it certainly does in animal studies, but clinical evidence for this is scant. Hemorrhagic shock alone is an unusual occurrence clinically.

Injured patients who are in shock at the time of arrival at the emergency department frequently have positive blood cultures and do less well [39]. It has not been determined whether this is a meaningful happening, contributing to death, or an epiphenomenon [40]. The evidence in man that hemorrhage per se leads to an increased incidence of infection is in part based upon circumstantial evidence, because of the association of trauma and tissue injury. Hemorrhage alone in humans with no contamination, no tissue injury and no other insult probably is infrequently associated with infection.

Trauma - and Persistent Inflammatory Cascades

The relationships of tissue injury and the inflammatory response have been studied extensively. Suffice it to say that there are indeed relationships between the acute phase response to elective surgery and accidental injury by mediators such as TNF, the interleukins and others. TNF has not been documented to increase after elective operations and may or may not be increased with accidental injuries. IL-6 levels increase later. IL-8 levels have been associated with nosocomial pneumonia. Roumen et al. found that the cytokine patterns varied in patients after major vascular operations, hemorrhagic shock and blunt trauma [41]. In nonsurvivors, there were higher plasma levels of TNF-α and IL-Iβ on admission. Patients with ruptured abdominal aneurysms had higher levels than those with trauma. With ARDS/MOF, there was a great increase in IL-6. In contrast, however, Rabinovici found that TNF-α levels did not correlate in trauma patients with injury severity score (ISS), the Glasgow coma scale, shock, MOF, or septic shock and, therefore, the levels and the response seemed to be unrelated [42]. Casey et al. [43] found that cytokine levels and endotoxin correlated with survival in patients with the sepsis syndrome.

Naturally occurring cytokine antagonists such as IL-1 receptor antagonists (IL-1ra) and soluble TNF receptors (STNFR-I) were elevated in critically ill patients [44]. STNFR-I levels were lower in patients who survived.

Altered Immune Response with Major Injury

Extensive studies by Faist et al. [45] and others have shown a major alteration in cellular immunity with major operations and with large injuries, with the finding that monocytes play a central role [46]. They found a deficit in IL-1, IL-2 and IL-8 production several days after injury [47]. There was excessive prostaglandin (PG) E_2 production and an increase in the production of IL-6. These abnormalities could be reversed by administration of cyclooxygenase inhibitors when combined with thymopentin-5 [1]. The changes in cytokines had a positive correlation with the severity of injury. These have been reviewed in great detail by Eugen Faist. In one of the early studies, Faist showed that the response of mononuclear cells to phytohemagglutinin was depressed by more than 30% for 5 - 7 days after injury and, eight of 11 patients with such a depression developed infectious complications. The addition of indomethacin to the in vitro cultures resulted in an enhancement back toward normal [48].

Is It Blood Transfusion or Shock That Increases the Risk of Infection After Trauma

It has been recognized that blood transfusions depress immune function, improve transplant graft survival and increase tumor recurrence in colon and head and neck cancer. Younes et al. [49] found that the most significant single factor that effected recurrence rate in patients who had complete resection of colorectal liver metastases was the number of hypotensive episodes during the operative procedure. This suggests that shock does indeed contribute to immune suppression and altered tumor dynamics. Waymack et al. found that blood transfusions administered 7 days before endotoxin challenge prolonged survival in animals, suggesting depression of immune function in a beneficial manner in that setting [50]. In another study, Waymack found that transfusions impaired cell mediated immunity and macrophage migration [51]. Thus they indicated that blood transfusion seemed to increase further the immunosuppression seen with trauma and surgery. In a third study, they found that transfusions adversely affected survival in animals that had been transfused and then received a burn wound painted with *Pseudomonas aeruginosa* bacteria [52]. They thought that this was due to exposure to non-self histocompatibility antigens. However, Cue and Malangoni and also Livingston [53,54] found that transfusion without shock did not impair the ability to fight an intradermal injection of *Staphylococcus aureus*, whereas hemorrhagic shock impaired this response. Nielsen [55] found that transfusion induced postoperative impairment of delayed hypersensitivity which could be prevented by perioperative ranitidine treatment. The reasons for this are unclear.

The Risk of Infection after Shock, Trauma and Blood Transfusions in Patients

It has been well documented that immune suppression occurs after blood transfusion alone. It occurs certainly with hemorrhage, and it occurs with trauma without shock. Thus, in injured patients, the risk of infection seems to increase, but it is hard to sort out what are the most important factors. In an extensive study of injured patients by Agarwal et al. [56], the incidence of infection was found to be significantly related to the mechanism of injury. However, blood transfusion in the injured patient was also an important, independent statistical predictor of infection. They could not relate its contribution to age, sex or the underlying mechanism or severity of injury. The ISS and the amount of blood received were, however, related and were both significant predictors of infection. Therefore, it is impossible to separate out which is the most important factor. Nichols et al. evaluated the risk of infection after penetrating abdominal trauma [57]. They found that the presence of shock on arrival at the hospital was found to increase the risk of infection when this factor was analyzed individually. However, the major associations with infection were increased age, injury to the left colon necessitating a colostomy, a larger number of units of blood or blood products administered, and the number of injured organs. When shock was added to this, it did not add predictive power. Thus it seems quite clear that shock, blood transfusion, tissue injury and the inflammatory response all contribute to the immunosuppression occurring in our patients. Although it is important scientifically to determine which factors have an influence, we must treat the whole patient by resuscitation and restoration of normal blood flow. Microcirculatory monitoring by measurement of gastric pH, tonometers in muscles, hepatic vein blood samples or coronary sinus blood lactate, and oxygen (O_2) content may be helpful to provide adequate resuscitation. Immunomodulation and other support mechanisms may also have an important role.

In conclusion, shock alters cell and organ function, eventually damages cells and organs and contributes to immune dysfunction. Shock also produces ischemia-reperfusion injury, the no-reflow problem and inadequate microcirculatory resuscitation and/or blood flow [58]. Trauma also produces these three factors along with tissue, cell and organ damage which contribute to immune dysfunction. Injured tissue produces mediator activation and the inflammatory cascade, which also contributes to immune dysfunction. These factors all seem additive in contributing to immune dysfunction, sepsis and/or MOF and the eventual possibility of death.

References

1. *Markewitz A, Faist E, Lang S, Endres S, Fuchs D, Reichart B (1993) Successful restoration of cell-mediated immune response after cardiopulmonary bypass by immunomodulation. J Thorac Cardiovasc Surg 105: 15-24*
2. *Sayeed MM, Baue AE (1973) Na-K transport in rat liver slices in hemorrhagic shock. Am J Physiol 224: 1265*
3. *Baue AE, Wurth MA, Chaudry IH, Sayeed MM (1973) Impairment of cell membrane transport during shock and after treatment. Ann Surg 178: 412-422*
4. *Chaudry IH, Sayeed MM, Baue AE (1973) Depletion and restoration of tissue ATP in hemorrhagic shock. Arch Surg 108: 208-211*
5. *Baue AE, Chaudry IH, Sayeed MM, Wurth MA (1974) Cellular alterations with shock and ischemia. Angiology 25: 16-20*
6. *Baue AE (1974) The energy crisis in surgical patients. Arch Surg 109: 349-350*
7. *Chaudry IH, Sayeed MM, Baue AE (1976) Alterations in high energy phosphates in hemorrhagic shock as related to tissue and organ function. Surgery 79: 666-668*
8. *Chaudry IH, Clemens MG, Baue AE (1981) Alterations in cell function with ischemia and shock and their connection. Arch Surg 116: 1309-1317*
9. *Barroso-Aranda J, Schmid-Schönbein GW, Zweifach BW, Engler RL (1988) Granulocytes and no-reflow phenomenon in irreversible hemorrhagic shock. Circ Res 63: 437-447*
10. *Stephan RN, Kupper TS, Geha AS, Baue AE, Chaudry IH (1987) Hemorrhage without tissue trauma produces immunosuppresion and enhances susceptibility to sepsis. Arch Surg 122: 62-68*
11. *Stephan RN, Conrad PJ, Janeway CA, Geha AS, Baue AE, Chaudry IH (1986) Decreased interleukin-2 production following simple hemorrhage. Surg Forum XXXVII: 73*
12. *Chaudry IH, Ayala A (1993) Immune consequences of hypovolemic shock and resuscitation. Cur Opin Anesthesiol 6: 385-392*

13. Chaudry IH, Ayala A (1993) Mechanism of increased susceptibility to infection following hemorrhage. Am J Surg 165: 59S-67S
14. Ertel W, Morrison MH, Ayala A, Chaudry IH (1991) Insights into the mechanisms of defective antigen presentation after hemorrhage. Surgery 110: 440-447
15. Ayala A, Perrin MM, Wagner MA, Chaudry IH (1989) Enhanced susceptibility to sepsis after simple hemorrhage. Arch Surg 125: 70-75
16. Meldrum DR, Ayala A, Ping W, Ertel W, Chaudry IH (1991) Association between decreased splenic ATP levels and immunodepression: amelioration with ATP-MgCl$_2$. Am J Physiol 261 (Regulatory Integrative Comp Physiol 30): R351-R357
17. Wang P, Zheng F, Morrison MH, Ayala A, Dean RE, Chaudry IH (1992) Mechanism of the beneficial effects of ATP-MgCl$_2$ following trauma - hemorrhage and resuscitation: downregulation of inflammatory cytokine (TNF, IL-6) release. J Surg Res 52: 364-371
18. Meldrum DR, Ayala A, Perrin MM, Ertel W, Chaudry IH (1991) Diltiazem restores IL-2, IL-3, IL-6, and IFN-r synthesis and decreases host susceptibility to sepsis following hemorrhage. J Surg Res 51: 158-164
19. Ertel W, Morrison MH, Ayala A, Chaudry IH (1993) Modulation of macrophage membrane phospholipids by n-3 polyunsaturated fatty acids increases interleukin 1 release and prevents suppression of cellular immunity following hemorrhagic shock. Arch Surg 128: 15-21
20. Ertel W, Morrison MH, Ayala A, Dean RE, Chaudry IH (1992) Interferon-r attenuates hemorrhage-induced suppression of macrophage and splenocyte functions and decreases susceptibility to sepsis. Surgery 111: 177-187
21. Ertel W, Morrison MH, Ayala A, Chaudry IH (1992) Chloroquine attenuates hemorrhagic shock-induced immunosuppression and decreases susceptibility to sepsis. Arch Surg 127: 70-76
22. Ertel W, Morrison MH, Meldrum DR, Ayala A, Chaudry IH (1992) Ibuprofen restores cellular immunity and decreases susceptibility to sepsis following hemorrhage. J Surg Res 53: 55-61
23. Ayala A, Meldrum DR, Perrin MM, Chaudry IH (1993) The release of transforming growth factor-β following haemorrhage: its role as a mediator of host immunosuppression. Immunology 79: 479-484
24. Barroso-Aranda J, Chavez-Chavez RH, Schmid-Schönbein GW (1992) Spontaneous neutrophil activation and the outcome of hemorrhagic shock in rabbits. Circ Shock 36: 185-190
25. Vedder NB, Winn RK, Rice CL, Chi EY, Artors KE, Harlan JM (1988) A monoclonal antibody to the adherence-promoting leukocyte glycoprotein CD 18, reduces organ injury and improves survival from hemorrhagic shock and resuscitation in rabbits. J Clin Invest 81: 939-944
26. Davis JM, Stevens JM, Peitzman A, Corbett WA, Illner H, Shires GT III (1983) Neutrophil migratory activity in severe hemorrhagic shock. Circ Shock 10: 199-204
27. Barroso-Aranda J, Schmid-Schönbein GW (1989) Transformation of neutrophils as indicator of irreversibility in hemorrhagic shock. Am J Physiol 257 (Heart Circ Physiol 26): H846-H852
28. Park BH, Fikbrig SM, Smithwick EM (1968) Infection and nitroblue-tetrazolium reduction by neutrophils. Lancet 2: 532
29. Abraham E, Chang YH (1984) Effects of hemorrhage on inflammatory response. Arch Surg 119: 1154-1157
30. Fink MP, Gardiner M, MacVittie TJ (1985) Sublethal hemorrhage impairs the acute peritoneal inflammatory response in the rat. J Trauma 25: 234-237
31. Deitch EA, Mancini M (1983) Complement receptors in shock and transplantation. Arch Surg 128: 1222-1226
32. Ayala A, Perrin MM, Meldrum DR, Ertel W, Chaudry IH (1990) Hemorrhage induces an increase in serum TNF which is not associated with elevated levels of endotoxin. Cytokine 2: 170-174

33. Abraham E, Freitas AA (1989) Hemorrhage produces abnormalities in lymphocyte function and lymphokine generation. J Immunol 142: 899-906
34. Esrig BC, Frazee L, Stephenson SF, Polk HC Jr, Fulton RL, Jones CE (1977) The predisposition to infection following hemorrhagic shock. Surg Gynecol Obstet 144: 915-917
35. Esrig BC and Fulton RL (1975) Sepsis, resuscitated hemorrhagic shock and "shock lung". Ann Surg 182: 218-227
36. Meyers JR, Meyer JS, Baue AE (1972) Does hemorrhagic shock damage the lungs? J Trauma 13: 509-518
37. Kock T, Duncker P, Roland A, Schiefer HG, Van Ackern K, Neuhoff H (1993) Effects of hemorrhage, hypoxia, and intravascular coagulation on bacterial clearance and translocation. Crit Care Med 21: 1758-1764
38. Collins JA, James PM, Bredenberg CE, Anderson RW, Heisterkamp CA, Simmons RL (1978) The relationship between transfusion and hypoxemia in combat casualties. Ann Surg 188: 513-520
39. Rush BF Jr, Soria J, Murphy TI et al (1988) Endotoxemia and bacteremia during hemorrhagic shock. Ann Surg 207: 549-554
40. Moore FA, Moore EE, Poggett RS et al (1992) Post-injury shock and early bacteremia. Arch Surg 127: 893-898
41. Roumen RMH, Hendriks T, van der Ven-Jongekrilg J et al (1993) Cytokine patterns in patients after major vascular surgery, hemorrhagic shock, and severe blunt trauma. Ann Surg 218: 769-776
42. Rabinovici R, Renz J, Esser KM, Vernick J, Feuerstein G (1993) J Trauma Serum tumor necrosis factor-alpha profile in trauma patients. J Trauma 35: 698-702
43. Casey LC, Balk RA, Bone RC (1993) Plasma cytokine and endotoxin levels correlate with survival in patients with the sepsis syndrome. Ann Intern Med 119: 771-778
44. Rogy MA, Coyle SM, Oldenburg HSA et al (1994) Persistently elevated soluble tumor necrosis factor receptor and interleukin-1 receptor antagonist levels in critically ill patients. J Am Coll Surg 178: 132-138
45. Faist E, Mewes A, Baker CC et al. (1987) Prostaglandin E_2 (PGE_2) dependent suppression of interleukin-2 (IL-2) production in patients with major trauma. J Trauma 27,8: 837-848
46. Faist E, Schinkel C, Zimmer S, Kremer JP, Von Donnersmarck GH, Schildberg FW (1993) Inadequate interleukin-2 synthesis and interleukin-2 messenger expression following thermal and mechanical trauma in humans is caused by defective transmembrane signalling. J Trauma 34: 846-854
47. Faist E, Storck M, Hültner L et al (1992) Functional analysis of monocyte activity through synthesis patterns of proinflammatory cytokines and neopterin in patients in surgical intensive care. Surgery 112: 362-372
48. Faist E, Kupper TS, Baker CC, Chaudry IH, Dwyer J, Baue AE (1986) Depression of cellular immunity after major injury. Arch Surg 121: 1000-1005
49. Younes RN, Rogatko A, Brennan MF (1991) The influence of intraoperative hypotension and perioperative blood transfusion on disease-free survival in patients with complete resection of colorectal liver metastases. Ann Surg 14: 107-113
50. Waymack JP, Fernandes G, Cappelli PJ et al (1991) Alterations in host defense associated with anesthesia and blood transfusions. Arch Surg 128: 59-62
51. Waymack JP, Raplen J, Garnett D, Tweddell JS, Alexander W (1986) Effect of transfusion on immune function in a traumatized animal model. Arch Surg 121: 50-55
52. Waymack P, Robb E, Alexander W (1987) Effect of transfusion on immune function in a traumatized animal model. Arch Surg 122: 935-939

53. Cué JI, Peyton JC, Malangoni MA (1992) Does blood transfusion or hemorrhagic shock induce immunosuppression? J Trauma 32: 613-617
54. Livingston DH, Malangoni MA (1988) An experimental study of susceptibility to infection after hemorrhagic shock. Surg Gynecol Obstet 168: 138-142
55. Nielsen HJ, Hammer JH, Moesgaard F, Kehlet H (1989) Ranitidine prevents postoperative transfusion-induced depression of delayed hypersensitivity. Surgery 105: 711-717
56. Agarwal N, Murphy JG, Cayten G, Stahl WM (1993) Blood transfusion increases the risk of infection after trauma. Arch Surg 128: 171-177
57. Nichols RL, Smith JW, Klein DB et al (311) Risk of infection after penetrating abdominal trauma. N Engl J Med 311(17): 1065-1070
58. Wang P, Hauptman JG, Chaudry IH (1990) Hemorrhage produces depression in microvascular blood flow which persists despite fluid resuscitation. Circ Shock 32:307-318

Human Volunteer Endotoxin Studies: A Useful Approach for the Understanding of Immunologic and Inflammatory Pathways

M.L. Rodrick, J.A. Mannick

There is a burgeoning consensus that the trigger for many of the metabolic and immunologic abnormalities noted after traumatic or thermal injury is bacterial endotoxin, either leaked directly from the gut into the portal circulation or produced by intestinal bacteria translocated from the gut in response to injury [1]. Because gram negative bacterial endotoxins are well-known stimuli of monocyte and macrophage cytokine and prostanoid production, it is logical to study the effects of small doses of bacterial endotoxin on metabolism, and on the activation of lymphocytes and monocytes in the circulating blood, including the production of cytokines and prostaglandins by these cells, in order to determine whether the effects of intravenous endotoxin mimic the abnormalities seen after serious injury in patients and in animal models.

For this reason our own laboratory and others [2, 3] have administered endotoxin to normal human volunteers over the past decade.

The volunteers for the endotoxin studies reported here were normal young men (mean age 33 years, range 28-39 years) judged healthy by history, physical examination, hematology, clinical studies and stress electrocardiogram. They were admitted 4 days before each study to the Clinical Research Center of the Brigham and Women's Hospital for acclimitization and evaluation. Written informed consent, which was reviewed and approved by the Brigham and Women's Hospital Committee for the Protection of Human Subjects from Research Risks, was obtained from all volunteers. The subjects were given a standard hospital diet and activity was limited to the Clinical Research Center. Ambulatory normal healthy volunteers were also studied at the same times as infused hospital volunteers. Two normal subjects of similar age were studied for each hospitalized volunteer. The volunteers in separate hospitalizations were given either an intravenous infusion of purified *Escherichia coli* endotoxin (4 ng/kg) and saline into an indwelling intravenous catheter or an infusion of saline alone. Venous blood samples were drawn from the volunteers before endotoxin or saline infusion and at varying intervals after infusion for the first 24 h. In other studies, volunteers received two doses of ibuprofen 800 mg orally 2 h before and at the time of endotoxin or saline infusion. In still other studies volunteers received an infusion of hydrocortisone 100 or 200 mg in saline with or without an accompanying endotoxin infusion.

Peripheral blood mononuclear cells (PBMCs) were harvested by centrifugation of heparinized venous blood samples diluted 1:2 in phosphate-buffered saline (PBS) on Ficoll-Hypaque for 35 minutes at 400 g. The interface cells were collected, washed three times and placed in Eagle's minimal essential medium containing glutamine, HEPES buffer and 5% fetal bovine serum (complete medium) (CM). The cells were counted for viability and observed with Turk's stain for morphology. Cells were always more than 95% viable but in some instances interface cells from the centrifugation were contaminated with myeloid cells and therefore estimation of mononuclear cells was made and cell counts adjusted accordingly so the total number of mononuclear cells per well of all cultures was similar.

PBMCs isolated as above were cultured in 220 µl/volume at 1×10^5 cells/well in 96-well flat-bottomed tissue culture plates containing CM. Phytohemagglutin (PHA) was added at a concentration of 6 µg/ml for 90 h at 37C in 5% CO_2 and wells were pulsed with 1 µCi/[^{3}H]Tdr during the last 18 h of culture. The cells were harvested and incorporated radioactivity was measured in a liquid scintillation counter. The counts per minute of triplicate cultures containing no mitogen were subtracted from the cultures with mitogen and this number was used in all calculations. Treated volunteers were compared with untreated volunteers and with themselves prior to endotoxin infusion. To avoid interassay variation, suppression of mitogenic response was calculated by the formula:

$$\% \text{ suppresion} = \frac{1 - \text{patient cpm}}{\text{control cpm}} \cdot 100$$

The sensitivity of PBMCs to the inhibitory effects of prostaglandin E_2 (PGE_2) was determined as previously described [4]. A total of 1×10^5 PBMCs were placed into culture with 200 µl CM containing 1 µg/µl indomethacin (to prevent de novo PGE_2 synthesis) and 0, 10^{-6}, 10^{-7}, or 10^{-8} molar PGE_2, followed by addition of 20 µl of the T-cell mitogen PHA (concentration 6 µg/ml). The cultures were incubated, pulsed and harvested and incorporated radioactivity determined as before. The percentage suppression for each concentration of PGE_2 was determined by the formula:

$$\% \text{ suppresion} = \frac{1 - \text{cpm of cultures with } PGE_2 + \text{Indo}}{\text{cpm of cultures of Indo only}} \cdot 100$$

The dose of PGE_2 that caused 50% inhibition was calculated by determining the two PGE_2 concentrations more than and less than 50% inhibition and extrapolating from these two points the concentration of PGE_2 that caused 50% inhibition.

For determination of PGE_2 production, PBMCs, 200 µl/well in CM at a concentration of 5×10^6/ml, were incubated in 96-well microtiter plates for 1 h at 37C. Nonadherent cells were removed by washing with FBS-free medium. Adherent cells were then cultured in FBS-free medium for 24 h with or without the addition of *E. coli* 055:B5 lipopolysaccharide (LPS, Sigma Chemical Corp., St. Louis, MO) at a concentration of 1.5 µg/ml. Supernatants were harvested and the PGE_2 concentration was measured by commercial radioimmunoassay.

Production of interleukin-2 (IL-2) was measured by culturing PBMC's at 1×10^5 cells/well in 200 ul volume for 24 hours in CM with or without 2.5 ug PHA/well. Indomethacin was added to some of the cultures at a final concentration of 1 µg/ml. Supernatants were collected and frozen at -70C until assayed. Interleukin-2 concentrations were determined by bioassay using CTLL-2 cells as described. IL-2 content of culture supernatants was calculated using a program provided by Dr. Brian Davis (Immunex, Seattle, Washington).

Generation of IL-1 and TNF-α and Bioassay of IL-1

PBMCs (200 μl cells at 5×10^6/ml) in MEM-FCS were allowed to adhere to flat-bottomed plastic microtiter plates for 1 h at 37C, 5% CO_2 and 95% air. Nonadherent cells were removed by washing three times in RPMI-1640 medium containing antibiotics, l-glutamine, and HEPES buffer as above without FCS, and the adherent cells were cultured as above for 24 h in 100 μl of the same medium in the presence of 1.0 μg/ml culture of LPS (E. coli 0.55:B5, Sigma, St. Louis, Mo., USA). Supernatant solutions were pooled from three or four wells, frozen and assayed for IL-1 as described previously [2, 4] using thymocytes from C3H/HeJ mice or assayed for IL-1β and TNF-α by ELISA as described below.

ELISA Method for IL-1 and TNF

In these assays goat antihuman lymphokine antibody in a previously determined appropriate dilution in 0.1 M carbonate buffer, pH 9.6, was added to wells of ELISA plates (Costar, Cambridge, Mass., USA) incubated overnight at 4C and washed in washing solution (PBS plus 0.05% Tween 20). Active sites on the plates were then blocked with 1% bovine serum albumin (BSA) in PBS for 1 h and washed as above. The samples to be tested were added in 100-μl volumes. The plates were incubated for 60 min at room temperature, washed three times and 100 μl rabbit anti-human lymphokine antibody appropriately diluted in PBS, 0.1% BSA and 0.1% normal goat serum was added per well. The plates were incubated for 1 h, washed and appropriately diluted alkaline phosphatase conjugated goat antirabbit immunoglobulin antibody in washing solution added to appropriate wells. Plates were again incubated for 60 min at room temperature and washed as above. The substrate, *para*-nitrophenylphosphate disodium, 1 mg/ml in substrate diluent (pH 9.8, 0.05 M sodium carbonate buffer with 1 mM $MgCl_2$,) was added, 100 μl/well, incubated at room temperature for 1 h and stopped by the addition of 100 μl 1N sodium hydroxide per well. The results were read at 405 nm in an ELISA reader. Standards of lymphokines and negative controls for antibodies and antigens were used in all assays. All assays were tested for sensitivity and specificity using recombinant cytokines and mixtures of cytokines to control for synergy. Data were obtained from standard curves generated by the ELISA reader software Softmax (Molecular Devices, Menlo Park, Ca., USA).

Statistical analysis was performed by using a normal probability plot to detect nonparametric data. Student's t-test was used for parametric data and the Mann Whitney U-test for non-parametric data.

Results

Volunteers uniformly experienced fever, malaise and tachycardia beginning shortly after endotoxin infusion. Significant blood pressure lowering was not observed. Clinical laboratory measurements demonstrated a prompt diminution in the circulating lymphocyte population and an increase in circulating PMN. Metabolic effects included elevation of serum cortisol, epinephrine and ACTH. Clinical symptoms abated and laboratory values returned to normal levels within 24 h.

Using a sensitive limulus lysate assay for plasma endotoxin, endotoxin could be found in the circulating blood of the volunteers a few minutes following endotoxin infusion but not thereafter. Measurements of the circulating plasma cytokines in the endotoxin-treated volunteers performed in another laboratory demonstrated an early peak in circulating TNF-α and IL-1β [5].

On the other hand, stimulation of adherent PBMCs in vitro with LPS demonstrated a profound depression in the production of IL-1β and TNF-α by PBMCs from endotoxin-treated volunteers as compared with saline-treated controls beginning within 1 h of endotoxin infusion [2]. An overshoot with increased production upon stimulation in vitro with LPS was seen in many volunteers at approximately 24 h (Fig. 1). Circulating PMNs showed a similar profound depression in IL-1β and TNF-α production beginning shortly after endotoxin infusion. These results coupled with early increased levels of circulating proinflammatory cytokines suggested a temporary exhaustion of cellular production following an initial intense stimulus with increased productive capacity manifest 24 h later.

After stimulation in vitro with the T-cell mitogen PHA, PBMCs from endotoxin-treated volunteers showed a profound suppression of proliferation and IL-2 production by 4 h after endotoxin infusion [2, 4]. Both proliferation and IL-2 production returned to normal 24 h after endotoxin infusion (Fig. 1). Similarly, PBMCs from endotoxin-treated volunteers showed a marked increased sensitivity to inhibition by PGE_2 at 4 h following endotoxin infusion, which disappeared by 24 h (Fig. 2). We have observed such an increase in sensitivity to PGE_2 by circulating PBMCs from patients with major burns [4]. The addition of indomethacin to the PBMC cultures stimulated with PHA partially restored the proliferative capacity of PBMCs from endotoxin-treated volunteers 24 h after endotoxin infusion. The addition of IL-2 to the same cultures completely restored the proliferative ability of these cells, thus indicating the presence of normally functioning IL-2 receptors. The addition of IL-1β had no effect [2].

Endotoxin stimulated cultures of adherent PBMCs from endotoxin-treated volunteers showed maintenance of PGE_2 at 4 h following endotoxin infusion and a marked increase in production of PGE_2 production at 24 h as compared with saline-treated controls (Table 1). Thus PGE_2 production in response to endotoxin was maintained in adherent PBMCs after endotoxin treatment despite marked reduction in proinflammatory cytokine production at this time interval.

Effects of Ibuprofen

Pretreatment of volunteers with ibuprofen prior to endotoxin infusion inhibited many of the clinical manifestations of endotoxin, including fever and malaise and resulted in a marked attenuation of the hormonal response to endotoxin [6].

Ibuprofen pretreatment abrogated the depression of circulating lymphocyte proliferation and IL-2 production seen following endotoxin infusion (Fig. 3). However, ibuprofen pretreatment had no effect whatsoever on the profound depression of TNF-α and IL-1β production by LPS-stimulated adherent PBMCs early after endotoxin infusion. Since endotoxin causes a temporary elevation in serum cortisol levels and ibuprofen pretreatment blunts this cortisol response, we performed further studies to try to separate the effects of cortisol from those of endotoxin by infusion of hydrocortisone or endotoxin or both into volunteers. We found that the circulating levels of PBMCs were significantly depressed following hydrocortisone infusion alone. This suppression was not as profound as that seen following endotoxin infusion, though the values were not statistically significantly different (Table 2). While the circulating numbers of PBMCs were depressed following hydrocortisone infusion, the

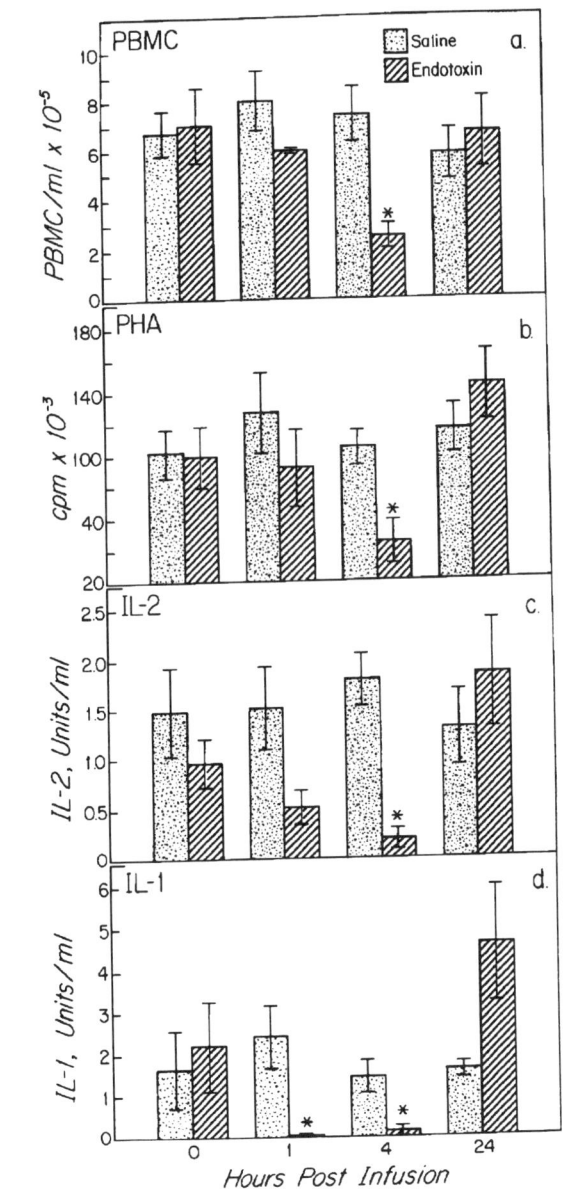

Fig. 1: *Effects of intravenous infusion of endotoxin on normal human volunteers. The effects of an infusion of saline are compared in each instance with the effects of infusion of endotoxin in saline. Marked diminution in the numbers of circulating PBMCs in the response to PHA stimulation with respect to proliferation and IL-2 production and in IL-1 production following stimulation by LPS in vitro were seen by 4 h following endotoxin infusion. (Reprinted with permission of J Clin Immunol [2])*

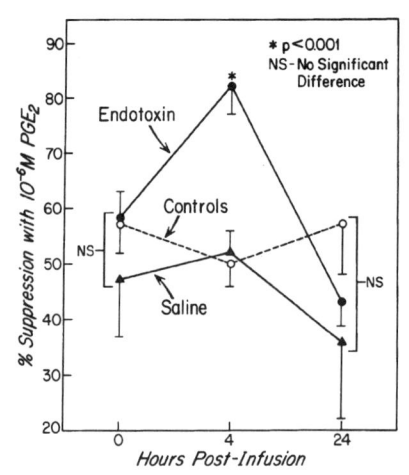

Fig. 2: Sensitivity of PBMCs to inhibition by PGE$_2$ in the proliferative response to PHA. Four hours after endotoxin infusion a marked increased sensitivity to PGE$_2$ was seen. Saline infusion produced no such effect and was similar to no treatment (controls). (Reprinted with permission of Ann Surg [4])

Table 1: PGE$_2$ synthesis (pg/ml)

	Infusion 0 h	Time after infusion (h)	
		4h	24h
Saline	5656 + 1845	2679 + 621	3471 + 525
Endotoxin	5043 + 641	4364 + 1423	9257 + 2857*
Ibuprofen +saline	5123 + 2376	4654 + 1451	3717 + 781
Ibuprofen + endotoxin	6094 + 2567	3750 + 812	6975 + 782*

*$p < 0.05$ compared with control infusion at same time.

Table 2: Results at 4 h post-infusion

Group	WBC x 10^3	Cortisol ug/dl	PBMC x 10^5/ml	PHA (cpm)	IL-2 (units/ml)	TNF-α (pg/ml)
Saline	6.9 + 0.8	10 + 1	13.7 + 2.4	115 741 + 24 109	1.18 + 0.32	1800 + 352
HC	9.9 + 1.2*	93.13*	4.6 + 0.7*	75 589 + 8314	0.64 + 0.20	1185 + 375
LPS	10.8 + 1.0*	32 + 1	2.9 + 0.6*	45 883 + 14 661*	0.08 + 0.06*	761 ± 370*
HC/LPS	15.7 + 1.3*	82 + 10	5.5 + 1.2	34 430 + 13 182	0.26 + 0.09*	1144 ± 375

*$p < 0.05$ vs. saline by the Mann-Whitney U-test.

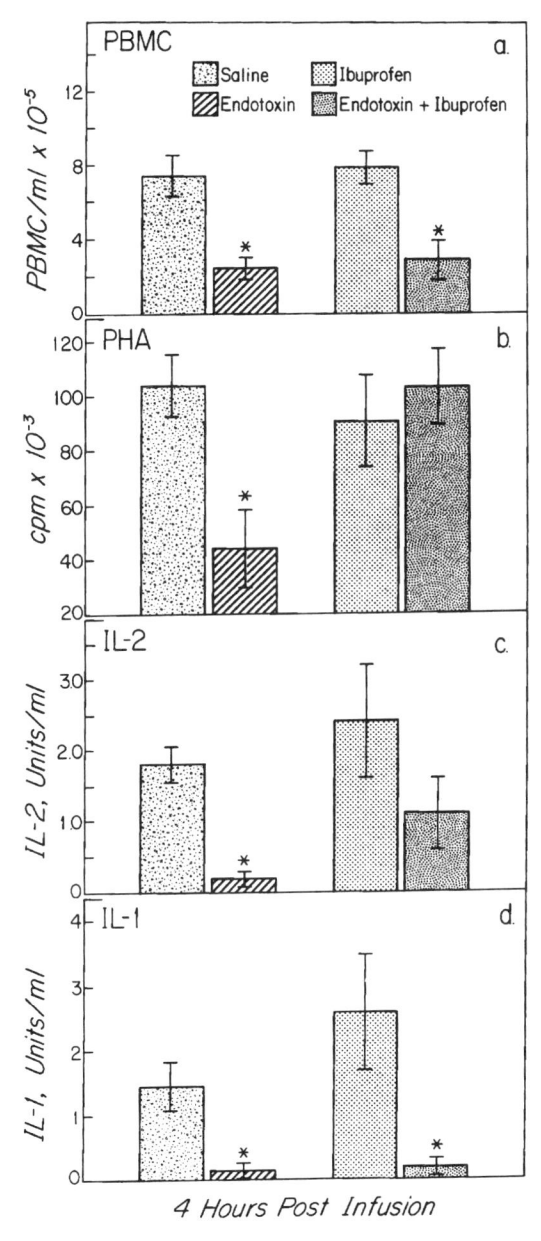

Fig. 3: Effect of ibuprofen pretreatment on the response of normal human volunteers to endotoxin. Ibuprofen treatment effectively abrogated the diminution of PHA response with respect to proliferation and IL-2 production seen after infusion of endotoxin alone. However, ibuprofen had no effect on the production of IL-1 by PBMCs in response to LPS stimulation. (Reprinted with the permission of J Clin Immunol [2])

proliferative response to the T-cell mitogen PHA was not significantly suppressed nor was the production of IL-2. The production of IL-1β and TNF-α was not significantly affected by hydrocortisone infusion. It should be noted that circulating levels of cortisol were higher following hydrocortisone infusion than following endotoxin in this group of volunteers. It was of interest that the infusion of hydrocortisone just prior to endotoxin blunted the inhibition of TNF-α and IL-1β production upon in vitro stimulation of adherent PBMCs 4 h following infusion. In fact, TNF-α production by adherent PBMCs from hydrocortisone and endotoxin-treated volunteers was not significantly different from those treated with saline alone. Hydrocortisone also completely blocked the increase in proinflammatory cytokine production seen 24 h after endotoxin infusion.

We have interpreted these results as indicating that increased levels of circulating cortisol are not responsible for the depression of T-lymphocyte activation seen following endotoxin exposure. Since this phenomenon can be overcome by inhibitors of prostaglandin synthesis, a pivotal role for PGE_2 is postulated. However, cortisol can blunt the initial inhibition of proinflammatory cytokine production seen following endotoxin infusion, and this phenomenon is not abrogated by inhibition of PGE_2 synthesis.

Discussion

Studies from our laboratory and those of other investigators have shown that the administration of a single dose of gram-negative bacterial endotoxin to normal human volunteers can reproduce many of the abnormalities of lymphocyte function noted after traumatic injury and burns. These abnormalities include diminished responsiveness of circulating T cells to stimulation of their receptors by mitogens along with diminished production of IL-2. We have also noted continued normal production of PGE_2 by stimulated adherent mononuclear cells from the circulating blood of the same endotoxin-treated individuals and excessive production at 24 h after endotoxin stimulation. These findings lend further credence to the idea that similar abnormalities in immune responsiveness that accompany serious injury are triggered by bacterial endotoxin leak from the gut or released from enteric organisms translocated from the gut. The fact that the abnormalities of T-cell function noted in endotoxin-treated volunteers could be abrogated by ibuprofen further highlights the role of prostanoid production in mediating these abnormalities [7].

A surprising finding in the present studies was that pro-inflammatory cytokine production by circulating adherent PBMCs and PMNs after stimulation in vitro with LPS was profoundly depressed in endotoxin treated volunteers early after endotoxin infusion. Since elevated plasma levels of inflammatory cytokines were noted in these individuals, we have interpreted these results as indicating temporary exhaustion of cytokine production by the appropriate cell populations obtainable from samples of circulating blood. Whether such exhaustion reflects a temporary suppression of gene transcription or is a post-transcriptional phenomenon remains to be determined by studies of messenger RNA expression in the circulating PBMC and PMN populations.

The results obtained in our laboratory are somewhat at variance with those obtained by other investigators utilizing the same model of endotoxin infusion in human volunteers. Other investigators have concluded that increased circulating cortisol levels are responsible for the diminished numbers of circulating PBMCs and inhibition of lymphocyte activation seen following endotoxin infusion [8, 9]. The experiments reported above in which hydrocortisone was administered alone or just prior to endotoxin suggest to us that cortisol is itself partly responsible for reducing numbers of circulating PBMCs but those lymphocytes left in the circulation appear to respond normally to T cell receptor stimulation, both with regard to proliferation and IL-2 production. Interestingly enough, administration of cortisol with endotoxin partly abrogated the profound suppression in proinflammatory cytokine production seen immediately following endotoxin infusion.

The question of involvement of complement activation in the phenomena observed after endotoxin infusion clearly must be addressed. While it is clear that endotoxin can activate complement by the alternative pathway, this appears to be a dose dependent phenomenon. The volunteers following endotoxin infusion were studied for complement activation by measurement of circulating anaphylotoxins and, as previously reported, no increase in levels of circulating C3a or C4a were found in these individuals, thus suggesting that there was no detectable complement activation after infusion of low doses of endotoxin [10]. However, it has also been clearly demonstrated that endotoxin can increase the expression of complement receptors on circulating monocytes and PMNs in the absence of serum [11] and such increased receptor expression, suggestive of profound activation of these cells, was characteristically seen following infusion of small amounts of endotoxin in the volunteers in the present study [10].

The fact that some of the abnormalities of metabolism, catabolic hormone production and lymphocyte activation seen in injured man were mimicked, at least temporarily, following endotoxin infusion in human volunteers does not necessarily mean that endotoxin is responsible for the abnormalities seen after injury. It has been remarkably difficult to demonstrate persistent or repeated elevations of circulating endotoxin in either the systemic [12] or portal [13] blood of injured man despite evidence from animal studies that translocation of gram negative bacteria is an invariable accompaniment to injury. However, these observations clearly suffer from defects of the techniques used for endotoxin measurement and the fact that local effects of endotoxin release by translocated bacteria clearly cannot be ruled out.

References

1. Maejima K, Deitch EA, Berg R (1984) Promotion by burn stress of the translocation of bacteria from the gastrointestinal tracts of mice. Arch Surg 119: 166-172
2. Rodrick ML, Moss NM, Grbic JT, Revhaug A, O'Dwyer ST et al (1992) Effects of in vivo endotoxin infusions on in vitro cellular immune responses in humans. J Clin Immunol 12(6): 440-450
3. Cannon JG, Tompkins RG, Gelfand JA, Michie HR, Stanford GG, vander Meer JWM et al. (1990) Circulating interleukin-1 and tumor necrosis factor in septic shock and experimental endotoxin fever. J Infec Dis 161: 79-84
4. Grbic JT, Mannick JA, Gough DB, Rodrick ML. The role of prostaglandin E_2 in immune suppression following injury. Ann Surg 214(3): 253-263
5. Michie HR, Manogue KR, Spriggs DR, Revhaug A, O'Dwyer S, Dinarello CA et al (1988) Detection of circulating tumor necrosis factor after endotoxin administration. N Eng J Med 318: 1481-1486
6. Revhaug A, Michie HR, Manson JMcK, Wattes JA, Dinarello CA, Wolff SM, Wilmore DW (1988) Inhibition of cyclooxygenase attentuates the metabolic response to endotoxin in humans. Arch Surg 123: 162-170
7. Faist E, Ertel W, Cohnert T et al. (1990) Immunoprotective effects of cyclooxygenase inhibition in patients with major surgical trauma. J Trauma 30: 8-17

8. Calvano SE, Albert JD, Legaspi A, Organ BC, Tracey KJ, Lowry SF, Shires GT, Antonacci AC (1987) Comparison of numerical and phenotypical leucocyte changes during constant hydrocortisone infusion in normal humans with those in thermally injured patients. Surg Gynecol Obstet 164: 509-520
9. Richardson RP, Rhyne CD, Fong Y, Hesse DG, Tracey KH, Marano MA, Lowry SF, Antonacci AC, Calvano SE (1989) Peripheral blood leucocyte kinetics following in vivo lipopolysaccharide (LPS) administration to normal human subjects. Ann Surg 210: 239-245
10. Moore FD Jr, Moss NA, Revhaug A, Wilmore D, Mannick JA, Rodrick ML (1987) A single dose of endotoxin activates neutrophils without activating complement. Surgery 102: 200-205
11. Davis CF, Moore FD, Jr, Rodrick ML, Fearon DT, Mannick JA (1987) Neutrophil activation after burn injury: contributions of the classic complement pathway and of endotoxin. Surgery 102: 477-484
12. Munster AM, Smith-Meek M, Dickerson C, Winchurch RA (1993) Translocation: Incidental phenomenon or true pathology? Ann Surg 218: 321-327
13. Moore FA, Moore EE, Poggetti R et al (1991) Gut bacterial translocation via the portal vein: a clinical perspective with major torso trauma. J Trauma 31: 629-639

Experimental and Clinical Aspects of Sepsis Associated with Obstructive Jaundice

B.J. Rowlands, M.I. Halliday, W.B.D. Clements, J.A. Kennedy

Introduction

Following surgical, endoscopic and radiological procedures, patients with obstructive jaundice have significant morbidity and mortality as a result of sepsis, wound failure, bleeding disorders and renal failure [1, 19]. Several factors have been implicated: for example, hypotension, impaired nutritional status, impaired immune function and the presence of toxic substances [25]. Wardle and Wright [27] reported an association between renal insufficiency and endotoxaemia in jaundiced patients, and since that time there has been increasing recognition of the role of circulating endotoxins in the development of complications in biliary obstruction [12]. Bile duct ligation (BDL) in experimental animals has been used to show that jaundice results in depressed wound healing, portal hypertension, liver structural damage, significant portal and systemic endotoxaemia, increased sensitivity to septic challenge, decreased reticuloendothelial function, depressed non-specific cell-mediated immunity, decreased bacterial trapping and clearance and increased bacterial translocation [6]. Biliary drainage remains the main therapeutic strategy in obstructive jaundice. Using the choledochovesical fistula model which provides sterile external biliary drainage, Diamond et al. [13] showed internal and external biliary drainage to be equally effective in reversing endotoxaemia. Using a choledochoduodenal fistula, other workers have shown that T-cell dysfunction returns to normal with internal biliary drainage [23, 24, 26].

Endotoxaemia in Biliary Obstruction

Two major factors contribute to the development of endotoxaemia: the absence of bile salts in the intestinal lumen and the impairment of Kupffer cell phagocytic function [4, 11]. The passage of viable resident bacteria and bacterial toxins from the intestinal lumen (bacterial translocation) occurs under a variety of experimental conditions, e.g. mucosal damage, bowel ischaemia, trauma, burns, systemic administration of endotoxin and obstructive jaundice. A cycle of events may exist where altered intestinal permeability (enhanced by circulating endotoxin and a lack of bile flow) results in increased portal endotoxaemia which exceeds the impaired Kupffer cell phagocytic function and facilitates spillover of endotoxin into the systemic circulation (Fig. 1). Using gnotobiotic animals, with negligible concentrations of intraluminal endotoxin, Greve et al. [14] have shown that endotoxaemia is directly responsible for the depression of cell-mediated immunity in biliary obstruction.

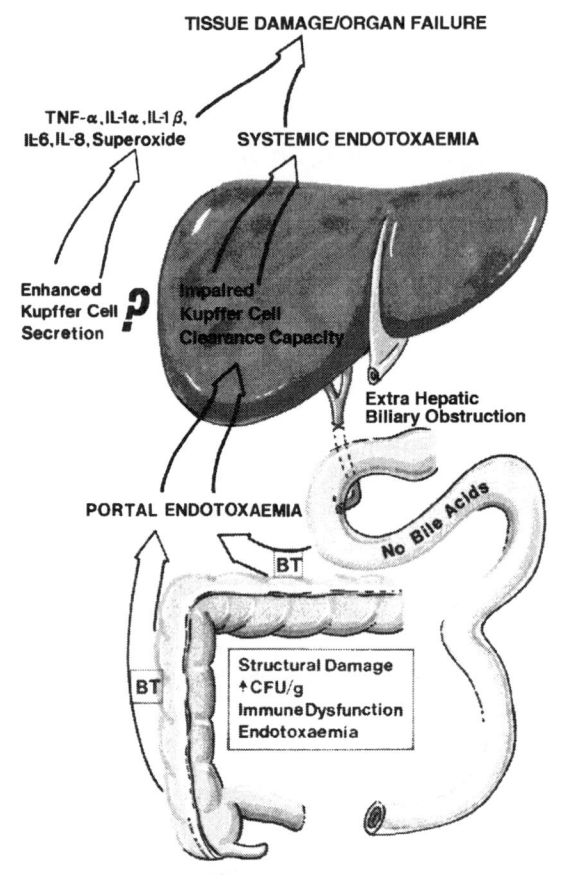

Fig. 1: Cycle of events associated with portal and systemic endotoxaemia and bacterial translocation from the gastrointestinal tract in obstructive jaundice

Kupffer Cell Function in Biliary Obstruction

There is marked functional heterogeneity within the mononuclear phagocyte system (MPS). Most investigations of the MPS have concentrated on phagocytic properties rather than other immunological functions, e.g. activation and secretion. The anatomical juxtaposition of the Kupffer cells and hepatocytes at the confluence of the portal venous drainage allows effective sequestration and elimination of all antigens, endotoxins and microorganisms derived from the gastrointestinal tract. Under normal conditions Kupffer cells are in a low grade state of activation due to small quantities of endotoxin which permeate the intact gastrointestinal barrier, but during sepsis and acute inflammation, Kupffer cells are highly activated and produce active inflammatory substances which mediate acute and sometimes deleterious pathophysiological reactions [22]. A paradoxical relationship exists between the benefits of control of systemic endotoxaemia and the harmful effects of production of inflammatory mediators. The regulation of this relationship in the cholestatic host is not known and macrophage activation may not be beneficial.

Cytokines in Biliary Obstruction

If endotoxaemia is central to the aetiology of complications in obstructive jaundice, there is little clinical or experimental evidence for the role of inflammatory cytokines. Increased urinary excretion of prostaglandins has been demonstrated in a canine model of biliary obstruction [28] and in rodents [18]. Bennelmans et al. [2] measured cytokine secretion in vitro by peritoneal macrophages harvested from mice with obstructive jaundice (BDL model) and observed high concentrations of spontaneous TNF-α and IL-6 production. Puntis et al. [20] harvested peripheral blood monocytes from cholestatic patients and showed an increased production of TNF-α to supraphysiological doses of lipopolysaccharide. Jiang et al. [15] have reported recently that neutrophils from patients with obstructive jaundice have raised oxidative responses which may be due to priming in vivo by cytokines such as IL-6, IL-8 and TNF-α. It is possible that excessive secretion of cytokines from Kupffer cells may be responsible for the development of the multiple organ dysfunction syndrome (MODS) in sepsis, fulminant hepatic failure and cirrhosis [10].

Immunomodulation of Kupffer Cells

Enhancement of host immune function may be achieved by nutritional, pharmacological and immunological means. Deficiencies of certain nutritional substrates lead to impairment of immune function [2] and dietary supplementation with ribonucleotides, n-3 polyunsaturated fatty acids and arginine [9] has been shown to promote immune function. Supplemental dietary regimens in animal models of sepsis and trauma have beneficial effects and in vivo data demonstrates immune enhancement when individual nutrients (e.g. L-arginine) are used in supraphysiological doses (500 mg/kg body wt.) [17]. Recently, Kennedy et al. [16] have shown that rodents with obstructive jaundice for 21 days have less weight loss and immune suppression than control animals when given drinking water supplemented by 1.8% L-arginine.

Investigation of the "Enterohepatic Axis" in Obstructive Jaundice

The structural and functional relationship between the gastrointestinal tract and the liver is important in the development of complications associated with obstructive jaundice. There is overwhelming evidence to support the presence of circulating endotoxin in biliary obstruction and its role in depression of cell-mediated immunity. Our working hypothesis of the sequence of events that follows the development of obstructive jaundice is illustrated in Fig. 2. The relationships between bowel permeability, bacterial translocation, endotoxaemia,

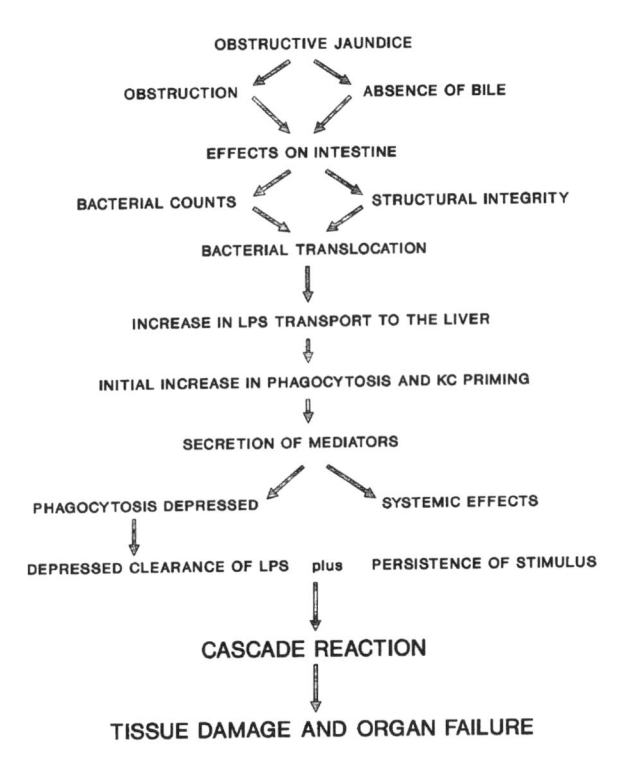

```
                    OBSTRUCTIVE JAUNDICE
                   ↙              ↘
        OBSTRUCTION              ABSENCE OF BILE
                   ↘              ↙
                   EFFECTS ON INTESTINE
                   ↙              ↘
        BACTERIAL COUNTS         STRUCTURAL INTEGRITY
                   ↘              ↙
                   BACTERIAL TRANSLOCATION
                            ⇓
            INCREASE IN LPS TRANSPORT TO THE LIVER
                            ⇓
         INITIAL INCREASE IN PHAGOCYTOSIS AND KC PRIMING
                            ⇓
                    SECRETION OF MEDIATORS
                   ↙              ↘
   PHAGOCYTOSIS DEPRESSED          SYSTEMIC EFFECTS
            ⇓
   DEPRESSED CLEARANCE OF LPS   plus   PERSISTENCE OF STIMULUS
                            ⇓
                     CASCADE REACTION
                            ⇓
             TISSUE DAMAGE AND ORGAN FAILURE
```

Fig. 2: Hypothesis of events leading to the development of multiple organ dysfunction syndrome (MODS) in obstructive jaundice

and Kupffer cell function have been investigated in our laboratories at Queen's University, Belfast. A better understanding of these mechanisms may lead to new therapeutic strategies employing nutritional, pharmacological or immunological manipulations that have the potential to reduce mortality and morbidity of obstructive jaundice.

Development and Validation of In Situ Hepatic Perfusion Technique [4]

This technique has been employed for many years in investigations of the biochemical and pharmacological aspects of hepatocyte function but has not been widely used in the study of non-parenchymal cells (Fig. 3). Thirty-five normal rats were perfused to validate the technique, confirm reproducibility and identify a reference range for Kupffer cell clearance capacity (KCCC) in normal healthy rats. Fluorescent particles appeared in the effluent in less than 1 min and equilibrated rapidly. The mean value was taken from ten readings throughout the period of the perfusion and the coefficient of variation ranged from 1.3% to 7.1%. Transmission electron microscopy confirmed the exclusive ingestion of latex particles by the Kupffer cell population. These perfusion experiments established a reference point for KCCC of 33.5% ± 2.26% (mean ± SEM).

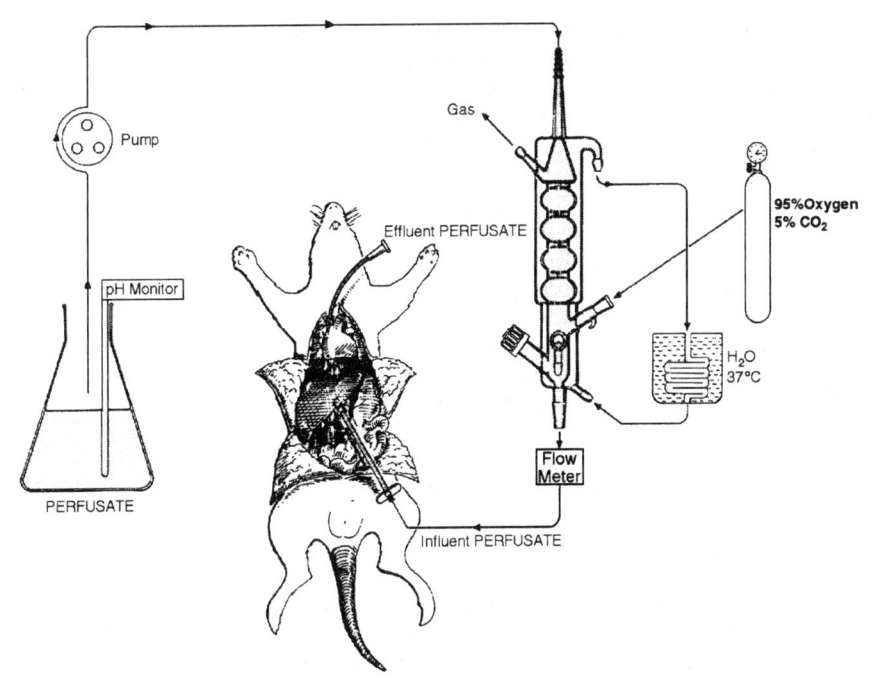

Fig. 3: Diagram of in situ hepatic perfusion technique used in experimental models of obstructive jaundice

The Effects of Extrahepatic Obstructive Jaundice on Kupffer Cell Clearance Capacity (KCCC) [4]

Control, sham operated (sham) and BDL Wistar rats (1, 2, 3 and 4 weeks BDL) were perfused. Plasma bilirubin, endotoxin and anticore glycolipid antibody (ACGA) concentrations were assayed. KCCC was calculated and expressed as percentage clearance of influent perfusate. Rats jaundiced for greater than 2 weeks had a significantly decreased KCCC. Significantly higher endotoxin concentrations and ACGA concentrations correlated positively with hyperbilirubinaemia. ACGA concentrations correlated strongly with system endotoxaemia and both were inversely correlated with duration of BDL. Maximal hyperbilirubinaemia preceded reduced KCCC. Impairment of Kupffer cell function may contribute to endotoxaemia associated with biliary obstruction. Laser scanning confocal microscopy was employed to quantitate Kupffer cell uptake and was compared to KCCC from perfusion studies. There was a strong inverse correlation between both techniques ($Rs=-0.875$, $p<0.0001$). The protocol was modified and a pilot study carried out using FITC (10 ng/mg) labelled endotoxin (*E. coli* 026:B6) as the probe to assess endocytosis of immunogenically active endotoxin. The BDL population ingested significantly less than controls (BDL 6.3%±0.45% vs. sham 21.2%±2.43%).

The Effects of Internal and External Biliary Drainage on KCCC Recovery in Jaundiced Rats [8]

Six groups of rats were studied using models of internal and external biliary drainage described by Diamond et al. [13] [BDL 3/52, sham, sham + choledochoduodenostomy

(CDD) 3/52, sham + choledochovesical fistula (CDVF) 3/52. BDL 3/52 + CDD 3/52. BDL 3/52 + CDVF 3/52]. KCCC returned to normal after a 3-week period of internal and external biliary drainage, although internal drainage was significantly more effective than external drainage. Bilirubin and anticore glycolipid concentrations normalised and both drainage groups had no significant systemic endotoxaemia.

The Effects of Extrahepatic Obstructive Jaundice on Intestinal Mucosal Integrity [7]

Using the protocol of Berg and Garlington [3], we have investigated the effects of extrahepatic obstructive jaundice on the microecology of the indigenous colonic flora and intestinal mucosal integrity in the rat model. Jaundiced rats have significantly increased bacterial translocation (BT) (sham 18% vs. BDL 56.3%, $p < 0.02$, Fisher's exact test), which correlates with increased plasma endotoxin and ACGA concentrations ($Rs = 0.56$, $p < 0.05$, Spearman's rank). There was no qualitative or quantitative difference in colonic luminal bacterial flora or intestinal structure between groups. Obstructive jaundice promotes translocation of enteric bacteria, despite there being no demonstrable change in intraluminal colonic flora or intestinal structure. This phenomenon may be induced by endotoxin, which perpetuates a cycle of bacterial translocation.

Morphometric Analysis of Kupffer Cells in Obstructive Jaundice [5]

This study determined morphometric changes in KC ultrastructure which might account for the diminution in phagocytosis seen in cholestasis. Three groups of Wistar rats were studied: control, sham and BDL. After 3 weeks animals were put to death and livers were "perfusion fixed" with 3% glutaraldehyde and processed for transmission electron microscopy and image analysis. In the BDL group Kupffer cell numbers were increased, biliary duct proliferation was evident and sinusoidal spaces were significantly compromised. Eleven nuclear and cytoplasmic parameters were measured and 6/11 were significantly different between the BDL group and controls. The most striking difference occurred in the extent of the intracellular lysosomal activity reflected in the lysosome number, lysosomal area and cytoplasm/nuclear ratio. Results suggest that Kupffer cells are activated and demonstrate enhanced phagocytosis during jaundice. This conclusion does not explain the reduction in KCCC in biliary obstruction.

Summary

These studies demonstrate the usefulness of a novel in situ hepatic perfusion technique for investigating Kupffer cell function. Preliminary conclusions from these experiments are (1) KCCC is depressed in biliary obstruction. (2) Biliary obstruction promotes translocation of enteric bacteria and endotoxin. (3) Three weeks of internal and external biliary drainage produce complete recovery of KCCC. (4) Electron microscopic appearances of Kupffer cells in biliary obstruction suggest activation of these cells. It is paradoxical that Kupffer cells appear activated at an ultrastructural level despite a decreased clearance capacity. In biliary obstruction, upon challenge with portal endotoxaemia, Kupffer cells may become primed and consequently activated to secrete proinflammatory cytokines. Further investigations are planned to elucidate the importance of Kupffer cell secretion in the pathophysiology of biliary obstruction and to evaluate the modulatory effects of biliary decompression on both these important parameters of Kupffer cell function. In addition, there is a need to assess the effects of nutritional, immunological and pharmacological manipulation as a potential strategy for future clinical use. A combination of these therapies may improve morbidity and mortality in clinical obstructive jaundice.

References

1. Armstrong CP, Dixon JM, Taylor TV, Davies GC (1984) Surgical experience of deeply jaundiced patients with bile duct obstruction. Br J Surg 71: 234-238
2. Bemelmans MHA, Gouma DJ, Greve JW, Buurman WA (1992) Cytokines, tumor necrosis factor and interleukin-6 in experimental biliary obstruction in mice. Hepatology 15: 1132-1136
3. Berg RD, Garlington AW (1979) Translocation of certain indigenous bacteria from the gastrointestinal tract to the mesenteric lymph nodes and other organs in a gnotobiotic mouse model. Infect Immun 23: 403-411
4. Clements WDB, Halliday MI, McCaigue M, Barclay RG, Rowlands BJ (1992) The effects of extrahepatic obstructive jaundice on Kupffer cell clearance capacity (KCCC). Arch Surg 128: 200-205
5. Clements WDB, Macartney R, Hamilton P, Cameron S, Toner P, Rowlands BJ (1992) Morphometric analysis of Kupffer cells in obstructive jaundice. Br J Pathol 169: 61
6. Clements WDB, Diamond T, McCrory DC, Rowlands BJ (1993) The effects of biliary drainage on obstructive jaundice: Experimental and clinical aspects. Br J Surg 80: 834-842
7. Clements WDB, Erwin P, Halliday MI, Barclay RG, Rowlands BJ (1993) Obstructive jaundice promotes bacterial translocation. Gut 34: S69
8. Clements WDB, Halliday MI, Barclay RG, Erwin P, McCaigue M, Rowlands BJ (1996) Biliary decompression promotes Kupffer cell recovery in obstructive jaundice. Gut (in press)
9. Daly JM, Lieberman MD, Goldfine J, Shou J, Weintraub F, Rosato EF, Lavin P (1992) Enteral nutrition with supplemental arginine, RNA, and omega-3 fatty acids in patients after operation: Immunologic, metabolic and clinical outcome. Surgery 112: 56-67
10. Deitch EA (1992) Multiple organ failure. Ann Surg 216: 117-134
11. Diamond T, Rowlands BJ (1989) Endotoxaemia in obstructive jaundice: the role of gastrointestinal bile flow. Surg Res Commun 5: 11-16
12. Diamond T, Rowlands BJ (1991) Endotoxaemia in obstructive jaundice. HPB Surgery 4: 81-94
13. Diamond T, Dolan S, Thompson RLE, Rowlands BJ (1990) Development and reversal of endotoxaemia and endotoxin related death in obstructive jaundice. Surgery 108: 370-375
14. Greve JW, Gouma DJ, Soeters PB, Buurman WA (1990) Suppression of cellular immunity in obstructive jaundice is caused by endotoxins: a study with germ free rats. Gastroenterology 98: 478-485
15. Jiang WG, Puntis MCA, Hallett MB (1994) Neutrophil priming by cytokines in patients with obstructive jaundice. HPB Surgery 7: 281-289
16. Kennedy JA, Kirk SJ, McCrory DC, Halliday MI, Barclay GR, Rowlands BJ (1994) Modulation of immune function and weight loss by L-arginine in experimental obstructive jaundice in the rat. Br J Surg 81: 1199-1201
17. Kirk SJ, Barbul A (1990) Role of arginine in trauma, sepsis, and immunity. J Parenter Enterol Nutr 14: 226S-229S
18. O'Neill PA, Wait RB, Kahng KU (1990) Obstructive jaundice and renal failure in the rat: the role of renal prostaglandins and the rennin/angiotensin system. Surgery 108: 356-362
19. Pain JA, Cahill CJ, Bailey ME (1985) Perioperative complication in obstructive jaundice: therapeutic considerations. Br J Surg 72: 942-945
20. Puntis MCA, Jiang WG, Thomas MA, Mathews N (1991) The effect of monocyte production of tumour necrosis factor in jaundice. Br J Surg 78: 759

21. Redmond HP, Shou J, Kelly CJ, Miller E, Daly JM. Immunosuppressive mechanisms in protein-calorie malnutrition. Surgery 110: 311-317
22. Rees RC (1992) Cytokines as biological response modifiers. J Clin Pathol 45: 93-98
23. Roughneen PT, Gouma DJ, Kulkarni AD, Fanslow WF, Rowlands BJ (1986) Impaired specific cell mediated immunity in experimental biliary obstruction and its reversibility by internal biliary drainage. J Surg Res 41: 113-125
24. Roughneen PT, Drath DB Kulkarni AD, Rowlands BJ (1987) Impaired nonspecific cellular immunity in experimental cholestasis. Ann Surg 206: 578-582
25. Su CH, Pleng FK, Lui WY (1992) Factors affecting morbidity and mortality in biliary tract surgery. World J Surg 16: 536-540
26. Thompson RLE, Hoper M, Diamond T, Rowlands BJ (1990) Development and reversibility of T lymphocyte dysfunction in experimental obstructive jaundice. Br J Surg 77: 1229-1232
27. Wardle EN, Wright NA (1970) Endotoxin and acute renal failure associated with obstructive jaundice. Br Med J 4: 472-474
28. Zambraska EJ, Dunn MJ (1984) The importance of renal prostaglandins in control of renal function after chronic ligation of the common bile duct in dogs. J Lab Clin Med 4: 549-559

Standardized Sheep Model for Multiple Organ Failure (MOF) After Severe Trauma

M. Grotz, G. Regel, A. Dwenger, H.-C. Pape, C. Hainer, R. Vaske, H. Tscherne

Introduction

Because of the successful treatment of early complications and increased survival time after severe multiple trauma, multiple organ failure (MOF) has become the most severe and most often lethal complication which follows this condition [1, 2]. In recent years numerous attemps have been made to develop a standardized animal model which reproduces MOF [5, 6]. This could be helpful for a better understanding of the pathophysiology and for verification of therapeutic regimens. The aim of this study was to develop a reproducible animal model in which the combination of several damaging mechanisms [hemorrhagic shock, operating trauma, administration of endotoxin (ET) and zymosan-activated plasma (ZAP)] lead to irreversible sequential failure of most of the parenchymal organs (multiple organ failure, MOF).

Materials and Methods

The study was performed according to the German Council's Guide for the Care and Use of Laboratory Animals (§8 Section 1, 18.8.1986).
Animal Preparation. Female adult merino sheep (25-30 kg body weight) were used for this study. On day 0 a central venous catheter was placed into the right external jugular vein. Anesthesia was initiated with 0.5 mg atropine and 3.5 mg/kg body weight pentobarbital. At this time a blood sample was taken for measurement of all biochemical parameters. Anesthesia was continued with a mixture of halothane, nitrous oxide and oxygen. An arterial and a venous catheter were inserted into the femoral vessels in addition to a Swan-Ganz thermodilution catheter (Baxter 93 A-131-9F, Edwards Critical-Care Division, Irvine, CA, U.S.A.) via the right external jugular vein into a pulmonary artery. In addition a urine catheter (Norta 10-No. 9285, BDF Beiersdorf, Hamburg, FRG) was inserted and connected to a collecting box. Hemorrhagic shock was induced by fractional bleeding to a mean arterial

pressure of 50 mmHg. For a further 2 h mean arterial pressure was kept at 50 mmHg. Withdrawal of total of 450-600 ml blood (22-24 ml/kg body weight) was necessary. The crystalloid solution was then infused until blood pressure and filling pressure reached normal levels. After this closed femoral nailing was performed according to the standardized AO-technique.

During the subsequent 10 days representitive parameters for organ function were measured once a day. on days 1 - 5 ZAP and endotoxin were administered every 12 h.

Zymosan-activated plasma (ZAP). First, 450 ml blood was centrifuged at 800 g for 10 min at room temperature. Plasma was then obtained and incubated with 3 mg/ml zymosan (Zymosan A, Sigma, sterilized at 120C, 1 atm for 20 min) for 30 min at 37C in a water bath. After 15 min of centrifugation at 800 g at room temperature the supernatant was frozen in 20-ml portions at -25C. Before administration ZAP was warmed to room temperature.

Endotoxin. An *E. coli* endotoxin preparation (serotype 055:B5, Sigma, USA; concentration 200 µg/ml) was used. A volume calculated to give 0.75 µg/kg bodyweight was diluted in a 10-ml syringe with 0.9% NaCl and injected simultaneously with the ZAP injection. During the experiment the animals received no further treatment and had free access to food and water. The animals were observed for a further 5 days. On day 10 histologic specimens were taken of all the representative organs.

Statistics

In Figs. 1 - 4 data are presented as mean values ± standard error of the mean (SEM). For statistical analysis the Wilcoxon test was used. Data were compared with baseline data.

Results

Cardiac function and hemodynamics. Cardiac index increased significantly in the late phase (day 1: 6.47 ± 0.41 ml/min m^2; day 10: 10.36 ± 0.79 ml/min m^2) (Fig. 1).

Pulmonary function. Arterial oxygen pressure declined significantly (day 1, 103.1 ± 1.6 mmHg; day 10: 89.8 ± 4.2 mmHg) (Fig. 2). At the same time pulmonary artery pressure showed a significant increase (day 1: 17.0 ± 0.7 mmHg; day 10: 28.8 ± 1.7 mmHg).

Liver function. Liver function was impaired, bilirubin levels showed a significant increase (day 1: 2.94 ± 0.34 µmol/l; day 10: 7.19 ± 0.91 µmol/l) (Fig. 3).

Kidney function. Creatinine clearance was low at day 1 (54.3 ± 7.4 ml/min), increased up to day 5 and deteriorated again significantly in the late phase over the entire period (day 2: 104.3 ± 26.8 ml/min; day 10: 53.1 ± 17.6 ml/min) (Fig. 4).

Sequence of MOF. First there was damage to lung and liver. Pulmonary artery pressure and bilirubin levels showed a significant increase on day 4. On day 7 there was resultant damage of the cardiac function with a significant increase in the cardiac index. Creatinine clearance decreased significantly on day 9, the damage to the kidney function being obvious.

Histology. Histologic changes were seen in all the representative organs (Figs. 5-7).

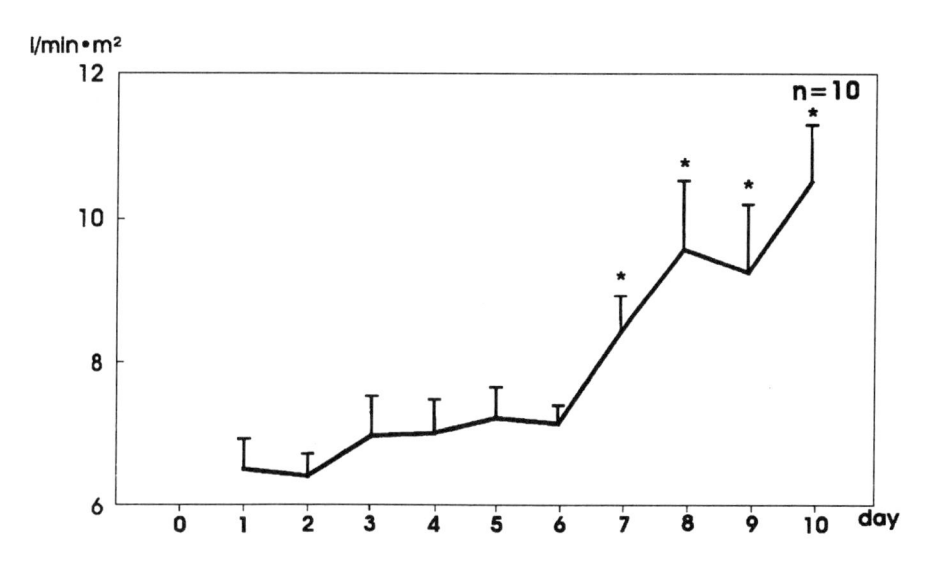

*Fig. 1: Cardiac index (CI) (l/min m^2): post-traumatic course days 1-10. *p<0.05*

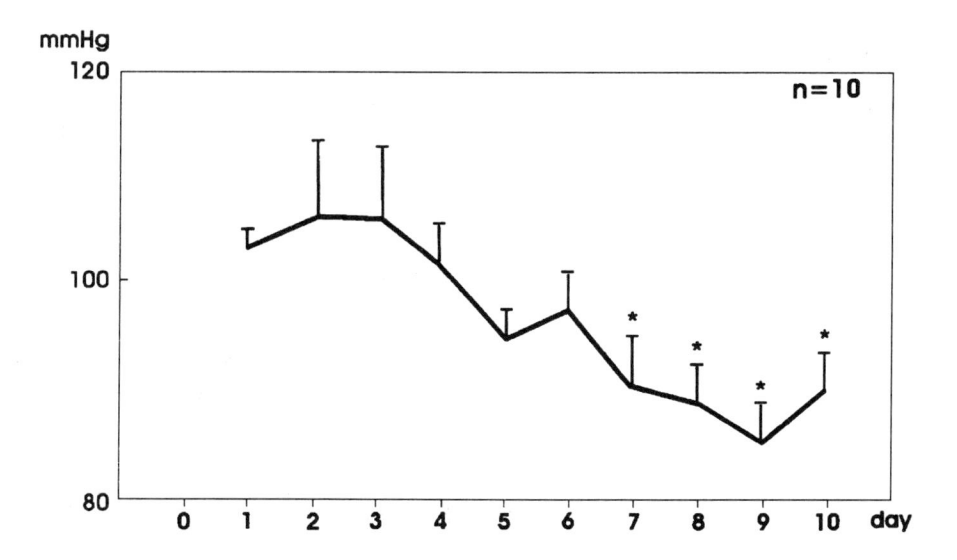

*Fig. 2: Arterial oxygen tension (PaO$_2$) (mmHg): post-traumatic course days 1-10. *p<0.05*

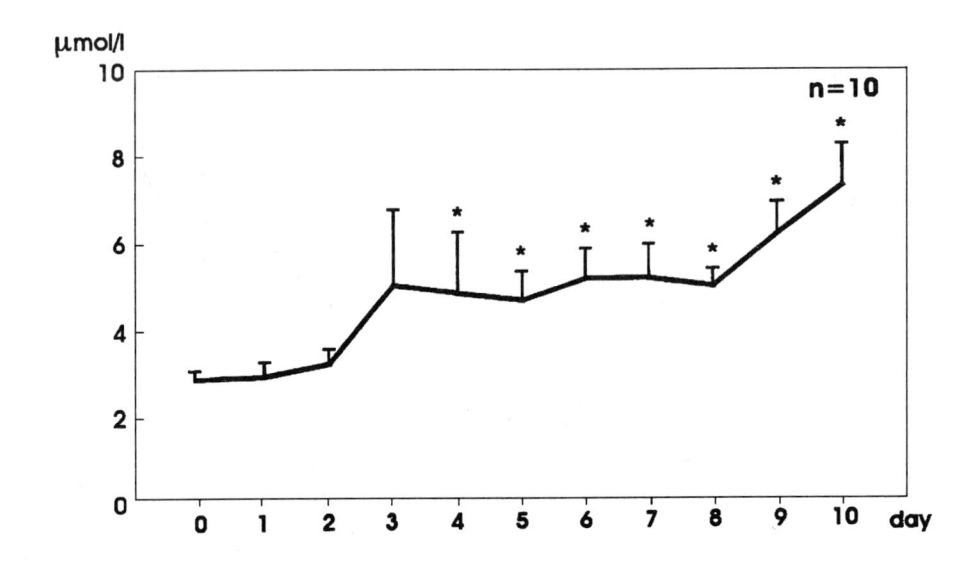

*Fig. 3: Serum bilirubin (Bili) (µmol/l): post-traumatic course days 1-10. *p<0.05*

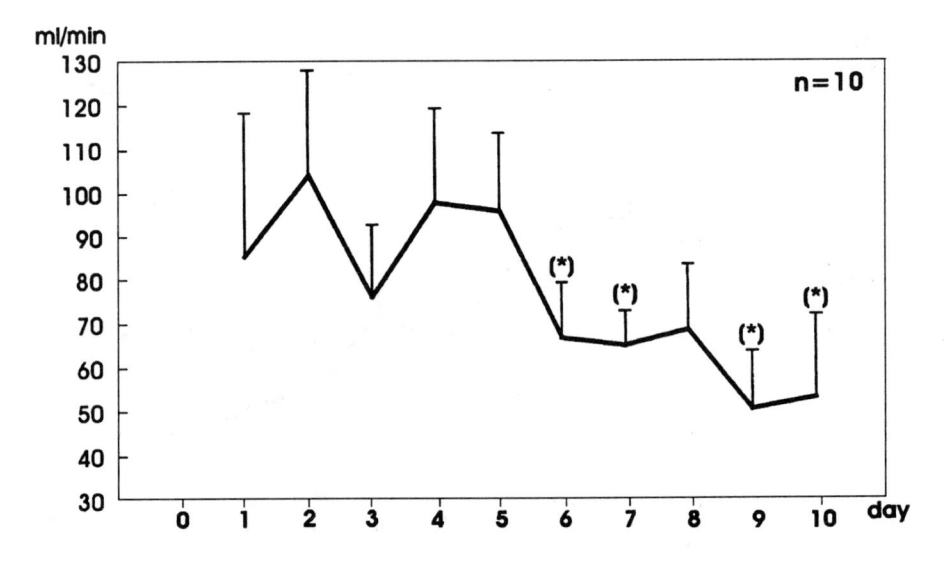

*Fig. 4: Creatinine clearance (CrCl) (ml/min): post-traumatic course days 1-10 *p<0.05*

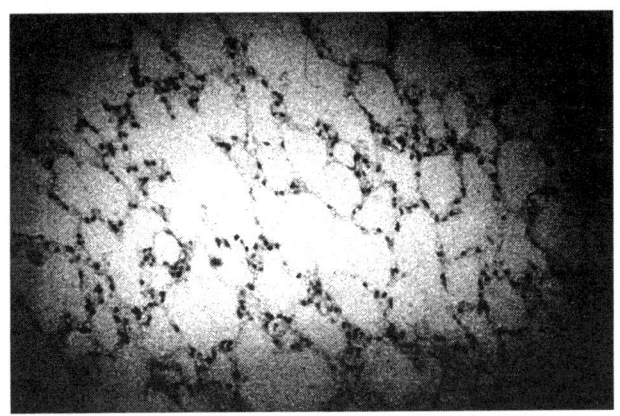

Fig. 5: Lung specimen: left apical lobe - showing high-degree perivascular edema and erythrodiapedesis

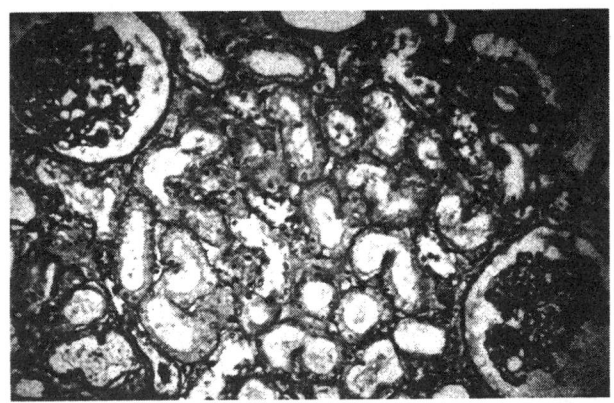

Fig. 6: Liver specimen: multifocal necrotic areas of parenchymal cells with accumulation of neutrophils.

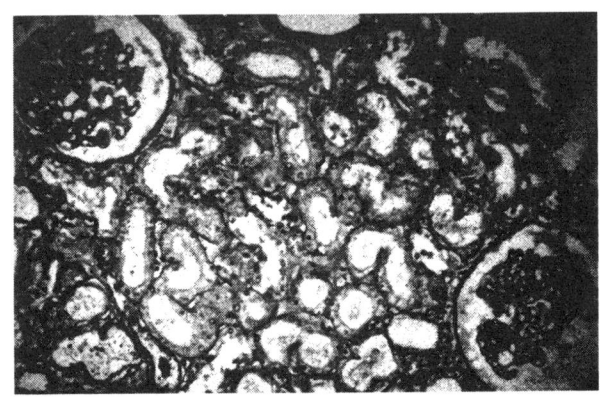

Fig. 7: Kidney specimen: great infarction of the glomerulus with extensive neutrophil infiltration

Discussion

Previous animal models of MOF

Goris et al. [5] described a rat model of MOF using intraperitoneal administration of zymosan, injected in a suspension of mineral oil. This caused a severe inflammatory response with an early increase in oxygen consumption, fever, dyspnea, tachycardia and diarrhea. In addition, there were histopathological changes in several organs [5, 10]. Comparison of this animal model with MOF after severe trauma in humans is difficult. MOF is caused by local peritonitis and not by shock, hypoxia and tissue damage. A rat model is less representative of mechanisms in humans. Nuytnick et al. [8] combined a 4-h infusion of zymosan-activated plasma with hypoxemia. This led to an increase in organ damage. Zimmermann et al. [11] showed with the combination of hemorrhagic shock and endotoxin administration histologic changes in lung, liver, bowel and kidney. The observation time was very short (1 h), so the results do not represent a typical MOF status. Hersch et al. [6] chose a different induction of MOF in sheep. After ligation and perforation of the intestine, damage to all the organ systems was seen after 3 days. Hemodynamic and pulmonary parameters deteriorated, and there was an increase in serum bilirubin. No significant decrease in kidney function was detected. Histologic specimens confirmed these results. The pathogenesis of this model is different from that of trauma in man. In the short observation period (3 days) the irreversible damage of organ function could not be proved.

Signs of organ damage

All the cardiac parameters reflected a hyperdynamic state. This was seen especially after day 7, leading to significant cardiac failure with an increase in cardiac index and decrease in systemic vascular resistance. Hersch et al. [6] found similar results after 24 and 48 h. In a small animal model Steinberg et al. [10] was only able to show an increase in the heart rate. Disturbances of pulmonary function were demonstrated in a decrease of arterial oxygen pressure over the entire period. Hersch et al. [6] showed in his 3-day model a similar course of lung failure. Goris et al. [5], however, reported clinical evidence of pulmonary failure and measured a decrease in oxygen consumption. Serum bilirubin levels represent the excretion function of the liver. A significant increase in bilirubin levels as in this sheep model could only be shown by Hersch et al. [6]. Steinberg et al. [10] determined the degree of liver damage by measuring cytochrome 450 levels postmortem. Continuous monitoring of this organ could not be initiated. The imediate decrease in creatinine clearence on day 1 is probably due to the hemorrhagic shock on day 0. After fluid resuscitation the kidney showed normal levels during the subsequent 4 days. In the late course renal function deteriorated again significantly. These results confirm Steinberg et al.'s [10] findings. Hersch et al. [6] was not able to show any change in kidney function in his model.

Sequence of Organ Damage

In this animal model representative organ parameters showed a similar course to that of MOF after multiple trauma in humans. In the literature the lung is found to be the first organ to fail [1, 2, 4, 7]. Faist et al. [3] postulated that there is no MOF without pulmonary failure. Liver failure is also often associated with generalized organ failure. In our patient population significant disturbances of organ function are regularly seen after 4 days [9]. The most interesting aspect in this model of MOF is that the induced injury during the first 5 days leads to irreversible and self-perpetuating deterioration of organ function in the last 5 days. So this animal model imitates the clinical situation of multiple trauma patients up to MOF and can be used fur further therapeutic investigations.

References

1. Baue AE (1975) Multiple, progressive, or sequential system failure: a syndrome for the 1970's. Arch Surg 110: 779-781
2. Border JR, Hasset J, La Duca J (1987) The gut origin septic state in blunt multiple trauma. Ann Surg 206: 427-448
3. Faist E, Baue AE, Dittmer H, Heberer G (1983) Multiple organ failure in polytrauma patients. J Trauma 23: 775-785
4. Fry DE, Pearlstein L, Fulton RL, Polk HC (1980) Multiple organ failure - the role of uncontrolled infection. Arch Surg 115: 136-190
5. Goris RJA, Boekholtz WKF, van Bebber IPT, Nuytinck JKS, Schillings PHM (1986) Multiple organ failure and sepsis without bacteria. Arch Surg 121: 897-901
6. Hersch M, Gnidec A, Bersten AD, Troster M, Rutledge FS, Sibbald WJ (1990) Histologic and ultrastructural changes in nonpulmonary organs during early hyperdynamic sepsis. Surgery 107: 397-410
7. McMenamy RH, Birkhahn R, Oswald G, Reed R, Rumph C, Vaidyanath N, Yu L, Cerra FB, Sorkness, R, Border JR (1981) Multiple system organ failure: I. The basal state. J. Trauma 21: 99-114
8. Nuytinck JK, Goris RJ, Weerts JG, Schillings PH, Stekhoven JH (1986) Acute generalized microvascular injury by activated complement and hypoxia: the basis of the adult respiratory distress syndrome and multiple organ failure? Br J Exp Pathol 67: 537-548
9. Regel G, Sturm JA, Pape HC, Gratz KF, Tscherne H (1991) Das Multiorganversagen (MOV). Ausdruck eines generalisierten Zellschadens aller Organe nach schwerem Trauma. Unfallchirurg 94: 487-497
10. Steinberg S, Flynn W, Kelley K, Bitzer l, Sharma P, Gutierrez C, Baxter J, Lalka D, Sands A, van Liew J, Hasset, Price R, Beam T, Flint L (1989) Development of a bacteria-independant model of the multiple organ failure syndrome. Arch Surg 124: 1390-1395
11. Zimmermann T, Laszik Z, Nagy S, Kaszaki J, Joo F (1989) The role of the complement system in the pathogenesis of multiple organ failure in shock. Prog Clin Biol Res 308: 291-297

Increased Cytokine Release in Severe Acute Pancreatitis Is Closely Related to the Development of Organ Failure

M. Ogawa, S. Ikei, H. Sameshima, K. Sakamoto, J. Yamashita

Acute pancreatitis is caused by different etiologic factors, but once pancreatic tissue is infected patients show a similar pattern of aggravation and organ failure. Buggy and Nostrant [1] reported that infectious complications were responsible for 80% of deaths in patients with acute pancreatitis. In the present review, we summarize our recent studies on the release of cytokines and activation of leukocytes (neutrophils and macrophages) in severe acute pancreatitis, and demonstrate that the increase in cytokine release in patients with septic complications is closely related to the development of organ failure in acute pancreatitis.

Hypercytokinemia and Organ Failure in Acute Pancreatitis

We recently treated 14 patients with acute pancreatitis (12 survived and 2 died). The patients were divided into three groups, with mild (eight), moderate (two) and severe (four) acute pancreatitis according to the criteria of the Research Group for Intractable Diseases of the Pancreas in Japan. The three groups represented different combinations of changes in biological parameters and organ function.

Figure 1 shows the serial changes in the serum level of interleukin-6 (IL-6), a crucial mediator for the host defense which is released by the stimulation of tumor necrosis factor (TNF), IL-1 or lipopolysaccharide (LPS) [2]. The serum level of IL-6 in patients with severe pancreatitis was significantly higher than that in patients in the mild group. IL-1β was detected only in two out of four severe cases, whereas TNF-α was detected in all the severe cases at the time of admission (Fig. 2). The changes in plasma polymorphonuclear leukocyte elastase (PMN-E) level in these groups are shown in Fig. 3. Plasma PMN-E in the severe group was significantly higher than in the mild group. Figure 4 shows the significant correlation between the peak levels of serum IL-6 and plasma PMN-E.

Most patients had complications of serious dysfunctioning of organs other than the pancreas. Figure 5 indicates the significant correlation between peak serum IL-6 level and number of organs showing failure. Acute pancreatitis itself was counted as one organ failure. There was also a significant correlation between peak plasma PMN-E level and number of failed organs (Fig. 6). In contrast, there was no significant correlation between peak serum pancreatic amylase level and number of organs showing failure. These results suggested that the release of cytokines and activation of neutrophils may be involved in the development of multiple organ failure (MOF) frequently seen in severe acute pancreatitis.

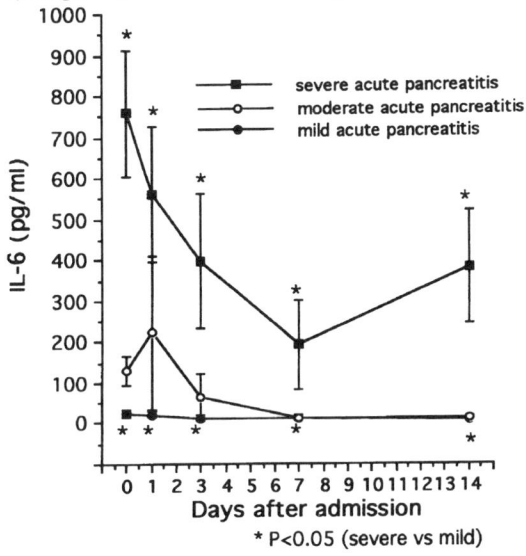

Fig. 1: Changes in IL-6 serum levels during the first 14 days after admission. Values are means ± SEM

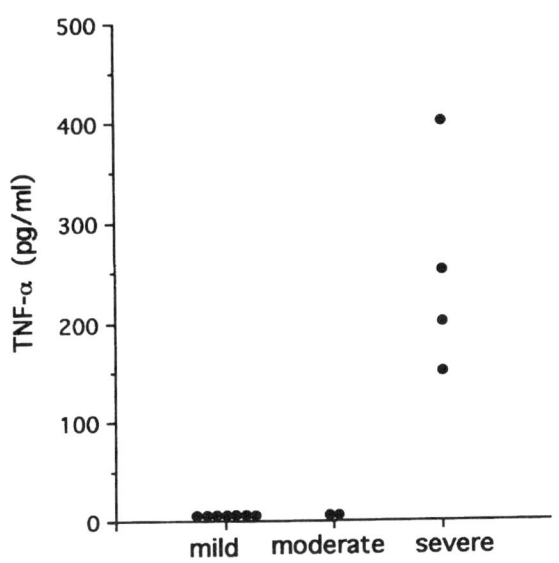

Fig. 2: Peak levels of serum TNF-α during the first 14 days after admission

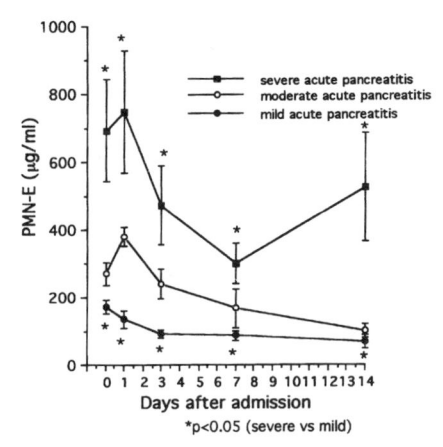

Fig. 3: Changes in PMN-E plasma levels during the first 14 days after admission. Values are means ± SEM

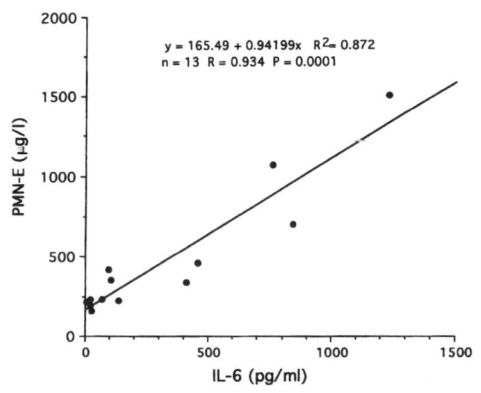

Fig. 4: Correlation between peak IL-6 serum levels and plasma PMN-E

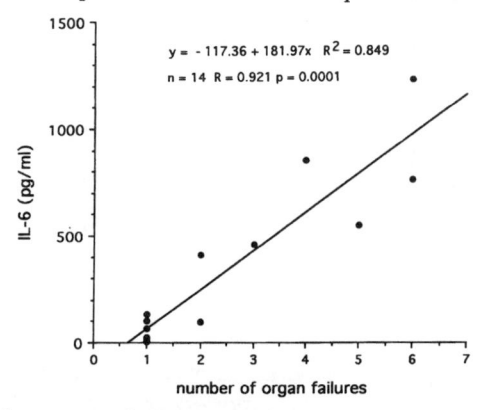

Fig. 5: Correlation between peak IL-6 serum levels and number of failed organs (acute pancreatitis counted as one organ failure)

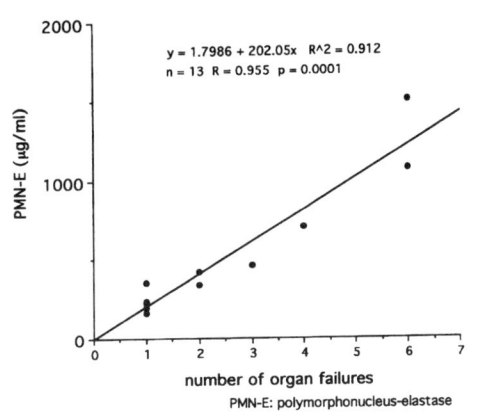

Fig. 6: Correlation between peak plasma PMN-E levels and number of organs failed (acute pancreatitis counted as one organ failure)

Priming of Macrophages in Mild Acute Pancreatitis

The hyperreactivity of macrophages was frequently reported from patients with major trauma [3] or the burn-sepsis model [4]. Recently, Sameshima et al. [5] demonstrated the hyperreactivity of peritoneal macrophage in the cerulein-induced pancreatitis model. TNF-α production by isolated peritoneal macrophages from rats with cerulein-induced pancreatitis was significantly increased compared with control rats following LPS stimulation (40.76 $\pm$ 4.03 vs. 0.415 $\pm$ 0.046 U/ml per milligram protein). This finding indicated that, even in mild, cerulein-induced pancreatitis, excessive macrophage stimulation is possible. It can be suggested that a large amount of cytokines will be secreted from macrophages, if infection is complicated under these circumstances. In fact, administration of a lethal dose of LPS to rats with cerulein-induced pancreatitis caused a significantly greater elevation of serum TNF-α activity than with controls administered LPS (Fig. 7).

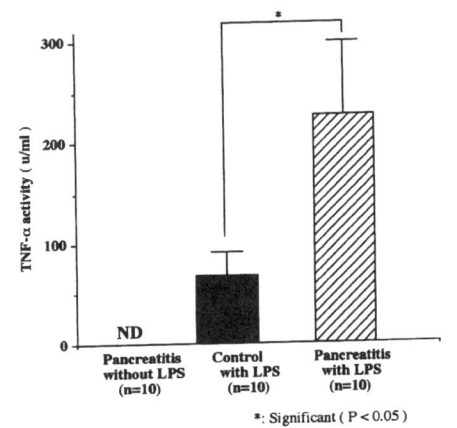

Fig. 7: Serum TNF-α activity 90 min after LPS administration to pancreatitis and normal rats. Values are means $\pm$ SEM. ND, not detectable

Cytokine Release and Development of Organ Failure in Acute Pancreatitis

Neutrophils migrate in response to various inflammatory mediators and are activated by those mediators. Marked and early neutrophil infiltration into the various vital organs, especially into the lung or liver, and neutrophil sequestration have been frequently reported after the administration of cytokines, indicating that it occurs during hypercytokinemia as seen in acute pancreatitis. The increase in plasma neutrophil elastase in patients with even mild acute pancreatitis indicates the partial activation of neutrophils.

Oka et al. [6] developed a coculture system of human neutrophils and a cultural human hepatoblastoma cell line, HuH-6, as normal hepatic cell substitutes, and demonstrated that neutrophils stimulated by cytokines can mediate cellular injury. Their results suggested infiltrated neutrophils in various vital organs can cause tissue injury by the stimulation of cytokines, resulting in dysfunction of these organs where no inflammation or bacteria exist. Our experiment revealed that LPS administration after induction of acute pancreatitis by cerulein increased mortality rate compared with controls administered LPS (50% vs. 20%) 24 h after LPS administration. Also, severe damage to the liver (evaluated by both histological findings and liver function tests) was induced by LPS administration in rats with pancreatitis and not in control rats [5].

Mechanism to Develop Organ Failure in Acute Pancreatitis Complicated by Infection

Infection is the most life-threatening complication in acute pancreatitis, because it often leads to the development of MOF. As seen in major trauma and burn, increased cytokine release and hyperreactivity of leukocytes (macrophages and neutrophils) occur in acute pancreatitis, leading neutrophils to infiltrate into the vital organs such as the lung or liver. When acute pancreatitis is complicated by infection, hyperreactive macrophages release a large amount of cytokines, which activate neutrophils as a second attacker. Utilizing proteolytic enzymes and oxidant, neutrophils attack and infiltrate vital organs, causing cellular damage and dysfunction of the vital organs (Fig. 8). MOF in acute pancreatitis with septic complications can be caused, at least in part, by the mechanism of cytokine release and leukocyte activation. Recent studies suggested that the modulation of cytokine release may be of great importance in the treatment of acute pancreatitis. Application of antibody, soluble receptor and receptor antagonist against inflammatory cytokines will give us a clue toward clarifying the complicated mechanisms involved in the development of MOF in severe acute pancreatitis.

References

1. Buggy BP, Nostrant TT (1983) Lethal pancreatitis. Am J Gastroenterol 78: 810-814
2. Kishimoto T (1989) The biology of interleukin 6. Blood 74: 1-10
3. Takayama TK, Miller C, Szabo G (1990) Elevated tumor necrosis factor-α production concomitant to elevated prostaglandin E_2 production by trauma patients' monocytes. Arch Surg 125: 29-35

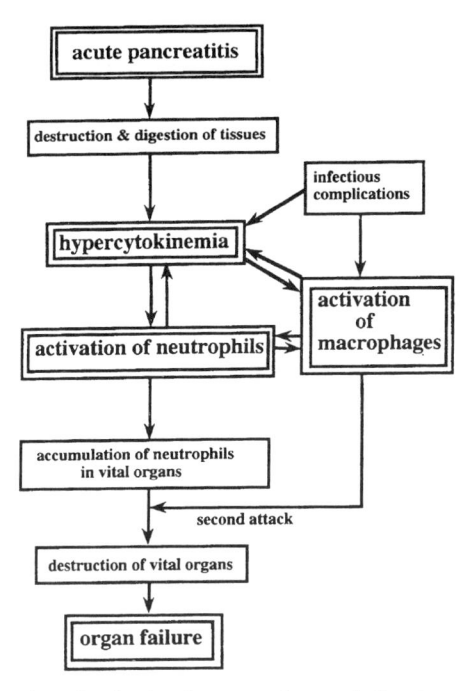

Fig. 8: Possible mechanisms for the development of organ failure in severe acute pancreatitis (working hypothesis)

4. O'Riordain MG, Collins KH, Pilz M, Saporoschetz IB, Mannick JA, Rodrick ML (1992) Modulation of macrophage hyperactivity improves survival in a burn-sepsis model. Arch Surg 127: 152-158
5. Sameshima H, Ikei S, Mori T, Yamaguchi Y, Egami H, Misumi M, Moriyasu M, Ogawa M (1993) The role of tumor necrosis factor-α in the aggravation of cerulein-induced pancreatitis in rats. Int J Pancreatol 14: 107-115
6. Oka Y, Murata A, Nishijima J, Ogawa M, Mori T (1993) The mechanism of hepatic cellular injury in sepsis: an in vitro study of the implication of cytokines and neutrophils in its pathogenesis. J Surg Res 55: 1-8

Severity of Multiple Organ Failure but not of Sepsis Correlates with Irreversible Platelet Degranulation

M. Gawaz, S. Fateh-Moghadam, G. Pilz, H.-J. Gurland, K. Werdan

Introduction

Sepsis is frequently associated with multiple organ failure (MOF), which is a leading cause of death among patients treated in intensive care units [15, 16]. It has been well recognized that multiple changes occur in the coagulation and fibrinolysis cascade in sepsis, leading to disseminated intravascular coagulation (DIC) and MOF [19]. There is increasing evidence that platelets play a major role in the pathophysiology of sepsis and MOF. Although enhanced platelet activation and formation of microaggregates in MOF have been attributed to impaired microcirculation and organ dysfunction [18, 19], the pathophysiological role of platelets in MOF is still poorly understood. This study focuses on functional changes of circulating platelets in patients with sepsis and MOF. Under normal conditions platelets circulate down the vascular tree in a resting state without interacting with each other. After activation platelets expose multiple adhesion receptors on their plasma membrane (fibrinogen receptor on GPIIb-IIIa, thrombospondin, p-selectin GMP-140, GP53, etc.) that play a crucial role in platelet aggregation or platelet interaction with other vascular cells, respectively [2, 6, 8, 13, 14, 23]. To elucidate the role of platelet glycoproteins these patients, we studied surface expression of membrane glycoproteins using flow cytometric techniques and a panel of platelet-specific monoclonal antibodies. Severity of disease was assessed by intensive care unit scoring systems including the sepsis-specific Elebute score [1, 17] as well as the non-sepsis-specific severity score of MOF, APACHE II [12].

Patients and Methods

Patients

Fourteen patients (nine female) with suspected or apparent sepsis or MOF were studied prospectively. The underlying diseases leading to submission were pneumonia ($n = 4$), chronic liver disease ($n = 2$), cardiac surgery ($n = 4$), and cardiovascular disease ($n = 4$). Mean age was 55.9 years (range 16 - 80 years), mean APACHE II score was 25.5 (range 4 - 46), and mean Elebute score was 12.7 (range 3 - 27). Mortality of the total study group was 43%. The APACHE II and Elebute scoring systems were used to characterize severity of MOF [12] or sepsis [1, 16], respectively. Patients of group I were characterized by moderate MOF with an APACHE II score of < 20, whereas group II included patients with severe MOF and an APACHE II score of ≥ 20. Patients with an Elebute score of ≥ 12 were classified as septic and patients with an Elebute score of < 12 were classified as nonseptic.

Platelet Flow Cytometric Analysis

Blood samples were taken from an arterial indwelling catheter and were anticoagulated with citrate (3.8%) containing an antiplatelet cocktail as previously described [2]. Platelet analysis was performed in platelet-rich plasma (PRP) by flow cytometric techniques [2, 4, 5, 9] and by using activation-specific monoclonal antibodies (mAbs). mAbs anti-CD41 and anti-CD42 (Dianova) recognize the complexed form of GPIIb-IIIa and the von Willebrand receptor GPIb, respectively. mAb anti-LIBS1 (generously provided by Dr. Mark Ginsberg, RISC, La Jolla) recognizes the fibrinogen receptor exposed on the activated form of GPIIb-IIIa [9]. mAbs anti-TSP, anti-CD62, or anti-CD63 (Dianova) bind to glycoproteins thrombospondin, GMP-140, and GP53, respectively, which remain associated with the platelet membrane after degranulation occurred.

Statistics

Results are given as mean ± standard error of mean deviation (mean ± SEM) for N observations. Significance was defined as $p < 0.05$ using Student's t-test for unpaired data.

Results

Effect of Sepsis in Platelet Membrane Glycoprotein

Anti-LIBS1 binding to circulating platelets was significantly increased in septic compared with nonseptic patients ($p<0.05$) (Fig. 1, Table 1). A significant correlation between anti-LIBS1 binding and Elebute score was observed ($r = 0.597$) (Fig. 2). In contrast, surface expression of glycoproteins GPIIb-IIIa, GPIb, TSP, GMP-140, or GP53, as assessed by mAb binding, was not significantly different in septic compared with nonseptic patients although platelets of septic patients tended to show higher surface expression of the granule glycoproteins TSP, GMP-140, or GP53 (Fig. 1, Table 1).

Effect of Multiple Organ Failure on Platelet Membrane Glycoproteins

Surface expression of TSP and GMP-140, respectively, was significantly increased in patients with severe MOF compared with patients suffering from moderate MOF ($p < 0.05$) (Fig. 3). Similar results were obtained for LIBS1 and GP53 surface expression although not to a statistically significant level (Fig. 3). Surface exposure of TSP ($r = 0.643$) or GMP-140 ($r = 0.611$) correlated well with APACHE II score (Fig. 4). No significant relationship between GPIIb-IIIa or GPIb surface expression and APACHE II score was found (Table 1).

Table 1: Sepsis, MOF, and platelet surface glycoproteins

	Nonseptic (Elebute<12)	Septic (Elebute ≥12)	p	Moderate MOF (APACHEII<20)	Severe MOF (APACHEII≥20)	p
CD41	798±8[a]	795±47	NS	798±8	797±40	NS
CD42	747±23	734±43	NS	753±23	733±37	NS
CD62	329±38	373±19	NS	316±30	372±43	<0.05
CD63	369+25	395+25	NS	365+23	392+26	=0.064
TSP	370+43	432+25	NS	358+45	426+54	<0.05
LIBS1	335+51	417+72	<0.05	342+49	390+82	NS
Platelet count ($\times 10^3/\mu l$)	236+240	91+73	NS	275+271	98+63	NS

[a]Mean intensity of immunofluorescence ± standard error of mean deviation

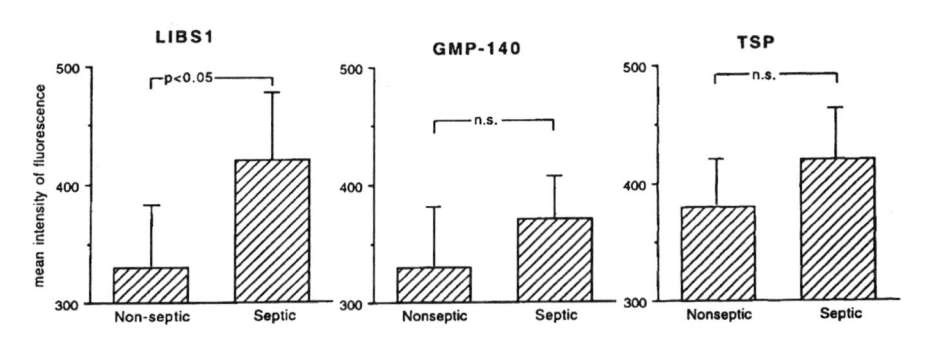

Fig. 1: Surface expression of fibrinogen receptor, p-selectin, and thrombospondin in septic patients. Elebute score of ≥ 12 indicates septic and < 12 nonseptic patients. Surface exposure of fibrinogen was determined by flow cytometric methods and by use of specific mAb

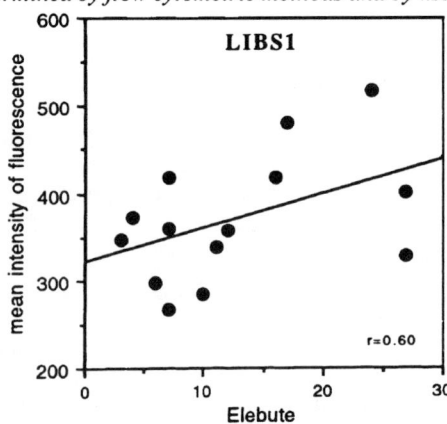

Fig. 2: Correlation between severity of sepsis as assessed by Elebute score and fibrinogen receptor activation (LIBS1 surface expression) on circulating platelets

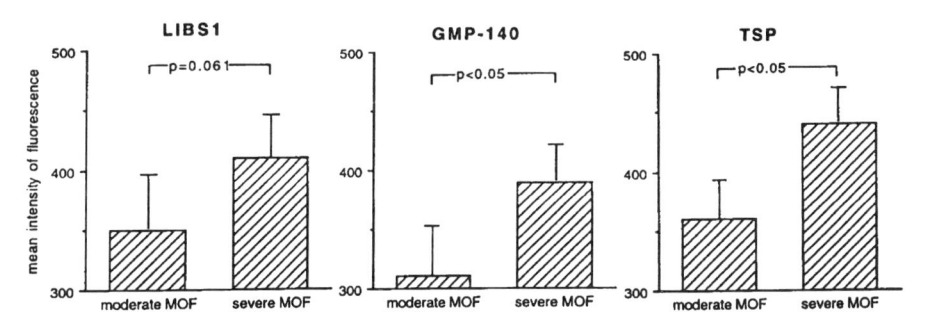

Fig. 3: Surface expression of fibrinogen receptor, p-selectin, and thrombospondin in patients with MOF. APACHE II score was used to assess severity of MOF. A score of <20 indicates the presence of moderate, ≥ 20 of severe MOF)

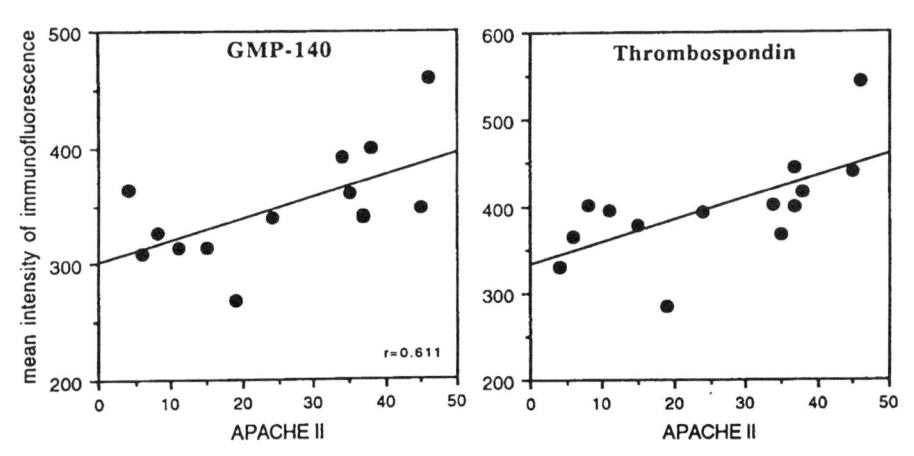

Fig. 4: Correlation between severity of MOF as assessed by APACHE II score and platelets degranulation (surface expression of GMP140 and TSP, respectively) on circulating platelets

Discussion

The present study shows that multiple changes in membrane glycoproteins occur on circulating platelets in patients with sepsis and MOF. In specific, platelets of septic patients reveal increased surface exposure of fibrinogen receptor activity that correlates well with severity of disease, but these patients do not show significant enhanced platelet degranulation. Multiple organ failure (MOF), however, is associated with an increased degranulation of granule-stored adhesion molecules such as thrombospondin (TSP), GMP-140, or GP53, which correlates significantly with severity of MOF. The increased platelets fibrinogen receptor activity in septic patients indicates that platelets circulate in a hyperaggregable state. In the course of the disease, platelets undergo release reaction and surface expresses multiple adhesion molecules that might play a role in impaired microcirculation and organ dysfunction, and thus in the development of MOF.

Abnormal platelet physiology has been well recognized in the pathogenesis of impaired microcirculation in MOF [10, 18, 21], which is frequently associated with sepsis [16]. Despite the large body of research done over the last decade, the underlying pathophysiological mechanisms are still poorly understood. Morphological analysis of tissue from organs involved in MOF revealed massive platelet aggregation and microembolization in the microvasculature [10, 20], Thus, an increased formation of circulation platelet microaggregates and release of platelet-derived products might contribute significantly to organ dysfunction in these patients.

The present study shows an increased fibrinogen receptor activity on circulating platelets in septic patients without a significantly increased release of granule-stored adhesion molecules. Since induction of the fibrinogen receptor requires platelet activation and represents the first but still reversible step of platelet aggregation [6, 8], we speculate that platelets become activated in the course of sepsis and circulate in a hyperactive state. It has been shown that increased platelet activation is associated with an enhanced risk of microthrombotic events and vessel occlusion in a variety of prethrombotic states [7]. Thus, circulating platelet microaggregates may be formed during the course of sepsis, which is still a reversible process as long as degranulation and subsequent surface expression of granule-store adhesion molecules does not occur. In our study we did not observe a significant increase of degranulation in septic patients. However, significant release of granule glycoproteins did occur in patients suffering from severe MOF. Thus, it is tempting to speculate that, although sepsis is not primarily associated with increased platelet degranulation, an enhanced exposure of adhesion glycoproteins on the surface of circulating platelets in the course of the disease might favor formation of irreversible stabilized microaggregates and interaction of platelets with other vascular cells such as leukocytes or endothelium [22]. The presence of platelet aggregates in the microvasculature may impair microcirculation and organ perfusion, which then initiates development of MOF.

This study does no address the nature of mediators involved in microcirculatory ischemia in patients with sepsis and MOF. However, the increased degranulation process in MOF indicates that besides adhesive glycoproteins biologically potent platelet-derived products are released into the circulation (thromboxane A_2, serotonin, ATP, growth factors, etc.) [22] that may aggravate microcirculatory disturbances by inducing vasoconstriction and endothelial injury.

The evaluation of platelet function in patients with sepsis presented here may be helpful in the early detection of platelet activation in these patients. Early recognition of platelet activation in the course of sepsis might be helpful in assessing the risk of microembolization, and thus development of MOF. Moreover, the flow cytometric methods described here might be useful in developing preventive and therapeutic strategies for septic patients with imminent MOF.

References

1. *Elebute EA, Stoner HB (1983) The grading of sepsis. Br J Surg 70: 29-31*
2. *Gawaz MP, Ward RA (1991) Effects of hemodialysis on platelet-derived thrombospondin. Kidney Int 40: 257-265*
3. *Gawaz MP, Loftus JC, Bajt ML, Frojmovic MM, Plow EF, Ginsberg MH (1991) Ligand bridging mediates integrin αIIbβ3 (platelet GPIIb-IIIa) dependent homotypic and heterotypic cell-cell interactions. J Clin Invest 88: 1128-1134*
4. *Gawaz MP, Bogner C, Gurland HJ (1993) Flow cytometric analysis of mepacrine-labeled platelets in patients with end-stage renal failure. Haemostasis 23: 284-292*

5. Gawaz MP, Dobos G, Späth M, Mujais S (1994) Impaired function of platelet membrane glycoprotein IIb-IIIa in end-stage renal disease. J Am Soc Nephrol (in press)
6. George JN, Nurden AT, Phillips DR (1984) Molecular defects in interactions of platelets with the vessel wall. N Engl J Med 311: 1084-1098
7. George JN, Pickett EB, Saucerman S, McEver RP, Kunicki TJ, Kieffer N, Newman PJ (1986) Platelet surface glycoproteins. Studies on resting and activated platelets and platelet microparticles in normal subjects, and observation in patients during adult respiratory distress syndrome and cardiac surgery. J Clin Invest 78: 340-348
8. Ginsberg MH, Loftus JC, Plow E (1988) Cytoadhesins, integrins, and platelets. Thromb Haemost 59: 1-6
9. Ginsberg MH, Frelinger AL, Lam SCT, Forsyth J, McMillan R, Plow EF, Shattil SJ (1990) Analysis of platelet aggregation disorders based on flow cytometric analysis of membrane glycoprotein IIb-IIIa with conformation-specific monoclonal antibodies. Blood 76: 2017-2023
10. Heffner JE, Sahn SA, Repine JE, (1987) The role of platelets in adult respiratory distress syndrome. Am Rev Respir Dis 135: 482-492
11. Knaus WA, Draper EA, Wagner DP, Zimmermann JE (1985) Prognosis in acute organ system failure. Ann Surg 202: 685-693
12. Knaus WA, Draper EA, Wagner DP, Zimmermann JE (1985) APACHE II: a severity of disease classification system. Crit Care Med 13: 818-829
13. Leung L, Nachman R (1986) Molecular mechanisms of platelet aggregation. Annu Rev Med 37: 179-186
14. Nieuwenhuis HK, Oosterhoutvon JJG, Rosemuller E, van Iwaarden, F, Sixma JJ (1987) Studies with a monoclonal antibody against activated platelets. Evidence that a secreted Mw 53,000 lysosome-like granule protein is exposed on the surface of activated platelets in the circulation. Blood 70: 838-845
15. Parker MM, Parrillo JE (1983) Septic shock: hemodynamics and pathogenesis. JAMA 250: 3324-3327
16. Parrillo JE, Parker MM, Natanson C, Suffredini AF, Danner RL, Connion RE, Ognigene FP (1990) Septic shock in humans. Advances in the understanding of pathogenesis, cardiovascular dysfunction, and therapy. Ann Intern Med 113: 227-242
17. Pilz G, Gurniak T, Bujdoso O, Werdan K (1991) A BASIC program for calculation of APACHE II and Elebute scores and sepsis evaluation in intensive care medicine. Comput Biol Med 21: 143-159
18. Saba TM, Fortune JB, Wallace JR (1992) Microaggregation hypothesis of multiple system organ failure. In: Frey DE (ed.) Multiple system organ failure - pathogenesis and management. Mosby-Yearbook, St. Louis
19. Saldeen T (1983) Clotting, microembolism, and inhibition of fibrinolysis in adult respiratory distress. Surg Clin North Am 63: 285-304
20. Schirmer WJ, Fry DE (1992) Microcirculatory arrest. In: Frey DE (ed.) Multiple system organ failure - pathogenesis and management. Mosby-Yearbook, St. Louis
21. Schneider RC, Zapol WM, Carvalho AC (1980) Platelet consumption and sequestration in severe acute respiratory distress syndrome. Am Rev Respir Dis 122: 445-451
22. Siess W (1989) Molecular mechanisms of platelet activation. Physiol Rev 69: 50-178
23. Stenberg PE, McEver RP, Shuman MA, Jacques YV, Bainton DF (1985) A platelet α-granula membrane protein (GMP-140) is expressed on the plasma membrane after activation. J Cell Biol 101: 88-885

Oxidative stress and Antioxidants in Clinical Sepsis

G. Sganga, G. Gangeri, D. Gui, M. Castagneto

Introduction

By sepsis or septic state we mean the systemic response of the organism to infection. Associated with the presence of the original septic focus is a pathophysiologic and symptomatologic response. Such a response is also seen with microorganisms in the circulation (bacteremia, septicemia) and their toxic by-products (endotoxemia) and with the effect of humoral mediators and the subsequent immune mechanisms, originally activated for host defense.

The septic process [sepsis, septic syndrome, septic shock, multiple organ dysfunction syndrome (MODS)] today represents the most frequent cause of death in postoperative surgical patient and in the multiple trauma patient. Despite recent therapeutic progress, the relative mortality lies between 30% and 80%. In the United States it is estimated that septicemia is ranked 13th in the causes of death, and that between 1969 and 1988 its incidence increased by 139%.

The aggressive surgical approach, which very often requires relaparotomy and laparotomy, and the use of antibiotics represent the best ways of controlling the septic focus.

However, recent pathophysiologic studies indicate the use of newer supportive therapies, directed to the diagnosis and prevention of the metabolic, biochemical, and immunobiological abnormalities induced by bacteria and their toxic products. These therapies are very important in slowing down the progression of the septic process, allowing traditional therapy to take effect successfully. The usefullness of the following measures is well known: parenteral nutrition to prevent metabolic dysfunctions, antiinflammatory antioxidative and antiprotease drugs to reduce cellular damage, anti-TNF and anti-PAF substances to prevent mediator activation, and monoclonal and polyvalent antibodies to enhance host's own defense capability. Alongside this variety of therapeutic alternatives there is a role for antioxidative drugs against reactive oxygen species (ROS) or the improvement of endogenous antioxidative activity.

Pathophysiology of Oxidative Damage

Free radicals are molecular species capable of existing independently that contain one or more unpaired electrons in their exterior orbit. Examples are superoxide ($O_2\text{-}^\circ$), thiol (RS°), trichloromethyl ($CCl_3^°$), and nitric oxide ($NO^{o!}$). They are strongly reactive because of their oxidant or reducing effect against other molecules. Oxygen free radicals (OFR) form sequential reduction of oxygen with single electrons; they can exist as unprotonated and protonated forms. The term "reactive oxygen species (ROS)" indicates all reactive species derived from reduction of oxygen, including both the radicals and the nonradical forms (Fig. 1). ROS are very toxic for biologic systems, since they produce severe damage to all biologic molecules.

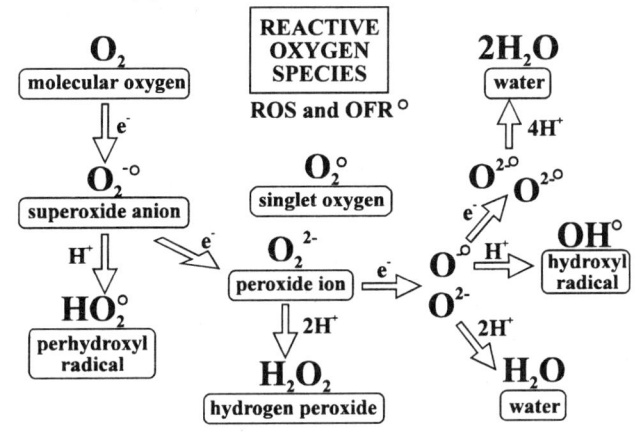

Fig. 1: Chemical generation of reactive oxygen species. ° indicates the radical forms of ROS

The main damage caused by ROS activity is peroxidation of membrane lipids, at cellular and subcellular levels, so-called lipoperoxidative damage. Once started by a hydroxyl radical this appears as a self-maintaining production chain, producing new radicals, lipid hydroperoxides, and cross-linking of fatty acids (Fig. 2). The consequences for cell viability include:
1. Disruption of membrane architecture fluidity
2. Inactivation of enzymatic activity (mostly ATPases)
3. Formation of new channels through the membrane with consequent ion escape (e.g. Ca^{2+} and iron)
4. Generation of highly cytotoxic products (e.g. aldehydes)
5. Damage to membrane-bound receptors
6. Alteration of red-cell deformability

Fig. 2: Self-maintaining process of fatty acid peroxidation and its consequences

ROS are continuously produced in the cells during metabolism (physiological production) as the consequence of chemical accidents (such as autoxidation of some molecules, leaks of single electrons from the mitochondrial respiratory chain or the microsomal electron carrier system), and enzymatic reactions (dismutation reactions, Haber-Weiss and Fenton chemical reactions). In the latter a major role is played by free metal ions, such as iron. ROS are produced in increased quantities in pathophysiologic conditions such as inflammation:
1. Through the activation of the phagocytes (circulating neutrophils, tissue macrophages) and through membrane-bound NADPH-reductase enzyme, as part of the mechanism for killing bacteria.
2. Through the well-known arachidonic cascade

Another pathophysiologic conditions is the ischemia-reperfusion syndrome caused by xanthine-oxidase. Indeed hypoxia leads to the conversion of xanthine dehydrogenase, which is NAD dependent on xanthine oxidase and is O_2 dependent, and an accumulation of hypoxanthine; on reoxygenation xanthine oxidase produces a burst of OFR.

All these mechanisms are common in shock, trauma, sepsis, and multiple organ failure syndrome (MOFS), leading to tissue injury by producing intracellular and/or intravascular damage or directly by inducing tissue damage (Fig. 3).

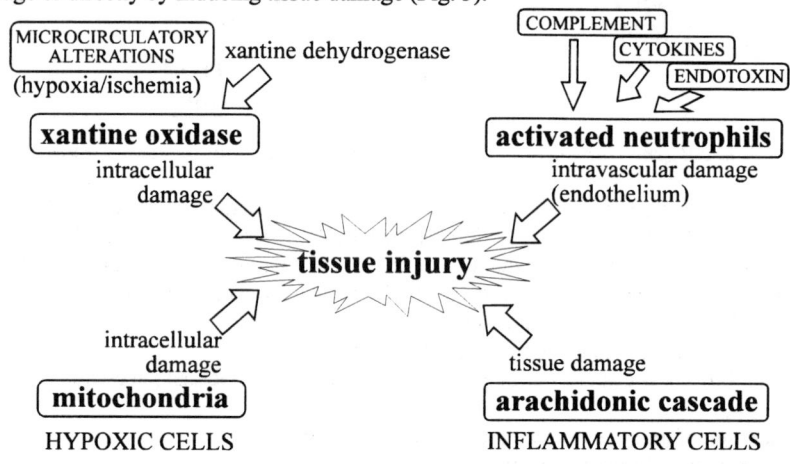

Fig. 3: Factors and mechanisms of tissue injury mediated by reactive oxygen species in sepsis, trauma, shock, and MOFS

Fortunately, cells have several mechanisms which prevent the oxidative damage induced by ROS, the so-called antioxidant defenses [6]. They can be differentiated into three systems:
1. Primary defenses, mainly useful for preventing or scavenging ROS, which include metal-ion sequestration mechanisms and the enzymatic antioxidants or scavenger enzymes [superoxide dismutase (SOD), catalase, other peroxidases, etc.]
2. Secondary defenses, mainly useful for blocking or eliminating the ROS, including the nonenzymatic antioxidants, which can be separated into hydrosoluble antioxidants (glutathione, vitamin C) and liposoluble antioxidants (vitamin E, carotene, coenzyme Q_{10})
3. Repair systems, which include increased protein synthesis, repair of DNA, degradation of protein damaged by radicals, and metabolization of lipid hydroperoxides

The oxidative damage found in a number of biochemical and pathophysiologic conditions results from an imbalance between pro-oxidants and antioxidants, in favor of the pro-oxidants [31]. Therefore, oxidative damage can be caused both from an overproduction of ROS sufficient to overcome antioxidant defenses, and a deficiency of any one of the antioxidant mechanisms. OFR-induced damage is found at the biochemical and cellular level. Its determination therefore in living organisms is unfortunately very difficult and can be undertaken indirectly by measuring bioproducts of the lipid peroxidation in different biologic samples. Also, controversial in the evaluation of oxidative damage is the type of compound selected as a marker of oxidative injury and the analytic method used for its detection.

The substances most frequently used to measure the presence and extension of OFR-induced lipid peroxidation are conjugated dienes, malondialdehyde (MDA), ethane, pentane, hydroxynonenal, and hydroperoxides. More specific and sensitive methods of measurement are liquid and gas chromatography, but they are expensive and time-consuming. Therefore, other analytic methods, which are less accurate and specific, such as the thiobarbituric acid reaction, are routinely used. These measurements can be carried our on tissue samples, red blood cell membranes, arterial and venous plasma, urine, and expired air.

The status of the antioxidant defenses can be assessed by measuring the activity of scavenger enzymes and the levels of hydrosoluble and liposoluble antioxidants in tissue samples, plasma and red blood cells, and from the use of bronchoalveolar lavage.

Oxidative Damage in Trauma, Shock, and Sepsis (Experimental Studies)

Several studies have been undertaken in the fields of trauma, hemorrhagic shock, sepsis, ARDS, and multiple organ failure to evaluate oxidative damage and antioxidant defenses. In spite of the different experimental models used (especially septic models), and the different biochemical approaches to the problem, these studies all confirmed the presence of increased lipoperoxidative products and a reduction in antioxidants at both the plasma and tissue level.

Oxidative Damage in Trauma, Shock, and Sepsis (Clinical Studies)

Clinical investigations of heterogenous groups of critically ill patients and the by-products of lipoperoxidation have produced little evidence of lipoperoxidative damage. Increased lipid hydroperoxides have been observed in blood-draining septic foci [12] in the following groups of patients:

1. In patients with head injuries, thiobarbituric acid reactive substances (TBARS) in jugular venous blood were elevated [3].
2. In patients with sepsis and a range of different MOF scores, plasma MDA concentration was increased and correlated with decreased red blood cell deformability [17].
3. In patients with sepsis and ARDS, plasma MDA concentration was increased, and plasma vitamin E concentration was decreased (probably as a consequence of malnutrition), with an inverse correlation between these two measurements [27]; and almost the same findings were reported in a heterogenous group of patients under intensive care [21].
4. In patients with circulatory shock of different etiology, erythrocytes showed a strong increase in the concentration of peroxidation-derived aldehydes and the presence of highly toxic 4-hydroxynonenal [24]. Other studies have reported evidence of increased lipoperoxidative by-products in surgical trauma [11], cardiogenic shock [24], and critically ill patients [33].

In spite of these reports Girotti failed to find an increase in lipoperoxidative products in the blood stream in injured patients in the early post-traumatic period [8].

Studies that have been carried out on the antioxidant defenses in critically ill patients have been controversial and have not presented unequivocal data:

1. In ARDS, plasma and red cell glutathione decreased [15].
2. In patients with sepsis, serum Mn SOD and catalase activity was higher in patients who subsequently developed ARDS {15].
3. Patients with sepsis and ARDS had increased serum catalase activity (more than patients with sepsis but without ARDS and controls). Serum glutathione peroxidase activity was the same in all three groups [14].
4. Patients with sepsis and ARDS had decreased levels of glutathione in alveolar fluid [22].
5. Tissue levels of CoQ_{10} are reduced in patients with circulatory shock [5].
6. During the uncomplicated postoperative course, acute phase response was accompanied by a transient decrease in leukocyte vitamin C concentration and in the plasma concentration of vitamin E [16].

In a recent study [7, 30] we evaluated the OFR-induced cellular damage and level of endogenous liposoluble antioxidants in a group of critically ill patients with sepsis admitted to our intensive care unit (ICU). To this end the plasma levels of conjugated dienes (CD), which represent the first product of oxidative damage to cellular membrane lipids, were measured together with the plasma levels of α-tocopherol and coenzyme Q_{10} (CoQ_{10}).

α-Tocopherol is the biologically active form of vitamin E, a well-known membrane-bound antioxidant; CoQ_{10} is a lipophilic molecule which plays a major role in mitochondrial energy production (as a component of the mitochondrial respiratory chain) and also acts as a powerful antioxidant agent. In 16 critically ill patients with sepsis (mean sepsis score = 19 ± 7; mean APACHE II score = 22 ± 4), we found an increase above the normal range of conjugated dienes in 60% of the measurements and a significant reduction of α-tocopherol and CoQ_{10}, respectively, in 86% and 100% of the measurements. Using linear regression analysis, a direct relationship was found between the plasma level of CoQ_{10} and cholesterol ($p < 0.001$), reflecting the common hepatic biosynthetic pathway, which was probably depressed. A direct relationship between CD and plasma uric acid and between vitamin E and CoQ_{10} was also observed, showing the possible source of OFR from xanthine-oxidase and the synergistic action of the two liposoluble antioxidants studied.

Antioxidative Therapy

Based on previous reports in our own experience, we consider it likely that, in patients with sepsis and MOFS, enhancing the endogenous antioxidant activity and administering exogenous antioxidant agents could have a synergistic pharmacologic effect. We define as antioxidant "any substance that, when present at low concentrations compared with those of an oxidizable substrate, significantly delays or prevents oxidation of that substrate" [10]. "Oxidizable substrate " includes almost everything found in living cells: lipids, proteins, carbohydrates, and nucleic acids. The functions of antioxidants as blockers of radical processes can be summarized as: (1) prevention of radical production, (2) scavengers and oxygen reactive species, (3) eliminators of radicals. Table 1 lists the natural antioxidants and artificial drugs with antioxidative properties which are available for therapy.

Table 1: Natural antioxidants and artificial drugs with antioxidative properties

Natural antioxidants	Antioxidant drugs
Enzymatic • Superoxide dismutase (SOD) • Catalase (CAT) Nonenzymatic (vitamins and vitamin-like compounds) • Vitamin C (ascorbate) • Glutathione (GSH) • Vitamin E (α-tocopherol) • Coenzyme Q_{10} (CoQ_{10}) • b-Carotene Cofactors (nutritional oligoelements) • Selenium (Se) • Manganese (Mn) • Zinc (Zn) • Copper (Cu)	• Deferoxamine • Lazaroids, 21-aminosteroids (U74006F) • Mannitol • AllopurinolDimethylthiourea (DMTU) • a-Mercatopropionylglycine (α-MPG) • Propylgallate (PG) • Butylated hydroxytoluene derivatives • N-Acetyldehydroalanines (AD 20) • Vitamin C and vitamin E analogs • Ebselen (PZ51)

The overall clinical objectives are the control of tissue injury, the improvement of organ dysfunction, and eventually a positive outcome. However, effects, nonenzymatic scavenging-type antioxidants have a potential pro-oxidative effect; indeed scavenger function leads to the generation of secondary radicals, the radical form of antioxidant, which in themselves can produce biologic damage. As for the lipoperoxidative damage, there are several experimental studies which have shown a beneficial effect of antioxidative therapy in shock, trauma, sepsis, and MOF [4, 25, 26, 28, 32, 34]; Table 2 summarizes some of the agents used and their beneficial effects. But again, in the clinical setting, there have been few reports of critically ill patients where some positive pharmacological effect has been proved [35].

Table 2: Antioxidants used in experimental studies and their beneficial effects

Antioxidants	Effects
Superoxide dismutase (SOD)	Reduces LPD, reduces gastric erosions, increases survival
Catalase	Reduces LPD, reduces histologic and physiologic lung damage
Glutathione	Reduces LPD
Vitamin E	Reduces LPD, prevents DIC
Coenzyme Q_{10}	Improves metabolic derangements and survival

LPD, lipoperoxidative damage

With blunt trauma, α-tocopherol and ascorbic acid improve PMN locomotory dysfunction [18]; with ARDS, intravenous N-acetylcysteine increases plasma and red cell glutathione and improves cardiopulmonary physiology [2]; in a heterogenous group of ICU patients, administration of different antioxidant mixtures resulted in poorly defined protection against free radical production and improved outcome [21]. In the study by Muizelaar et al. [19] the administration of superoxidase dismutase was well tolerated and led to an improvement in outcome after severe head injury.

Finally, nutrition certainly plays a critical role in increasing antioxidant defenses and particularly with regard to endogenous antioxidants or are direct oxygen scavengers, being mainly natural agents with several other beneficial actions and no side effects. Nutrients with antioxidant activity are reported in Table 3.

The prospects for research in this field look very promising and we await more knowledge on the complex pathophysiology of OFR damage. Indeed experimental and clinical studies are testing newly synthesized drugs; many scientists are focusing their interest on a new class of steroids (21-aminosteroids or lazaroids), which have proved to be potent inhibitors of iron-dependent lipid peroxidation and to prevent radical damage to the central nervous system after an ischemic insult. More clinical trials are necessary to define their antioxidant properties and to demonstrate an improvement in outcome.

Table 3: Nutrients and their mechanisms of antioxidant activity. Nutrition plays a critical role in maintaining endogenous antioxidants defenses. A number of nutrients are components of the primary endogenous antioxidants or are direct oxygen scavengers.

Nutrient	Mechanism
Vitamin C	Direct cytosolic antioxidant
Vitamin E	Direct antioxidant, lipid protection
β-Carotene	Direct antioxidant, lipid protection
Zinc	Constituent of SOD in cytosol
Manganese	Constituent of SOD in mitochondria
Copper	Constituent of SOD and of ceruloplasmin
Iron	Constituent of catalase
Selenium	Constituent of glutathione peroxidase
Glutamine	Substrate for endogenous glutathione

Conclusions

Considering the current state of research in this field, it is very difficult to draw definite conclusions, but we would like to put forward some experimental and clinical studies in this area.
1. Antioxidants cannot distinguish radical that play a physiologic role from those that cause cellular damage.
2. Antioxidants may intrinsically have a pro-oxidant action.
3. Which biomolecule is the antioxidant supposed to protect? An inhibitor of lipid peroxidation may not be useful to protect proteins or DNA.
4. Is the compound in sufficient concentration and mainly in the right place?
5. Which is the mechanism of its action - scavenging OFR, preventing their formation, or repairing the damage?
6. Finally, we have to be very careful when using antioxidants to avoid the cellular damage being greater than beneficial effect.

In conclusion, however, we are quite confident that more research in this field and further knowledge will give a better chance of survival to patients with sepsis.

References

1. Bast A, Haenen GR, Doelman CJ (1991) Oxidants and antioxidants: state of the art. Am J Med 91: 2S-13S
2. Bernard GR (1991) N-Acetylcysteine in experimental and clinical acute lung injury. Am J Med 91: 54S-59S
3. Bochicchio M, Latronico N, Zani DG, Mariotti M, Morandini L, Acquarolo AM, Candiani A (1990) Free radical-induced lipoperoxidation and severe head injury. A clinical study. Intensive Care Med 16: 444-447
4. Castillo M, Toledo-Pereyra LH, Gutierrez R et al. (1991) Peritonitis after cecal perforation. An experimental model to study the therapeutic role of antibiotics associated with allopurinol and catalase. Am Surg 57: 313-316
5. Corbucci GG, Gasparetto A, Candiani A, Crimi G, Antonelli M, Bufi M, De Blasi RA, Cooper MB, Gohil K (1985) Shock-induced damage to mitochondrial function and some cellular antioxidant mechanisms in humans. Circ Shock 15: 15-26
6. Di Mascio P, Murphy ME, Sies H (1991) Antioxidant defense system: the role of carotenoids, tocopherols, and thiols. Am J Clin Nutr 53: 194S-200S
7. Gangeri G, Sganga G, Lippa S, Colacicco G, Landolfi E, Forte E, Carducci P, Gui D, Castagneto M (1994) Endogenous antioxidant deficiency in trauma and sepsis. Clin Intensive Care S5(2): 73
8. Girotti MJ, Khan N, McLellan BA (1991) Early measurement of systemic lipid peroxidation products in the plasma of major blunt trauma patients. J Trauma 31: 32-35
9. Goode HF, Webster NR (1993) Free radicals and antioxidants in sepsis. Crit Care Med 21: 1770-1776
10. Halliwell B (1991) Reactive oxygen species in living systems: source, biochemistry, and role in human disease. Am J Med 91: 14S-22S
11. Keen RR, Stella LA, Flanigan DP, Lands WEM (1990) Differences between mixed venous levels of plasma hydroperoxides following thoracic and abdominal operations. Free Radic Biol Med 9: 485-494
12. Keen RR, Stella LA, Flanigan DP, Lands WEM (1991) Differential detection of plasma hydroperoxides in sepsis. Crit Care Med 19: 1114-1119
13. Kretzschmar M (1994) Role of oxygen free radicals in the pathophysiology of sepsis. In: Reinhart K, Eyrich K, Sprung C (eds.) Sepsis. Springer, Berlin, Heidelberg, New York, pp. 122-135
14. Leff JA, Parsons PE, Day CE et al. (1992) Increased serum catalase activity in septic patients with the adult respiratory distress syndrome. Am Rev Respir Dis 146: 985-989
15. Leff JA, Parsons PE, Day CE et al. (1993) Serum antioxidants as predictors of adult respiratory distress syndrome in patients with sepsis. Lancet 341: 777-780
16. Louw JA, Werbeck A, Louw ME, Kotze TJ, Cooper R, Labadarios D (1992) Blood vitamin concentrations curing the acute-phase response. Crit Care Med 20: 934-941
17. Machiedo GW, Powell RJ, Rush BF, Swisloski NI, Dikdan G (1989) The incidence of decreased red blood cell deformability in sepsis and the association with oxygen free radical damage and multiple-system organ failure. Arch Surg 124: 1386-1389
18. Manderazo EG, Woronick CL, Hickingbotham N et al. (1991) A randomized trial of replacement antioxidant vitamin therapy for neutrophil locomotory dysfunction in blunt trauma. J Trauma 31: 1142-1150

19. Muizelaar JP, Marmarou A, Young HF et al. (1993) Improving the outcome of severe head injury with the oxygen radical scavenger polyethylene glycol-conjugated superoxide dismutase: a phase II trial. J Neurosurg 78: 375-382
20. Oxidants and antioxidants: pathophysiologic determinants and therapeutic agents (1991) Proceedings of a symposium. Am J Med 91: 1S-141S
21. Ortolani O, Biasiucci M, Trebbi A, Cianciulli M, Cuocolo R (1987) Antioxidant drugs and shock therapy. 1st Vienna Shock Forum, pp. 271-280
22. Pacht ER, Timerman AP, Lykens MG, Merola AJ (1991) Deficiency of alveolar fluid glutathione in patients with sepsis and the adult respiratory distress syndrome. Chest 100: 1397-1403
23. Peck MD, Alexander JW (1991) Survival in septic guinea pigs is influenced by vitamin E, but not by vitamin C in enteral diets. JPEN 15: 433-436
24. Poli G, Biasi F, Chiarpotto E, Dianzani MU, De Lula A, Esterbauer H (1989) Lipid peroxidation in human diseases: evidence of red oxidative stress after circulatory shock. Free Radical Biol Med 6: 167-170
25. Powell RJ, Machiedo GW, Rush BF Jr, Dikdan GS (1991) Effect of oxygen-free radical scavengers on survival in sepsis. Am Surg 57: 86-89
26. Powell RJ, Machiedo GW, Rush BF Jr, Dikdan GS (1991) Oxygen free radicals: effect on red cell deformability in sepsis. Crit Care Med 19: 732-735
27. Richard C, Lemonnier F, Thibault M, Couturier M, Auzepy P (1990) Vitamin E deficiency and lipoperoxidation during adult respiratory distress syndrome. Crit Care Med 18: 4-9
28. Robinson MK, Rounds JD, Hong RW, Jacobs DO, Wilmore DW (1990) Glutathione deficiency increases organ dysfunction after hemorrhagic shock. Surgery 112: 140-147
29. Schiller HJ, Reilly PM, Bulkley GB (1993) Tissue perfusion in critical illnesses. Antioxidant therapy. Crit Care Med 21: S92-102
30. Sganga G, Gangeri G, Castagneto M (1994) Lipoperoxidative damage and antioxidative therapy in sepsis and MODS. In: Hammerle A (ed.) MODS - multiple organ dysfunction syndrome. Springer, Vienna, New York (in press)
31. Sies H (1991) Oxidative stress: from basic research to clinical application. Am J Med 91: 31S-38S
32. Sharpe MD, Mustard RA, Finley RR, Rutledge FS, Sibbald WJ (1990) Failure of therapy with 2,3-dihydroxybenzoic acid to modify the course of sepsis-induced lung injury. J Appl Physiol 69: 1893-1902
33. Takeda K, Shimada Y, Amano M, Sakai T, Yoshiya I (1982) Lipid peroxidation in critically ill patients. Anesthesiology 57: A117
34. Tanaka H, Broaderick P, Shimazaki S et al. (1992) How long do we need to give antioxidant therapy during resuscitation when its administration is delayed for two hours? J Burn Care Rehabil 13: 567-572
35. Youn YK, LaLonde C, Demling R (1991) Use of antioxidant therapy in shock and trauma. Circ Shock 35: 245-249

Expression of c-*fos* protein in Brain and Endotoxin Levels in Plama Following Occlusion of Superior Mesenteric Artery of Rat

T. Hase, T. Tani, H. Oka, T. Yokota, M. Kodama, H. Kimura, I. Tooyama

Introduction

In humans, the occlusion of the superior mesenteric artery (SMA occlusion) is a progressive and lethal disease accompanied initially by hypovolemic shock and acute renal failure, subsequently by endotoxemia and sepsis, and finally by multiple organ failure [1]. In serious cases of sepsis, neurologic dysfunctions including mental status abnormalities such as alteration of consciousness, seizures and convulsion are often seen [2, 7, 14]. Therefore, there should be some functional alterations and damages in the central nervous system, about which little is yet known. The present study aimed to clarify how the central nervous system is affected under sepsis following SMA occlusion in a rat model. We employed c-*fos* expression as a marker of brain activation, and possible changes in c-*fos* expression in brain were assessed in relation to levels of plasma endotoxin, which is thought to be an important factor in the production of various symptoms in sepsis and multiple organ failure.

Materials and Methods

c-fos Immunohistochemistry

SMA Occlusion and Tissue Preparations. Thirty male Wistar rats weighing 200-250 g were used. Under general anesthesia with sodium pentobarbital (50 mg/kg), clipping of the SMA was performed in 24 rats. Six animals had laparotomy and abdominal closure as a sham operation. Two, 4, 6 and 8 h after surgery, six animals at each time were perfused under deep anesthesia through the left ventricle with 80 ml 0.01 M phosphate-buffered saline (pH 7.4) and then with 300 ml of a fixative containing 4% paraformaldehyde, 0.35% glutaraldehyde and 0.2% picric acid in 0.1 M phosphate buffer (pH 7.4). The coronal blocks of the brain were postfixed for 2 days in a fixative containing 4% paraformaldehyde and 0.2% picric acid in

0.1 M phosphate buffer at 4°C and placed for at least 48 h in 0.1 M phosphate buffer (pH 7.4) containing 15% sucrose and 0.1% sodium azide at 4°C.

c-*fos* immunostaining. The sections were stored in a free floating state for 4 days in 0.1 M phosphate-buffered saline (pH 7.4) containing 0.3% Triton X-100 (PBST). Serial sections at 200-μm intervals were processed for avidin-biotin-peroxidase complex immunohistochemistry. The sections were incubated for 4 days with c-*fos* antibody (Cambridge Research Biochemical, Cambridge, UK, diluted 1 : 10 000) at 4°C, for 2 h at room temperature with biotinylated anti-sheep IgG (Vector Lab, USA, diluted 1 : 1000). The peroxidase activity was demonstrated by incubating sections with 0.02% 3,3'-diaminobenzidine, 0.005% H_2O_2 and 0.3% nickel ammonium sulfate.

Measurement of the Plasma Endotoxin Level

In five male Wistar rats weighing 200-250 g SMA clipping was performe under general anesthesia. The blood was drawn before the operation and 2, 4, 6 and 8 h after SMA clipping. Plasma endotoxin was measured with the chromogenic limulus method after preparation by the new PCA method.

Results

Macroscopic Findings

The ischemic change was observed in the rat intestine 2 h after SMA clipping. After 8 h, the intestines were dilated with a change to dark color, and infiltration of dark-red-colored and badly-smelling ascites. In addition, the body hair of the rats was bristle-like and the peripheral skin of the extremities was cyanotic. In summary, intestinal necrosis, panperitonitis, a massive sympathetic response and peripheral circulatory disturbance were observed in rats 8 h after SMA clipping.

c-fos Immunohistochemistry

In sham-operated rats, weak c-*fos* immunoreactivity was detected in neuronal nuclei. Positive nuclei were scattered in the Pa, So and LHb (see legend to Fig. for key to abbreviations). c-*fos* immunoreactivity was significantly increased in neuronal nuclei of certain brain regions 2, 4, 6, and 8 h after SMA clipping. Immuno-reactivity was detected in the cell nuclear region. Positive neurons were recognized as being scattered in rat nuclei after 2 and 4 h, after 6 h they were abundant, and the most predominant after 8 h. The neuronal cell bodies containing immunoreactivity were localized in specific areas of the brain, including the SFO, Pa, So, PVA, Pe, LHb, VMH, Ce, LC, NTS, and X from rostrally to caudally (Fig. 1). The most predominant immunoreactivity was observed in the Pa, So and LHb. However, no immunoreactivity was detected in the neocortex, hippocampus and striatum.

Plasma Edotoxin Level

The mean endotoxin level in plasma 0, 2, 4, 6, and 8 h after treatment were 6.48 ± 5.57, 15.0 ± 4.37, 10.0 ± 4.18, 14.4 ± 3.52 and 58.4 ± 28.6 pg/ml respectively. Endotoxin levels were low and stable after 2, 4, and 6 h, but with a drastic change to an increase after 8 h (Figs. 2, 3).

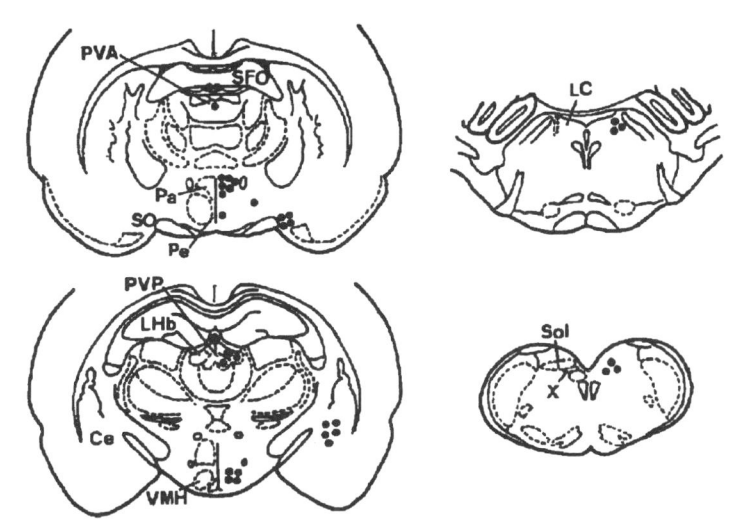

Fig. 1: The specific nuclei containing c-fos immunoreacivity in the study were widely distributed not only in the brain stem, hypothalamus and circumventricular organs but also in the limbic system. The expression sites are indicated by the solid circles.
Abbreviations: (1) Brainstem: LC, locus coeruleus; X, dorsal motor nucleus of vagus; NTS, nucleus tractus solitarius; (2) Hypothalamus: Pa, hypothalamic paraventricular nucleus; Pe, hypothalamic periventricular nucleus; So, hypothalamic supraoptic nucleus; VMH, hypothalamic ventromedial nucleus; (3) Limbic system: PVA, thalamic paraventricular anterior nucleus; PVP, thalamic paraventricular posterior nucleus; LHb, lateral habenular nucleus; Ce, central amygdaloid nucleus; (4) Circumventricular organ: SFO, subfornical organ

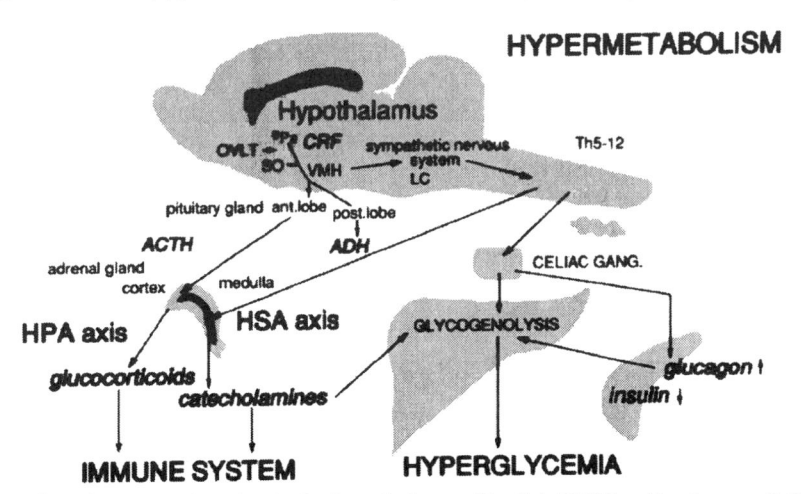

Fig. 2. The c-fos expression sites in the hypothalamus (Pa, So), VMH and brain stem (LC) are involved in the HPA (hypothalamus-pituitary gland-adrenal cortex) axis and HSA (hypothalamus-sympathetic nervous system-adrenal medulla) axis, respectively. Both axes affect not only the cardiovascular and respiratory system but also the immune and metabolic

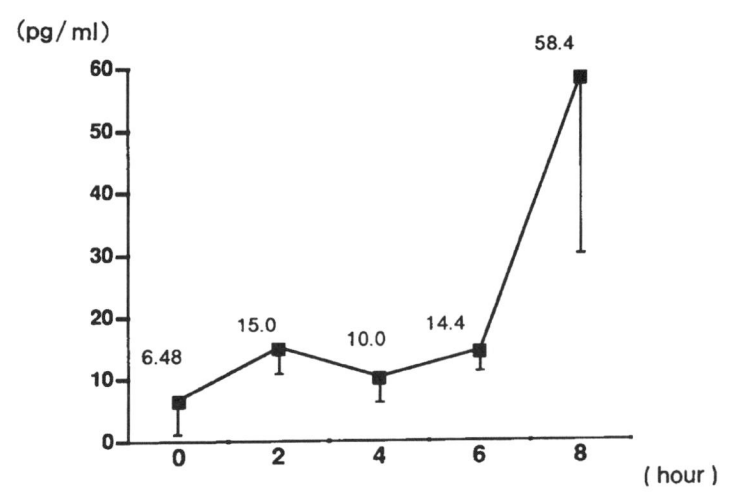

Fig. 3: The plasma endotoxin levels were low and stable after 2, 4, 6 h but drastically changed to an increase after 6 h

Discussion

The present study demonstrated that c-*fos* expression was increased in specific nuclei of rat brain in SMA occlusion of rat, and that the initial expression precedes the elevation of plasma endotoxin levels. This indicates that specific neuronal function of the central nervous system may be activated as a pathophysiologic response to occlusion of SMA in a phase earlier than the endotoxemia stage.

c-*fos* is one of the immediate early genes whose expression is low or undetectable in quiescent cells but is activated transiently by extracellular stimulation [10]. Therefore, these genes have been observed to be a marker of the activated neuron [5, 9]. According to previous reports, stimulation of c-*fos* expression in the central nervous system can be classified into three types: (1) growth factors [9], electrical stimulation [11] and seizures [8]; (2) brain injury such as ischemia [6, 13], brain destruction [3] and amputation in the neuronal tract [12]; and (3) nociceptive stress including peritoneal stimulation on injection of hyperosmolar NaCl, restriction and nociception of skin [20].

Firstly, brain ischemia during hypovolemia is the most likely cause of the increment of c-*fos* expression in the present experiment. However, Jørgensen reported that c-*fos* expression after brain ischemia was mainly detected in the hippocampus (CA, dentate gyrus), and Taniguchi also reported c-*fos* expression in the hippocampus of rat brain with hypoxia. In our experiment, there was no c-fos expression in the hippocampus. Therefore, c-*fos* expression in SMA occlusion cannot be explained by brain ischemia or hypoxia. Secondly, peritoneal stimulation and nociceptive stimulation is the next explanation for the present c-*fos* expression. Ceccatelli reported that c-fos expression was observed in Pa of the hypothalamus, locus caeruleus, ventral nucleus of the medulla oblongata and NTS associated with the nociceptive stimulation. Although these areas are included in our c-*fos* expression sites, c-*fos* was more widely expressed in our experiment than in their report. This difference in c-fos expression may account for the difference in the pathophysiologic response to peritoneal nociceptive activation and SMA occlusion.

To clarify how the central nervous system is involved in endotoxemia and sepsis, it is worthwhile to analyze the c-*fos* expression sites physioanatomically. The expression sites in this study are categorized as follows: (1) brain stem; NTS, X, LC; (2) hypo-thalamus: Pa, So, Pe, VMH; (3) circumventricular organs: SFO; and (4) limbic system: Ce, LHb and PV thalamic nucleus. The NTS and X are involved in autonomic regulation of the cardiovascular, respiratory and gastrointestinal function. Pa and So in the hypothalamus have a neuroendocrine function including the so called hypothalamo hypophyseal tract, which is involved in the HPA (Hypothalamus-pituitary gland-adrenal cortex) axis. For example, through this axis antidiuretic hormone, synthesized in Pa and So, is secreted into the general circulation.

The stimulation of VMH produces an excitation of the sympathetic nervous system through so called HSA (hypothalamus-sympathetic nervous system-adrenal medulla) axis. The excitation of the HSA axis causes hypersecretion of glucagon and suppression

of insulin secretion in the pancreas to induce gluconeogenesis, deamination and an increase in DNA synthesis in the liver (Fig. 3). Circum-ventricular organs have fenestrated capillaries and because of their permeability they are said to be outside the blood-brain barrier. The SFO has a receptor for angiotensin II which induces antidiuretic hormone (ADH) secretion from the hypothalamus to increases body water. These physiological theories regarding c-*fos* expression sites in the treated rat brain provide a good explanation for the pathophysiological response observed in patients with SMA occlusion.

Interestingly, c-*fos* immunoreactivity was observed in the limbic system in addition to that mentioned above in rats with SMA occlusion. This indicates that limbic function such as control of emotion and behavior is stimulated in endotoxemia and sepsis following SMA occlusion, and suggests that these changes are linked to the etiology of mental abnormalities in sepsis.

Acknowledgement

This study was supported by a grant-in-aid from the Ministry of Education, Sceince and Culture (0680703).

References

1. Amit P, Ronald NK, Robert JS (1992) *Pathophysiology of mesenteric ischemia. Surg Clin North Am* 72: 31-41
2. Bolton CF, Young GB (1989) *Neurological complications in critically ill patients*. In: Amminoff MJ (ed.) *Neurology and General Medicine*. Churchill, New York
2a. Ceccatelli S, Villar MJ, Goldstein M, Hökfelt T (1989) Expression of c-*fos* immunoreactivity in transmitter-characterized neurons after stress. Proc Natl Acad Sci USA 86: 9569-9573
3. Dragunow M, Robertson HA (1988) Localization and induction of c-*fos* protein like immunoreactive material in the nuclei of adult mammalian neuron. Brain Res 40: 252-260
4. Greenberg ME, Ziff EB, Greene LA (1986) Stimulation of neuronal acetylcholine receptors induces rapid gene transcription. Science 234: 80-83

5. James I, Morgan, Tom C (1989) Stimulus-transcription coupling in neurons: role of cellular immediate-early gene. TINS 12: 459-462
6. Jørgensen MB, Deckert J, Wright DC, Gehlert DR (1989) Delayed c-fos proto-oncogene expression in the rat hippocampus induced by transient global cerebral ischemia: an in situ hybridization study. Brain Res 484: 393-398
7. Marneros A, Rohde A (1987) Psychopathology of mental disorders due to infections in the antibiotics era. Psychopathology 20: 129
8. Morgan JI, Cohen DR, Hempstead JL, Hoiit V (1987) Mapping patterns of c-fos expression in the central nervous system after seizure. Science 237: 192-197
9. Morgan S, Michael E, Greenberg (1990) The regulation and function of c-fos and other immediate early genes in the nervous system. Neuron 4: 477-485
10. Müller R, Brave R, Bruck HJ, Cerren T (1984) Induction of c-fos gene protein by growth factors precedes activation of c-myc. Nature 312: 716-720
11. Sagar SM, Sharp FR, Curren T (1988) Expression of c-fos protein in brain: metabolic mapping at the cellular level. Science 240: 1328-1331
12. Sharp FR, Griffith J, Gonzalez MF (1989) Trigeminal nerve section induces fos-like immunoreactivity (FLI) in brainstem and decreases FLI in sensory cortex. Mol Brain Res 6: 217-220
13. Taniguchi T, Fukunaga R, Terai K, Tooyama I, Kimura H (1994) Biphasic expression of c-fos protein in rat hippocampus following transient in vivo hypoxia. Brain Res 640: 119-125
14. Thomas PB, Michael CS (1993) Neurologic complications of critical medical illness. Crit Care Med 21: 98-103

Acute Hypoxemia Due to Prostacyclin Release During Major Abdominal Surgery

A. Brinkmann, Ch.-F. Wolf, E. Kneitinger, D. Berger, M. Rockemann, M. Büchler, H. Wiedeck, W.Seeling, M.Georgieff

Abdominal mesenteric traction (MT) results in decreased mean arterial pressure, systemic vascular resistance, and increased cardiac output. This response is induced by a considerable release of prostacyclin (PGI_2) [4, 7, 15, 16], which has been reported to originate from the pulmonary vascular bed [8]. It has been hypothesized that MT is also accompanied by an increased pulmonary shunt (Qs/Qt) [14, 17], resulting in arterial hypoxemia [15]. In conscious healthy humans, the pulmonary shunt or venous admixture (Qva/Qt) amounts to only 1%-2% of cardiac output. During anesthesia, shunt increases to an average of about 10% [11]. Since pulmonary vasodilation by prostacyclin increases venous admixture, we investigated the gas exchange effects of traction on mesentery root during two different major abdominal operations (infrarenal aortic and pancreatic surgery) in a prospective placebo controlled study with intravenous ibuprofen.

Methods

After approval by the Human Investigation Review Board, we studied 52 patients in a prospective, randomized double-blinded protocol who were scheduled for infrarenal aortic reconstructive surgery ($n=26$) or pancreatic resection ($n=26$). Ibuprofen (400 mg i.v.) or a placebo equivalent was administered 15 min before skin incision. Anesthesia was maintained with N_2O 65%-70%, enflurane 0.4%-0.5% in O_2 combined with supplemental thoracic epidural anesthesia (0.25% bupivacaine, sensory blockade T4-L1). Pulmonary artery thermodilution and radial artery catheters were placed after induction of anesthesia. Mesenteric traction was applied in a uniform fashion. After incision of the peritoneum the surgeon performed an extensive exploration of the abdominal cavity terminated by eventration of the small bowel. Baseline values preceded the incision of the peritoneum. Further assessments followed 5, 15, 30, 45, 90 and 180 min after mesenteric traction. The plasma concentrations (PC) of 6-keto-$PGF_{1\alpha}$ (stable metabolite of PGI_2) were determined in arterial blood by radioimmunoassay. At all points in time we recorded hemodynamic parameters and measured arterial and mixed venous blood gases. Pulmonary vascular resistance (PVR), Horovitz oxygenation index (paO_2/FiO_2) [6] and Qs/Qt were calculated by standard formulae.

Statistical analyses were performed using ANOVA and Student's t-test after log(x) transformation. We analyzed the effects of ibuprofen, surgical procedure and repeated measurements. The preliminary data are given as means ± SEM or as notched box and whisker plots displaying the 10th, 25th, 50th, 75th and 90th percentiles. The notches represent 95% confidence bands about the median. An α-value of $p < 0.05$ was considered significant, applying the Bonferroni adjustment.

Results

Patients in the treatment and control groups were comparable with regard to sex, age, height, weight and American Society of Anesthesiologists (ASA) classification of physical status. Mean pulmonary arterial pressure (MPAP) only tended to decrease after mesenteric traction in the placebo group. However, PVR significantly decreased after MT in untreated patients ($n = 26$) (Table 1). There was a substantial rise in pulmonary shunt after mesenteric traction in the placebo group (Fig. 1), resulting in a notable drop in paO$_2$ (Fig. 2) and Horovitz oxygenation index (Table 1). These changes were accompanied by a marked increase of 6-keto-PGF$_{1\alpha}$ PC up to 180 min after mesenteric traction in arterial blood of untreated patients (Table 1). Although there was no difference in 6-keto-PGF$_{1\alpha}$ PC between the two surgical procedures, the increase in pulmonary shunt (Fig. 2) and the drop in paO$_2$ (Fig. 4) as well as changes in Horovitz oxygenation index were more prominent in patients undergoing infrarenal aortic surgery. Patients in the aorta group showed a higher ASA status (pancreas group ASA II, $n = 16$; ASA III, $n = 10$; aorta group ASA II, $n = 7$; ASA III, $n = 19$; $p < 0.01$ aorta versus pancreas). Moreover, patients in the aorta group were significantly older than patients who underwent pancreatic resection (pancreas group, 55 ± 2.3 years; aorta group, 65 ± 2.7 years; $p < 0.01$ pancreas versus aorta). Ibuprofen-pretreated patients ($n = 26$) demonstrated a stable pulmonary shunt and paO$_2$ while 6-keto-PGF$_{1\alpha}$ remained within the normal range.

Discussion

Our data clearly indicate that the response to MT not only consists of relevant hemodynamic alterations, but in addition includes a critical rise in pulmonary shunt, resulting in a significant decrease in paO$_2$. Abdominal MT is followed by a considerable release of prostacyclin, which lasts about 2 - 3 h. A splanchnic vascular source for PGI$_2$ release seems to be likely, but could not be proved from our current data. The prostacyclin generating capacity of the gastrointestinal tract is greater than that of other organs [9]. Ninety-five percent of prostaglandins escaping the local metabolism are inactivated by the lung in a single circulation, thus preventing entry into the general circulation. Prostacyclin represents an exception to this rule, as its pulmonary metabolism is very low and therefore could serve as a potent circulating hormone [3, 9]. Moreover, PGI$_2$ may be converted to the biologically active metabolite 6-keto-PGE$_1$. Prostacyclin and 6-keto-PGE$_1$ develop potent vasodilative effects in both the systemic and the pulmonary circulation [9] and inhibit hypoxic pulmonary vasoconstriction [10].

Table 1: 6-Keto-PGF$_{1\alpha}$ plasma concentrations, PVR, MPAP, and Horovitz oxygenation index before and 180 min after abdominal MT comparing the ibuprofen-treated with the control group.

	Before MT	5 min after MT	15 min after MT	30 min after MT	45 min after MT	90 min after MT	180 min after MT
6-Keto-PGF$_{1\alpha}$ arterial concentration (ng/l)							
Ibuprofen	59±0.7	103±12	86±11	106±24	89±15	71±6.3	71±5.3
Placebo	60±1.4	2274±284[a]	2059±263[a]	1313±177[a]	888±142[a]	490±103[a]	286±58[a]
PVR (dyn s/cm^5)							
Ibuprofen	121±9.7	119±12	119±13	123±10	123±7.8	146±15	137±10
Placebo	130±11	92±7.8[c]	86±7.6[b]	84±6.7[b]	105±11	106±10[d]	121±9.6
MPAP (mmHg)							
Ibuprofen	21.6±0.7	22.7±1.4	22.2±1.3	20.4±1.1	20.8±1.1	21.5±0.8	23.3±1.1
Placebo	23.9±0.9	20.9±0.8	20.9±0.7	20.8±0.9	20.2±0.9	19.9±0.7	22.4±0.9
Horovitz index							
Ibuprofen	369±16	348±17	354±17	370±16	383±15	402±17	387±17
Placebo	375±23	302±21[d]	293±22[c]	290±22[b]	312±22[c]	354±21	397±21

Mean ± SEM. Mesenteric traction (MT), mean pulmonary arterial pressure (MPAP), pulmonary vascular resistance (PVR), Horovitz oxygenation index (paO$_2$/FiO$_2$)
[a] $p < 0.0001$, [b] $P < 0.001$, [c] $p < 0.01$, [d] $p < 0.05$ placebo versus ibuprofen.

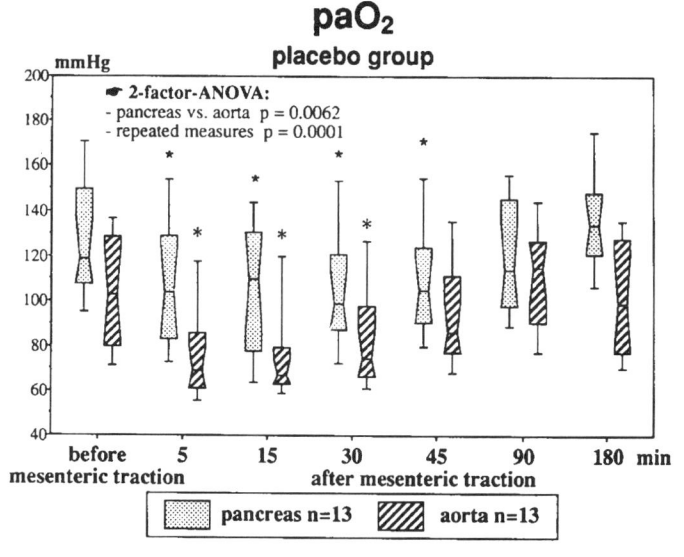

*Fig. 1: Pulmonary shunt before and 180 min after abdominal MT comparing the ibuprofen-treated (n=26) with the control group (n = 26). *$p<0.001$ placebo versus ibuprofen*

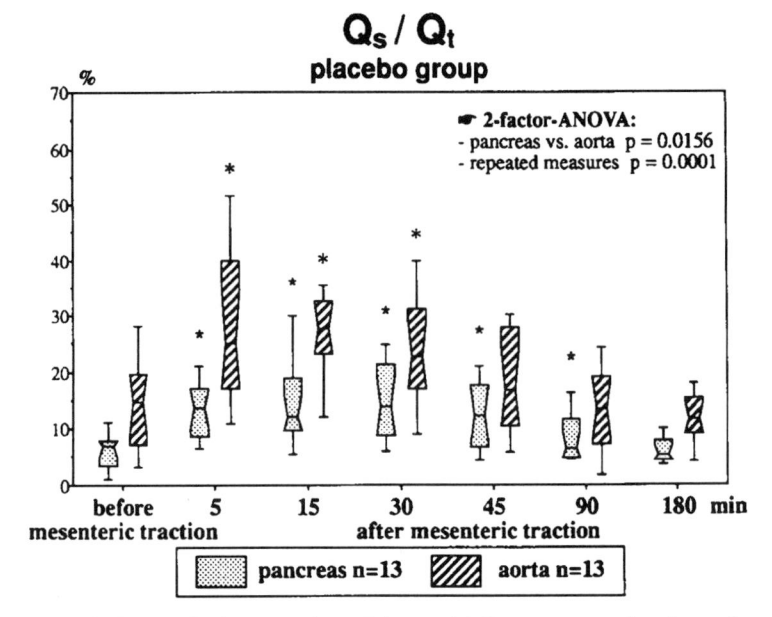

Fig. 2: PaO₂ before and 180 min after abdominal MT comparing the ibuprofen-treated (n=26) with the control group (n=26). *p<0.01 placebo vs. ibuprofen

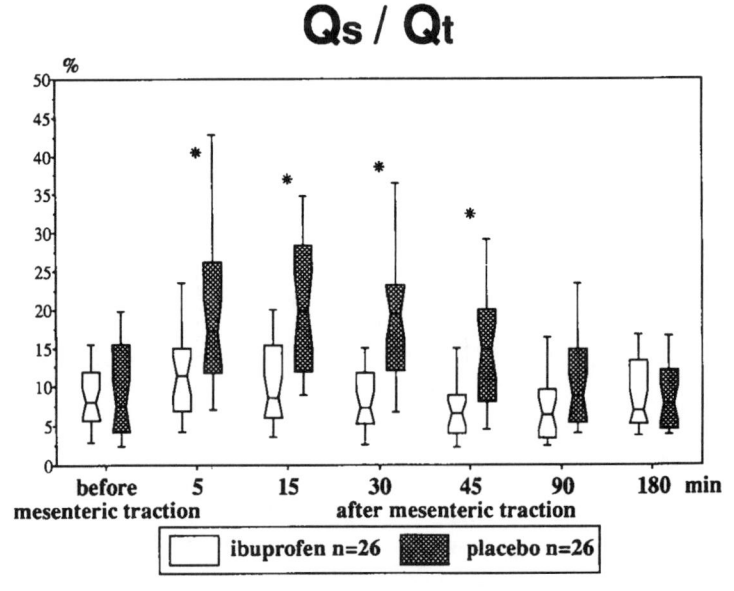

Fig. 4: PaO₂ before and 180 min after abdominal MT in untreated patients (n=26) comparing the aorta with the pancreas group. *p<0.005 vs. before MT (pancreas); *p<0.0006 vs. before MT (aorta)

paO₂

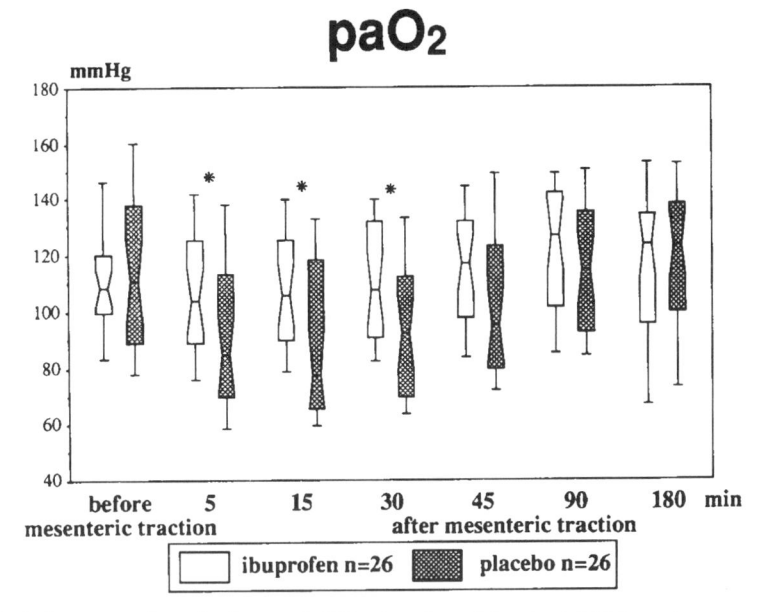

Fig. 3: Pulmonary shunt before and 180 min after abdominal MT in untreated patients (n=26) comparing the aorta with the pancreas group. *p<0.001 vs. before MT (pancreas); ⁺p<0.0002 vs. before MT (aorta)

As a consequence of prostacyclin release pulmonary venous admixture demonstrated a substantial increase after mesenteric traction in untreated patients. The pretraction values of about 5%-10% of cardiac output are very similar to those confirmed by the current literature [11]. The increased venous admixture during anesthesia is due partly to an increase in true pulmonary shunt (due to compression atelectasis), and partly to increased distribution of perfusion to areas of low ventilation/perfusion ratios [1]. The latter component increases with age [11]. The reduction in functional residual capacity (FRC) during anesthesia is explained by the reduction in lung volume, which appears to be mainly due to loss of end-expiratory tone in the diaphragm [2, 5]. During infrarenal aortic reconstructive surgery, Seeling et al. [14] documented an increase in pulmonary shunt from 9.5% to 20% after small bowel eventration. In our study the ibuprofen-pretreated patients showed a stable pulmonary shunt with no relevant changes in paO$_2$, thus indicating an action mediated by prostacyclin.

In acute respiratory distress syndrome (ARDS) patients infusion of prostacyclin leads to a diffuse dilation of the pulmonary vasculature. In those patients inert gas analysis demonstrated an increased right-to-left shunt alone or the combination of shunt and perfusion of lung regions with low ventilation/perfusion ratios [12, 13]. This mismatch between ventilation and perfusion potentially compromises partial pressure of arterial oxygen [13].

Patients who underwent infrarenal aortic surgery were particularly susceptible to clinically relevant changes in pulmonary shunt and paO$_2$ following a substantial release of prostacyclin into the systemic circulation. This could be due to frequently occurring concomitant pulmonary disorders in patients with vascular diseases. Compared with patients who underwent pancreatic resection, patients in the aorta group demonstrated more prominent alteration of pulmonary shunt, paO$_2$ and Horovitz oxygenation index during the whole observation period.

A 30%-40% inspired oxygen concentration is usually adequate to provide an acceptable paO_2 during uncomplicated anesthesia [11]. However, the deterioration of ventilation and perfusion mismatch of the lung induced by prostacyclin may lead to a clinically relevant impairment of pulmonary gas exchange during major abdominal surgery. Patients with major cardiopulmonary dysfunctions possibly benefit from perioperative cyclooxygenase inhibition.

References

1. Bindslev L, Hedenstierna G, Santesson J, Gottlieb I, Carvallhas A (1981) Ventilation-perfusion distribution during inhalation anaesthesia. Effects of spontaneous breathing, mechanical ventilation and positive end-expiratory pressure. Acta Anaesthesiol Scand 25: 360-371
2. Dueck R, Prutow RJ, Davies NJ, Clausen JL, Davidson TM (1988) The lung volume at which shunting occurs with inhalation anesthesia. Anesthesiology 69: 854-861
3. Dusting GJ, Moncada S, Vane JR (1978) Disappearance of prostacyclin (PGI_2) in the circulation of the dog. Br J Pharmacol 62: 414-415
4. Gottlieb A, Skrinska VA, O'Hara P, Boutros AR, Melia M, Beck GJ (1989) The role of prostacyclin in the mesenteric traction syndrome during anesthesia for abdominal aortic reconstructive surgery. Ann Surg 209: 363-367
5. Hedenstierna G (1988) Causes of gas exchange impairment during general anaesthesia. Eur J Anaesthesiol 5: 221-231
6. Horovitz JH, Carrico ChJ, Shires GT (1974) Pulmonary response to major injury. Arch Surg 108: 349-355
7. Hudson JC, Wurm WH, O'Donnel TF Jr, Kane FR, Mackey WC, Su YF, Watkins WD (1990) Ibuprofen pretreatment inhibits prostacyclin release during abdominal exploration in aortic surgery. Anesthesiology 72: 443-449
8. Huval WV, Lelcuk S, Allen PD, Mannick JA, Shepro D, Hechtman HB (1984) Determinants of cardiovascular stability during abdominal aortic aneurysmectomy (AAA). Ann Surg 199: 216-222
9. Kadowitz PJ, Lippton HL, McNamara DB, Wolin MS, Hyman AL (1984) Cardiovascular actions of prostaglandins. In: Antonaccio M (ed.) Cardiovascular pharmacology. 2nd ed. Raven, New York, pp. 453-474
10. Kubo K, Kobayashi T, Kusama S, Sakai A, Ueda G (1985) Effects of prostacyclin (PGI_2) on hypoxic pulmonary vasoconstriction in the conscious adult sheep. Jpn Circ J 49: 685-691
11. Nunn JF (1993) Applied respiratory physiology, 4th ed. Butterworth-Heinemann, London, pp. 407-414
12. Radermacher P, Santak B, Wüst HJ, Tarnow J, Falke KJ (1990) Prostacyclin for the treatment of pulmonary hypertension in the adult respiratory distress syndrome: Effects on pulmonary capillary pressure and ventilation-perfusion distributions. Anesthesiology 72: 238-244
13. Rossaint R, Falke KJ, Lopez F, Slama K, Pison U, Zapol WM (1993) Inhaled nitric oxide for the adult respiratory distress syndrome. N Engl J Med 328: 399-405
14. Seeling W, Ahnefeld FW, Grünert A, Heinrich H, Lotz P, Rosenberg G, Wieser E (1986a) Aortofemoraler Birfurkationspypass. Der Einfluss des Anaesthesieverfahrens (NLA, thorakale kontinuierliche Katheterperidualanaesthesie) auf Kreislauf, Atmung und Stoffwechsel, Homöostase und Sauerstofftransport. Anaesthesist 35: 80-92
15. Seeling W, Heinrich H, Oettinger W (1986b) The eventration syndrome: prostacyclin liberation and acute hypoxemia due to eventration of the small intestine. Anaesthesist 35: 738-743
16. Seltzer JL, Goldberg ME, Larijani GE, Ritter DE, Starsnic MA, Stahl GL, Lefer AM (1988) Prostacyclin mediation of vasodilation following mesenteric traction. Anesthesiology 68: 514-518
17. Seltzer JL, Ritter DE, Starsnic MA, Torjman M, Marr AT, Schieren H (1991) Pulmonary shunt (Qs/Qt) is increased by abdominal mesenteric traction. Anesthesiology 75 Suppl: A118

Prostacyclin Mediates Increased Oxygen Consumption and Arterial Hypoxemia, Preserves Cardiac Index, and Prevents Platelet Aggregation During Graded Bacteremia

J.G. Gallucci, J.V. Quinn, D. Woolley, G. Seidel, G.J. Slotman

Introduction

Prostacyclin (PGI_2) has been implicated as a causative agent of hemodynamic dysfunction and cardiopulmonary failure during septic shock [1-3]. Endothelial damage, increased capillary permeability, and acute hypoxemia in sepsis may also be mediated by PGI_2 [4-6]. Exogenously administered PGI_2 exacerbates chemically induced tissue edema [7]. These results suggest a proinflammatory role for PGI_2 in acute disease states.

An extensive further body of research, however, has identified potentially beneficial effects of PGI_2 during sepsis and inflammation [8-11] In experimental studies of acute respiratory failure and septic shock, therapeutically administered PGI_2 has uniformly decreased pulmonary vascular resistance [12, 13], has maintained cardiac output [8, 14], has increased oxygen transport [10], and has attenuated sepsis-induced tissue damage [11]. After oleic acid injection and during bacteremia and endotoxemia, PGI_2 infusion preserves normal platelet function [14-16].

The paradox between the apparently adverse physiologic properties of endogenous PGI_2 and its potential benefits when administered exogenously during septic shock and/or the systemic inflammatory response syndrome (SIRS) [17] indicates that the role of PGI_2 in critical illnesses remains ill-defined. The present study was undertaken in order to determine the hemodynamic events and derangements of end-organ function for which the involvement of PGI_2 is necessary during graded bacteremia. This was achieved by infusing a specific antibody which bound circulating PGI_2 in bacteremic animals.

Materials and Methods

Seventeen adult swine were anesthetized, and underwent tracheostomy and insertion of pulmonary artery, arterial, and peripheral venous catheters. Animals were ventilated on room air at rates sufficient to maintain PCO_2 in the range of 35 - 45 mmHg. After a 60 min control period, a 4-h experimental period began in which the animals were studied in three groups: anesthesia control (AC; $n = 6$) - infusion of saline vehicle only; septic control (SC; $n = 6$) - continuous intravenous infusion of *Aeromonas hydrophila* (1.0×10^9/ml) at rates that were increased incrementally from 0.2 ml/kg per hour to 4.0 ml/kg per hour over 3 h (graded bacteremia); prostacyclin antibody (PGA; $n = 5$) - graded bacteremia plus continuous infusion of a rabbit anti-PGI_2 antibody at 50 ml/h i.v. beginning after 2 h of graded bacteremia.

Mean systemic (MAP) and pulmonary artery (PAP) pressures, arterial blood gases, including PO_2, mmHg, arterial (SaO_2) and mixed venous (SvO_2) hemoglobin oxygen saturation (percentage) and cardiac output by the thermodilution method were measured at the end of the control period (baseline), and hourly during the 4-h experiment. At these same intervals, cardiac index (CI) (l/min), oxygen delivery (DO_2), and oxygen consumption (VO_2) (ml/min), and oxygen extraction ratio (ER) (percentage) were calculated.

At baseline and hourly intervals thereafter, platelet aggregometry (PLT) (% maximum aggregation) was measured using fresh platelets collected from experimental animals at the indicated intervals and a standard ADP aggregation stimulus. Plasma levels of prostaglandin 6-keto F1α (6-keto), the stable metabolite of PGI_2 (pg/ml) were measured at baseline and hourly intervals during the experimental period by ELISA, using commercially available reagents and standard laboratory techniques.

The anti-PGI_2 antibody used in this experiment was obtained from Dr.Lawrence Levin of Brandeis University. The antibody was engineered specifically to react with 5,6-dihydroprostaglandin I_2, which enables it to bind endogenously released PGI_2 [18]. Dose-response studies of the anti-PGI_2 antibody, in which it specifically antagonized the physiologic effects of exogenous PGI_2, verified physiologically the antibody's ability to bind PGI_2 [19]. The 50 ml/h rate of i.v. antibody infusion used in this study was chosen on the basis of preliminary experiments using adult swine, in which this infusion rate prevented systemic hypotension when exogenous PGI_2 was infused at a rate of 0.7 µg/kg per hour.

Statistical analysis was carried out by analysis of variance. The 95% confidence interval ($p<0.05$) was used to determine statistical significance.

Results

As seen in Table 1, compared with septic controls, anti-PGI_2 antibody treatment of septic animals resulted in decreased CI, VO_2, 6-keto levels, and decreased in vitro platelet aggregation responsiveness. Anti-PGI_2 antibody administration caused arterial PO_2 and SaO_2 to increase significantly. Intergroup differences in MAP, PAP, ER, and PO_2 were not statistically significant.

Discussion

The results of this study demonstrate that PGI_2 is necessary for the development of arterial hypoxemia, high oxygen consumption, and high CI during graded bacteremia. Prostacyclin also downregulates increased intravascular platelet aggregation in sepsis. The data indicate, however, that PGI_2 is not required for the development of systemic hypotension in septic shock.

The finding that endogenous prostacyclin exacerbates sepsis-induced acute respiratory failure is consistent with previous clinical studies in which arterial PO_2 correlated directly with increasing plasma PGI in critically ill patients without ARDS, but corresponded inversely to arterial PO_2 in established noncardiogenic pulmonary edema [5, 6]. Significantly increased arterial PO_2 and SaO_2 in septic animals receiving anti-PGI_2 antibody indicate that prostacyclin mediates alveolar-capillary membrane dysfunction in graded bacteremia. Whether this is a direct pro-inflammatory effect of PGI_2, or secondary to physiologic vasodilatation and increased delivery of pro-inflammatory reactants to the tissue bed, is not clear from the data.

Table 1: Cardiopulmonary function, platelet aggregation, and prostacyclin during graded bacteremia

Time		MAP	PAP	CI	PO_2	SaO_2
0 h	PGA	90±8	24±5	5.9±0.4	87.6±6	97±0.8
	SC	90±17	25±3	7.2±0.3	88±7	97±0.6
4 h	PGA	44±16*	43±7*	2.2±1.2**,*	62±8**,*	89±4**,*
	SC	51±15*	44±3*	2.7±0.5*	54±10*	83±7.0*
Time		VO_2	O_2ER	DO_2	PLT	6-Keto
0 h	PGA	187±32	0.40±0.20	838±132	100±0.0	100±4.5
	SC	202±22	0.23±0.03	871±122	100±0.0	136±28
4 h	PGA	165±29**	0.41±0.23	306±130*	21±9.0**,*	1237±670**,*
	SC	227±24	0.62±0.07*	368±51*	43±22*	8043±2710*

**$p < 0.05$ vs. (SC); *$p < 0.05$ vs. 0 h, ANOVA.

Decreased oxygen consumption during graded bacteremia with anti-PGI_2 antibody infusion suggests that high VO_2 in sepsis is also mediated by prostacyclin. The metabolic significance of this observation, however, is not welldefined, as anti-PGI_2 antibody did not change oxygen delivery or the oxygen extraction ratio in this model. These data may represent a physiologic dose-response study consistent with previous investigations in which exogenous prostacyclin reduced PO_2 and increased oxygen consumption.

Although infusion of anti-PGI_2 antibody in bacteremic animals significantly reduced CI, compared with septic control swine, the results suggest that prostacyclin is not the sole physiologic factor responsible for the characteristic hemodynamics of sepsis. Since CI fell significantly from baseline in both the septic control and septic anti-PGI_2 antibody groups of this study, it is probable that additional factors other than prostacyclin are involved. It may also be that the role of endogenous prostacyclin, and its dynamic equilibrium with thromboxane A_2 [5, 6, 9], during graded bacteremia, may be different than the therapeutic actions of exogenous prostacyclin in other experimental [9, 21] and clinical [11, 22] acute inflammatory states. Furthermore, the actions of PGI_2 in sepsis may differ from its role in other acute stress states, such as cardiopulmonary bypass [23, 24], where inflammation is not such an important component.

Under physiologic conditions, the degree to which circulating platelets aggregate it is determined largely by the flux of a dynamic equilibrium between prostacyclin and thromboxane A_2 [25-28]. During graded bacteremia, the balance is shifted toward an increased thromboxane A_2/prostacyclin ratio, resulting in increased in-vivo platelet aggregation, which is reflected subsequently in decreased platelet responsiveness upon in-vitro analysis. The involvement of prostacyclin in maintaining platelet homeostasis was unmasked by infusion of the PGI_2 antibody, which caused increased in vivo platelet aggregation.

Prostacyclin does not mediate systemic hypotension in this model of graded bacteremia, manifested in the absence of significant differences between treatment groups in mean arterial pressure. Considering that increased plasma PGI is associated with hypotension in patients with septic shock [1] and has been inversely cross-correlated with mean arterial pressure in this graded bacteremia model [9], it may be that vasoactive factors in addition to prostacyclin are also involved in the pathophysiology of bacteremic shock.

Exogenous prostacyclin is known to decrease hypoxic pulmonary vasoconstriction [29]. The acute pulmonary hypertension of graded bacteremia, however, was not affected by anti-PGI_2 antibody infusion, indicating that PGI_2 is not necessary for this phenomenon to occur.

Infusion of anti-PGI_2 antibody in a porcine model of graded bacteremia revealed that PGI_2 exacerbates arterial hypoxemia, prevents increased platelet aggregation, and preserves CI during systemic sepsis. Prostacyclin appears to mediate increased oxygen consumption in this model, but is not necessary for the development of systemic hypotension. In spite of its potent vasodilatory effects, endogenous PGI_2 does not attenuate increased pulmonary artery pressure induced by bacteremia.

Conclusions

. PGI_2 exacerbates arterial hypoxemia during graded bacteremia.
: PGI_2 prevents increased platelet aggregation.
. PGI_2 preserves cardiac index.
. Increased oxygen consumption in septic shock is mediated by PGI_2.
. In this model, PGI_2 is not necessary for decreased mean arterial pressure.
. Endogenous PGI_2 does not attenuate increases in pulmonary artery pressure during graded bacteremia.

References

1. Slotman GJ et al. (1986) Interactions of prostaglandins, activated complement, and granulocytes in clinical sepsis and hypotension. Surgery 99(6): 744-750
2. Petrak RA et al. (1989) Prostaglandins, cyclo-oxygenase inhibitors, and thromboxane synthetase inhibitors in the pathogenesis of multiple system organ failure. Crit Care Clin 5(2): 303-314
3. Bernard GR et al. (1991) Prostacyclin and thromboxane A_2 formation is increased in human sepsis syndrome. Am Rev Respir Dis 1095-1101
4. Steinberg SM et al. (1983) Prostacyclin in experimental septic acute respiratory failure. J Surg Res 34: 298-302
5. Slotman GJ et al. (1985) Thromboxane and prostacyclin in clinical acute respiratory failure. J Surg Res 39: 1-7
6. Slotman GJ et al. (1986) Prostaglandin and complement interaction in clinical acute respiratory failure. Arch Surg 121: 271-274
7. Ford-Hutchinson AW et al. (1979) PGI_2: a potential mediator of inflammation. Prostaglandins 16(2): 253-258
8. Hanly PJ et al. (1986) Role of prostacyclin and thromboxane in the circulatory changes of acute bacteremic Pseudomonas pneumonia in dogs. 1-3 Am Rev Respir Dis 137: 700-706

9. Slotman GJ et al. (1985) Thromboxane, prostacyclin and the hemodynamic effects of graded bacteremic shock. Circulatory Shock 16: 395-404
10. Pittet JF et al. (1990) Prostacyclin but not phentolamine increases oxygen consumption and skin microvascular blood flow in patients with sepsis and respiratory failure. Chest 98: 1467-1472
11. Bihari DJ et al. (1988) The therapeutic value of vasodilator prostaglandins in multiple organ failure associated with sepsis. Intensive Care Med 15: 2-7
12. Yun-Chao SU et al. (1989) Relation of TXA_2 and PGI_2 to the difference in hypoxic pulmonary vasoconstriction between different strains of cats. J Tongi Med Univ 9(3): 148-152
13. Archer SL et al. (1986) ZK 36-374, A stable analog of prostacyclin prevents acute hypoxic pulmonary hypertension in the dog. J Am Coll Cardiol 8: 1189-1194
14. Slotman GJ et al. (1979) Hemodynamic effect of prostacyclin (PGI_2) in acute hypoxic respiratory failure. Surg Forum 30: 177-179
15. Svartholm E et al. (1989) Thromboxane A2-receptor blockade and prostacyclin in porcine Escherichia coli shock. Arch Surg 124: 669-672
16. Ditter H et al. (1988) Beneficial effects of prostacyclin in a rabbit endotoxin shock model. Thromb Res 51: 403-415
17. Bone RC et al. (1992) Definitions of sepsis and organ failure and guidelines for the use of innovative therapies in sepsis. Chest 101: 1644-1655
18. Pace-Asciak CR et al. (1980) Antibodies to 5,6-dihydroprostaglandin I_2 trap endogenously produced prostaglandin I_2 in the rat circulation. Biochim Biophys Acta 620: 186-192
19. Pace-Asciak CR et al. (1980) PGI_2-specific antibodies administered in vivo suggests against a role for endogenous PGI_2 as a circulating vasodepressor hormone in the normotensive and spontaneously hypertensive rat. Prostaglandins 20(6): 1053-1060
20. DeBacker D et al. (1993) Relationship between oxygen uptake and oxygen delivery in septic patients: effects of prostacyclin versus dobutamine. Crit Care Med 21(1): 1658-1664
21. Steinberg SM et al. (1983) Prostacyclin in experimental septic acute respiratory failure. J Surg Res 34: 298-302
22. Richardson A et al. (1984) Use of prostacyclin and ultrafiltration in adult respiratory distress syndrome. Intensive Care Med 10: 107-109
23. Chelly J et al. (1982) Hemodynamic and metabolic effects of prostacylcin after coronary surgery. Circulation 66: 45-49
24. Yhikorkala O et al. (1981) Increased prostacyclin and thromboxane production in man during cardiopulmonary bypass. J Thorac Cardiovasc Surg 82: 245-247
25. Oettinger W et al. (1987) Profiles of endogenous-prostaglandin $F_2\alpha$, thromboxane A_2 and prostacyclin with regard to cardiovascular and organ functions in early septic shock in man. Eur Surg Res 19: 65-77
26. Myers SI et al. (1993) Endotoxic shock has differnetial effects on renal and splanchnic eicosanoid synthesis. Prostaglandins Leukot Essent Fatty Acids 49: 509-513
27. Schirmer WJ et al. (1987) Effects of ibuprofen, indomethacin, and imidazole on survival in sepsis. Curr Surg 102-105
28. Moncada S et al. (1979) Pharmacology and endogenous roles of prostaglandin endoperoxides, thromboxane A_2 and prostacyclin. Pharmacol Rev 30: 293
29. Welte M et al. (1993) PGI_2 aerosol versus nitric oxide for selective pulmonary vasodilation in hypoxic pulmonary vasoconstriction. Europeean Surg Res 25: 329-340

Significance of Sinusoidal Lining Cells and of Humoral Factors on Hepatocytic Function Following Sepsis and Major Surgery

K. Hirata, T. Ohmura, H. Yamaguchi, T. Matsuno, K. Yamashiro, T. Katsuramaki, M. Mukaiya, X.A. Ming, R. Denno

Introduction

Chronic sepsis due to severe infection during the perigastrointestinal operation period in humans induces profound suppression of cell function and cell kinetics. In patients with severe sepsis, renal and/or respiratory dysfunction(s) with a hyperdynamic state have been observed, which have rarely been followed by irreversible hepatic failure. Though the stereotyped response of the liver to hepatic failure has been well reported [1] (Fig. 1)., little is known about the mechanisms of cholestasis which are characteristic of hepatic failure. Cholestatic liver disease is one form of liver injury that carries the threat of cirrhosis or follows extrahepatic bile duct obstruction and/or intrahepatic metabolic abnormalities [2]. The pathogenesis of the cholestasis which develops during sepsis is based on the infectious toxemia, i.e., endotoxemia, bacteremia, etc. Although our knowledge of the sinusoidal lining cell response and hepatic parenchymal cell degeneration during sepsis continues to grow, little is known about the effect of sinusoidal lining cell response to cholestasis. To investigate this relationship, we designed in vivo and in vitro systems to examine hepatotoxicity as a result of the reaction between endotoxin and individual sinusoidal lining cells.

Results and Discussion

Biopsy Findings of Hepatic Changes in Patients with Sepsis and Cholestasis

Microscopic examinations were performed in patients with clinically defined sepsis. These patients underwent hepatectomy or pancreatoduodenectomy and suffered from cholestasis induced by the postoperative infection. Though significant hepatic regeneration must generally occur after hepatectomy (Fig. 2), poor regeneration in the patients with cirrhosis and/or sepsis was observed (Fig. 3). The sinusoidal dilatation and the increase in infiltrating cells in the sinusoid are well-known and common histological findings in such patients with cholestasis (Fig. 4). Ultrastructural observations sometimes indicate intrasinusoidal cell aggregations, which consist of Kupffer cells, polymorphonuclear cells, platelets, esosinophils, etc. with a fibrin-like appearance (Fig. 5); and significant degeneration of parenchymal hepatocytes has been found to occur with such sinusoidal changes. The dilatation of sieves and pores of the endothelial cells and their exfoliation from the sinusoidal wall has been observed. Such insufficient circulation might induce the dilatation of the space of Disse.

Kinetics of Kupffer Cells

The responsiveness of Kupffer cells to external stimulation (i.e., operation and/or infection) has been reported as being the result or the cause of sequential biochemical reactions [3, 4]. The first step is the interaction between hepatic parenchymal cells and Kupffer cells with the response of specific and nonspecific receptor(s) or binding site(s) to external stimulus [5]. That one of the functions of differentiated may be suppressed by the incubation medium between Kupffer cells and a lipopolysaccharide has been suggested by in vitro experiments (Fig. 6). This is followed by many regulatory steps of signaling in stimulated Kupffer cells, which are repeated until the final stage of Kupffer cell function is reached, during which the regulation of cell-cell interactions by signal transmission or autostimulation occurs in vivo with the release of several signal molecules, i.e., interleukins (1, 2-6), interferons (α, β), tumor necrosis factor-α, transforming growth factor-β, prostaglandins (D, E, F), thromboxane A_2, prostacyclin, leukotriene B, platelet-activating factor, inorganics, etc. [6-9] (Fig. 7). The regulation of Kupffer cells on sinusoidal lining cells is schematically outlined in Fig. 7. One of morphological results observed in the sequence of interactions with Kupffer cells and other cells is the aggregations of intrasinusoidal cells [10]. Such reactions are thought to be started by the release of signal molecules. Under the stimulation of Kupffer cells by lipopolysaccharide in vitro, platelet aggregations around a Kupffer cell have been observed in culture with serum-containing medium. The quantitation of platelet-activating factor released from various intrasinusoidal cells by the stimulation of lipopolysaccharide has been studied in vitro (Fig. 8) and IL-6 secretion has also been studied.

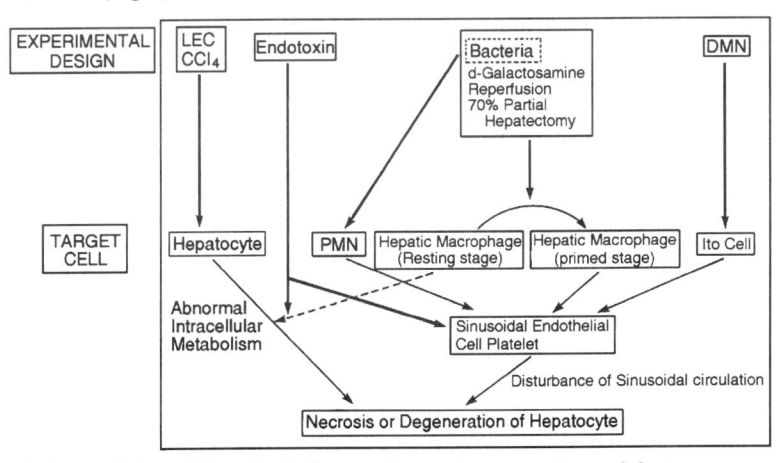

Fig. 1: Schema of the cell kinetics in liver under various experimental designs.

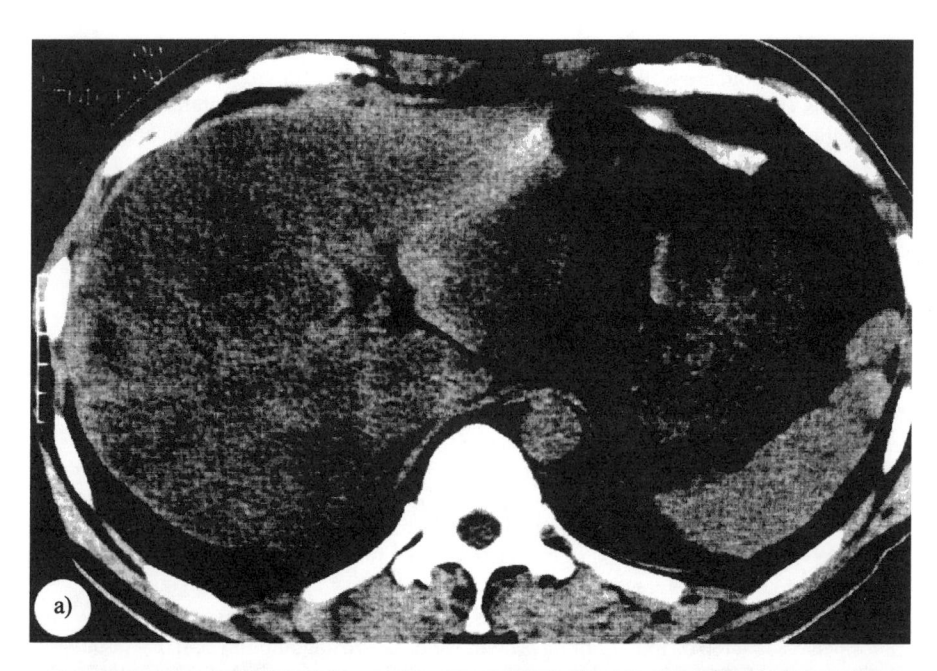

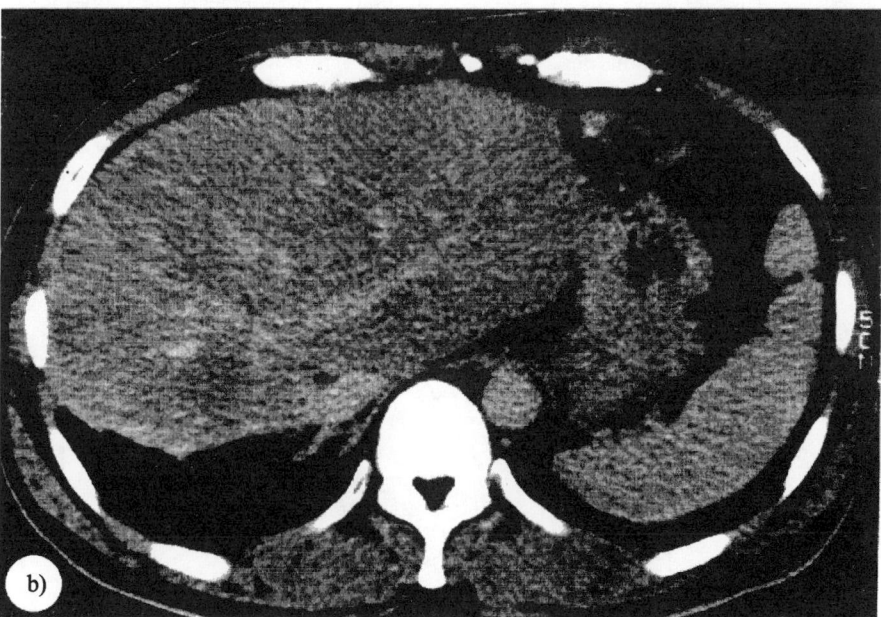

Fig. 2 a, b: Right lobectomy of the liver for biliary carcinoma of the hepatic hilar region. a) Preoperative liver; b) postoperative liver. Regeneration in the postoperative course is easily observed

Fig. 3 a, b: Right lobectomy of the liver for biliary carcinoma of the hepatic hilar region. The postoperative complication of a peritoneal abscess is observed, which was insufficiently controlled by drainage tubes. Poor regeneration is observed. a) Preoperative liver. b) Postoperative liver

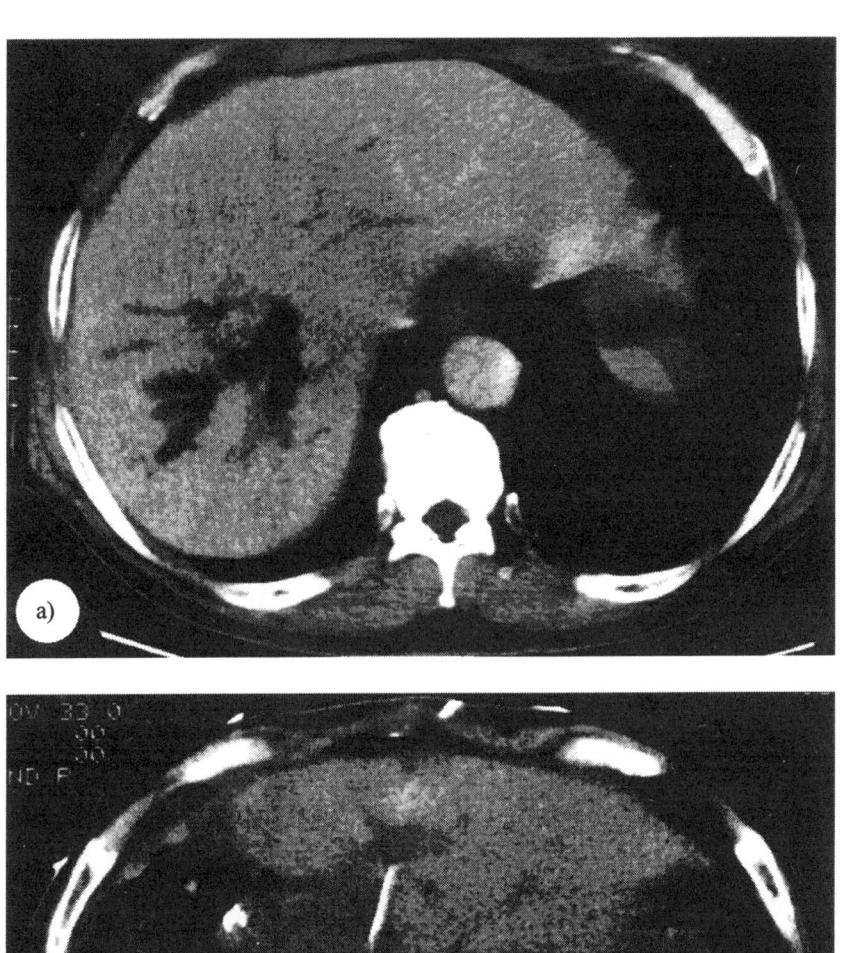

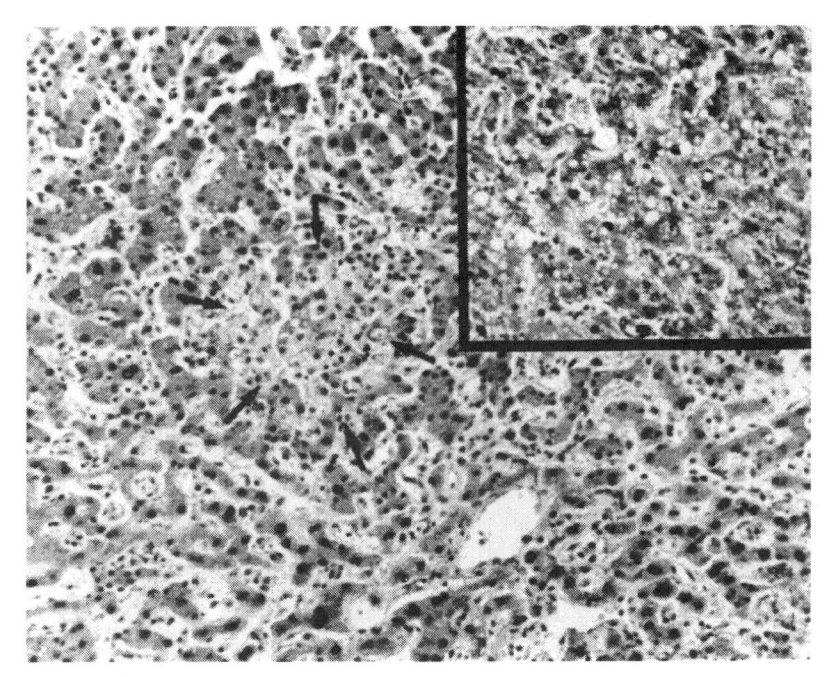

Fig. 4: Microscopic view of the liver in severe sepsis. Significant dilatation of sinusoids and spotty degeneration of hepatocytes is observed. The upper right corner indicates massive necrosis of the hepatocytes

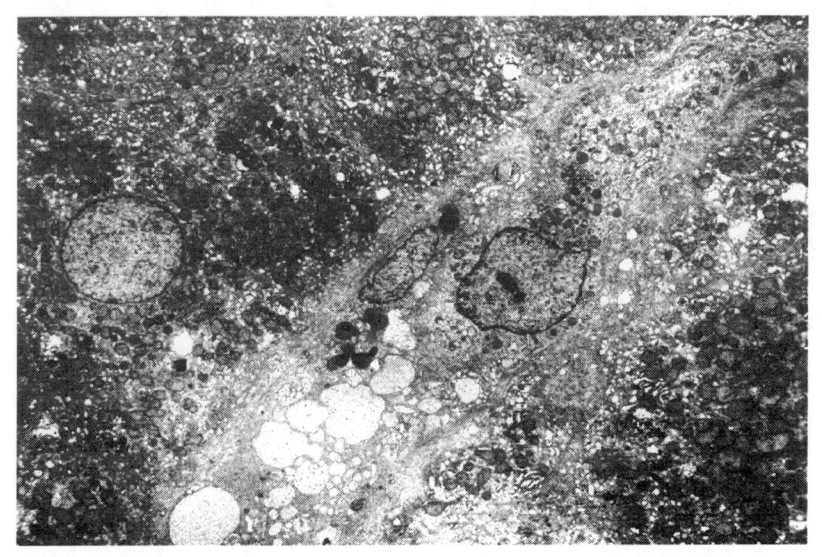

Fig. 5: Electron microscopic observation of sinusoids. Massive aggregations of sinusoidal lining cells and anoxic changes in hepatocytes are seen

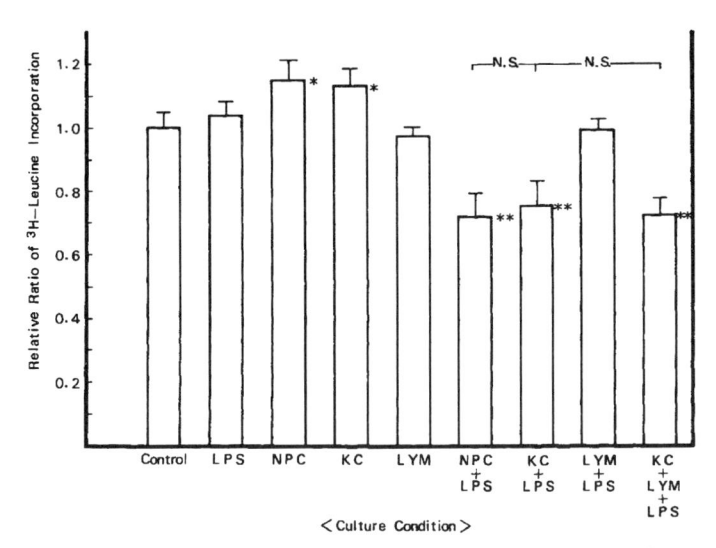

*Fig. 6: Incorporation of tritiated leucine in hepatocytes under various culture conditions. LPS, lipopolysaccharide; NPC, nonparenchymal cell; KC, Kupffer cell; Lym, lymphocyte. Co-culture time is 24 h and the last 4-h period was utilized for the incorporation of tritiated leucine in hepatocytes. *$p<0.05$; **$p<0.01$*

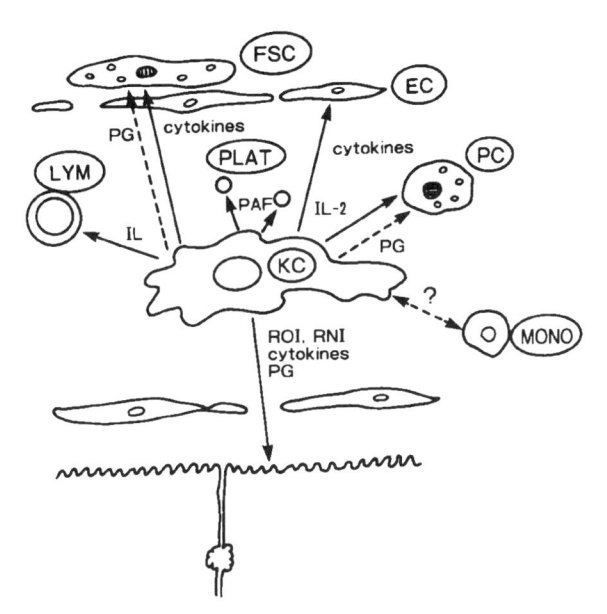

Fig. 7: Schema of the Kupffer cell kinetics for sinusoidal lining cells including cytokines, superoxides, etc. FSC, fat-storing cell; EC, endothelial cell; Lym, lymphocyte; PLAT, platelet; PC, pit cell; KC, Kupffer cell; MONO, monocyte; PG, prostaglandins; IL, interleukin; ROS, reactive oxygen species; RNS, reactive nitrogen species

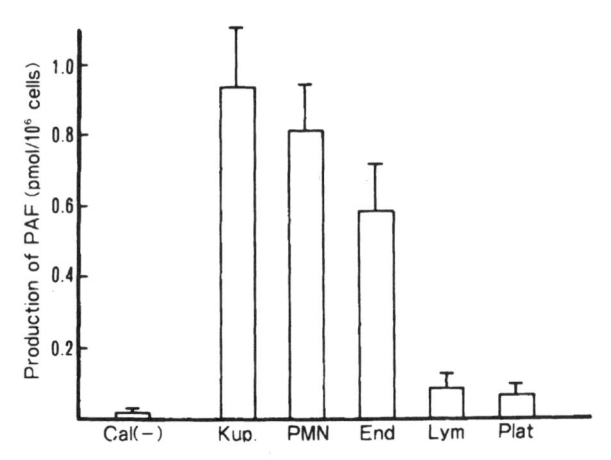

Fig. 8: Production of platelet aggregation factor (PAF) in the isolated mesenchymal cells stimulated by a lipopolysaccharide

Kupffer cells produced the highest cell count in four types of cells, and dexamethasone significantly suppressed the production of IL-6 by LPS-stimulated Kupffer cells. The control mechanism between various cell-cell interactions and various signal molecules, i.e., the change in mRNA in these molecules, etc., requires clarification in the near future.

Kinetics of Sinusoidal Endothelial Cells

Hepatic microcirculation is best understood in terms of the lobule, the basic anatomical unit of the liver (Fig. 9). The blood in the lobule starts at its periphery via the hepatic artery and the portal vein. Blood enters the sinusoids, the specialized capillaries of the liver, and flows into the central vein at the lobule's center. During the removal or the addition of substances through the sinusoids, oxygen consumption and several types of metabolic products are created. This unique structure and function of the sinusoids depends mainly on sinusoidal endothelial cells. In contrast to other capillary endothelial cells, the sinusoidal endothelial cells have no basement membrane, no fibroblastic cell and no muscle cell and possess pores approximately 0.1 μm in diameter (Fig. 10), which are arranged in clusters of sieve plates. Through these fenestrations, the endothelial cells influence the filtration of particles from the blood to parenchymal cells and vice versa. Recent investigations have suggested that the size of sieve plates and/or pores are influenced by the cytokines [11] (Fig. 11) or the contact of intrasinusoidal macrophages with the endothelial cells. Under such conditions, the selective exchanges of nutritional substances between the blood in the sinusoid and the space of Disse cannot be performed selectively and, paralleling this dysfunction, the intrasinusoidal cell aggregations have been suspected to be due to the functional and morphological changes at the endothelial cell surface. Therefore, the sinusoidal endothelial cells have the important role of facilitating the exchange and transport from/into the bloodstream and also the maintenance of elasticity of sinusoidal wall and blood viscosity (Fig. 12). However, a novel monoclonal antibody (SE-1) which specifically reacts with rat hepatic sinusoidal endothelial cells has been reported by Ohmura, one of coauthors of this article [12].

Immunohistochemical staining of the liver tissues clearly demonstrates that immunoreactivity for SE-1 was detected only in endothelial cells and not in other cells of the major organs, i.e., brain, lung, liver, spleen, small intestine, adrenal gland, bone marrow and aorta. The reaction products showed a significant presence on the cell surface of sinusoidal endothelium (Fig. 13). In the liver of septic or acute hepatotoxic models in rat, the regular arrangement of SE-1 staining showed significant changes. Moreover, the morphological changes were electron microscopically observed to occur under severe conditions. The functions of the antigen recognized by SE-1 are still not known but clarification of SE-1 function(s) will aid the recognition of pathophysiological conditions of the liver.

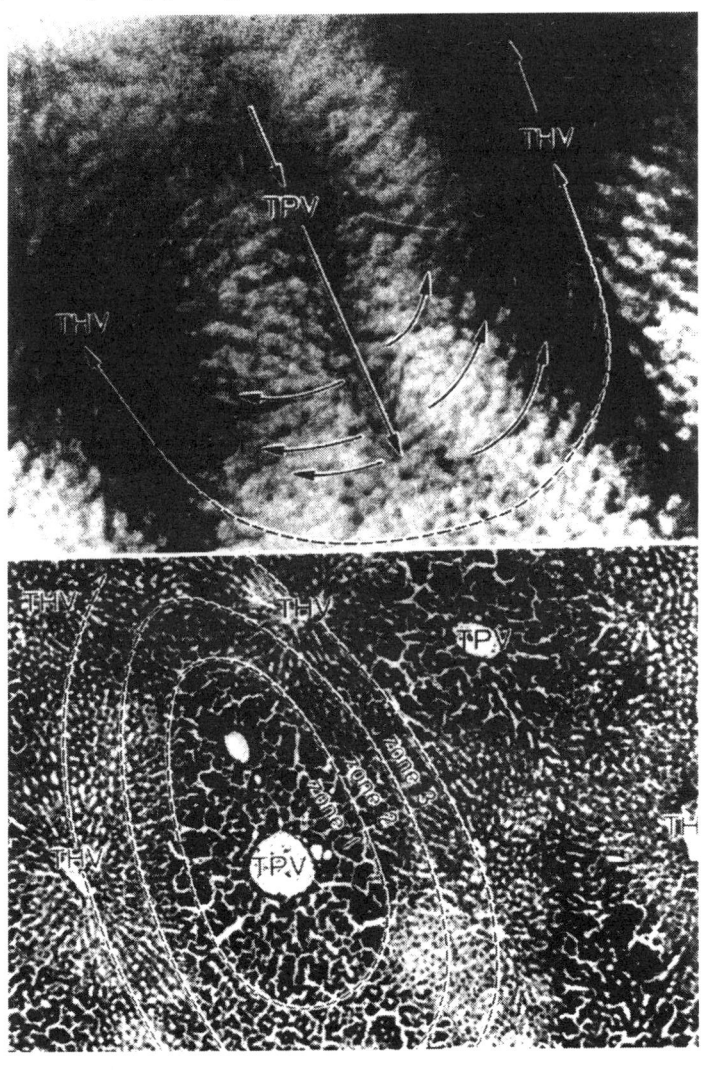

Fig. 9: Hepatic microcirculation in the lobulus. THV, total hepatic vein; TPV, total portal vein. A lobule was divided into three according to distance from the central vein

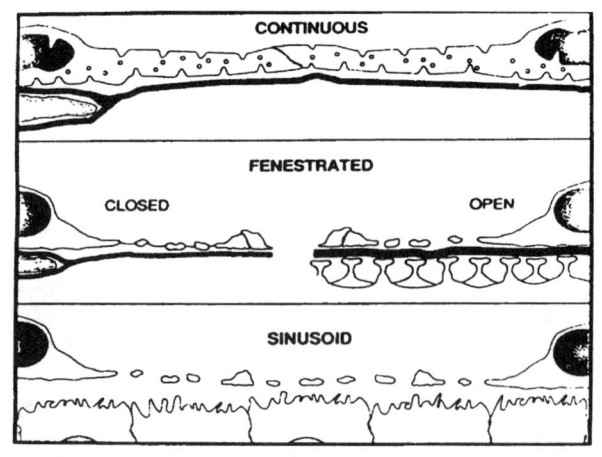

Fig. 10: Diagram of capillary types. The lowest is the sinusoid of the liver

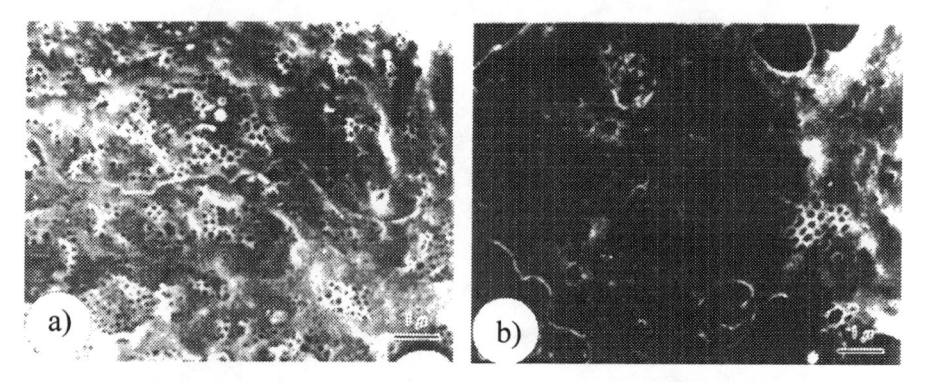

Fig. 11 a, b: Scanning electron microscopic view of sinusoidal endothelial cells. These were stimulated by IL-1 (a) and TNF-a (b). Significant change in the endothelial cells was observed stimulated by TNF-a

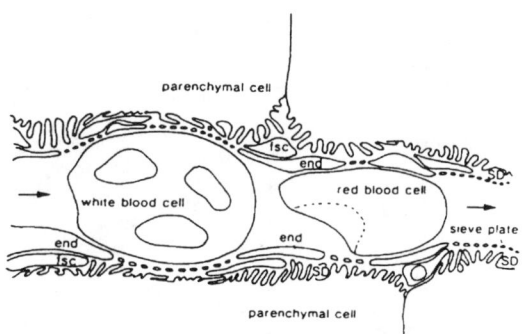

Fig. 12: Blood stream flow and the sinusoidal structure. Note the elasticity of the sinusoidal endothelial cells and of the hepatic microvilli. ISC, interstitial cell; end, endothelial cell; fsc, fat-storing cell; SD, space of Disse

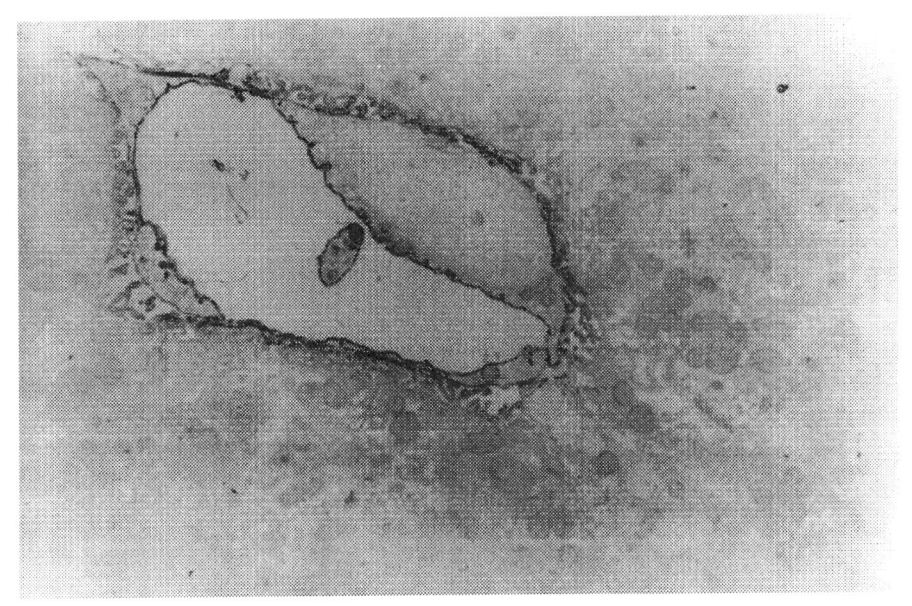

Fig. 13: Strongly positive staining of the endothelial cell surface by a new monoclonal antibody which has been named SEC-1

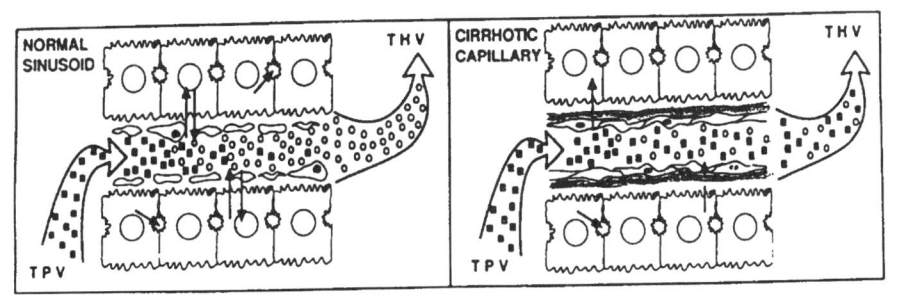

Fig. 14: Diagram of the proposed effect of capillarization of hepatic function showing abnormal accumulation of basal matrix under the sinusoidal endothelium. THV, total hepatic vein; TPV, total portal vein

In Japan, most patients who have undergone hepatectomy for hepatocellular carcinoma show cirrhotic changes of the liver, which is considered a high-risk condition for operation. Sinusoidal capillarization in the cirrhotic liver has recently become well known [13] (Fig. 14). This phenomenon is detected from the appearance of the basal lamina just under the sinusoidal endothelial cells in the space of Disse [4]. This abnormal layer interferes with the transport of substances and the oxygenation of the hepatic parenchymal cells, etc. Though the fenestrae in the sinusoidal endothelial cell are characteristic, the regulation of the formation of the fenestrae is still unknown. Damage to the structure of the fenestrae during acute episodes has been observed and the mechanisms of this are currently being studied. Future research on the effect of external stimulation of the sinusoidal endothelial cells in cirrhotic liver is required.

Kinetics of Pit Cells

The pit cell has been recognized as the large granular cell in the sinusoid, which is a resident cell in the blood stream which originates from the blood marrow [14] (Fig. 15). The pit cell, which is isolated by the perfusion method, has been used in an analysis of the characteristics of the surface marker concerning the immune response. Characteristics such as natural killer activity, expression of Ia antigens and antigen-specific T-dependent immunity have suggested that this cell plays an important role in the locoregional immune system [15]. The number of receptors of anticancerous activity and anti-foreign substances activity are certainly increasing. Our interpretation is that pit cells recognize exogenous antigens in association with class II histocompatibility antigens (Ia antigens) on the surface of an antigen-presenting cell (APC) or that pit cells have the role of an APC [16]. In mouse, the ability of a population of macrophages to present antigen correlates with the proportion of macrophages that express Ia. Pit cells, when activated, might secrete lymphokines that recruit Ia-positive macrophages from the bone marrow. Thus, pit cells can recruit additional functional APCs to amplify the immune response. Our preliminary experimental data have suggested that rat mononuclear phagocytic cells may undergo a similar reaction. The greater the increase in I-a positive cells among the isolated pit cells, the more severe the infection (Fig. 16). The same result was obtained in rats indicated by the appearance of $\gamma\delta T$ cells (Fig. 17). Such data indicate an inhibitory pathway which is involved in the regulation of macrophage Ia antigen expression, and may explain, in part, the reported immunosuppressive effects of LPS.

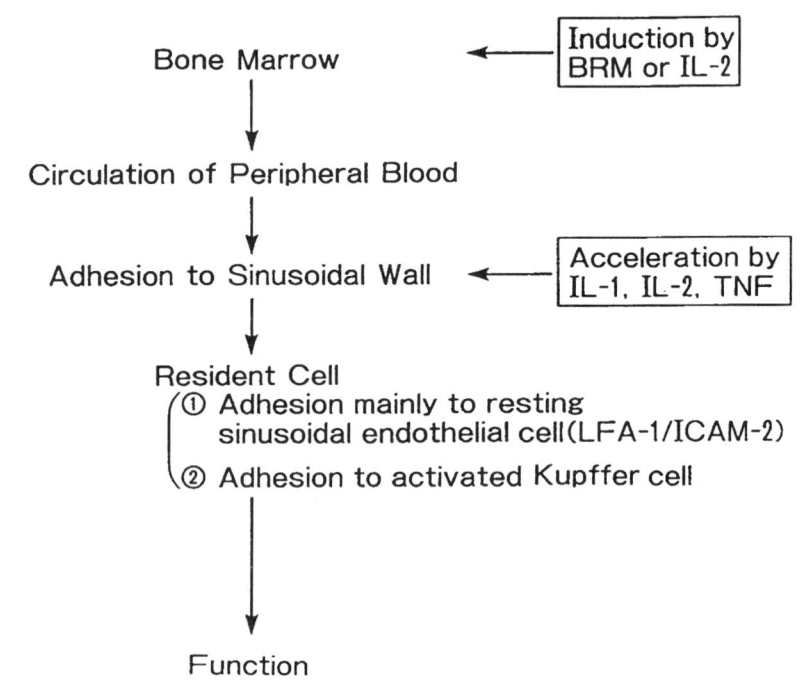

```
Bone Marrow  ←——— Induction by BRM or IL-2
    ↓
Circulation of Peripheral Blood
    ↓
Adhesion to Sinusoidal Wall  ←——— Acceleration by IL-1, IL-2, TNF
    ↓
Resident Cell
   ① Adhesion mainly to resting
      sinusoidal endothelial cell(LFA-1/ICAM-2)
   ② Adhesion to activated Kupffer cell
    ↓
Function
```

Fig. 15: Origin of the pit cell and its control mechanism

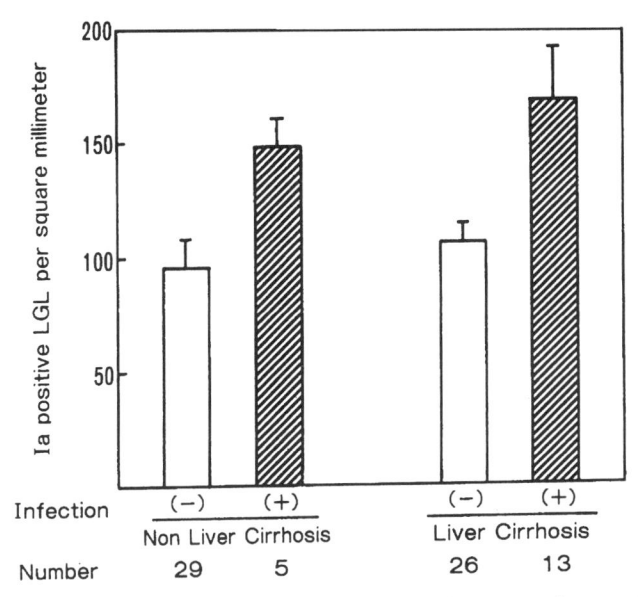

Fig. 16: Appearance of Ia-positive large granular lymphocytes in liver with or without cirrhosis. Many more cells were counted in patients with infection

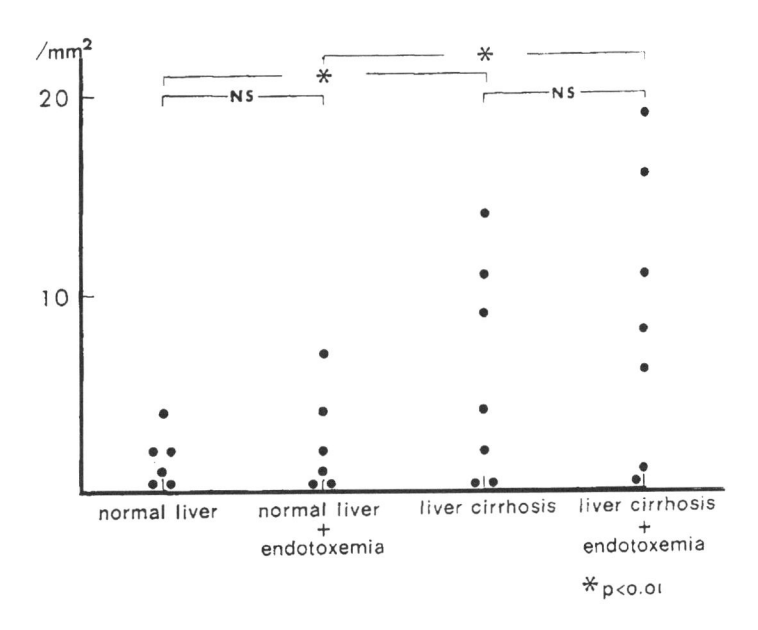

Fig. 17: γδT lymphocyte count in the liver. Liver cirrhosis and/or endotoxemia induced an increase of γδT lymphocytes in the liver.

Kinetics of Ito Cells (Fat-Storing Cells)

Fat-storing cells are nonparenchymal cells of mesenchymal origin situated in the space of Disse, between the endothelial lining and the parenchymal cells. During hepatic toxicosis or inflammation, the presence of fat-storing cells is no longer restricted to the space of Disse. In the are of inflammation or the neighboring mechanically injured area, many fat-storing cells can be found in close proximity to damaged hepatic parenchymal cells, with locally infiltrated Kupffer cells and other inflammatory cells. Activated myofibroblast-like cells express a wide variety of connective tissue molecules than quiescent cells and nearly every connective tissue molecule is expressed at a higher level. Using in situ hybridization, specific mRNA transcripts for several basement membrane matrix, proteoglycans, etc., were found in quiescent cells in significant numbers in myofibroblast-like cells. Such characteristics suggested the association of hepatic fibrogenesis and tissue repair [17] (Fig. 18).

Activation of fat-storing cells might be induced by the factors secreted by activated Kupffer cells [18]. Results from several studies have supported the presence of this mechanism because of the proliferation of Kupffer cells near the injured area which has been observed and because the conditioned medium utilized in Kupffer cell cultures has an effect on the proliferation of fat-storing cells, collagen or proteoglycan synthesis, etc. These phenomena can be explained by the regulation of both paracrine stimulation and autocrine stimulation. With the former, it has been reported that platelet-derived growth factor and tumor growth factor-β (TGF-β), which are part of the spectrum of other cytokines and mitogenic factors, modulate the proliferation and functions of fat-storing cells. Similar phenomena have been reported with regard to interleukin -Iα, tumor necrosis factor-α, epidermal growth factor (EGF), and insulin-like growth factor (IGF) [19]. The expression of EGF-α and TGF-β cell surface receptor in fat-storing cells has also been observed.

In summary, it is clear that the changes in or modulation of intrasinusoidal lining cells are linked to the dysfunction of hepatic parenchymal cells in sepsis, etc. Moreover, the regeneration after hepatectomy or hepatic partial necrosis is subject of a high degree of control by the fine network relationship between the cells with stimulant. Future work will be required to elucidate the essential pathophysiology of irreversible hepatic failure and discover better methods of treatment.

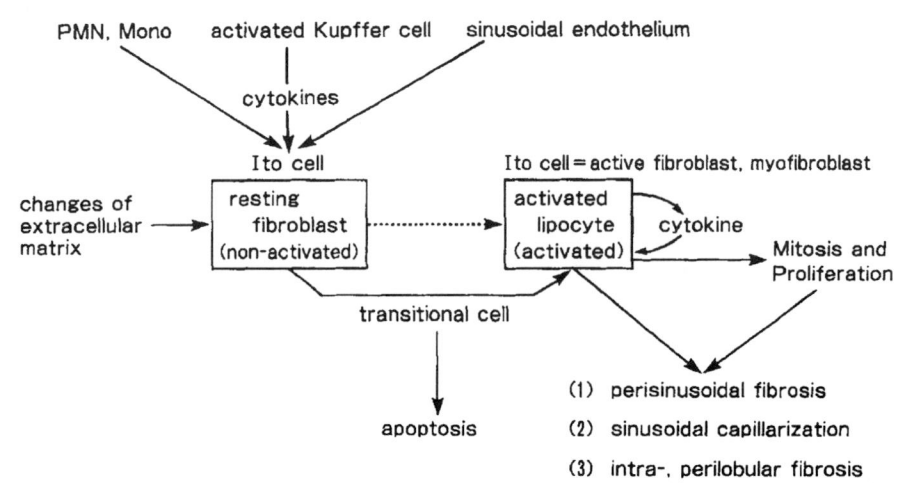

Fig. 18: Activation and roles of Ito cells

References

1. Philips MJ et al. (1986) Mechanisms of cholestasis. Lab Invest 54: 593-608
2. Frey GH, Gauldie J (1988) The acute phase response of the liver in inflammation. In: Popper H, Schaffne F (eds.) Progress in liver disease. Saunders, Philadelphia
3. Grun M et al. (1977) Biological significance of altered von Kupffer cells function in experimental liver disease. In: Wisse E, Knook DL (eds.) Kupffer cells and other sinusoidal cells. Elsevier/North-Holland, Amsterdam, pp. 437-446
4. Caldwell-Kenkel JC et al. (1991) Kupffer cell activation and endothelial cell damage after storage of rat livers: effects of reperfusion. Hepatology 13: 83-95
5. Van Furth R et al. (1985) New perspectives on the kinetics of mononuclear phagocytes. In: Van Furth R (ed.) Mononuclear phagocytes: characteristics, physiology and function. Nijhoff, Dordrecht, pp. 201-208
6. Callery MP et al. (1991) Kupffer cell tumor necrosis factor-α production is suppressed during live regeneration. J Surg Res 50: 515-519
7. Stephen W et al. (1991) In vivo biologic and immunohistochemical analysis of interleukin-1 and tumor necrosis factor during experimental endotoxemia. Am J Pathol 138: 395-402
8. Kobayashi S, Clements MG (1992) Kupffer cell exacerbation of hepatocyte hypoxia/reoxygenation injury. Circ Shock 37: 245-252
9. Ayla A et al. (1992) Differential effects of hemorrhage on Kupffer cells: decreased antigen presentation despite increased inflammatory cytokine (IL-1, IL-6 and TNF) release. Cytokine 4: 66-75
10. Yamada S et al. (1989) Intravascular coagulation in the development of massive hepatic necrosis induced by Corynebacterium parvum and endotoxin in rats. Scand J Gastroenterol 24: 293-298
11. Matsuura T et al. (1992) Studies on the cultured liver endothelial cells: ultrastructures revealed by the ultra high resolution scanning electron microscopy and the polymerization replica method and effects of TNF (in Japanese). In: Tanikawa I (ed.) Progress in hepatic sinusoidal cell studies. Kokusai Isho, Tokyo, pp. 119-123
12. Ohmura T et al. (1993) Establishment of a novel monoclonal antibody SE-1 which specifically reacts with rat hepatic sinusoidal endothelial cells. J Histochem Cytochem 41: 1253-1257
13. Schaffner F, Popper H (1963) Capillarization of hepatic sinusoids in man. Gastroenterology 44: 239-242
14. Wisse E et al. (1976) The pit cell: distribution of a new type of cell occurring in rat liver sinusoids and peripheral blood. Cell Tissue Res 173: 423-435
15. Steeg PS et al. (1982) Regulation of murine macrophage Ia antigen expression by an immune interferon-like lymphokine: inhibitory effects of endotoxin. J Immunol 129: 2402-2407
16. Vanderkerken et al. (1990) Characterization of a phenotypically and functionally distinct subset of large granular lymphocytes (pit cells) in rat liver sinusoids. Hepatology 12: 70-75
17. Ballardini G et al. (1989) Correlation between Ito cells and fibrinogenesis in an experimental model of hepatic fibrosis. A sequential stereological study. Liver 3: 58-63
18. Greerts A et al. (1984) Kinetic aspects of Kupffer and fat-storing cell behaviour during the induction of liver fibrosis by chronic CCl_4 intoxication. In: Van Bezooyen C (ed.) Pharmacological, morphological and physiological aspects of liver aging. Rijswijk (The Netherlands): TNO Rijswijk, pp. 85, 91
19. Yamamoto M, Enzan H (1975) Morphology and function of Ito cell (fat-storing cell) in the liver. Recent Adv Reticuloendothelial System Res 15: 54-75

Section 6:

Mechanisms of Inflammatory Lung Injury and Strategies for Counterregulation

New Concepts in Septic ARDS: Initiation by Synergism Between Nontoxic Doses of Lipopolysaccharide and Platelet-Activating Factor

R. Rabinovici, L.F. Neville, G. Feuerstein

Introduction

A most severe consequence of sepsis is the development of microvascular lung injury (adult respiratory distress syndrome, ARDS), which is the leading cause of deaths in these patients [1]. Although inroads have been made into understanding the pathophysiology of septic lung injury, which have been facilitated by expression cloning of a number of inflammatory mediators such as cytokines [2] and adhesion molecules [3], little progress has been made in the development of an effective pharmacotherapy to combat septic lung injury. This lack of progress would indicate a failure in understanding both the nature of its initial trigger and the mechanisms by which different inflammatory mediators interact with each other to elicit ARDS.

The most favored concept in the pathophysiology of septic ARDS is that the production of highly inducible proinflammatory mediators which mediate tissue injury are triggered by the release into the systemic circulation of massive amounts of bacterial endotoxin lipopolysaccharide (LPS). Nevertheless, several considerations would cast doubt on the validity of this hypothesis. First, the basis of this postulate was provided by animal models of septic lung injury induced by the administration of large doses of LPS or live bacteria, which fail to parallel the clinical settings of sepsis-induced lung injury. Second, all clinical trials with anti-LPS monoclonal antibodies, which were developed as a direct consequence of these animal models, failed to demonstrate protection against sepsis (for review see [4, 5]).

Based upon these considerations, we hypothesized that septic ARDS may be precipitated not via massive doses of LPS but rather as a result of interactions amongst minuscule doses of LPS and rapidly induced inflammatory mediators. Such an example of a rapidly induced de novo synthesized, proinflammatory mediator is platelet-activating factor (PAF), which has been implicated in septic lung injury [6, 7].

Interactions Between Minuscule Doses of Lipopolysaccharide and Platelet-Activating Factor Trigger ARDS-Like Injury In Vivo

It has been shown that PAF exerts a key role in the development of septic lung injury and synergizes with LPS in augmenting the in vitro production of other mediators implicated in the pathogenesis of septic ARDS, such as tumor necrosis factor-α (TNF-α) [8,10]. Therefore, the effect of various combinations of minuscule doses of LPS and PAF on lung injury were evaluated in vivo. Parameters of lung injury included lung edema, myeloperoxidase (MPO) activity, serum TNF-α and electron microscopy of pulmonary tissue.

The combined administration of noninjurious doses of LPS (0.1 µg/kg, i.v. bolus) and PAF (1 pmol/kg/min over 60 min) elicited a profound lung permeability defect evidenced by elevated water content (Fig. 1) and increased protein and polymorphonuclear leukocyte (PMN) accumulation in bronchoalveolar lavage (BAL) fluid. Also, there was leukocyte sequestration in lung tissue, as assessed by increased MPO activity. Furthermore, electron microscopy of lung sections prepared from LPS-PAF challenged rats indicated pronounced neutrophil sequestration and adherence to endothelium (Fig. 2) [11]. In accord with these latter findings, northern blots of total RNA derived from lungs of LPS-PAF challenged rats revealed up-regulation of ELAM-1 mRNA (Fig. 3), an inducible ligand that mediates neutrophil adherence [3, 12]. Enhanced hybridization was observed both 1 and 3 h post LPS-PAF challenge, indicating its highly inducible nature. None of these effects were observed from rats challenged with the single LPS or PAF paradigms. The effects of PAF in this model were receptor-specific, since they were abrogated by BN 50739, a PAF receptor antagonist [13], and not induced by a combination of LPS and lyso-PAF, the inactive metabolite of PAF [11]. Furthermore, PAF appeared to prime for the effect of LPS and not vice versa, since LPS given prior or after PAF infusion failed to elicit lung injury [11]. However, the precise relationships between LPS and PAF in the induction of lung injury still remain to be resolved and should be investigated using monocytes or macrophages in culture.

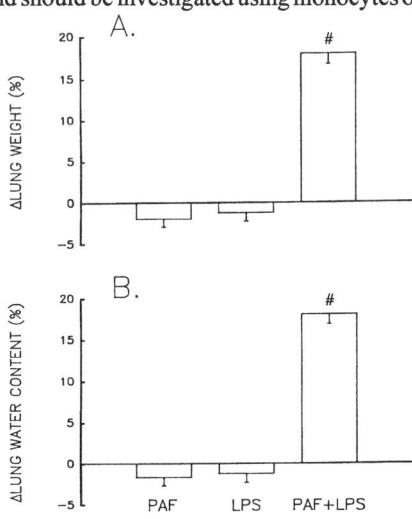

Fig. 1 a, b: Priming effect of platelet-activating factor (PAF) on endotoxin-induced elevation of lung weight (a) and water content (b). LPS, lipopolysaccharide; change vs. control; # p<0.01

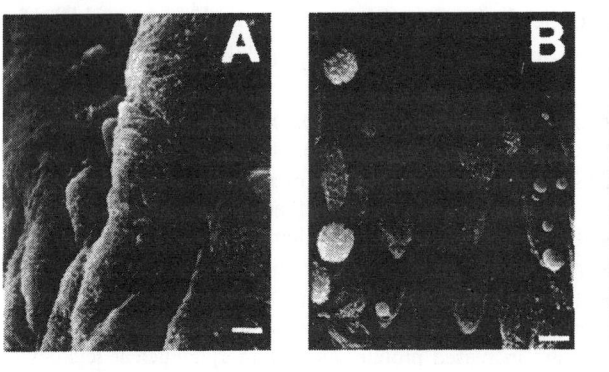

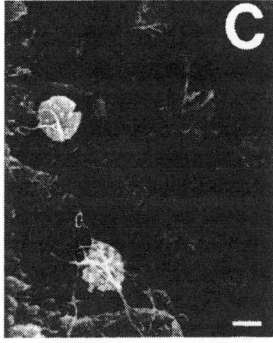

Fig. 2 a-c: Scanning electron micrograph of the luminal surface of a pulmonary venule from rats given a) platelet-activating factor (PAF), b) lipopolysaccharide (LPS), or c) the LPS-PAF combination. Note that the endothelium in (a) is devoid of adherent leukocytes or platelets, whereas few platelets (small arrows) and leukocytes (large arrows), probably neutrophils, are adherent to endothelium in (b). In contrast, the endothelium in (c) is covered by adherent leukocytes (large arrows) and platelets (small arrows) embedded in branching fibrin (f) strands. The surface of the leukocytes in (c) is thrown into numerous blebs, evidence of activation. Bar, 6 µm

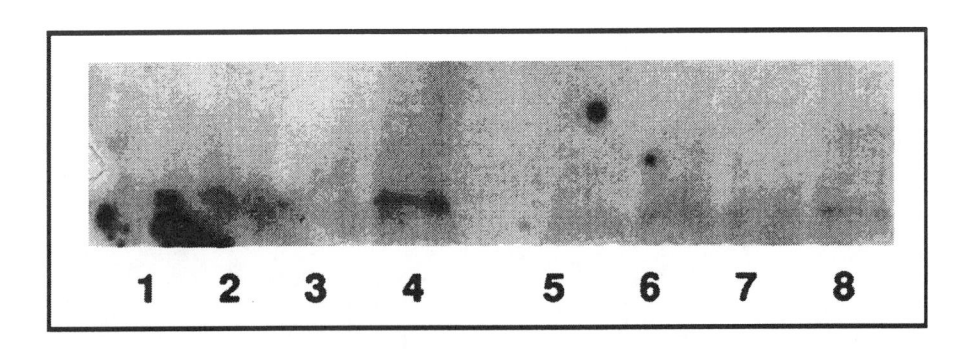

Fig. 3: Lipopolysaccharide-platelet-activating factor (LPS-PAF) induces ELAM-1 mRNA accumulation in lung tissue. Total RNA was extracted [23] from lungs of rats challenged with LPS-PAF or various controls at 1 h (lanes 1-4) or 3 h (lanes 5-8) after drug treatment. Note the enhanced ELAM-1 mRNA signal solely from LPS-PAF treated rats in lanes 4 and 8. Lanes 1 and 5, controls; lanes 2 and 6, LPS; lanes 3 and 7, PAF; lanes 4 and 8, LPS-PAF

A Second Lipopolysaccharide-Platelet-Activating Factor Challenge Further Exacerbates the ARDS-Like Lung Injury

Since a single challenge of minuscule LPS-PAF was found to induce lung injury highly reminiscent of the early stages of ARDS [11], we further hypothesized that fulminant ARDS-like lung injury may be produced by a repeated LPS-PAF challenge. Rats subjected to an identical dose of LPS-PAF 4 h after the primary one exhibited severe lung injury comprising many pathophysiological and histological features of clinical ARDS [14]. These included severe pulmonary edema, proteinaceous exudates within alveoli indicative of interstitial pneumonia not observed in the single LPS-PAF paradigm. The mortality and persistent elevation of serum TNF-α following the second LPS-PAF challenge (Fig. 4) also indicated the development of fulminant ARDS-like lung injury.

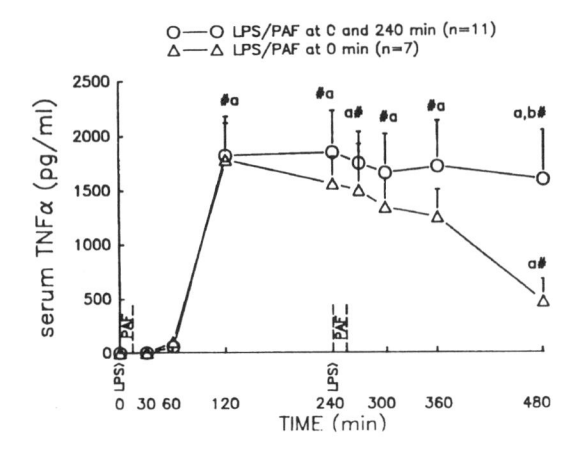

Fig. 4: Serum tumor necrosis factor-α (TNF-α) response to the double lipopolysaccharide-platelet activating factor (LPS-PAF) stimulus. Note the persistent elevation of serum TNF-α at approximately 2000 pg/ml 8 h after the primary bolus dose of LPS + PAF. #Significance at $p < 0.05$; a, vs. basal value; b, vs. all other groups

Tumor Necrosis Factor-α Is a Pivotal Mediator in Lipopolysaccharide-Platelet-Activating Factor - Induced Lung Injury

Based on numerous studies implicating TNF-α in the pathogenesis of septic shock and septic lung injury [10, 15, 16], serum TNF-α levels from LPS-PAF challenged rats were determined using a "sandwich" ELISA [11]. Whereas serum TNF-α remained at undetectable levels in rats challenged with either LPS or PAF alone, the combined LPS-PAF regimen elicited a robust and monophasic increase in serum TNF-α (Fig. 5). A central role for TNF-α in mediating LPS-PAF induced lung injury was confirmed by the protective effect afforded by anti-TNF-α monoclonal antibody (mAb) against the development of lung injury. Rats pretreated (10 min) with hamster anti-mouse TNF-α mAb (25 mg/kg) prior to the LPS-PAF stimulus effectively attenuated all parameters of lung injury

(Table 1) [14, 17]. Furthermore, the potent effect of TNF-α in up-regulating ELAM-1 in endothelial cells in culture (Fig. 6) [12] would indicate that newly synthesized TNF-α exerts a key role in the induction of ELAM-1 in lung endothelial cells, based upon the northern blot data (Fig. 3).

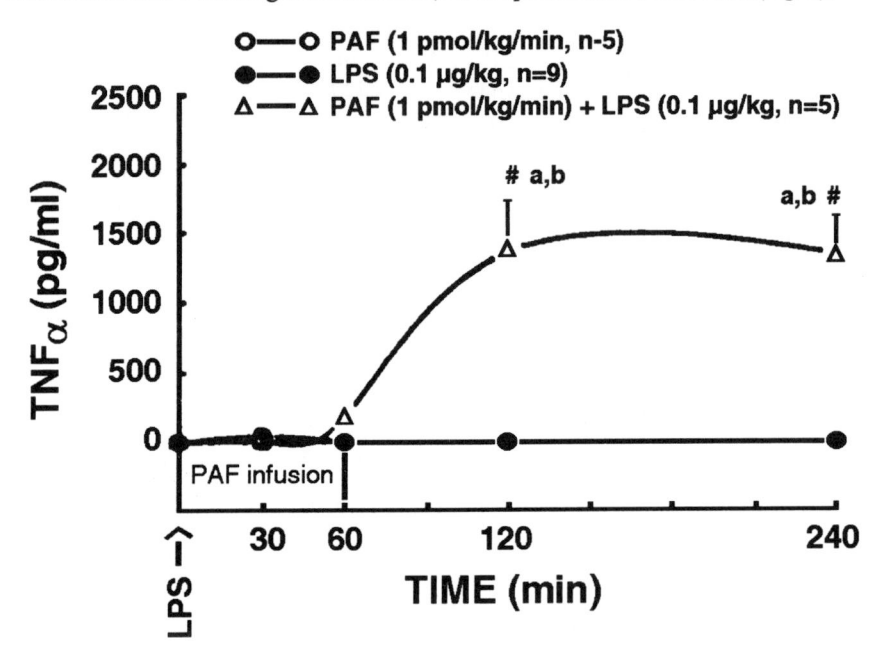

Fig. 5: Effect of platelet-activating factor (PAF) (1 pmol/kg per min) on tumor necrosis factor-α (TNF-α) response to endotoxin. Note the lack of effect of either lipopolysaccharide (LPS) or PAF alone, yet the combination of these otherwise subtoxic doses elicits a robust serum TNF-α response. #$p < 0.01$; a vs. basal value; b vs. all other groups

Table 1: Effect of pretreatment with anti-tumor necrosis factor-α monoclonal antibody (n=10) on lipopolysaccharide-platelet activating factor-induced lung injury and mortality

	Anti TNF-α mAb + LPS-PAF	IgG + LPS-PAF
Wet lung weight[a]	+6±8	+41±6*
Wet-dry lung weight[a]	+8±10	+37±6*
Protein concentration	-3±6	+35±7*
Mortality h[b]	10	60**

TNF-α, tumor necrosis factor-α; mAb, monoclonal antibody; LPS, lipopolysaccharide; PAF, platelet-activating factor; *p<0.05; **p<0.05 vs. anti-TNF-α mAb + LPS/PAF group; IgG, nonspecific IgG.
[a]Percent change vs. negative control group (IgG vehicle + LPS/PAF vehicle).
[b]Percent at 4 h.

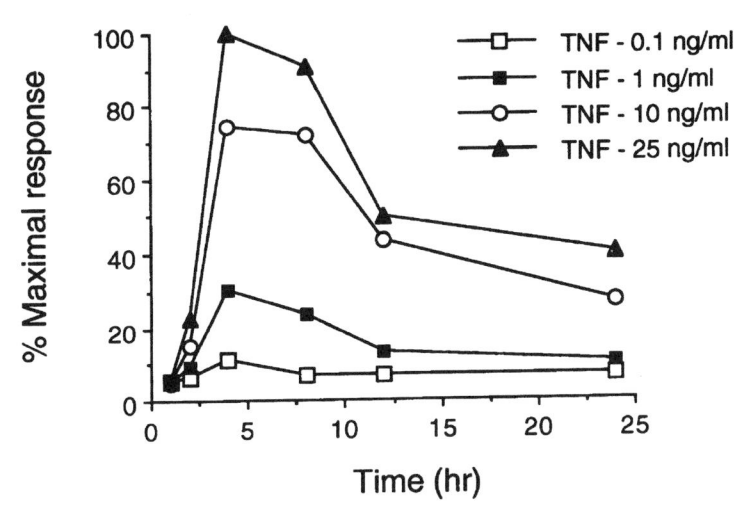

Fig. 6: Dose-response and time course of tumor necrosis factor (TNF-α) stimulated up-regulation of ELAM-1 in human aortic arch-derived endothelial cells. Endothelial cells were challenged with human recombinant TNF-α (0.1 ng - 25 ng/ml) from 1 h to 24 h and surface expression of ELAM-1 determined by ELISA using mouse anti-human ELAM-1 monoclonal antibody as the primary antibody followed by goat anti-mouse, peroxidase-linked IgG as the secondary

Is Tumor Necrosis Factor-α the Sole Mediator of Lipopolysaccharide-Platelet-Activating Factor Induced Lung Injury?

Based on the elevation of TNF-α levels in the serum of LPS-PAF challenged rats [11, 14, 17] together with the striking protective effect of anti-TNF-α mAb in preventing LPS-PAF induced lung injury [14, 17], TNF-α would appear to be central in the development of lung injury in this model.

Nevertheless, due to a multicytokine involvement of lung injury in previous animal models [18], the presence of other cytokines in the LPS-PAF model was examined. Due to the unavailability of commercially available rat cytokine probes (e.g., monoclonal antibodies) to enable peptide quantitation, northern blots were performed on total RNA isolated from lungs of rats challenged with LPS-PAF paradigm. An increased hybridization signal (ten-fold as compared to controls) for TNF-α mRNA was observed (Fig. 7). Interestingly, a much greater signal (at least 100-fold enhancement) was observed for interleukin (IL)-1 β and IL-6 mRNA derived solely from LPS-PAF treated rats (Fig. 7).

Lung histopathological findings of LPS-PAF treated rats revealed adherence of neutrophils to the endothelium of pulmonary venules (Fig. 2). This phenomenon would indicate the likely involvement of a rat, IL-8-like chemotactic factor responsible for promoting neutrophil infiltration [19]. To address this issue, Northern blots were probed at high stringency with KC. KC, which shares 64% amino acid homology with human gro [20], a member of the IL-8 subfamily of chemokines and itself a potent chemotactic molecule [21], produced a striking hybridization signal to RNA extracted from lungs of LPS-PAF treated rats (Fig. 7).

CYTOKINE mRNA INDUCTION IN ARDS-LIKE LUNG INJURY

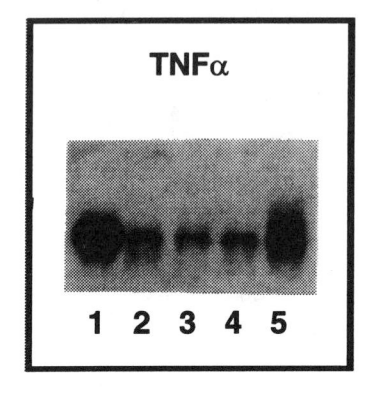

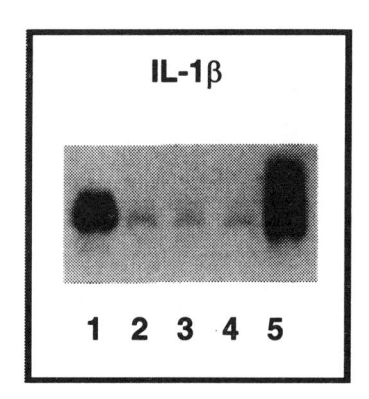

TNFα

1 2 3 4 5

IL-1β

1 2 3 4 5

1. **LPS** - stimulated macrophages
2. PAF vehicle - LPS vehicle
3. **PAF** - LPS vehicle
4. PAF vehicle - **LPS**
5. **PAF** - **LPS**

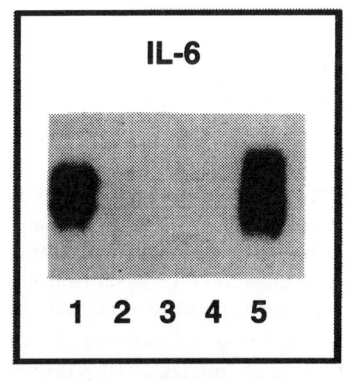

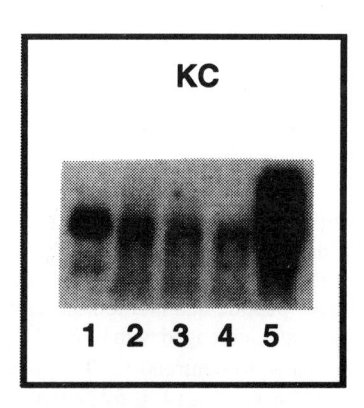

IL-6

1 2 3 4 5

KC

1 2 3 4 5

Fig. 7: Lipopolysaccharide-platelet-activating factor (LPS-PAF) administration to rats causes up-regulation in lung tumor necrosis factor-α (TNF-α), interleukin (IL)-1 β, IL-6 and KC mRNA levels. Northern blots were performed on total RNA isolated from: LPS (100 ng/ml)-stimulated peritoneal macrophages (positive control, lanes 1), and lungs from rats challenged with LPS vehicle-PAF vehicle (lanes 2), LPS vehicle-PAF (lanes 3), LPS-PAF vehicle (lanes 4) and LPS-PAF (lanes 5). RNA was hybridized to random-prime prepared ^{32}P-labeled cytokine cDNA probes, washed and taken for autoradiography. Note the pronounced and selective induction of all cytokines solely form LPS-PAF challenged rats (lanes 5)

Furthermore, recent studies with the novel and highly selective complement inhibitor soluble complement receptor 1 (sCR1) supported a role of complement in the LPS-PAF model of lung injury [22]. In these studies, pretreatment with sCR1 prevented lung edema and the increase in BAL fluid cell count and protein concentration. Also, sCR1 attenuated the deposition of C3 and C5b-9 to lung vessels. Interestingly, there was no effect on lung MPO activity and serum TNF-α. Therefore, in addition to the central role of TNF-α in mediating LPS-PAF induced lung injury, our data clearly support the involvement of a multimediator network which leads to tissue injury.

Future Goals and Directions

As described above, a multicytokine involvement would appear to prevail in the genesis of septic lung injury and ARDS. To further confirm this concept, the kinetics of appearance of TNF-α, IL-1 β, IL-6 and IL-8 in the serum of LPS-PAF treated rats should be investigated to determine the mechanisms of interaction between these different cytokines. Establishing suitable bioassays for the rat interleukin members would facilitate such studies. Also, further studies using specific inhibitors of cytokine production or action could help to dissect the individual role of each cytokine in promoting lung injury thereby promoting more effective therapeutic strategies to combat this grave condition. In vitro studies using alveolar macrophages will give insight into the mechanisms of LPS-PAF interactions. Furthermore, the pronounced elevation in lung cytokine mRNA levels from LPS-PAF treated rats could lend itself to identifying new members of the cytokine family by adopting either subtractive cDNA library or differential expression display methodologies over a specific time course following LPS-PAF administration.

Our model described herein provides a new experimental paradigm to confirm our hypothesis that lung injury is elicited by interactions amongst minute doses of LPS and inflammatory mediators. It should be noted that this paradigm may not imply the sole involvement or relative contribution of PAF in the genesis of septic lung injury. Instead, the model serves as an example that such interactions may indeed result in microvascular lung injury. Further investigations of interactions between rapidly induced inflammatory mediators and LPS should be ensued and may provide clues to the physiological triggering and progression of ARDS. Insights into such interactions could provide new target sites for pharmacological intervention in septic lung injury.

References

1. Demling RH (1990) Current concepts on the adult respiratory distress syndrome. Circ Shock 30: 297-310
2. Shaw AR (1991) Molecular biology of cytokines: an introduction. In: The cytokine handbook. Academic, New York, pp. 19-46
3. Bevilacqua MP, Stengelin S, Gimbrone MA Jr, Seed B (1989) Endothelial leukocyte adhesion molecule 1: an inducible receptor for neutrophils related to complementary regulatory proteins and lectins. Science 243: 1160-1165
4. Neugebauer EA, Holaday JW (eds.) Handbook of mediators in septic shock. CRC, Boca Raton
5. Baumgartner JD (1992) Anti-endotoxin antibodies: a critical appraisal. In: Lamy M, Thijs LG (eds.) Mediators of sepsis. Springer, Berlin, Heidelberg, New York, pp. 315-328
6. Chang SW, Feddersen CO, Hensen PM, Voelkel NF (1987) Platelet-activating factor mediates hemodynamic changes and lung injury in endotoxin-treated rats. J Clin Invest 79: 1498-1509

7. Chang SW, Fernyak S, Voelkel NF (1990) Beneficial effect of platelet activating factor antagonist, WEB 206, on endotoxin-induced lung injury. Am J Physiol 257: 153-158
8. Dubois C, Bissonnette E, Rola-Pleszczynski M (1989) Platelet activating factor (PAF) enhances tumor necrosis factor production by alveolar macrophages: prevention by PAF receptor antagonists and lipoxygenase inhibitors. J Immunol 143: 964-970
9. Bonavida B, Mencia-Huerta JM, Braquet P (1990) Effects of platelet activating factor on peripheral blood monocytes: induction and priming for TNF secretion. J Lipid Mediators 2: 65-76
10. Mathison JC, Wolfson E, Ulevitch RJ (1988) Participation of tumor necrosis factor in mediation of gram negative bacterial lipopolysaccharide-induced injury in rabbits. J Clin Invest 81: 1925-1937
11. Rabinovici R, Esser KM, Lysko PG, Yue TL, Griswold DE, Hillegass LM, Bugelski PJ, Hallenback JM, Feuerstein GZ (1991) Priming by platelet activating factor of endotoxin-induced lung injury and cardiovascular shock. Circ Res 69: 12-25
12. Benjamin C, Dougas I, Chi-Rosso G, Luhowskyj S, Rosa M, Newman B, Osborn L, Vassallo C, Hession C, Goelz S, McCarthy K, Lobb R (1990) A blocking monoclonal antibody to endothelial-leukocyte adhesion molecule 1 (ELAM-1) Biochem Biophys Res Commun 171: 348-353
13. Rabinovici R, Yue TL, Farhat M, Smith EF II, Esser KM, Slivjak M, Feuerstein GZ (1990) Platelet activating factor (PAF) and tumor necrosis factor-α (TNF-α) interactions in endotoxemic shock: studies with BN 50739, a novel PAF antagonist. J Pharmacol Exp Ther 255: 256-263
14. Rabinovici R, Bugelski PJ, Esser KM, Hillegass LM, Vernick J, Feuerstein GZ (1993) ARDS-like lung injury produced by endotoxin in platelet activating factor primed rats. J Appl Physiol 74: 1791-1802
15. Stephens KE, Ishizaka A, Larrick JW, Raffin TA (1988) Tumor necrosis factor causes increased pulmonary permeability and edema: comparison to septic acute lung injury. Am Rev Respir Dis 137: 1364-1370
16. Ferrari-Baliviera E, Mealy K, Smith RJ, Wilmore DW (1989) Tumor necrosis factor induces adult respiratory distress syndrome in rats. Arch Surg 124: 1400-1405
17. Rabinovici R, Bugelski PJ, Esser KM, Hillegass LM, Griswold DE, Vernick J, Feuerstein GZ (1993) Tumor necrosis factor-α mediates endotoxin-induced lung injury in platelet activating factor-primed rats. J Pharmacol Exp Ther 267: 1550-1557
18. Dinarello CA (1992) Blocking cytokines in infectious diseases. In: Lamy M, Thijs LG (eds.) Mediators of sepsis. Springer, Berlin, Heidelberg, New York, pp. 362-376
19. Matsushima K, Baldwin ET, Mukaida N (1992) Interleukin-8 and MCAF: novel leukocyte recruitment and activating cytokines. In: Kishimoto T (ed.) Interleukins: molecular biology and immunology. Karger, Basel. Chem Immunol 52: 236-265
20. Oquendo P, Alberta J, Wen D, Graycar JL, Derynck R, Stiles CD (1989) The platelet-derived growth factor-inducible gene encodes a secretory protein related to platelet α-granule proteins. J Biol Chem 264: 4133-4137
21. Sager R (1990) GRO as a cytokine. In: Molecular and cellular biology of cytokines. Wiley-Liss, New York, pp. 327-332
22. Rabinovici R, Grace Yeh C, Hillegass LM, Griswold DE, DiMartino MJ, Vernick J, Fong KL, Feuerstein GZ (1992) Role of complement in endotoxin/platelet-activating factor-induced lung injury. J Immunol 149: 1744-1750
23. Chomczynski P, Sacchi N (1987) Single step method in RNA isolation by acid guanidinium thiocyanate-phenol-chloroform extraction. Anal Biochem 162: 156-159

Neutrophil Function and Lung Injury in a Standardized Sheep Model of Multiple Organ Failure

A. Dwenger, M. Grotz, H.-C. Pape, C. Hainer, G. Schweitzer, G. Regel

Study Objectives

In recent years multiple organ failure (MOF) has become the main cause of late death after severe trauma, with a more than 75% lethal outcome [1-4, 7]. After several efforts to develop an appropriate animal model for pathophysiological and therapeutic studies of MOF [8, 10, 12 15], only now has a standardized large animal model been established which mimics the post-traumatic development of sequential irreversible MOF [9, 13].This model includes combined injuries of pathophysiological importance which are found in multiple trauma patients. This report focuses on the behavior of blood and alveolar neutrophils during lung failure in this sheep model of MOF.

Materials and Methods

This sheep model [13] combined hemorrhagic shock (MAP = 50 mmHg for 2 h) and closed femoral nailing with a standardized AO technique [11] at day 0, 12-h injections of *Escherichia coli* endotoxin (serotype 055:B5, Sigma, Deisenhofen, FRG) and zymosan-activated autologous plasma (3 mg zymosan A/ml plasma for 30 min and 37°C; zymosan from Sigma) on days 1 - 5 (injections of 0.75 µg endotoxin + 0.7 ml zymosan-activated plasma/kg body wt.) and further monitoring of hemodynamics, and lung, liver and kidney functions on days 6-10. Using the citrated venous blood (daily collection) and bronchoalveolar lavage fluid (BALF) of ten merino sheep (20-30 kg weight), the following parameters were determined before treatment (day 0), 12 h after the last injection (day 6) and after MOF development (day 10) [5, 6]: neutrophil (PMN) count in blood and BALF, epithelial lining fluid (ELF)/plasma ratio of albumin concentrations, zymosan-induced (stimulated) and noninduced (spontaneous) chemiluminescence response (CL) of blood- and BALF-isolated neutrophils, plasma bilirubin concentrations, plasma and urine creatinine concentrations, and plasma and BALF urea concentrations.

Results

Figure 1 shows examples of the time-dependent alterations of organ functions during MOF development: significant increases in cardiac index (heart) and plasma bilirubin concentration (liver) as well as significant decreases in creatinine clearance (kidneys) and oxygenation ratio (lung). The neutrophil counts of blood and ELF (calculated from BALF according to Rennard [14]) and the distribution of neutrophils and alveolar macrophages in the BALF are shown in Fig. 2. Figure 3 depicts the spontaneous and stimulated (as a measure of neutrophil metabolic capacity and surface receptor expression) photon emission of blood (a, b) and alveolar (c) neutrophils, and compares the chemiluminescence response of blood-derived and simultaneously BALF-derived neutrophils (d). In Fig. 4 the ELF/plasma ratio of albumin concentrations (as a biochemical marker of the lung capillary permeability damage) and the plasma albumin concentration (as a marker of the general permeability damage and the inflammation-induced synthesis reduction) are shown.

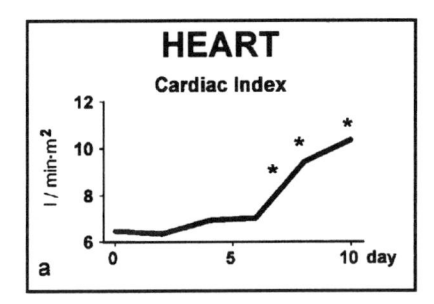

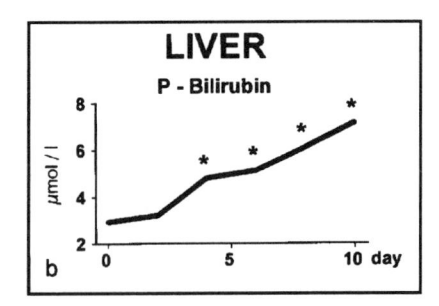

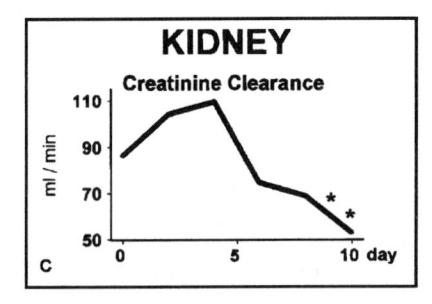

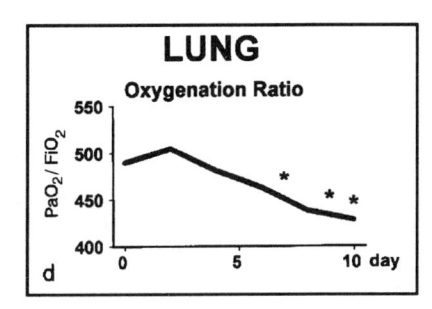

Fig. 1 a-d: Cardiac index (a), plasma bilirubin concentration (b), creatinine clearance (c), and oxygenation ratio (d) during MOF development in sheep ($\bar{x}$; n=10). *p<0.05; Wilcoxon's test; data vs. data of day 0

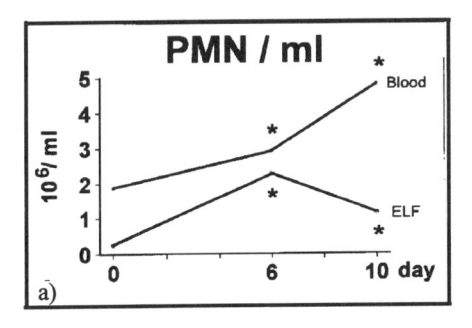

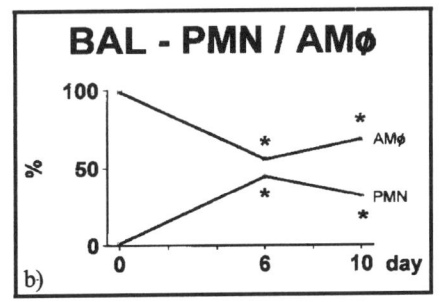

*Fig. 2 a, b: Neutrophil count in blood and epithelial lining fluid (ELF) (a), and distribution of neutrophils (PMN) and alveolar macrophages (AMø) in BALF (b) during MOF development in sheep ($\bar{x}$; n=10). *p<0.05; Wilcoxon's test; data vs. data of day 0*

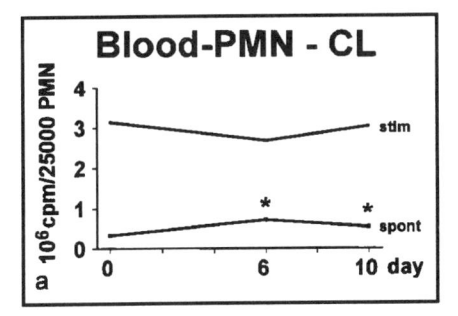

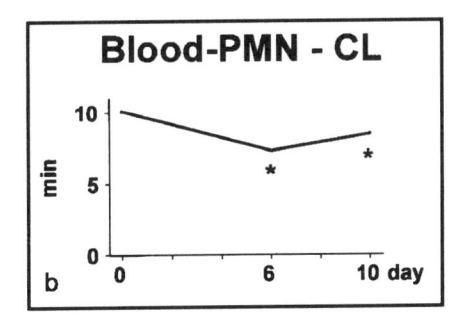

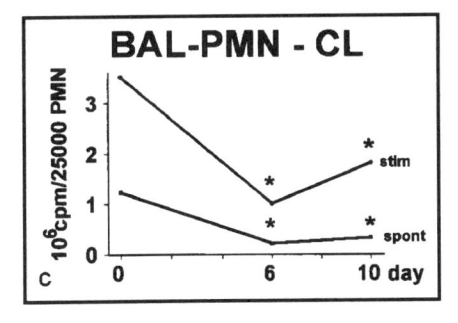

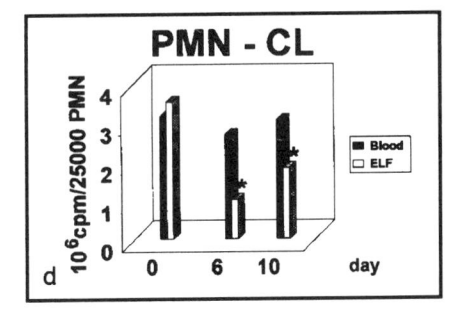

*Fig. 3 a-d: Chemiluminescence (CL) response after zymosan administration (stim) and basic response (spont) of neutrophils isolated from blood (a), time to reach the maximum zymosan-induced CL response (b), CL response upon zymosan (stim) and basic response (spont) of neutrophils isolated from BALF (c), and comparison of CL response after zymosan administration of neutrophils isolated from blood and BALF simultaneously (d) during MOF development in sheep ($\bar{x}$; n=10). *p<0.05; Wilcoxon's test; data vs. data of day 10 (a-c). *p<0.05; Mann-Whitney test; blood vs. ELF data (d)*

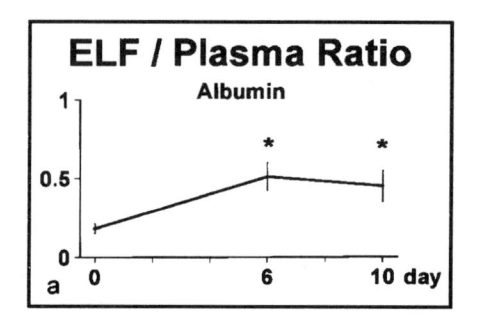

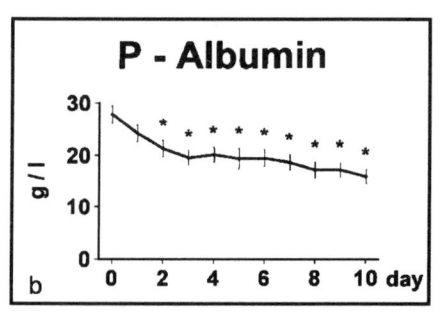

*Fig. 4 a, b: Ratio of albumin concentrations in ELF and plasma (a), and plasma albumin concentration (b) during MOF development in sheep ($\bar{x} \pm SEM$; n=10). *$p<0.05$; Wilcoxon's test; data vs. data of day 10*

Discussion

The results demonstrate that there was an increased migration of neutrophils into the alveoli during MOF development. An in vivo activation of blood neutrophils could be seen from the spontaneous photon emission and C3b receptor increase on neutrophils. Simultaneous comparisons of the zymosan-induced chemiluminescence response of the neutrophils isolated from blood and BALF gave evidence for the loss of metabolic capacity of neutrophils during their passage from the capillary into the alveolar space. This decrease was in parallel to the increase in the ELF/plasma ratio of albumin concentrations, demonstrating increased lung capillary permeability damage. In conclusion, the experimental results provide evidence that the lung failure of the MOF model described was caused by classical neutrophil-mediated pathomechanisms.

References

1. Baue AE (1975) Multiple, progressive, or sequential system failure: a syndrome for the 1970s. Arch Surg 110: 779-781
2. Border JR, Chenier R, McMenamy RH, La Duca J, Seibel R, Birkhahn R, Yu L (1976) Multiple systems organ failure: muscle deficit with visceral protein malnutrition. Surg Clin North Am 56: 1147-1167
3. Crump JM, Duncan DA, Wears R (1988) Analysis of multiple organ system failure in trauma and non-trauma patients. Am Surg 54: 702-708
4. DeCamp MM, Demling RH (1988) Posttraumatic multisystem organ failure. JAMA 260: 530-534
5. Dwenger A, Schweitzer G, Regel G (1986) Bronchoalveolar lavage fluid and plasma proteins, chemiluminescence response and protein contents of polymorphonuclear leukocytes from blood and lavage fluid in traumatized patients. J Clin Chem Clin Biochem 24: 73-88

6. Dwenger A, Regel G, Ellendorff B, Schweitzer G, Funck M, Limbrock H, Sturm JA, Tscherne H (1990) Alveolar cell pattern and chemiluminescence response of blood neutrophils and alveolar macrophages in sheep after endotoxin injection. J Clin Chem Clin Biochem 28: 163-168
7. Fry DE, Pearlstein L, Fulton RL, Polk HC (1980) Multiple organ failure - the role of uncontrolled infection. Arch Surg 115: 136-140
8. Goris RJA, Boekholtz WKF, van Bebber IPT, Nuytnick JKS, Schillings PHM (1986) Multiple organ failure and sepsis without bacteria. Arch Surg 121: 897-901
9. Grotz RJA, Remmers D, Dwenger A, Pape HC, Hainer C, Regel G (1994) A standardized sheep-model for multiple organ failure after severe trauma. Clin Int Care 5(Suppl): 31
10. Hersch M, Gnidec A, Bersten AD, Troster M, Rutledge FS, Sibbald WJ (1990) Histologic and ultrastructural changes in pulmonary organs during early hyperdynamic sepsis. Surgery 107: 397-410
11. Pape HC, Dwenger A, Regel G, Schweitzer G, Jonas M, Remmers D, Krumm K, Neumann C, Sturm JA, Tscherne H (1992) Pulmonary damage after intramedullary femoral nailing in traumatized sheep - is there an effect from different nailing methods? J Trauma 33: 574-581
12. Pape HC, Dwenger A, Regel G, Schweitzer G, Remmers D, Pape D, Sturm JA (1993) Haemorrhagic shock, endotoxin and complement activation induce late organ failure in sheep. Theor Surg 8: 21-28
13. Regel G, Grotz M, Pape HC, Dwenger A, Hainer C, Tscherne H (1996) Multiple organ failure after severe trauma: a standardized model in sheep. In: Faist E (ed.) MOF, MODS and SIRS - concepts, clinical correlates and therapy. Pabst Science, Lengerich
14. Rennard SI, Basset G, Lecossier D, O'Donnell KM, Pinkston P, Martin PG, Crystal RG (1986) Estimation of volume of epithelial lining fluid recovered by lavage using area as marker of dilution. J Appl Physiol 60: 532-538
15. Steinberg S, Flynn W, Kelley K et al. (1989) Development of a bacteria-independent model of the multiple organ failure syndrome. Arch Surg 124: 1390-1395

Anti-inflammatory Effects of the Neuropeptide a-Melanocyte Stimulating Hormone in Systemic Inflammation

A. Catania, D. McCoy, K. Carnes, A. Macaluso, G. Ceriani, J. Biltz, J.M. Lipton

Introduction

Inflammatory reactions are clearly pivotal in may disorders and have important secondary influences in many more [2]. Inflammation can occur in barrier tissues such as the skin or gut or in deep tissues such as the joints in arthritis. Inflammation can also present as a systemic disorder in endotoxemia, septic shock, and adult respiratory distress syndrome (ARDS). Recent evidence indicates that the neuropeptide α-melanocyte stimulating hormone (α-MSH) inhibits such reactions in animal models of inflammatory responses [1]. Experiments in which different methods and treatments were used indicate that α-MSH reduces the effects of cytokines that mediate host responses. α-MSH inhibits fever and inflammation induced by recombinant interleukin-1 β (IL-1β), interleukin-6 (IL-6), and tumor necrosis factor-α (TNF-α) given individually and by endogenous pyrogen, which contains cytokines [3]. Intraperitoneal injection of α-MSH in mice blocks migration of neutrophils into subcutaneous sponges treated with IL-1, TNF, or complement C5a [4]. This result suggests that α-MSH inhibits cytokine-induced neutrophil chemotaxis. Although the extent of involvement in systemic inflammation is much greater than in more localized forms of inflammation, it is believed that mediators (e.g., cytokines) are shared. Therefore, we tested the influences of α-MSH, alone or in combination with an agent that inhibits bacterial growth, in models of systemic inflammation.

Adult Respiratory Distress Syndrome

The adult respiratory distress syndrome is marked by increased vascular permeability of the lung to neutrophils. In this condition, the cellular component of the intra-alveolar exudate includes red blood cells, macrophages, neutrophils and, occasionally, eosinophils. However, there is evidence supporting a central role for neutrophils in the pathogenesis of the disease

[5]. Indeed, neutrophils and their secretory products accumulate in the lungs of humans with ARDS and neutrophil depletion protects lungs of animals in many models of ARDS [5].

To test the influence of α-MSH on experimental ARDS, the peptide was administered to rats after intratracheal infusion of endotoxin (*Salmonella typhi*, 500 μg in 0.25 ml saline). Three groups (n=10 each) received either: (1) intratracheal infusion of endotoxin plus i.p. injections of α-MSH (100 μg in 0.2 ml saline) at 0, 2, and 4 h postendotoxin treatment; (2) intratracheal endotoxin infusion plus saline injections; (3) control intratracheal saline infusion plus i.p. saline injections. Six hours after endotoxin administration the trachea was cannulated and the cannula was secured with silk thread. Cell medium (12 ml) was used to wash the pulmonary tree (injected and withdrawn five times); both the bronchoalveolar lavage (BAL) fluid and whole blood from the jugular vein were transferred to test tubes for analysis in a Sysmex CC-130 cell counter. The BAL data showed that α-MSH treatment inhibited endotoxin-induced white blood cell (WBC) migration into the pulmonary tree ($p<0.05$) of rats given endotoxin. The WBC count was similar in the BAL of rats given endotoxin plus α-MSH and in those who received intratracheal injection of saline. Circulating WBC counts were markedly lower in groups given either endotoxin or endotoxin plus α-MSH compared to controls ($p<0.01$). However, there was no difference in WBC count between the two endotoxin-treated groups. The results indicate that α-MSH inhibits WBC migration in experimental lung injury but does not prevent endotoxin-induced reduction in circulating WBC.

Cecal Ligation and Puncture

In further experiments we tested the hypothesis that α-MSH, administered alone or in combination with an inhibitor of gram-negative bacterial growth, increases survival in a model of peritonitis/endotoxemia/septic shock. Cecal ligation and puncture were performed under sodium pentobarbital anesthesia (75 mg/kg, i.p.) in female BALB/c mice (16-20 g) that were then randomly assigned (15-17 mice per group) to receive at time 0 and 3 h later: control saline injections i.p., injections of α-MSH (100 μg), gentamicin sulfate (10 mg/kg), or both α-MSH and gentamicin. One ml of normal saline was given s.c. to each animal for fluid replacement. Both α-MSH and gentamicin treatments administered singly improved survival (approximately 40% at 48 h compared to 12% in saline treated controls); when given in combination survival was even greater (75%).

These data show that α-MSH can improve survival in experimental septic shock. It appears that the salutary effects of the peptide and of gentamicin can occur together. These findings suggest that the anticytokine α-MSH molecule might be useful for treatment of systemic inflammation, perhaps particularly when used in combination with agents that inhibit bacterial growth.

Acknowledgements

Supported by National Institute of Neurological and Communicative Disorders and Stroke Grant NS 10046 and NATO Collaborative Research Grant 900467.

References

1. Catania A, Lipton JM (1993) α-Melanocyte stimulating hormone in the modulation of host reactions. Endocr Rev 14: 564-576
2. Gallin JI, Goldstein IM, Snyderman R (1992) Inflammation: basic principles and clinical correlates. Raven, New York
3. Hiltz ME, Catania A, Lipton JM (1992) α-MSH peptides inhibit acute inflammation induced in mice by rIL-1, rIL-6, rTNF-α and endogenous pyrogen but not that caused by LTB4, PAF and rIL-8. Cytokine 4: 320-328
4. Mason MJ, Van Epps D (1989) Modulation of IL-1 tumor necrosis factor, and C5α-mediated murine neutrophil migration by α-melanocyte-stimulating hormone. J Immunol 142: 1646-1651
5. Simon RH, Ward PA (1992) Adult respiratory distress syndrome. In: Gallin JI, Goldstein IM, Snyderman R (eds.) Inflammation: basic principles and clinical correlates. Raven, New York, pp. 999-1016

Unreamed Femoral Nailing Reduces Lung Function Impairment and Increased Inflammatory Response in Polytrauma Patients

H.-C. Pape, A. Dwenger, D. Remmers, G. Regel

Introduction

Primary fixation of long bone fractures, preferably by intramedullary stabilization, represents an important principle in the treatment of multiply injured patients [1, 3]. However, it has recently been reported that there is an increased risk of pulmonary impairment if a reamed femoral nailing procedure is done in patients at high risk of adult respiratory distress syndrome (ARDS) [4, 6, 7]. The reaming process was thought to be responsible for the problems observed by causing a piston-like effect to the intramedullary cavity with subsequent intravasation of bone marrow fat [5]. We therefore investigated whether the effects of primary ($\leq$24 h) reamed vs. unreamed intramedullary femoral nailing on lung function are comparable in patients with multiple trauma.

Methods

The inclusion criteria were: (a) multiple trauma total ISS > 18 points; (b) no severe thoracic trauma (ISS $_{thorax}\leq$ 2) (c) midshaft femur fracture; primary ($\leq$ 24 hours) femur stabilization. There were two groups of patients. Group RFN was submitted to femoral nailing after reaming of the medullary canal (standard AO). In group UFN a small diameter, solid nail was inserted without reaming.
The following parameters were evaluated:
1. Lung function: oxygen ratio (PaO_2/FiO_2)
2. Pulmonary hemodynamics: pulmonary artery pressure (mmHg)
3. Polymorphonuclear leukocyte mediator: elastase (μg/l)
4. Coagulation: platelet count (x 1000/ml)

Statistics

A paired and unpaired t test with a significance level $p < 0.05$ was used to evaluate the intra- and intergroup differences.

Results

Group UFN ($n = 31$) had a mean ISS of 25.0 points and group RFN ($n = 28$) had a mean ISS of 24.1 points. Lung function remained stable in UFN patients but deteriorated in RFN patients from 353 ± 24 (PaO$_2$/FiO$_2$) preoperatively to 260 ± 28 (PaO$_2$/FiO$_2$) postoperatively ($p < 0.05$) (Fig. 1).

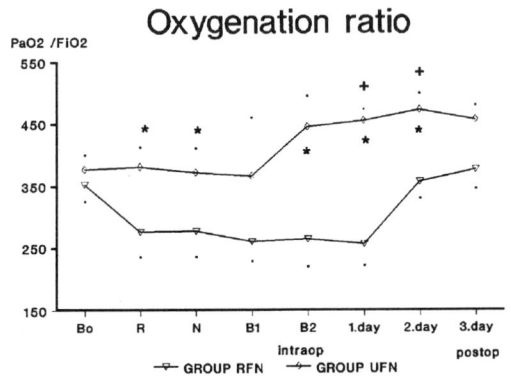

Fig. 1: Perioperative change of oxygenation in patients undergoing the intramedullary stabilization for a femoral shaft fracture. RFN, reamed femoral nailing; UFN, unreamed femoral nailing

Pulmonary artery pressure (Pap) did not change during surgery in UFN patients. In RFN patients Pap increased from 27.2 ± 3.1 mmHg preoperatively to 36.3 ± 4.1 mmHg ($p < 0.05$) upon reaming and normalized 1 h following insertion of the nail (Fig. 2).

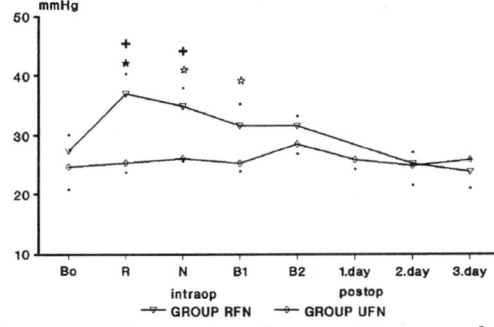

Fig. 2: Intraoperation pressure increase in patients receiving reamed femoral nailing

Total platelet count showed no change in the UFN group but dropped transiently in the RFN group (Fig. 3).
Serum elastase levels were determined from central venous blood and showed no significant change from baseline in UFN patients, whereas in RFN patients a significant increase from baseline was measured (Fig. 4).

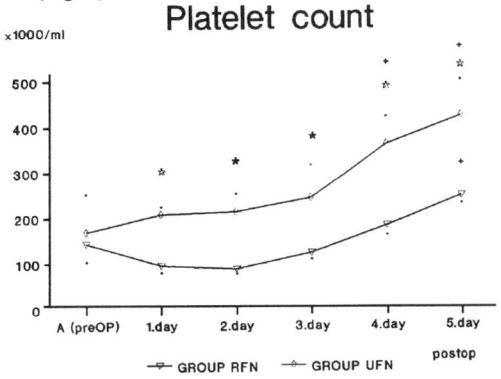

Fig. 3: Deterioration of platelet count was significantly worse in patients submitted to reamed femoral nailing

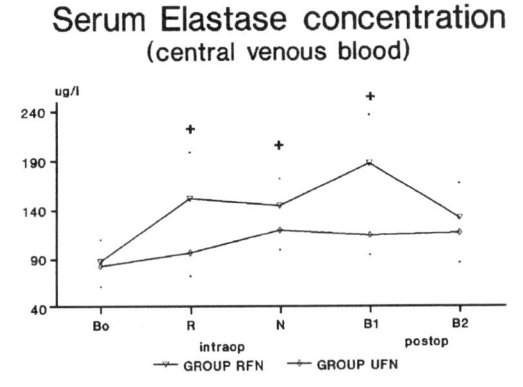

Fig. 4: Only in patients submitted to reamed femoral nailing an increase in elastase concentration was measured

Conclusions

Our results revealed a transient disturbance of pulmonary function along with activation of neutrophils and impairment of the coagulation system in RFN patients only. These changes were not seen in patients undergoing the unreamed procedure.
Femoral nailing after reaming represents a potential risk with respect to lung function disturbances. This might trigger the development of ARDS especially in patients prone to

this complication (additional lung contusion, borderline patients). For ethical reasons, these high risk patients were not included in the present study. Exclusion of these patients might partly explain why the changes seen were transient - in borderline patients a higher rate of ARDS might have been present.

In summary, in borderline patients, unreamed femoral nailing might offer an alternative by allowing primary intramedullary stabilization without the risk of adverse effects to the lung.

References

1. Bone LB, Johnson KD, Weigelt J et al. (1989) Early versus delayed stabilization of fractures - a prospective randomized study. J Bone Joint Surg (Am) 71-A 3: 336
2. Dwenger A, Regel G (1986) Pathomechanisms of the adult respiratory distress syndrome (ARDS) - chemiluminescence analysis of polymorphonuclear leukocytes. Fresenius Z Anal Chem 324: 360-361
3. Johnson KD, Codambi A, Seibert GB (1985) Incidence of ARDS in patients with multiple musculoskeletal injuries: effect of early operative stabilization of fractures. J Trauma 25: 375-384
4. Nast-Kolb D, Waydhas Ch, Jochum M et al. (1990) Günstigster Operationszeitpunkt für die Versorgung von Femurschaftfrakturen bei Polytrauma? Chirurg 61: 259-265
5. Pape H-C, Auf'm'Kolk M, Paffrath T et al. (1993) Primary intramedullary fixation in polytrauma patients with associated lung contusion - a cause of posttraumatic ARDS? J Trauma 34: 540-548
6. Pape H-C, Regel G, Tscherne H (1994) Der "Borderline patient" - Beeinflussung der Prognose des polytraumatisierten Patienten durch den Operationszeitpunkt der Sekundäroperation? Hefte Unfallheilkunde 232: 86-88
7. Wenda K, Ritter G, Degreif J et al. (1988) Zur Genese pulmonaler Komplikationen nach Marknagelosteosynthesen. Unfallchirurg 91: 432-435

Evidence for Involvement of IL-8 in Lung Injury after Esophagectomy

K. Sakamoto, H. Arakawa, T. Ishiko, S. Mita, M. Ogawa

Decreased oxygenation developing after major surgery was thought to be due to hypoventilation, blood shunting in the lung or low ventilation/blood flow ratio. In patients undergoing esophagectomy with a right thoracotomy and extensive lymphadenectomy, a major operation with much associated surgical stress, and whose respiration after surgery is supported by mechanical ventilation, lung injury, characterized by decreased oxygenation is often observed on the second to fourth postoperative day. However, in the absence of obvious complications such as pneumonia, heart failure, overhydration, atelectasis, pneumothorax or hypoventilation, the mechanism causing the lung injury remains unclear. Among the cytokines, interleukin-8 (IL-8) has been shown to be the most powerful neutrophil chemoattractant and activator in vitro [1] and in vivo [2, 3]. Hence IL-8 may have a crucial role in the development of lung injury after esophagectomy.

Here, we elucidate the involvement of IL-8 in the deterioration of pulmonary oxygenation after esophagectomy.

Postoperative Change in Pulmonary Oxygenation after Esophagectomy

The alveolar-arterial oxygen tension difference ($AaDO_2$) was serially measured in 17 patients to evaluate the deterioration of pulmonary oxygenation after surgery. Without exception, the $AaDO_2$ in all patients deteriorated postoperatively (Fig. 1). The mean $AaDO_2$ was lower (235 ± 15 mmHg) just after surgery and increased steadily afterward to reach a maximum (327 ± 23 mmHg) on the third postoperative day. Then, the mean $AaDO_2$ decreased gradually (Table 1). Thus pulmonary oxygenation deteriorated without any obvious complication after esophagectomy.

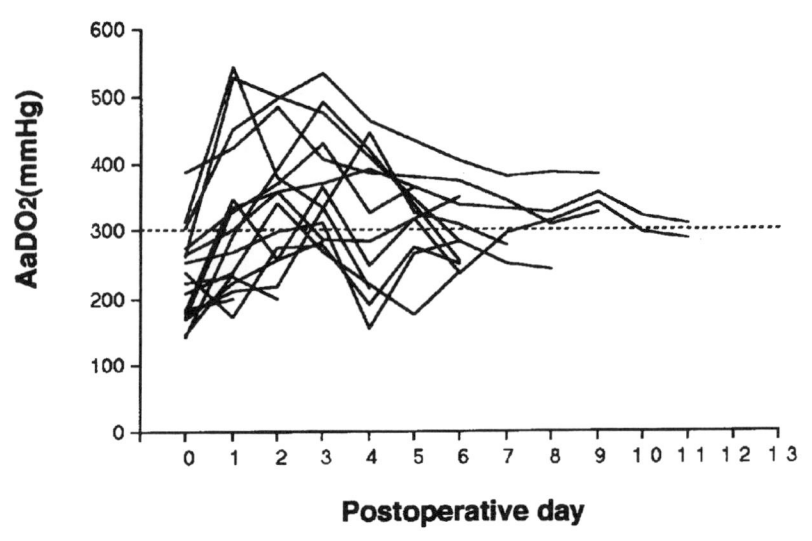

Fig. 1: Postoperative changes in AaDO2 in 17 patients who underwent esophagectomy

Table 1: Postoperative change in mean $AaDO_2$ in 17 patients who underwent esophagectomy

	Postoperative day						
	1	2	3	4	5	6	7
Mean $AaDO_2$ (mmHg)	310±33	344±24	372±23	304±33	348±32	290±30	309±25
Incidence of peak $AaDO_2$	35% (6)	17% (3)	35% (6)	11% (2)	0 (0)	0 (0)	0 (0)

$AaDO_2$, alveolar-arterial oxygen tension difference; Parentheses indicate the number of patients in whom the $AaDO_2$ value reached a peak

Postoperative Changes in Leukocyte/Neutrophil Elastase and Interleukin-8 in the Lung

The strong neutrophil chemoattractant and activator activities of IL-8 [1] and the involvement of neutrophil elastase (NE) in the pathogenesis of lung injury [4] led us to investigate whether neutrophils are recruited to the lung and activated and whether IL-8 levels are increased in the lung after surgery.

Bronchoalveolar lavage fluid (BALF) samples from the 17 patients were obtained from a single segment (S_4 or S_5) of the right and left lung through a flexible fiber optic bronchoscope. The total cell count on the third day was about threefold greater ($2983 \pm 853 \times 10^3$ cells/ml). The number of neutrophils detected on the first day ($123 \pm 54 \times 10^3$ cells/ml) was markedly increased by about tenfold ($1561 \pm 477 \times 10^3$ cells/ml) on the third day. Alveolar macrophages were predominant on the first day but increased only slightly ($1413 \pm 478 \times 10^3$

cells/ml) by the third postoperative day. Thus, the proportion of neutrophils increased from 10% to 50% by the third day, while that of alveolar macrophages decreased from 80% to 50% (Fig. 2). These results indicate that the increase in total cell count was attributed to neutrophils. Similar results were observed in both the right and left lungs.

The concentration of NE in BALF rose and reached a maximum level on the third day in both the right and left lungs (right, 1636 ± 662 µg/l; left, 1554 ± 772 µg/l). On the third day, elevated NE (more that 164 µg/l) was found in 80% of the right lung samples and 70% of the left lung samples. Furthermore, a high NE level (more than 500 µg/l) was seen in 53% (range:

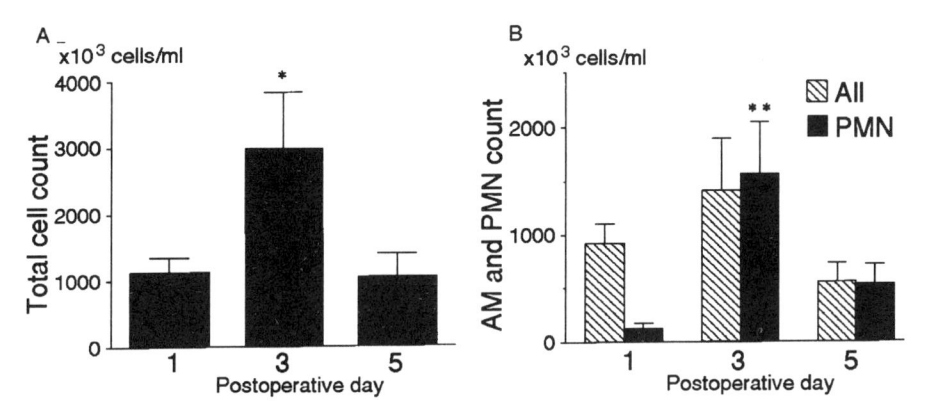

*Fig. 2 a, b: Postoperative change in bronchoalveolar lavage fluid (BALF) count in patients who underwent esophagectomy. A Total cell count; B alveolar macrophage (AM) and polymorphonuclear leukocyte (PMA) count; *p < 0.05 compared to the value on the first postoperative day; **p < 0.01 compared to the value on the first postoperative day*

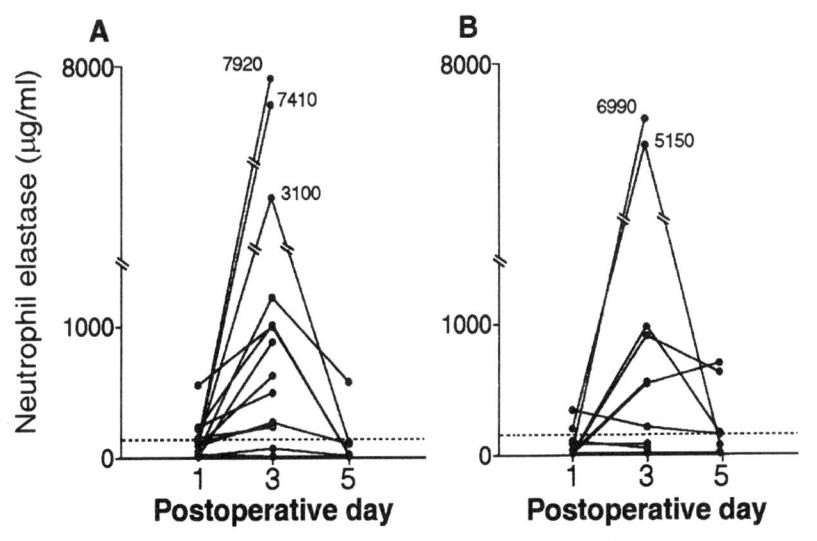

Fig. 3 a, b: Postoperative change in the concentration of neutrophil elastase in bronchoalveolar lavage fluid (BALF) in patients who underwent esophagectomy. a Right lung; b left lung

630 - 7920 µg/l) of the right lung BALFs and in 60% (range: 550 - 6990 µg/l) of the left lung BALFs (Fig. 3).

In most of the patients examined, the concentration of IL-8 in BALF also increased and reached a maximum level (right: 2149 ± 825 pg/ml, left: 2769 ± 1206 pg/ml) on the third day as did the NE level and the neutrophil count in both the right and left lungs. On the third day, IL-8 (> 96 pg/ml) was detected in 100% of the right lung samples and in 100% of the left lung samples. An even greater level (more than 1000 pg/ml) was detected in 62% (range: 1028 - 5575 pg/ml) and in 60% (range: 4470 - 6000 pg/ml) of the right and left lung BALFs, respectively. A high IL-8 level was seen only in the right lung on the first day in two patients (6000 pg/ml and 1000 pg/ml) (Fig. 4). This is probably due to the direct injury caused by the operative procedure since the right lung is the operative side. In contrast, IL-1β, tumor necrosis factor-α (TNF-α), and IL-6 could not be detected in BALF during the course examined.

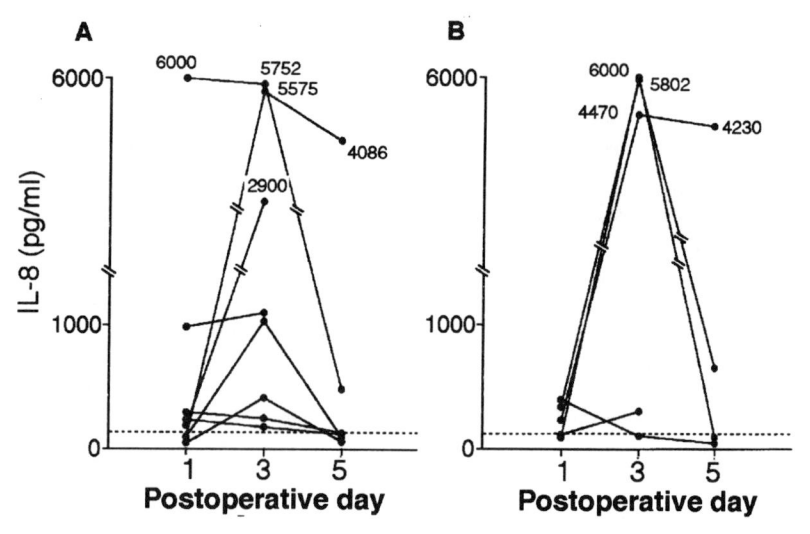

Fig. 4 a, b: Postoperative change in the concentration of interleukin-8 (IL-8) in bronchoalveolar lavage fluid (BALF) in patients who underwent esophagectomy. a Right lung; b left lung

Thus elevated concentrations of neutrophils, NE and IL-8 were observed on the third postoperative day in both the right and left lungs, indicating that these phenomena do not originate from direct trauma to the lung.

Correlations among Interleukin-8, Neutrophil Elastase, Neutrophil Count and $AaDO_2$

It is important to learn how neutrophils are recruited to the lung and how they accumulate there and are activated. Thus, we studied the relationship between IL-8, NE, and neutrophil count. There were significant relationships among the neutrophil count, NE and IL-8 in all

BALF samples evaluated. A significant correlation was found between the concentrations of IL-8 and NE ($r = 0.836$, $p = 0.0001$). The neutrophil count correlated with the concentration of both NE ($r = 0.678$, $p = 0.0001$) and IL-8 ($r = 0.552$, $p = 0.0007$). There were also significant correlations between AaDO2 values and the neutrophil count ($r = 0.572$, $p=0.0018$), and the concentration of NE ($r = 0.421$, $p = 0.0105$), or IL-8 ($r = 0.337$, $p=0.0234$). In contrast to the BALF neutrophil count, however, there was no significant correlations between alveolar macrophage count and the concentrations of IL-8 and NE, or the AaDO2 values (data not shown).

In conclusion, major surgical trauma such as esophagectomy may induce recruitment of neutrophils to the lung and cause lung injury. IL-8 is increased in the lung and is an important mediator of neutrophil recruitment and activation in the lung.

References

1. Yoshimura T, Matsushima K, Tanaka S, Robin SE, Appella E, Oppenheim JJ, Leonard EJ (1987) Purification of a human monocyte-derived neutrophil chemotactic factor that has peptide sequence similarity to other host defense cytokines. Proc Natl Acad Sci USA 84: 9233-9237
2. Colditz I, Zwahlen R, Dewald B, Baggiolini M (1989) In vivo inflammatory activity of neutrophil activating factor, a novel chemotactic peptide derived from human monocytes. Am J Pathol 134: 755-760
3. Rampart M, Damme JV, Zonnekeyn L, Herman AG (1989) Granulocyte chemotactic protein/interleukin-8 induce plasma leakage and neutrophil accumulation in rabbit skin. Am J Pathol 135: 21-25
4. Tanaka H, Sugimoto H, Yoshioka T, Sugimoto T (1991) Role of granulocyte elastase in tissue injury in patients with septic shock complicated by multiple-organ failure. Ann Surg 213: 81-85

Ischemia/Hypoxia-Induced Cell Damage Mediated by Enhanced Receptor-Ligand Interaction of Tumor Necrosis Factor-Alpha (TNF-α)

H. Gerlach, M. Gerlach, T. Kerner, C. Heid, S. Seiler, D. Keh, K.J. Fulke, J. Falke

Introduction

Hypoxemia is a frequent feature of disorders of the circulating system, especially those associated with ischemic organ failure as seen during septic events. Periods of ischemia followed by reperfusion produce endothelial damage and tissue edema in peripheral organs. This damage requires the vascular adherence and migration of neutrophils, which are activated after ischemia during the reperfusion phase, producing oxygen radicals at the surface of the vascular endothelial cells, thus causing the junctional complexes between adjacent cells to become more permeable to plasma proteins. After adherence of the neutrophils, combined with endothelial cell edema and "ruffling," vascular resistance and microvascular filtration pressure increases, promoting edema, insufficient microperfusion and organ failure [1].

The macrophage-derived cytokine tumor necrosis factor-α (TNF-α) plays a central role in the regulation of endothelial cell physiology. TNF-α was shown to mediate symptoms such as hypotension, disseminated intravascular coagulation, and multiple organ failure during septic shock [12]. TNF-α is able to influence endothelial cell physiology in order to enhance permeability, and to induce procoagulant while suppressing cell surface anticoagulant activity [5-7]. Together with the promotion of leukocyte adhesion, these mechanisms contribute to perivascular inflammation and edema, which finally ends in deterioration of microcirculation and in organ dysfunction.

Considering the pathophysiology of ischemia/reperfusion-induced vascular damage, the interaction of cytokines with endothelial cells, and concomitant clinical findings demonstrating elevated cytokine levels in hypoxic patients as well as in experimental ischemia/reperfusion models [3], the question arose whether TNF-α contributes to the pathogenesis of deteriorating organ function after ischemia/reperfusion periods, which had been ascribed to direct cellular damage.

Hypoxia and TNF

The effects of low concentrations of oxygen on cellular functions are quite complex, including changes in a spectrum of cellular properties ranging from redirection of protein synthesis with the expression of oxygen-regulated proteins to the production of α_1-adrenergic receptors and mitogens/inhibitors for smooth muscle growth. Thus, concomitant with the well-known hypoxia-mediated enhancement of glycolysis and suppression of aerobic metabolism, biosynthetic processes and changes in receptor expression are set into motion which can actively modulate cellular phenotype.

Of the many changes in homeostatic mechanisms in hypoxia, two are of particular clinical importance: increased vascular permeability and a prothrombotic tendency [10]. These effects are also induced by TNF-α [2], and further studies could demonstrate that the specific binding of TNF-α to the endothelial cell is a crucial regulatory factor [4]. It was shown that hypoxia induces enhanced binding of TNF-α to specific receptors on the endothelial cell surface in a time- and dose-dependent manner (Figs. 1-3) [8]. Hypoxia is able to modulate receptor affinity; this was demonstrated for α_1-adrenergic receptors on cardiac monocytes, probably mediated by specific long-chain acylcarnitines [9]. Whereas this seems to be a unique mechanism for myocytes, the effect of low environmental oxygen tension on the endothelial cell physiology is probably more unspecific. Several studies demonstrated that oxygen regulates endothelial cell growth and permeability. Together with our own findings of a correlation between growth and TNF-α receptor affinity [4], these data lead to the hypothesis that enhanced TNF-α binding of endothelial cells during hypoxia is a secondary effect due to perturbed integrity of the endothelial monolayer followed by biochemical conversion of the TNF-α receptor protein from the low-affinity to the high-affinity state. The molecular base for this conversion cannot be defined by the present studies, but other groups found that for TNF-α receptors as well as for other cytokine receptors, post-translational phosphorylation of the binding protein by intracellular kinases is crucial for regulation of receptor affinity [11]. At least, neither xanthine dehydrogenase/xanthine oxidase-dependent mechanisms nor de novo protein synthesis is involved in upregulation of receptor affinity, as shown by experiments with blocking agents.

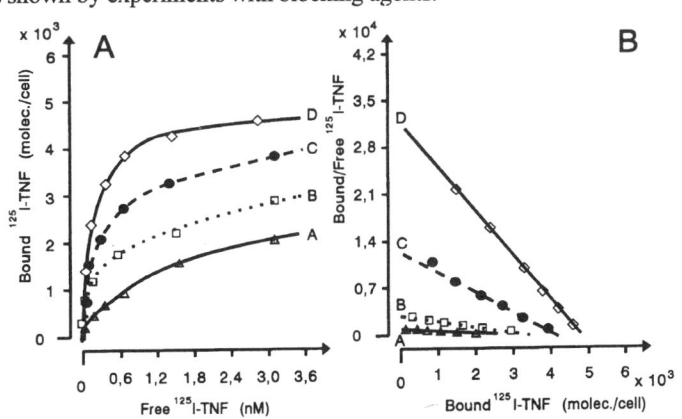

Fig. 1 a, b: TNF-α binding to endothelial cells after a 12-h hypoxia. a, Normotoxic control cells: B, 14% O_2; C 8% O_2; D, 2% O_2; a, original binding curves. b, Scatchard plot. Hypoxia changes affinity and number of binding sites for TNF-α in a significant manner (ANOVA: $p < 0.05$)

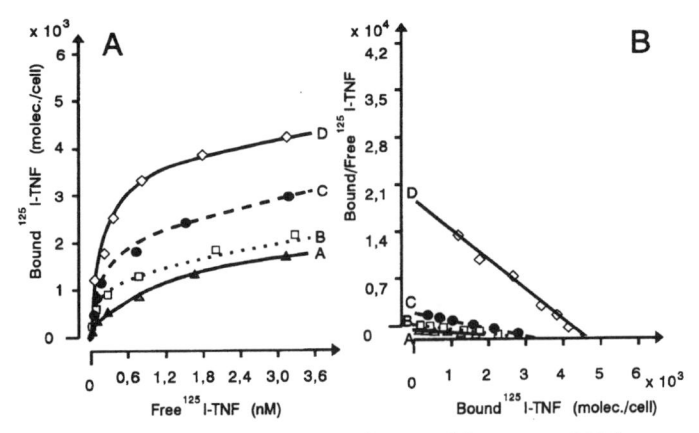

Fig. 2 a, b: TNF-α binding to endothelial cells after a 12-h hypoxia and 12-h reoxygenation. a, Normotoxic control cells: B, 14% O_2; C, 8% O_2; D, 2% O_2; a, original binding curves. b, Scatchard plot. Hypoxia changes affinity and number of binding sites for TNF-α in a significant

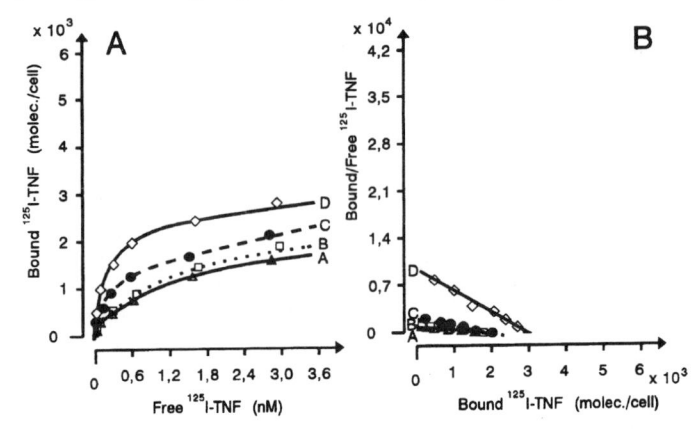

Fig. 3 a, b: TNF binding to endothelial cells after a 12-h hypoxia and 24-h reoxygenation. a, Normotoxic control cells: B, 14% O_2; C, 8% O_2; D, 2% O_2; a, original binding curves. b, Scatchard plot. Hypoxia changes affinity and number of binding sites for TNF-α in a significant manner (ANOVA: $p<0.05$)

Reoxygenation and TNF

In vitro studies with human monocytes showed that a hypoxic atmosphere is not able to induce synthesis or release of TNF-α, whereas reoxygenation after hypoxia initiated a significant increase in TNF-α [8]. The molecular mechanisms for these phenomena are mostly unclear, but there is at least one pathway which was found to play a central role in the pathogenesis of oxygen radical-dependent mechanisms: the xanthine dehydrogenase/xanthine oxidase pathway. Hypoxia and/or ischemia were found to inhibit the cellular Ca^{2+} pump, which is followed by an increase in intracellular Ca^{2+} and in unspecific protease activity; the proteases convert the enzyme xanthine dehydrogenase (XD) to xanthine oxidase

(XO). In this way, nucleotide metabolism is influenced: instead of OH⁻ ions as degradation product, O_2^- ions appear during oxidation of hypoxanthine to xanthine, which - after a biochemical cascade generating free O_2 radicals - initiates activation of lipid peroxidases and gene-regulating proteases, and inhibits second messenger systems such as cyclic nucleotides (cAMP) during subsequent reperfusion or reoxygenation periods, thus leading to membrane disintegration and a changed pattern of intracellular protein synthesis. This mechanism seems to be involved in upregulation of cytokine synthesis and expression, since several drugs (superoxide dismutase, catalase, pentoxifylline, cycloheximide), each of which is blocking XD/XO-dependent induction of protein synthesis on a different level, were shown to reduce induction of TNF-α and IL-1 synthesis during reoxygenation.

Clinical Consequences

The relevance of the interaction between cytokines and oxygen tension is emphasized by results from animal studies: experiments demonstrated a synergism between hypoxia and septic shock in respect of lethality [8]. LPS was used as a lethal drug, and hypoxia shifted the virtual dose-response curve to the left, i.e., the LD_{50} of LPS under normoxic conditions is higher than under hypoxic conditions. Considering pathogenesis of LPS-induced septic shock, which is mediated by TNF-α, the results underline the hypothesis that low oxygen tension leads to enhanced sensitivity of target cells for TNF-α. Furthermore, it was shown that the use of specific antisera against TNF-α in animals is able to reduce the ischemia/reperfusion-induced tissue damage significantly [10]. Initial clinical studies with anti-TNF-α antisera is patients seem to underline a protective effect. The possible relevance of these findings for future application in diagnostics and therapy is emphasized by several reports from other groups: especially for protection of reoxygenation/reperfusion injuries, e.g., during transplantations, the importance of cytokine-dependent mechanisms was recognized, and the clinical use of blocking agents such as pentoxifylline, applied successfully in in vitro as well as in in vivo models, is under discussion [13]. The question whether these agents might also help to improve the tolerance of inner organs against hypoxic damage cannot be answered so far.

Conclusions

Hypoxia and reoxygenation as a main characteristic of both ischemia and reperfusion are able to induce many changes in the biology of cells, including the enhanced synthesis of proteins. Synthesis and expression of cytokines such as TNF-α, followed by specific cytokine-target cell interaction, are a main characteristic of the so-called host response. The possible involvement of cytokines in hypoxia-related alterations of cell and organ function implies an influence of the environmental oxygen tension on the pathogenesis of host response. This might take place at the level of cytokine synthesis and expression, which means that hypoxia and/or reoxygenation stimulate monocytes to induce cytokine synthesis, or at the level of cytokine-target cell interaction, i.e., hypoxia and/or reoxygenation either regulate the sensitivity of target cells for cytokines or exert an amplifying effect on the target cell-derived reaction on cytokines.

It was demonstrated that isolated human monocytes respond to varying environmental oxygen tensions by induction of synthesis and expression of TNF-α. The induction does not take place under continuous normoxic or hypoxic conditions, but is recorded after reoxygenation following a hypoxic phase. De novo synthesis of TNF-α is necessary, and oxygen radicals obviously play an important role, since addition of "scavenger" drugs significantly reduces cytokine expression. Hypoxia, in contrast, induces enhanced binding of TNF-α to specific receptors on the endothelial cell surface in a time- and dose-dependent manner by a mechanism which is not dependent on oxygen radicals.

In conclusion, the proposed involvement of cytokine-dependent pathways in pathogenesis of organ dysfunction and multiple organ failure after hypoxia/ischemia and reoxygenation/reperfusion may provide a basis for understanding the initiation of hypoxic vascular injury, as manifested by an increased permeability and prothrombotic tendency. Future in vitro and in vivo studies should facilitate the identification and elevation of protective agents, which may ultimately prove useful in clinical medicine, and thus merit further attention.

References

1. Adkins WK, Taylor AE (1990) Role of xanthine oxidase and neutrophils in ischemia-reperfusion injury in rabbit lung. J Appl Physiol 69: 2012-2018
2. Brett J, Gerlach H, Nawroth P, Steinberg S, Godman G, Stern D (1989) Tumor necrosis factor/cachectin increases permeability of endothelial cell monolayers by a mechanism involving regulatory G proteins. J Exp Med 169: 1977-1991
3. Colletti LM, Remick DG, Burtch GD, Kunkel SL, Strieter RM, Campbell DA Jr (1990) Role of tumor necrosis factor-alpha in the pathophysiologic alterations after hepatic ischemia/reperfusion injury in the rat. J Clin Invest 85: 1936-1943
4. Gerlach H, Lieberman H, Bach R, Godman G, Brett J, Stern D (1989) Enhanced responsiveness of endothelium in the growing/motile state to tumor necrosis factor/cachectin. J Exp Med 170: 913-1931
5. Gerlach H, Esposito C, Stern D (1990) Modulation of endothelial hemostatic properties: an active role in the host response. Annu Rev Med 41: 15-24
6. Gerlach H, Clauss M, Ogawa S, Stern D (1992) Modulation of endothelial coagulant properties and barrier function by factors in the vascular environment. In: Simionescu N, Simionescu M (eds.) Endothelial cell dysfunction. Plenum, New York, pp. 525-545
7. Gerlach H, Clauss M, Ogawa S, Kao J, Ryan J, Stern D (1993) Cytokines and coagulation. In: Oppenheim JJ, Rossio JL, Gearing AJH (eds.) Clinical application of cytokines: role in pathogenesis, diagnosis and therapy. Oxford University Press, New York, pp. 293-300
8. Gerlach H, Gerlach M, Clauss M (1993) Relevance of tumor necrosis factor-α and interleukin-1-α in the pathogenesis of hypoxia-regulated organ failure. Eur J Anaesthesiol 10: 273-285
9. Heathers G, Yamada K, Kander E, Corr P (1987) Long-chain acylcarnitines mediate the hypoxia-induced increase in alpha$_1$-adrenergic receptors on adult canine myocytes. Circ Res 61: 735-746
10. Ogawa A, Gerlach H, Esposito C, Pasagian-Macaulay A, Brett J, Stern D (1990) Hypoxia modulates the barrier and coagulant function of cultured bovine endothelium. J Clin Invest 85: 1090-1098
11. Olson TS, Lane MD (1989) A common mechanism for posttranslational activation of plasma membrane receptors? FASEB 3: 1618-1624
12. Sherry B, Cerami A (1988) Cachectin/tumor necrosis factor exerts endocrine, paracrine and autocrine control of inflammatory responses. J Cell Biol 107: 1269-1277
13. Williams JH, Heshmati S, Tamadon S, Guerra J (1991) Inhibition of alveolar macrophages by pentoxifylline. Crit Care Med 19: 1073-1078

Pathomechanisms and Therapeutic Aspects of Pseudomonas Aeruginosa Cytotoxin-Induced Pulmonary Microvascular Injury: Studies on Isolated Perfused Rabbit Lungs

T. Koch, H.P. Duncker, J. Fisahn, F. Lutz, and H. Neuhof

Introduction

Bacterial sepsis and adult respiratory distress syndrome (ARDS) in critically ill patients is still linked with a high mortality rate [13, 17]. Although gram-negative aerobic rods are the predominant infectious agent, the course of ARDS is often complicated by nosocomial pneumonia caused by *Pseudomonas aeruginosa* [2, 12]. The lung seems to be the primary target organ for bacterial endo- and exotoxins. During the last decade intensive investigations have been made on endotoxins and on the development of specific antibodies, whereas very little is known about the pathophysiological impact of exotoxins and their therapeutic actions. Of the different *P. aeruginosa* exotoxins (e.g., toxin A), cytotoxin is regarded as an important virulence factor [5]. In vitro studies have shown that cytotoxin is released in micromolecular concentrations after phage conversion from various *P. aeruginosa* strains [10]. The toxin is an acidic protein with a molecular mass of 28 kDa, which primarily acts on a variety of target cell membranes to create discrete hydrophilic transmembrane pores [9, 20]. According to recent studies, the toxic effects of cytotoxin are initiated by the high affinity to binding sites of integral membrane proteins [7, 11]. The binding of cytotoxin to these channel proteins causes functional pores of approximately 1 nm radius, which increases the permeability for small molecules in mammalian cells. Subsequent pore-related calcium flux has been suggested as a primary trigger of cell-specific arachidonic acid (AA) metabolism as well as the release of histamine and lysosomal enzymes form neutrophils [6, 19]. Besides the direct cytotoxicity, the induction of proinflammatory mediators might thus distribute and amplify the toxic effects of this bacterial agent. The aim of this study was to evaluate the effects of cytotoxin on pulmonary vascular reaction and mediator release. In view of the prophylactic and therapeutic consequences the inhibitory effects of cyclooxygenase blocker and of the platelet-activating factor (PAF) antagonist WEB 2086 on cytotoxin-induced microvascular injury were tested in the isolated perfused rabbit lung. Furthermore, the kinetics of lipid mediator release and the development of pulmonary edema was studied after pretreatment with specific antibodies and unspecific immunoglobulins in the presence of cytotoxin.

Materials and Methods

The Lung Model

The techniques of preparing and perfusing isolated rabbit lungs
have been previously described in detail [8]. Standard breed rabbits of either sex weighing 3050±196 g (mean±SD) were anesthetized with pentobarbital sodium (60-80 mg/kg) and anticoagulated with heparin-sodium 1000 IU/kg body weight (BW). The isolated lungs were suspended from an electronic weight balance (Hottinger, Baldwin Meßtechnik Type U1, Darmstadt, FRG) in a tempered (37C) and humidified chamber, and were perfused with cell- and plasma-free Krebs-Henseleit-hydroxyethyl starch buffer solution (KHHB) at a constant flow of 200 ml/min in a recirculating system (circulating volume 200 ml). Ventilation was performed with 4% CO_2 in air [frequency 25/min, tidal volume 30 ml, positive end expiratory pressure (PEEP) 0.5-1.0 cm H_2O]. The pulmonary artery pressure (PAP), airway pressure (AP), and weight of the isolated lung, as parameters of edema formation, were recorded continuously. Initially, the lungs were perfused with KHHB solution, using low flow rates in the opened circulatory system to remove the remaining blood in the vascular bed. The perfusion fluid was then exchanged for fresh buffer via two separate perfusion circuits 2 min after the beginning of the extracorporeal circulation and 30 min later, after the flow was increased to 200 ml/min. The KHHB perfusion was able to maintain the integrity of the microcirculation for more than 5 h in our model, as verified by ultrastructural studies.

Experimental Protocol

Thirty-six lung preparations were randomly assigned to six groups of six each. Following a 30-min equilibration period, the first perfusate sample was drawn for measurements of baseline values. Thereafter, *P. aeruginosa* cytotoxin (approximately 0.4 mg/kg BW) was injected into the pulmonary artery, yielding a final concentration of 6 µg/ml in the perfusion fluid. Six of these experiments served as controls. Further samples were taken after 5, 15, 30, 60, and 120 min for determination of arachidonic acid metabolites, lactate dehydrogenase (LDH) and potassium concentrations. The same procedure was carried out in other experiments in which WEB 2086 (5×10^{-8} M, $n = 6$) or diclofenac (10 µg/ml, $n = 6$) was injected into the perfusion fluid 5 min prior to cytotoxin. Furthermore, the pretreatment with specific antitoxin (325 µg/ml, $n = 6$) and unspecific immunoglobulin (Venimmun, Behring) (7.5mg/ml, $n = 6$) as well as the combination of unspecific immunoglobulin, WEB 2086, and diclofenac ($n = 6$) was tested. The arterial pressure and the weight gain as an indicator for edema formation were continuously monitored during the 120-min perfusion phase. In additional pilot experiments, using the same protocol as described, effects on vascular resistance, permeability, and mediator release due to the various inhibitors ($n = 3$) and the immunoglobulin preparations (Venimmun, Behring, $n = 3$; antitoxin, $n = 3$) in the absence of *P. aeruginosa* cytotoxin could be excluded.

Radioimmunoassay of TXB$_2$ and 6-Keto PGF$_{1\alpha}$

Thromboxane B$_2$ (TXB$_2$) and 6-keto-PGF$_{1\alpha}$ were assayed serologically from 100 µl recirculating KHHB as stable hydrolysis products of thromboxane A$_2$ and prostacyclin by radioimmunoassay according to the method described by Peskar et al. [15]. Radioactivity was quantified with a Philips PW 4700 liquid scintillation counter. Results were obtained by standard constructed dose-response curves. The cross-reactivity of TXB$_2$ antiserum with prostaglandin D$_2$ was 2.7%, and 0.05% with 6-keto-PGF$_{1\alpha}$, PGE$_2$, PGE$_1$, PGF$_{1\alpha}$, 13,14-dihydro-15-keto PGE$_2$, and 13,14-dihydro-15-keto PGE$_{2\alpha}$ respectively. The cross-reactivity of 6-keto-PGF$_{1\alpha}$ antiserum was 0.05% with TXB$_2$ and the above-mentioned prostaglandins. *Potassium and lactate dehydrogenase (LDH)* were determined according to standard procedures.

Materials

A cell- and plasma-free perfusion medium was used in order to avoid the complex interactions with different circulating cells, which may have masked direct effects on vascular tone and mediator release. The perfusate consisted of a Krebs-Henseleit buffer solution with additional human albumin (Rhodalbumin 20%, Merieux, Leimen, FRG) in order to maintain a colloid oncotic pressure of between 23 and 25 mmHg, yielding final concentrations of albumin 20 g/l, Na$^+$ 138 mmol/l, K$^+$ 4.5 mmol/l, Mg^{2+} 1.33 mmol/l, Cl$^-$ 135mmol/l, Ca^{2+} 2.38 mmol/l, glucose 12 mmol/l, and HCO$_3$- 12 mmol/l. The osmolality was approximately 330 mosm/kg (Mikro-Osmometer, Roebling Meβtechnik, Berlin, FRG). The pH of the buffer solution was adjusted to 7.4 with 1 M NaHCO$_3$. The PAF antagonist WEB 2086 (C$_{22}$H$_{22}$ClN$_5$O$_2$S; mol. wt., 455.97) was a gift from Boehringer Ingelheim (Ingelheim, FRG). Diclofenac sodium (Voltaren) was purchased from Ciba-Geigy (Wehr, FRG). Rabbit anti-TXB$_2$ and rabbit anti-6-keto-PGF$_{1\alpha}$ were purchased from Paesel (Frankfurt, FRG), ^{3}H-labeled TXB$_2$ and ^{3}H-labeled-6-keto-PGF$_{1\alpha}$ from New England Nuclear (Dreieich, FRG), and goat anti-rabbit antibodies from Calbiochem-Behring (Frankfurt, FRG).

Preparation of Cytotoxin from P. aeruginosa

The cytotoxin was prepared from autolysate of *P. aeruginosa* strain 158 as described previously by [8a]. The preparation was free of lipid and carbohydrate moieties. No enzymatic activities of proteases, lipases, lecitinases, alkaline phosphatase, sphingomyelinase, phospholipase C and D, and ADP ribosyltransferase were detectable in the preparation. The toxin was about 98% pure as judged by sodium dodecyl sulfate-polyacrylamide gel electrophoresis. Portions of the toxin were stored at -20°C in phosphate-buffered saline (0.01 M sodium phosphate, 0.14 M sodium chloride, 0.003 M KCL, 0.001 M MgCl$_2$, pH 7.4).

Preparation of Antitoxin

Antibodies to cytotoxin were produced in rabbits and partially purified with ammonium sulfate and chromatography with DEAE cellulose. One milligram of antibodies inhibited the activity of 31±4 µg cytotoxin in the slide adhesion test ($n = 3$).

Statistical Analysis

Data are presented as means ± standard error of the mean (SEM). Differences between groups were tested by one-way analysis of variance (ANOVA) followed by an LSD multiple-comparison procedure. Significance was accepted at $p < 0.05$.

Results

Under baseline conditions, lung weight and vascular tone remained constant and only insignificant amounts of histamine or cyclooxygenase products of AA were detectable in the recirculating buffer. Injection of cytotoxin into the perfusion fluid caused a gradual increase in vascular resistance resulting in a maximum increase in PAP of 11 ± 1.9 mmHg 105 min after cytotoxin administration. PAP increased from 6.2 ± 0.5 (baseline value) up to 17 ± 2 mmHg (Fig. 1). The pressure reaction was accompanied by a delayed onset of edema formation, reaching a mean weight gain of 15.2 ± 3.04 g after 120 min. This was paralleled by a significant increase in prostacyclin generation and a continuous release of K^+ and LDH (Table 1). There was excessively enhanced thromboxane synthesis due to cytotoxin exposure resulting in final concentrations of 1133 ± 648 pg/ml. Pretreatment with WEB 2086 or diclofenac significantly ($p < 0.001$) attenuated the pressure response and edema formation evoked by cytotoxin (Figs. 1, 2). The generation of cyclooxygenase products was significantly reduced by administration of WEB 2086 and completely suppressed by administration of diclofenac prior to cytotoxin. Potassium and LDH, however, were only slightly reduced in the latter groups. The addition of the unspecific immunoglobulin preparation alone induced an acute transient pressure increase within the first 5 min (approximately 9 mmHg), but mean PAP values as well as the weight gain indicating edema formation remained below those of the control group in the continuing observation period (Fig. 3). In contrast to the previous groups LDH as a marker for cell lysis was significantly reduced in the presence of the immunoglobulins. Almost complete inhibition of the pressure reaction, the edema formation, and the metabolic alterations was achieved mainly by the combination of immunoglobulin, WEB 2086, and diclofenac and to a lesser extend by the specific toxin antibody (Figs. 3, 4).

Discussion

Pseudomonas aeruginosa cytotoxin seems to be a potent shock-producing agent which causes deleterious circulatory and metabolic effects comparable to those of endotoxin [14]. The current results demonstrate the effects of *P. aeruginosa* cytotoxin on lung vasculature and support the hypothesis that besides endotoxin other bacterial products, grouped as pore-formers [1], might be relevant for the development of septic organ failure. Since the purified cytotoxin was free of LPS [8a], effects due to endotoxin could be excluded. Circulatory disturbance and alterations in vascular resistance were found in various organs after intravenous injection of cytotoxin in rats [5]. The lung appears to be the predominant target organ for cytotoxin with respect to an early impairment of pulmonary gas exchange. The main effect of cytotoxin on pulmonary vasculature is the increase in vascular resistance with pulmonary hypertension and the enhanced permeability. Preliminary electron microscopic studies of cytotoxin-exposed rabbit lungs revealed an

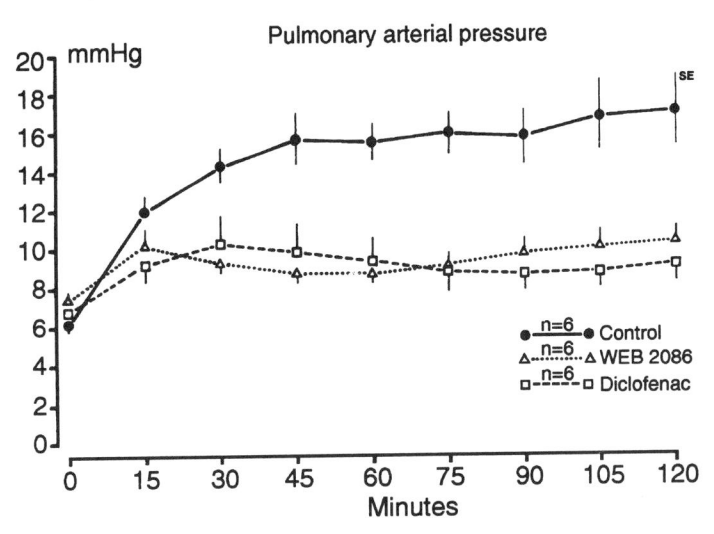

Fig. 1: Pulmonary arterial pressure (mean ± SE) following P. aeruginosa cytotoxin administration (6 μg/ml) in the absence (control, n = 6) and presence of inhibitors (diclofenac 10 μg/ml, n = 6 or WEB 2086 $5x10^{-8}$ M, n = 6). The cytotoxin-induced pressure increase was significantly attenuated by injection of diclofenac and WEB 2086 prior to cytotoxin administration ($p < 0.001$ vs. control at the time points 30-120 min, ANOVA)

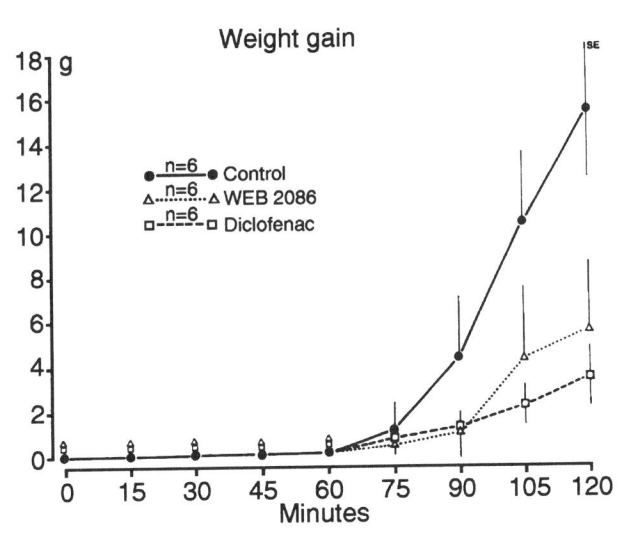

Fig. 2: Weight gain (mean ± SE) of the isolated lungs after cytotoxin administration in the control group (without inhibitors, n = 6) and after pretreatment with diclofenac (10 μg/ml, n=6) and WEB 2086 ($5x10^{-8}$ M, n = 6). Cytotoxin injection caused a delayed edema formation which was significantly reduced in the presence of diclofenac and WEB 2086 ($p<0.001$ at 120 min)

Table 1: Release of thromboxane B_2 (TXB_2) 6-keto-$PGF_{1\alpha}$, LDH, and potassium (K^+) into the perfusate after administration of P. aeruginosa (6 µg/ml) in the absence (control) or presence of inhibitors, respectively, after pretreatment with antitoxin or Venimmun and the combination of Venimmun, diclofenac, and WEB 2086. Data are means ± SEM.

Time (min) after cytotoxin (6 µg/ml)	Control (n=6)	Diclofenac 10 µg/ml (n=6)	WEB 2086 5×10^{-8} M (n=6)	Antitoxin 325 µg/ml (n=6)	Venimmun 7.5 mg/ml (n=6)	Venimmun + Diclofenac + WEB 2086 (n=6)
TXB_2 (pg/ml)						
0 (baseline)	25±5	ND	23±4	19±3	21±4	ND
5	77±16	ND	27±6	21±2	30±6	ND
15	87±18	ND	34±7	28±5	42±7	ND
30	182±62	ND	41±10**	36±7**	64±10	ND
60	612±101	ND	72±27**	57±19**	93±26**	ND
120	1133±648	ND	150±48**	136±33**	250±81*	ND
6-keto $PGF_{1\alpha}$ (pg/ml)						
0 (baseline)	176±26	82±4	107±14	52±25	103±8	89±3
5	191±32	96±5	111±11	74±16	145±15	77±8
15	221±40	100±4	125±18	113±14	181±16	76±4
30	357±106	102±6*	153±13	148±25	243±22	77±4*
60	588±125	58±21**	295±32*	225±31*	344±38	77±5**
120	1045±141	57±21**	597±54*	483±74*	827±163	83±5**
LDH (U/l)						
0 (baseline)	3±0.5	3±0.7	2±0.3	3±0.6	3±0.4	2±0.3
5	11±1.5	12±1.7	9±0.9	9±0.7	7±0.7	6±0.9
15	27±3.4	26±4.2	25±2.5	23±3.5	11±0.7**	13±1.9*
30	51±5.8	48±9.2	40±2.5	37±4.3	18±1.2**	22±3.7*
60	79±9.2	73±19	64±4.5	58±4.2	30±2.6**	38±5.4*
120	134±15.6	107±27	101±3.6	93±10.9	49±4.3**	58±8.2*
K^+ (mmol/l)						
0 (baseline)	4.56±0.09	4.43±0.1	4.54±0.05	4.49±0.01	4.41±0.01	4.61±0.05
5	4.79±0.08	4.83±0.18	4.82±0.1	4.69±0.05	4.86±0.07	4.92±0.07
15	5.17±0.08	4.89±0.19	5.22±0.06	5.11±0.07	5.19±0.12	5.19±0.11
30	5.53±0.1	5.29±0.22	5.31±0.15	5.25±0.08	5.49±0.05	5.44±0.11
60	5.76±0.14	5.44±0.17	5.56±0.11	5.36±0.05*	5.54±0.11	5.71±0.10
120	6.36±0.15	5.72±0.18*	5.84±0.11*	5.60±0.06**	5.84±0.12*	5.96±0.06*

ND not detectable; *$p<0.05$; **$p<0.001$ vs. control by ANOVA and consequential LSD multiple-range test.

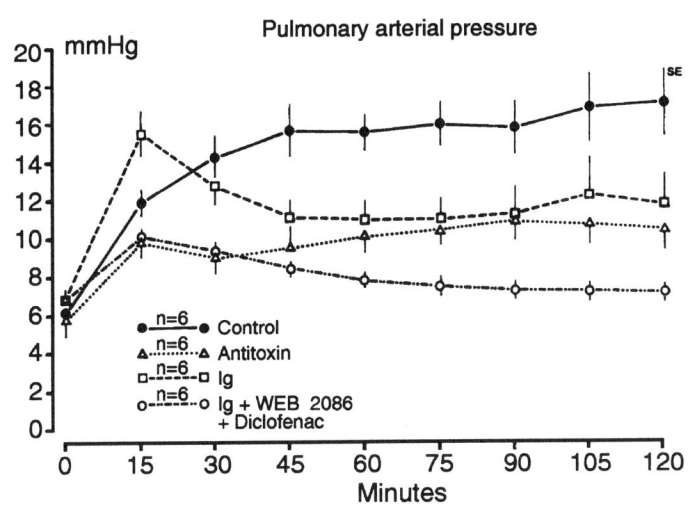

Fig. 3: Pulmonary arterial pressure after pretreatment with antitoxin (325 µg/ml, n = 6), unspecific immunoglobulin (Ig, 7.5 mg/ml, n = 6) and the combination of Ig, WEB 2086 and diclofenac (n = 6) compared with untreated controls (n = 6). Addition of the unspecific immunoglobulin preparation induced an acute transient pressure increase within the first 5 min (approximately 9 mmHg), but mean PAP values remained below those of the control group in the continuing observation period. Antitoxin and the combination of Ig, diclofenac and WEB 2086 significantly ($p<0.001$) suppressed the cytotoxin-induced pressure reaction

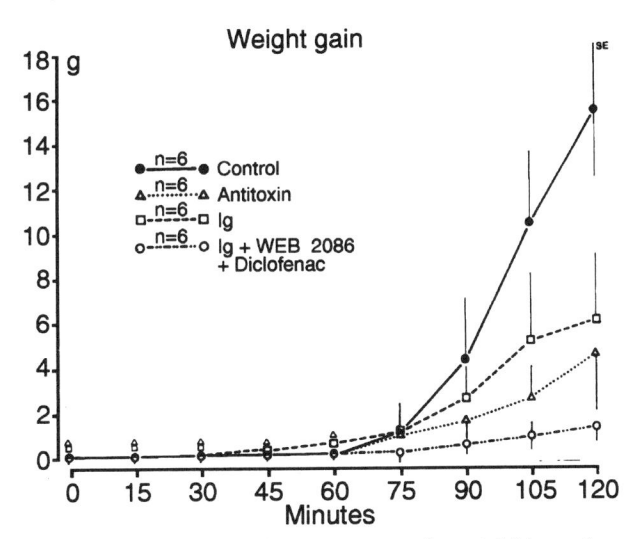

Fig. 4: Weight gain after cytotoxin administration without inhibitors (control) and after pretreatment with antitoxin, unspecific immunoglobulin (Ig), and the combination of Ig, diclofenac, and WEB 2086. Weight gain was significantly ($p < 0.001$) reduced by pretreatment with either antitoxin or Ig and almost completely prevented by the combination of Ig, diclofenac, and WEB 2086

excessive destruction of endothelial and epithelial cells and massive edema formation of the interstitial space, which correlate well with the impaired respiratory function. To what extend the pore-forming toxin directly activates smooth muscle cells of the pulmonary vessels by increasing Ca^{2+} influx, and whether other vasoconstrictors such as thromboxane and PAF are involved is unknown. The present study was designed to investigate the pathomechanisms of cytotoxin effects on lung vasculature. The concentration of P. aeruginosa cytotoxin used in the current experiments corresponds to those in other systems (range 5-50 µg/ml) [6, 14, 20], but is probably higher than it can be expected in the circulation in vivo. It has to be kept in mind, however, that far higher local concentrations must be expected to arise upon lung tissue invasion by this gram-negative rod, such as under conditions of nosocomial pneumonia with P. aeruginosa. According to previous experimental studies on lung and liver preparations [4, 18] there was a progressive increase in vascular resistance and an enhanced edema formation associated with an enhanced thromboxane generation after cytotoxin administration. Kinetics of lipid mediator release and inhibitory effects of cyclooxygenase blockers suggest a contributory role of these AA-derived products in the development of cytotoxin induced lung vascular injury. The protective effects of the PAF-receptor antagonist WEB 2086 provide evidence that PAF is also involved in cytotoxin-induced vascular reaction. In agreement with previous studies on isolated lungs [18], the acute pressure reaction within the first minutes, however, was not significantly attenuated by inhibition of both lipid mediators thus implicating an additional pathogenic mechanism. Since the initial effect of cytotoxin is a rapid increase in cell membrane permeability for water and small molecules, AA metabolism and PAF synthesis is presumably activated via secondary Ca^{2+} influx. This hypothesis was supported by the unaltered K^+ and LDH release after pretreatment with diclofenac and WEB 2086, which reflects an impaired cell integrity probably due to toxin-induced pore generation.

The high mortality rate of nosocomial infections, in spite of extended antibiotic therapy, has forced the development of immunological therapeutics. The use of specific antibodies in the case of bacterial infection was supported by the observation of an enhanced pulmonary clearance of P. aeruginosa in animals, which were systemically immunized with gram-negative organisms [3]. Furthermore, in previous studies it was shown that high serum titers of antibodies against P. aeruginosa could be correlated with a better outcome in patients [16]. Antibodies against cytotoxin were firstly used in recent animal studies [14] in which the cytotoxin-induced deleterious circulatory and metabolic effects and the lethal outcome could be successfully prevented. In the present study, the cytotoxin effects on vascular tone and permeability as well as LDH release were significantly suppressed by pretreatment of antitoxin or unspecific immunoglobulins, but complete inhibition of vascular reaction and metabolic alterations was achieved by the administration of immunoglobulins in combination with diclofenac and WEB 2086. The neutralization of cytotoxin prior to binding to the membrane channel proteins by specific or unspecific immunoglobulins might explain their protective effects. The activation of PAF and AA metabolites is presumably induced via cytotoxin-induced Ca^{2+} influx after transmembrane pore formation. In conclusion, cytotoxin may thus well contribute to the development of prolonged lung microvascular injury in states of P. aeruginosa sepsis or ARDS complicated by this infectious agent. The systemic or local administration of cytotoxin antibodies or even unspecific immunoglobulins in combination with PAF-antagonist and diclofenac appears to be a promising therapeutic approach in the case of infection with cytotoxin-producing strains.

References

1. Bhakdi S, Tranum-Jensen J (1988) Damage to cell membranes by pore-forming bacterial cytolysins. Prog Allergol 40: 1-43
2. Cryz SJ (1985) New insight into the epidemiology, pathogenesis and therapy of Pseudomonas aeruginosa infections. Eur J Clin Microbiol 4: 153-155
3. Dunn MM, Toews GB, Hart D, Pierce AK (1985) The effect of systemic immunization on pulmonary clearance of Pseudomonas aeruginosa. Am Rev Respir Dis 131: 426-431
4. Frimmer M, Scharmann W (1975) Toxicity of a highly purified leucocidin from Pseudomonas aeruginosa in perfused rat livers. Naunyn Schmiedebergs Arch Pharmacol 288: 123-132
5. Frimmer M, Neuhof H, Scharmann W, Schischke B (1976) Cardiovascular reactions induced by leukocidin from Pseudomonas aeruginosa. Naunyn Schmiedebergs Arch Pharmacol 294: 85-89
6. Grimminger F, Walmrath D, Walter H, Lutz F, Seeger W (1991) Induction of vascular injury by pseudomonas aeruginosa cytotoxin in rabbit lungs is associated with the generation of different leukotrienes and hydroxsyeicosatetraenoic acids. J Infec Dis 163: 362-370
7. Jungblut R, Grimmig M, Leidolf R, Lutz F (1992) Solubilization of the binding protein from Ehrlich ascites cells and erythrocytes to Pseudomonas aeruginosa cytotoxin. Biol Chem Hoppe Seyler 373: 93-100
8. Koch T, Duncker HP, Rosenkranz S, van Ackern K, Neuhof H (1992) Alterations of filtration coefficients in pulmonary edema of different pathogenesis. J Appl Physiol 73(6): 2396-2402
8a. Lutz F (1979) Purification of a cytotoxic protein from Pseudomonas aeruginosa. Toxicon 17: 467-475
9. Lutz F, Seeger W, Schischke B, Weiner R, Scharmann W (1989) Effects of a cytotoxic protein from Pseudomonas aeruginosa on phagocytic and pinocytic cells: In vitro and in vivo studies. Toxicon 3 Suppl: 257-260
10. Lutz F, Alberti U, Leidolf R, Weiss R (1989) Enzyme-linked immunosorbent fluorescence assay for quantitating the cytotoxin production by clinical Pseudomonas aeruginosa isolates. Naunyn Schmiedebergs Arch Pharmacol 339: R19
11. Lutz F, Mohr M, Grimmig M, Leidolf R, Linder D (1993) Pseudomonas aeruginosa cytotoxin-binding protein in rabbit erythrocyte membranes. An oligomer of 28 kDa with similarity to transmembrane channel proteins. Eur J Biochem 217: 1123-1128
12. McManus AT, Mason AD, McManus WF, Pruitt BA (1985) Twenty-five-year review of Pseudomonas bacteremia in a burn center. Eur J Clin Microbiol 4: 219-223
13. Montgomery AB, Stager MA, Carrico CJ, Hudson LD (1985) Causes of mortality in patients with the adult respiratory distress syndrome. Am Rev Respir Dis 132: 485-489
14. Neuhof H, Lutz F, Meier E, Reichwein A, Koch T, Duncker HP (1996) Systemic and pulmonary response to pseudomonas aeruginosa cytotoxin in rabbits and its prevention by specific antibodies. Appl Cardiopulm Pathophysiol (in press)
15. Peskar BA, Steffens C, Peskar PM (1979) Radioimmunoassay of 6-keto-prostaglandin F1-alpha in biological material. In: DaPrada M, Peskar BA (eds.) Radioimmunoassay of drugs and hormones in cardiovascular medicine. Elsevier/North-Holland, Amsterdam, pp. 239-248

16. Pollack M, Young LS (1979) Protective activity of antibodies to exotoxin A and lipopolysaccharide at the onset of Pseudomonas aeruginosa septicemia in man. J Clin Invest 63: 276-286
17. Rinaldo JE, Roger RM (1986) Adult respiratory distress syndrome. N Engl J Med 315: 578-579
18. Seeger W, Walmrath D, Neuhof H, Lutz F (1986) Pulmonary microvascular injury induced by Pseudomonas aeruginosa cytotoxin in isolated rabbit lungs. Infect Immun 52: 846-852
19. Suttorp N, Seeger W, Uhl J, Lutz F, Roka L (1985) Pseudomonas aeruginosa cytotoxin stimulates prostacyclin production in cultured pulmonary artery endothelial cells: membrane attack and calcium influx. J Cell Physiol 123: 64-72
20. Suttorp N, Hessz T, Seeger W, Wilke A, Koob R, Lutz F, Drenckhahn D (1988) Bacterial exotoxins and endothelial permeability for water and albumin in vitro. Am J Physiol 255: C368-C376

Inhaled Nitric Oxide in Acute Lung Injury

R. Rossaint, H. Gerlach, R. Kuhlen, K. Falke

Introduction

In 1980, Furchgott and Zawadski [8] reported that vascular endothelium is involved in the regulation of the tone of vascular smooth muscle cells. They demonstrated that acetylcholine only dilates arteries if the endothelium of the arteries is intact. The authors postulated that the vasodilation must be mediated by an unstable humoral factor, later known as the endothelium-derived relaxing factor (EDRF). In 1987, two independent research groups published results which implied that nitric oxide (NO) accounts for the vasodilatatory action of EDRF [15, 25]. This gas, previously considered to be merely an atmospheric pollutant, is synthesized in mammalian cells by oxidation of one of the two terminal guanidino nitrogen atoms of L-arginine. Subsequent division of the oxidized L-arginine into NO and citrulline occurs [25, 26]. This process is endothelial cell calcium- and calmodulin-dependent, and is catalyzed by an enzyme, termed "intrinsic" or "constitutive" NO synthase [20-22]; pulsatile flow characteristics [28] and shear stress [32] stimulate the generation of NO by this NO synthase. Due to the lipophilic characteristic of the formed NO, it rapidly diffuses from the vascular endothelium to vascular smooth muscles. In smooth muscle cells NO acts locally by activating soluble guanulate cyclase and, thereby, the gas produces smooth muscle relaxation [3]. Whereas normal blood pressure homeostasis is dependent on this basal NO synthesis [29, 34], inappropriate vasodilation or shock may occur due to cytokine- or endotoxine-induced overproduction of NO [12, 16, 23], which then is produced by an isoform of the NO synthase, the "inducible" NO synthase.

In contrast to septic shock with overproduction of NO, pulmonary hypertension in patients with acute lung injury and with chronic obstructive lung disease, and in newborns with primary pulmonary hypertension may be diseases associated with a relative or absolute lack of endogenous NO production within the pulmonary vasculature.

Physiology of Inhaled NO

In humans, NO is produced by the upper respiratory tract as demonstrated by Kobzig et al. [18] using immunocytochemical and histochemical methods. In volunteers and patients,

Gerlach et al. [10] measured NO concentrations in different parts of the upper airway. The highest concentrations were in the nose [0.649 ± 0.109 parts per million (ppm)], whereas, in intubated patients the NO concentration was < 0.01 ppm. This suggests that the NO synthesized predominantly in the nasopharynx is normally inhaled and resorbed by the lower respiratory tract. Here it may take part in the physiological regulation of the ventilation-perfusion ratio.

If NO is inhaled, 50%-80% of the inhaled NO is resorbed [35, 37]. NO freely diffuses from the alveoli into the surrounding lung tissue and nearby blood vessels. In blood, NO becomes inactivated within seconds by binding to hemoglobin, since NO has a high affinity to the hemoglobin molecule. Nitrosyl-hemoglobin (NOHb) is produced and, in the presence of oxygen, oxidized into methemoglobin, from which ferrous Hb is rapidly regenerated by methemoglobin reductase in red blood cells with nitrate as a by-product [14, 24]. The metabolism of the inhaled NO after its conversion to nitrate is identical to that of nitrate taken up via foodstuffs [37]. Most of the nitrate is excreted by the kidneys in urine.

Selective Pulmonary Vasodilation by Inhaled NO

Intravenously infused vasodilators have been used to reduce pulmonary hypertension, but due to their general vasodilator effects on the systemic and pulmonary circulation they may also decrease mean systemic arterial pressure and impair pulmonary gas exchange by increasing perfusion to unventilated lung areas. Based on the properties of NO, inhalation of gaseous NO may induce selective pulmonary vasodilation. As a gas, it reaches the pulmonary blood vessels from the abluminal surface adjacent to the ventilated airways. Thereby, in contrast to intravenous vasodilators, inhaled NO may increase perfusion of ventilated lung regions.

The first report presenting data on inhaled NO came from Higenbottam and coworkers in 1988 [13], who observed dilatory effects of inhaled NO on the pulmonary vasculature in patients with primary pulmonary hypertension, however, in contrast to the infusion of prostacyclin, they found no systemic vasodilation during NO inhalation [13]. Three years later, inhaled NO was also shown to dilate selectively in a dose dependent manner the pulmonary circulation in awake, spontaneously breathing lambs which were acutely vasoconstricted either by an infusion of the stable thromboxane endoperoxide analogue U46619 or by breathing a hypoxic gas mixture [5, 6]. Moreover, hypoxic pulmonary vasoconstriction in mechanically ventilated sheep was completely abolished by breathing 20 ppm NO without impairing gas exchange [27]. These results could be confirmed in human volunteers breathing a hypoxic gas mixture: hypoxia-induced pulmonary hypertension could be resolved by addition of 40 ppm NO to the hypoxic gas without any effect on systemic arterial pressure or cardiac output [7]. Also in patients with pulmonary hypertension of various etiology [1, 11, 27], short-term inhalation of NO was shown to produce a selective vasodilatory effect.

Therapeutic long-term and successful administration of NO was reported in newborns with persistent pulmonary hypertension [17, 30]. The increased pulmonary vascular resistance causes right-to-left shunting of blood across the patent ductus arteriosus and foramen ovale, which may result in critical hypoxemia [19]. Whereas intravenously infused vasodilators will not only dilate the pulmonary but also the systemic vasculature and, thereby, facilitate blood flow through the intracardiac and intrapulmonary shunt, causing a further reduction of the already compromised PaO_2 [19], inhaled NO induced a selective vasodilation of pulmonary blood vessels which reduced pulmonary hypertension and increased pulmonary blood flow and, thus, the PaO_2 [17, 30]. Moreover, long-term NO inhalation has been used for treatment of critical postoperative hypertension after cardiac surgery [2, 33], again showing its beneficial selective pulmonary vasodilatatory effect.

Inhaled NO in Acute Lung Injury

In 1991, administration of NO was found to reduce pulmonary hypertension in a patient with severe acute respiratory distress syndrome (ARDS) [4]. Surprisingly, the authors observed beside a selective pulmonary vasodilation an increase in PaO_2. Stimulated by this observation, they investigated the effects of short-term (40 min) inhalation of low concentrations of the gas NO in nine consecutive patients with severe ARDS [31]. The patients inhaled 18 ppm NO followed by 36 ppm NO before or after an intravenous infusion of 4 ng/kg per min prostacyclin (PGI_2). Systemic and pulmonary hemodynamics, blood gases and the ventilation/perfusion ratio were measured before, during and after administering each vasodilator. In this study, 18 ppm NO lowered pulmonary artery pressure by an average of 7 mmHg and to the same extent as the intravenous infusion of PGI_2. Whereas PGI_2 caused mean arterial pressure to fall and cardiac output to rise, these parameters remained unchanged during NO inhalation. Furthermore, in contrast to PGI_2, NO inhalation brought about a clear improvement in pulmonary oxygenation, and the PaO_2/F_IO_2 ratio increased significantly from 152 ± 75 mmHg to 199 ± 23 mmHg (mean ± SE). An increase in the NO concentration from 18 to 36 ppm displayed neither a further reduction in pulmonary artery pressure nor a further decrease in the intrapulmonary shunt. The analysis of the ventilation/perfusion ratio using the multiple inert gas elimination technique, a technique which allows the characterization of pulmonary gas exchange with respect to ventilation/perfusion distribution in a 50 compartment lung model [36], showed that the improved oxygenation was due to a reduction in the intrapulmonary shunt with a redistribution of the pulmonary blood flow benefitting ventilated and, due to inhaled NO, selectively vasodilated lung regions (Fig. 1). Using the same protocol, Rossaint et al. [31] investigated the effect of inhaled NO on right ventricular ejection fraction as assessed by the thermodilution technique. In ten patients with acute lung injury, inhaling 18 ppm NO reduced the mean pulmonary artery pressure by 5 ± 1 mmHg, increased right ventricular ejection fraction from $28\% \pm 2\%$ to $32\% \pm 2\%$, decreased right ventricular end-diastolic volume index from 114 ± 6 to 103 ± 8 ml/m^2 and right ventricular end-systolic volume index from 82 ± 4 to 70 ± 5 ml/m^2. Infusion of PGI_2 reduced PAP by 4 ± 2 mmHg, increased right ventricular ejection fraction from $29\% \pm 2\%$ to $32\% \pm 2\%$; and right ventricular end diastolic and end systolic volume indices did not change significantly. Whereas cardiac index remained constant during inhalation of NO, it increased from 4.0 ± 0.5 to 4.5 ± 0.5 l/min per square meter during infusion of PGI_2. This study, using a new approach to selective pulmonary vasodilation by inhaling NO, revealed that an increase in right ventricular ejection fraction is not necessarily associated with a rise in cardiac index.

To our knowledge, only one study exists which has investigated the effects of long-term NO inhalation in ARDS patients [31]. This study included seven patients, who inhaled 5 - 20 ppm NO between 3 and 53 days. A short daily interruption of the NO inhalation led to a reproducible rise in pulmonary artery pressure and an equally reproducible fall in PaO_2. No tachyphylaxia or other side effects, especially any increased formation of methemoglobin, were described in this study.

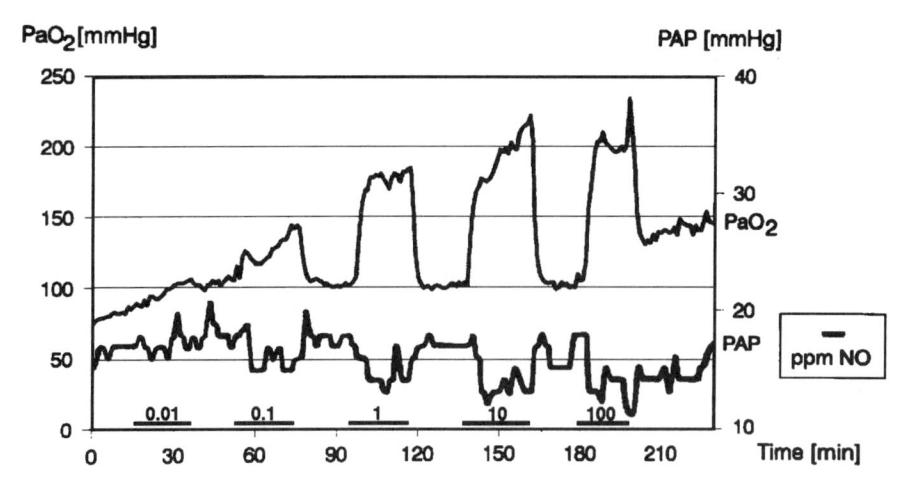

Fig. 1: Example of a continuous recording of PaO_2 (upper line, left y-axis) and mean pulmonary artery pressure (PAP, lower line, right y-axis) during brief periods of inhalation of 0.01, 0.1, 1, 10, and 100 ppm NO in a 22-year old man suffering from ARDS. The curves are reprinted using commercially available graphic software after transfer of the original data from an intraarterial blood gas monitor (PB 3300, Puritan Bennett, Carlsbad, CA, USA) and the hemodynamic monitor, respectively. Inhalation periods with the inspired NO concentration are indicated above the x-axis

Dose-Response Relationships of Inhaled NO

The same group investigated dose-response relationships between the concentration of inhaled NO and PaO_2 as well as between inhaled NO and pulmonary artery pressure in patients with acute lung injury [9]. Analysis of the dose-responses demonstrated that the effect of NO on PaO_2 was significant at 0.1 ppm, whereas the effect of NO on pulmonary artery pressure was only significant at concentrations of 1 ppm and more. The idealized dose-response curves for PaO_2 and pulmonary artery pressure showed different patterns: The improvement in oxygenation with 50% maximal response (ED_{50}) at about 0.1 ppm showed a maximum at 10 ppm NO and, at the highest tested concentration (100 ppm), drifted back towards the baseline data, whereas PAP presented a continuous, dose-dependent downwards tendency with an ED_{50} of approximately 2-3 ppm NO. In two of the patients included in this study, the authors found that 40% of the maximal achieved increase in PaO_2, which was recorded at 1 ppm, was reached at 0.01 ppm [9]. These data demonstrate that significant improvement of PaO_2 in patients with ARDS is induced by doses of NO which are much lower than those used in earlier studies and which are similar to those measured in the free atmosphere. Furthermore, using 100 ppm NO or more, the PaO_2 decreases back towards the baseline. This observation may be based on a diffusion of NO at high concentrations not only to ventilated but also to nonventilated lung areas. Thereby, intrapulmonary shunt increases and arterial oxygenation deteriorates. This presumption is confirmed by the further decrease in pulmonary artery pressure at these high NO concentrations. Therefore, clinicians need to decide whether they predominantly want to reduce the patients pulmonary artery pressure or to increase the PaO$_2$. Moreover, since both parameters in severe ARDS are influenced by NO over a range from 10 ppb to at least 100 ppm (Fig. 1), it is difficult to determine an "optimal" concentration for the individual patient, especially as the dose-response relationship may differ from day to day. Furthermore, we suppose that these different dose-relationships and problems with the determination of the "optimal" concentration also exist in other diseases with pulmonary hypertension.

For unknown reasons, some patients with severe ARDS showed no improvement in oxygenation nor a reduction in pulmonary artery pressure. However, we observed that some of these initial nonresponders demonstrated significant increases in PaO$_2$ or a reduction of pulmonary hypertension during inhalation of NO a few days later. So far, we have not been able to explain the day-to-day variations in dose-response relationship in an individual patient or the change from a nonresponder to a responder.

References

1. *Adnot S, Kouyoumdjian C, Defouilloy C et al. (1993) Hemodynamic and gas exchange responses to infusion of acetylcholine and inhalation of nitric oxide in patients with chronic obstructive lung disease and pulmonary hypertension. Am Rev Respir Dis 148: 310-316*
2. *Berner M, Beghetti M, Ricou B, Rouge JC, Pretre R, Friedli B (1993) Relief of severe pulmonary hypertension after closure of a large ventricular septal defect using low dose inhaled nitric oxide. Intensive Care Med 19: 75-77*
3. *Brenner BM, Troy JL, Ballermann BJ (1989) Endothelium-dependent vascular responses. Mediators and mechanisms. J Clin Invest 84: 1373-1378*
4. *Falke K, Rossaint R, Pison U et al. (1991) Inhaled nitric oxide selectively reduces pulmonary hypertension in severe ARDS and improves gas exchange as well as right heart ejection fraction: a case report. Am Rev Respir Dis Suppl 143: A248*
5. *Fratacci MD, Frostell CG, Chen TY, Wain JCJ, Robinson DR, Zapol WM (1991) Inhaled nitric oxide. A selective pulmonary vasodilator of heparin-protamine vasoconstriction in sheep. Anesthesiology 75: 990-999*
6. *Frostell C, Fratacci MD, Wain JC, Jones R, Zapol WM (1991) Inhaled nitric oxide. A selective pulmonary vasodilator reversing hypoxic pulmonary vasoconstriction. Circulation 83: 2038-2047*
7. *Frostell CG, Blomqvist H, Hedenstierna G, Lundberg J, Zapol WM (1993) Inhaled nitric oxide selectively reverses human hypoxic pulmonary vasoconstriction without causing systemic vasodilation. Anesthesiology 78: 427-435*
8. *Furchgott RF, Zawadzki JV (1980) The obligatory role of endothelial cells in the relaxation of arterial smooth muscle by acetylcholine. Nature 288: 373-376*
9. *Gerlach H, Rossaint R, Pappert D, Falke KJ (1993) Time-course and dose-response of nitric oxide inhalation for systemic oxygenation and pulmonary hypertension in patients with adult respiratory distress syndrome. Eur J Clin Invest 23: 499-502*
10. *Gerlach H, Rossaint R, Pappert D, Knorr M, Falke K (1994) Autoinhalation of nitric oxide after endogenous synthesis in the nose. Lancet 343: 518-519*
11. *Girard C, Lehot JJ, Pannetier JC, Filley S, Ffrench P, Estanove S (1992) Inhaled nitric oxide after mitral valve replacement in patients with chronic pulmonary artery hypertension. Anesthesiology 77: 880-883*

12. Hibbs JBJ, Westenfelder C, Taintor R et al. (1992) Evidence for cytokine-inducible nitric oxide synthesis from L- arginine in patients receiving interleukin-2 therapy. J Clin Invest 89: 867-877
13. Higenbottam T, Pepke-Zaba J, Scott J, Woolman P, Coutts C, Wallwork J (1988) Inhaled "endothelium derived-relaxing factor" (EDRF) in primary hypertension (Abstr) Am Rev Respir Dis 137: 107
14. Ignarro LJ, Lippton H, Edwards JC et al. (1981) Mechanism of vascular smooth muscle relaxation by organic nitrates, nitrites, nitroprusside and nitric oxide: evidence for the involvement of S-nitrosothiols as active intermediates. J Pharmacol Exp Ther 218: 739-749
15. Ignarro LJ, Buga GM, Wood KS, Byrns RE, Chaudhuri G (1987) Endothelium-derived relaxing factor produced and released from artery and vein is nitric oxide. Proc Natl Acad Sci USA 84: 9265-9269
16. Kilbourn RG, Griffith OW (1992) Overproduction of nitric oxide in cytokine-mediated and septic shock. J Natl Cancer Inst 84: 827-831
17. Kinsella JP, Neish SR, Shaffer E, Abman SH (1992) Low-dose inhalational nitric oxide in persistent pulmonary hypertension of the newborn. Lancet 340: 819-820
18. Kobzig L, Bredt DS, Lowenstein CJ et al. (1993) Nitric oxide synthase in human and rat lung: immunocytochemical and histochemical localization. Am J Respir Cell Mol Biol 9: 371-377
19. Levin DL, Heymann MA, Kitterman JA, Gregory GA, Phibbs RH, Rudolph AM (1976) Persistent pulmonary hypertension of the newborn infant. J Pediatr 89: 626-630
20. Mayer B, Schmidt K, Humbert R, Bohme E (1989) Biosynthesis of endothelium-derived relaxing factor: a cytosolic enzyme in porcine aortic endothelial cells Ca^{2+} dependently converts L-arginine into an activator of soluble guanylyl cyclase. Biochem Biophys Res Commun 164: 678-685
21. Moncada S, Palmer RM, Higgs EA (1991) Nitric oxide: physiology, pathophysiology, and pharmacology. Pharmacol Rev 43: 109-142
22. Mulsch A, Bassenge E, Busse R (1989) Nitric oxide synthesis in endothelial cytosol: evidence for a calcium-dependent and a calcium-independent mechanism. Naunyn Schmiedebergs Arch Pharmacol 340: 767-770
23. Ochoa JB, Curti B, Peitzman AB et al. (1992) Increased circulating nitrogen oxides after human tumor immunotherapy: correlation with toxic hemodynamic changes. J Natl Cancer Inst 84: 864-867
24. Oda H, Kusumoto S, Nakajima T (1975) Nitrosyl-hemoglobin formation in the blood of animals exposed to nitric oxide. Arch Environ Health 30: 453-456
25. Palmer RM, Ferrige AG, Moncada S (1987) Nitric oxide release accounts for the biological activity of endothelium-derived relaxing factor. Nature 327: 524-526
26. Palmer RM, Rees DD, Ashton DS, Moncada S (1988) L-Arginine is the physiological precursor for the formation of nitric oxide in endothelium-dependent relaxation. Biochem Biophys Res Commun 153: 1251-1256
27. Pison U, Lopez FA, Heidelmeyer CF, Rossaint R, Falke K (1993) Inhaled nitric oxide selectively reverses hypoxic pulmonary vasoconstriction without impairing pulmonary gas exchange. J Appl Physiol 74: 1287-1292
28. Pohl U, Holtz J, Busse R, Bassenge E (1986) Crucial role of endothelium in the vasodilator response to increased flow in vivo. Hypertension 8: 37-44
29. Rees DD, Palmer RMJ, Moncada S (1989) Role of endothelium-derived nitric oxide in the regulation of blood pressure. Proc Natl Acad Sci USA 86: 3375-3378
30. Roberts JD, Polander DM, Lang P, Zapol WM (1992) Inhaled nitric oxide in persistent pulmonary hypertension of the newborn. Lancet 340: 818-819

31. Rossaint R, Falke KJ, Lopez F, Slama K, Pison U, Zapol WM (1993) Inhaled nitric oxide in adult respiratory distress syndrome. N Engl J Med 328: 399-405
32. Rubanyi GM, Romero JC, Vanhoutte PM (1986) Flow-induced release of endothelium-derived relaxing factor. Am J Physiol 250: H1145-H1149
33. Sellden H, Winberg P, Gustafsson LE, Lundell B, Böök K, Frostell CG (1993) Inhalation of nitric oxide-reduced pulmonary hypertension after cardiac surgery in a 3.2-kg infant. Anesthesiology 78: 577-580
34. Vallance P, Collier J, Moncada S (1989) Effects of endothelium-derived nitric oxide on peripheral arteriolar tone in man. Lancet 2: 997-1000
35. Wagner HM (1970) Absorption von NO und NO_2 in MIK- und MAK-Konzentrationen bei der Inhalation. Staub Reinhalt Luft 30: 380-381
36. Wagner PD, Saltzman HA, West JB (1974) Measurement of continuous distributions of ventilation-perfusion ratios: theory. J Appl Physiol 36: 588-599
37. Yoshida K, Kasama K (1987) Biotransformation of nitric oxide. Environ Health Perspect 73: 201-205

Effect of Nitric Oxide Synthase Inhibitors on Pulmonary Shunt Volume and Cytokines in Human Septic Shock

J. Schilling, R. Bürki, H. Joller, M. Lachat, D. Gyurech, S. Geroulanos

Introduction

Nitric oxide (NO) is synthesized by endothelial and vascular cells from the amino acid L-arginine by the action of different isoforms of the enzyme nitric oxide synthase (NOS). This inflammatory-mediator-dependent mechanism is involved in the regulation of vascular tone and plays an important role in host defense mechanisms. Nowadays this arginine-NO cascade is believed to be responsible for the prolonged vasodilatation and the resistance to cathecholamines in human septic shock. N^G-Monomethyl-L-arginine (L-NMMA) is a synthetic and naturally occurring inhibitor of the enzyme NOS. In addition to previous reports on the cardiovascular effects of this inhibitor in human septic shock [1-3], we describe a case in which changes in immunological parameters and pulmonary shunt volume were observed.

Patient and Methods

A 68-year-old woman went into severe septic shock due to a retrospectively documented *Candida* and *Pseudomonas aeruginosa* infection complicated by adult respiratory distress syndrome (ARDS) within 9 days of abdominal surgery. Despite conventional therapy, the patient's condition deteriorated. Before stopping all therapeutic measurements it was decided to inhibit NOS. The study protocol was approved by the ethical committee of the Department of Surgery of our institution. Informed consent of the legal representatives of the patient was obtained. After administration of two boli of 200 mg L-NMMA (Department of Pharmacy, Zurich; Director, G. Folkert) a continuous infusion of 0.05 mg/kg per minute was initiated. Before and 90 min after the first bolus, during the continuous infusion, blood samples for immunological measurements were taken and processed together. Pulmonary shunt volume was observed before the administration of L-NMMA, and at intervals of 60 and 140 min postadministration.

Results

As expected, mean arterial blood pressure rose (from 62 to 134 mmHg), heart rate remained stable (126-118 beats/min), systemic vascular resistance increased (from 225 to 354 dyne s/cm^5), cardiac output decreased (from 17 to 15.2 l/min) and cardiac index declined (from 9.94 to 8.63 l/min per square meter) (Table 1). We report here a controversial observation: after blocking NO synthesis, pulmonary shunt volume decreased from 54.1% to 35.4% within 1 h and to 36.6% after 140 min. Decreases were also noted for immunoglobulins A, G, and M (3.2 to 2.9, 8.1 to 7.6, 1.1 to 0.9 g/l), C-reactive protein (111.1 to 105.6 mg/l), interleukin-1 (0 pg/ml), soluble interleukin-2 (2128 to 1983 units/ml), and α_1-antitrypsine (3.86 to 3.83 g/l), whereas complement factor C-3c and C-4 (0.54 to 0.50, 0.22 to 0.23 g/l) did not change significantly. In contrast neopterine increased during the 90 min from 16.51 to 32.55 ng/ml, tumor necrosis factor alpha (TNF-α) from 24.16 to 36.61 pg/ml, and interleukin-6 from 61.9 to 98.2 pg/ml.

Table 1: Hemodynamics

Time (hours)	HR	MAP	SVR	CO	CI	PCWP	PaO2	Qs/Qt1
13:00	126	62	225	17.0	9.94	16	10.0	54.06
13:05[a]	127	68						
13:10	126	115						
13:15	125	86	354	15.1	8.83	25		
13:18	123	81						
13:28	122	134						
14:00	123	68	269	14.8	8.65	20		
14:10	122	65					11.1	35.36
14:35	121	92						
14:55	122	70	236	15.2	8.88	19		
15:20	120	71					14.7	36.63

[a]First administration of L-NMMA of 200 mg; 13:20 hours second administration of 200 mg and from 13:30 hours continuous administration of 0.05 mg/min per kilogram.

HR, heart rate (min); MAP, mean arterial pressure (mmHg); SVR, systemic vascular resistance (dyne s/cm^5); CO, cardiac output (l/min); CI, cardiac index (l/min per square meter); PCWP, pulmonary capillary wedge pressure (mmHg); PaO$_2$ = arterial partial oxygen pressure in kilopascals; Qs;Qt1, pulmonary shunt volume in percent.

Discussion

In three episodes of septic shock with prolonged and therapy-resistant states of hypotension at our institute, including one episode complicated by ARDS, L-NMMA successfully reversed hypotension [1, 3]. As L-NMMA is metabolized to L-citrulline and in turn L-citrulline is metabolised to L-arginine, the substrate of NO [4], blood gas analyses of NO may be of great value in surveillance of patients in septic shock. Moreover, interpretation of clinical results using L-NMMA may again become more important.

It is noteworthy that, in these three cases, we isolated three completely different types of pathogen (*Candida*, *Pseudomonas aeruginosa*, and multiresistant coagulase-negative staphylococci). This observation suggests that endotoxin alone is not the main factor triggering the development of hypotension in septic shock by the NO pathway.

In many trials of ARDS and pulmonary hypertension, controlled inhalation of NO is reported to be beneficial by reducing pulmonary resistance. We observed after blocking NO synthesis that pulmonary shunt volume decreased. Interpretation of these findings is complex and controversial. Thus, a combination of controlled local NO administration and a partial systemic NO synthesis blockade may improve this new approach in the handling of patients with severe ARDS, septic shock and pulmonary hypertension in the future.

Conclusion

In patients with septic shock, blocking NO as an intervention at the end of a not yet fully understood cascade may be of value in the therapy of hypotension in septic shock and might have a major influence on pulmonary shunt volume and intercell communication.

References

1. Geroulanos S, Schilling J, Cakmakci M, Jung H, Largiadèr F (1992) Inhibition of NO synthesis in septic shock (Letter) Lancet 339: 435
2. Petros A, Bennett D, Vallance P (1991) Effect of nitric oxide synthase inhibitors on hypotension in patients with septic shock. Lancet 338: 1557-1558
3. Schilling J, Cakmakci M, Bättig U, Geroulanos S (1993) A new approach in the treatment of hypotension in human septic shock by N^G-monomethyl-L-arginine, an inhibitor of the nitric oxide synthetase. Intensive Care Med 19: 227-231
4. Hecker M, Mitchell JA, Harris HJ, Katsura M, Thiemermann C, Vane JR (1990) Endothelial cells metabolize N^G-monomethyl-L-arginine to L-citrulline and subsequently to L-arginine. Biochem Biophys Res Commun 167(3): 1037-1043

Extracorporeal Lung Support in Severe ARDS

R. Rossaint, D. Pappert, K. Lewandowski, K. Falke

Introduction

The adult respiratory distress syndrome (ARDS) is an acute and severe alteration in lung structure and function characterized by hypoxemia, reduced respiratory compliance, and diffuse radiographic infiltrates [2]. Since its first description by Ashbaugh et al. in 1967 [2], the mortality rate of this syndrome has remained above 50% despite extensive clinical and laboratory research efforts [6, 24, 25]. Among other unknown factors, this high mortality may be influenced by the disease itself as well as by iatrogenic factors such as ventilator settings with high airway pressures and high inspiratory oxygen concentrations (FIO_2). In the progression of ARDS high mean airway pressures as well as high FIO_2 may be required to ensure adequate arterial oxygen partial pressures (PaO_2). Both factors are considered to be harmful to the lung [3, 15]. Therefore, today's therapeutic approaches seek for a reduction in peak airway pressure and application of less enriched oxygen mixtures. Conventional concepts used are pressure- and/or volume-limited ventilation with positive end-expiratory pressure (PEEP) and acceptance of an increased partial pressure of carbon dioxide, positioning including prone position, differential lung ventilation, and avoidance of fluid overload [19]. In addition, the inhalation of low concentrations of nitric oxide has recently been described to increase PaO_2 and to decrease pulmonary artery pressure [21]. However, should these therapeutic interventions fail to improve pulmonary gas exchange, extracorporeal lung support has been advocated in the treatment of patients with severe, but potentially reversible, acute respiratory failure. This technique potentially allows both the FIO_2 and the peak airway pressures to be reduced, when pulmonary gas exchange is partly taken over by the extracorporeal support system. Assuring lung rest and minimizing the potential damage of mechanical ventilation is considered to provide a better environment for lung healing and/or to buy time for causal therapy [9].

History of Extracorporeal Lung Support in Severe ARDS

In the 1950s, silicon polymer membranes, permeable to oxygen and carbon dioxide, were developed for extracorporeal gas exchange. In contrast to the "bubble oxygenators", which had been used in cardiac surgery until that time, in which gas exchange was achieved by direct contact between gas bubbles and blood, oxygenators separating the blood and gas phases by membranes did not lead to severe hemolysis over time. Therefore, this development was the basis for consideration of extracorporeal support systems for the treatment of ARDS. In the 1960s, Kolobow et al. [13] started to investigate the long-term use of membrane oxygenators in animals, aiming at a method for temporary augmentation of deficient pulmonary gas exchange in patients with acute respiratory failure. In lambs, the extracorporeal support of up to 16 days which was achieved was still limited not only by technical problems, but also by septic complications, platelet loss, and coagulation disequilibrium over time [13]. After single, unsuccessful applications in patients, Hill et. al. in 1972 [11] reported the first successful treatment with extracorporeal membrane oxygenation (ECMO) in a 24-year-old man, suffering from severe acute respiratory failure after traumatic disruption of the aorta and multiple fractures. After 3 days of ECMO, the patient's lung function had improved and the patient could be weaned from extracorporeal bypass. Soon other centers, both in the United States and in Europe, reported the successful use of extracorporeal support for patients with ARDS [10, 23]. Within a few years, ECMO has been applied as a supportive therapy worldwide in about 150 patients with ARDS, with a 10% - 15% survival rate [10].

The success of Hill and coworkers as well as others was the basis for a prospective and randomized multicenter study, termed the US National-ECMO Study, which attempted to demonstrate a therapeutic breakthrough in the treatment of ARDS using ECMO, when compared with conventional treatment. The study was initiated in 1974 and planned to involve a total of 300 patients. Patients were included if they fulfilled the following criteria: (1) fast entry: PaO_2 < 50 mmHg for more than 2 h at a FIO_2 of 1.0 and PEEP > 5 cm H_2O and (2) slow entry: maximal therapy for 48 h, PaO_2 < 50 mmHg for more than 12 h at a FIO_2 of 0.6, PEEP > 5 cm H_2O and a venous admixture (Q_{VA}/Q_T) > 30% at a FIO_2 of 1.0 and PEEP > 5 cm H_2O. In 1976, the study was terminated after 90 patients had been included, when survival rates in both groups appeared to be less than 10% and unlikely to be significantly different with 300 patients studied. The final report confirmed the preliminary results and demonstrated a 90% mortality rate with no difference between the two groups [27]. The project was later accused of having had a poor study design. The therapeutic approach to ARDS concerning ventilator therapy, patient selection, and therapeutic strategies was not completely standardized and the participating centers were free to choose their own veno-arterial bypass system and type of oxygenator (Kolobow, Lande-Edwards, Bramson, and General Electric-Pierce). Furthermore, the veno-arterial perfusion route potentially induces inadequate perfusion to the lungs and, thereby, an insufficient oxygen supply as well as microthrombosis. However, the reduction in pulmonary blood flow resulting in a decrease in pulmonary artery pressures and shunt perfusion was thought to be advantageous for the recovery of the lung. From today's point of view, the defined minimum duration of ECMO may also have been too short, since extracorporeal support was allowed to be terminated after 5 days when no improvement of pulmonary function was detectable. Later studies showed that an average bypass time of 20 days may be required for the lungs to heal [18]. If the main potential benefit of ECMO is to keep the lungs at rest, then this goal also was not pursued during the US National ECMO Study: The continuous positive pressure ventilation in patients treated with extracorporeal support did not essentially differ from that in the conventionally treated patients.

The study results discouraged most researchers and clinicians from pursuing the concept of ECMO in severe ARDS, except for Kolobow and coworkers, who thought that some of the problems were due to the severity and irreversibility of the underlying disease, which was mostly viral or bacterial pneumonia. The study had shown that the technique of ECMO itself was safe and reliable over an extended period.

In 1977, Kolobow et al. [14] first described the possible separation of gas exchange into oxygenation and decarboxylation. They hypothesized that ventilation is mainly required for the removal of CO_2 from the lung, which is a function of tidal volume and frequency of breathing. They demonstrated in lambs that oxygenation without ventilation can be achieved only by intratracheally providing an amount of oxygen equal to the amount consumed, also called aventilatory mass flow or apneic ventilation. In these animals, extracorporeal removal of all the CO_2 produced was possible using a new kind of spiral coil membrane lungs. The formation of atelectasis could be prevented by providing 2-4 breaths/min. While the clinical application of ECMO was no longer pursued in the United States, as a consequence of the discouraging outcome from the US National ECMO Study, Gattinoni et al. [8] transferred his results from animal research to clinical applicability after his return to Milan. He combined the concept of extracorporeal CO_2 removal ($ECCO_2R$) with a ventilatory strategy, consisting of low ventilatory frequency (3-5 breaths/min) with a long expiratory phase, reduced peak pressures (< 45 cmH_2O) and increased PEEP (15-25 cmH_2O) to keep mean airway pressures constant. An additional continuous flow of oxygen (1-2 l/min) was administered through a small catheter, placed proximal to the carina to compensate for the oxygen consumption during the long expiratory phase. Thereby, oxygenation was mainly achieved by the patient's lungs. Indeed, using this strategy of low-frequency, positive pressure ventilation with extracorporeal CO_2 removal ($LFPPV-ECCO_2R$) allowed the lung to rest and avoided excessively high airway pressures by a reduction in peak pressures. CO_2 removal, which is physiologically achieved by ventilation, was separated from the need for oxygenation and accomplished by the use of the extracorporeal membrane lungs. Whereas the efficacy of extracorporeal oxygen transfer is mainly dependent on the blood flow through the extracorporeal membrane lungs, premembrane oxygen saturation, contact time of the erythrocytes, and hemoglobin concentration, decarboxylation is mainly determined by the sweep gas flow through the oxygenator and its surface area. Therefore, $ECCO_2R$ allowed a reduction of bypass blood flow compared with ECMO. Extracorporeal blood flow was restricted to 25% - 30% of total cardiac output. As originally advocated by Kolobow, Gattinoni chose for the extracorporeal bypass the venovenous access. In contrast to veno-arterial ECMO, cardiopulmonary blood flow is not compromised with this technique, as the net influx equals net outflux. Central venous pressures are not affected and exact monitoring of volume status is possible; cardiac output is completely dependent on cardiac performance and not influenced by the amount of extracorporeal blood flow. Lung restitution may be enhanced by the prepulmonary oxygenation of blood flow. Arterial embolic complications with tissue loss or necrosis, as observed with the veno-arterial bypass technique, may be avoided and the risk of pulmonary microthrombosis due to reduced blood flow or incomplete oxygenation depending on the placement of the cannulas is absent.

The first clinical experiences with this technique by the group of Gattinoni et al. [8] in Milan, followed by Falke et al. [7] and the group of Lennartz [12] in Germany, were very promising and showed an improved survival rate of up to 52%, when patients were selected according to the inclusion and exclusion criteria of the US National ECMO Study. The major problem during this time was bleeding and coagulation disorders due to an inactivation and destruction of platelets and activation of the coagulatory system by the surface of the extracorporeal system. Thrombocytopenia was common after initiation of the extracorporeal perfusion, possibly resulting from platelet trapping in the oxygenator. Systemic heparinization, necessary to prevent the system from clotting and to avoid thromboembolic episodes, was shown to induce thrombocytopenia and increase the risk of heparin induced uncontrollable hemorrhage. Diffuse bleeding from the cannulation sites as well as spontaneous hemorrhage was common, in some cases catastrophic, eventually leading to the patient's death. In 58 patients undergoing extracorporeal respiratory support, Uziel and coworkers reported 11 patients who underwent surgery during bypass and developed life threatening bleeding problems. Eight of these patients died, accounting for a 13.8% mortality rate [26], exceeded by a recent report of a 17.4% mortality rate caused by severe bleeding [5].

A solution to these problems was the development of a covalently bound heparin coating of the inner surface of extracorporeal equipment, thus minimizing the activation of the coagulatory system (Carmeda, Sweden). Its clinical use was first described by Bindslev and coworkers [4]. Heparinized membrane oxygenators, connectors, cannulas, and tubing theoretically allowed the extracorporeal system to run heparin free. Bleeding problems were reported to be reduced when compared with non-surface-heparinized systems and even major surgical interventions may be performed without an increased risk of uncontrolled bleeding [20].

Actual Procedures Using Extracorporeal Lung Support

Who Should Be Treated with Extracorporeal Lung Support?

The criteria which should be fulfilled before treatment with extracorporeal lung support starts, in general, still follow those the US National ECMO Study, even if they differ slightly between centers. Today, the decisions are more clinically oriented, using extracorporeal lung support as a last resort life support therapy. The criteria used in our center are shown in Table 1. However, even if we use as slow entry criteria the pathophysiological data shown in Table 1, we essentially perform a trend analysis to decide whether a patient should be treated with extracorporeal lung support. Patients with immunosuppression, cancer, end-stage chronic pulmonary diseases, irreversible neurologic damage, and diseases of the coagulation system are excluded from treatment with extracorporeal lung support.

Table 1: Criteria for treatment with extracorporeal lung support

Fast entry criteria are met, when despite maximal therapy for more than 2 h: $\quad PaO_2 < 50$ mmHg at FIO_2 1.0 PEEP > 10 cm H_2O
Slow entry criteria are met when three out of four of the following criteria are fulfilled after 24 - 120 h of maximal therapy: $\quad -PaO_2/FIO_2 < 150$ mmHg with PEEP ≥ 10 cm H_2O $\quad -Q_S/Q_T > 30\%$ at FIO_2 10 $\quad -$Extravascular lung water (EVLW) ≥ 15 ml/kg $\quad -$Total lung compliance ≤ 30 ml/cmH_2O

Bypass and Cannulation Technique

Today, extracorporeal lung support is usually performed using a veno-venous bypass technique. Blood is drained via one or two spring wire reinforced cannulas introduced through the femoral veins, with one cannula placed in the vena cava inferior and possibly a second cannula advanced to the iliacal bifurcation. The blood is passively drained, either into a collapsible reservoir equipped with a servo switch which controls the pump, or in tubings connected to pressure transducers for low pressure downregulation avoiding, high negative pressures in the drainage system. From here, the blood is actively pumped by an almost occlusive roller pump or, alternatively, by a centrifugal pump through the oxygenators back to the patient. For safety reasons and to facilitate membrane replacement, two roller or centrifugal pumps and membrane lungs may be used in parallel. The membrane oxygenators are ventilated with an oxygen/nitrogen mixture controlled by a flowmeter and an oxygen blender. The oxygenated and decarboxylated blood is then returned to a cannula introduced from the right jugular vein and advanced to the vena cava superior. For safety reasons the venous return has to be observed by a bubble detector, preventing inadvertent air embolization in the case of circuit disruption or leaks in negative pressure areas. The blood temperature is extracorporeally regulated by heat exchangers. Continuous monitoring of mixed venous oxygen saturation in the patient and oxygen saturation in the venous tract of the bypass gives precise information about the efficacy of the extracorporeal system.

During venovenous extracorporeal circulation, part of the venous return may recirculate through the system, depending on the ratio of extracorporeal to systemic blood flow and cannula placement. Almost total extracorporeal lung assist can be achieved only when the return cannula is placed into the right ventricle. Whereas until 1989 insertion of the cannulas was always performed by surgical exposure of the veins, today access to the bypass veins can easily be established by the percutaneous cannulation technique using a modified Seldinger technique.

The original concept of $ECCO_2R$ with LFPPV has to be modified in some patients, if pulmonary oxygen transfer capability is so severely reduced that additional oxygen transfer across the membrane lung is necessary to maintain adequate blood oxygenation. In these patients, extracorporeal blood flow has to be increased to achieve a higher extracorporeal O_2 transfer. The new cannulation technique, using percutaneous venous access with spring wire reinforced, thin walled cannulas, allows extracorporeal blood flows up to 40% - 60% of cardiac output, e.g., up to 4 l/min with a 21F cannula (Biomedicus) for venous return.

Oxygenators

Two types of membrane oxygenators are currently used in Europe, the Kolobow membrane lung (SciMed, Minneapolis, MN) and the microporous heparinized membrane lung (Medtronic Maxima, Anaheim, CA). The Kolobow oxygenator is a spiral silicone rubber membrane lung with an excellent long-term performance, in some instances for more than 3 weeks [18]. However, since the development of surface heparinization by Carmeda (Carmeda BioActive Surface, Stockholm, Sweden), microporous polypropylene hollow-fiber oxygenators are the most commonly used oxygenators today. But other internally heparin-coated systems are also available. The long-term use of hollow-fiber oxygenators is often complicated by an increasing plasma leakage over time across the membrane pores and a decrease in gas exchange capability. How these problems are linked to the patients' condition has not yet been evaluated, but they may be related to the adsorption of phospholipids to the membrane surface. Thus, the coating of the hydrophobic layer with hydrophilic components possibly results in a facilitated passage of plasma proteins across the membrane. Anecdotally, we experienced a reduced life span of oxygenators in patients with severe sepsis or liver failure, requiring a replacement of the oxygenators every 24 - 48 h, whereas in the same patient, when no sepsis and no liver failure was present, we used the same type of oxygenator for up to 3 weeks. A newly developed heparin coating (ECLA3) for microporous hollow-fiber oxygenators looks promising. Although the life span of silicon rubber oxygenators is superior to that of other types of oxygenators, they are not yet commercially available with surface heparinization.

Anticoagulation

The use of surface-heparinized equipment allows systemic heparinization to be limited low-dose anticoagulation to avoid clotting in areas of blood flow reduction due to diameter changes between connector and tubing or the collapsible reservoir. In case of an inadvertent pump stop, heparinization prevents disastrous irreversible clotting of the oxygenators. Anticoagulation is monitored every 4 h and an activated clotting time (ACT) around 120 - 150 s or activated partial thromboplastin time (APTT) in the upper normal range is desirable. Antithrombin III (ATIII) levels are kept at 80% - 100%. This approach even allows major surgical interventions without interruption of the bypass. In our institution 41 ECMO-treated patients underwent 104 thoracotomies or sternotomies for chest tube insertion, lung surgery or cardiac tamponade. Four patients underwent a laparotomy, and in 4 patients osteosynthesis of the pelvis and major fractures was necessary. None of the patients developed catastrophic bleeding complications in major surgery during ECMO. However, using this anticoagulatory regimen we observed that extracorporeal perfusion for more than 3 weeks is often associated with a formation of clots in the extracorporeal system in regions of reduced blood flow.

Whereas in the US National ECMO Study the requirement for blood replacement averaged 2500 ml, the use of both surface-heparinized devices and the percutaneous cannulation technique resulted in an overall reduction of blood replacement. Pesenti et al. [18] demonstrated a significantly reduced need for blood components when comparing patients treated with the surgical cannulation technique, percutaneous cannulation and heparinized equipment.

Ventilator Regimen and Adjunctive Strategies

During extracorporeal support, ventilator settings are adjusted to the decreased necessity of pulmonary gas exchange and focussed on the prevention of further structural damage by high FIO_2, large tidal volumes and/or high peak pressures. This may be achieved either using low frequency positive pressure ventilation with an additional continuous flow of oxygen administered through a small catheter just above the carina as described by Gattinoni or modifying this concept slightly. In our institution the patients are routinely ventilated in the pressure controlled mode. Respiratory rate is limited to < 10/min, I/E ratios 1:2 to 1:1, and pressure control is set to a maximum of 30 - 35 cmH_2O. Optimal PEEP is determined from periodically obtained pressure/volume curves, if no bronchopleural fistula is present. In the course of the disease, FIO_2 is adjusted to keep the PaO_2 at 60 - 65 mmHg.

Besides ventilatory support, other adjunctive types of therapeutic measures or concepts such as inhalation of low concentrations of nitric oxide, dehydration when fluid overloading is present, prone position, and physiotherapy are applied to achieve a further improvement of pulmonary gas exchange properties. Fiberoptic bronchoscopies are performed frequently to clear mucous plugs or secretions producing atelectases.

Disconnection from Extracorporeal Lung Support

In our institution, we daily test the maximum achievable PaO_2 with a ventilator and an artificial lung FIO_2 of 1.0. When PaO_2 increases during these daily tests to 250-300 mmHg, the patient is allowed to breath more and more spontaneously in the pressure support mode with the pressure still limited to a maximum of 30 - 35 cmH_2O. When PaO_2 further increases during the daily tests to 350-400 mmHg, gas flow through the membrane lungs can be stopped. Finally, disconnection from bypass is performed, if the patient proves under these conditions to be able to maintain adequate gas exchange via the natural lungs ($PaO_2 > 60$ mmHg at FIO_2 0.4 - 0.6 and $PaCO_2 < 70$ mmHg with the pressure further limited to a maximum of 35 cmH_2O). Using a percutaneous cannulation technique the catheters can be removed as for other intravenous lines without surgical repair of the veins.

Results

When ARDS was first described by Ashbaugh and coworkers, the mortality rate was 58% [2]. These results were confirmed by the "Additional Data Collection" group of the US National ECMO Study [17], exceeded by a 90% mortality rate in the final report [27]. More recent studies showed that the overall mortality rate was between 59% and 65% without ECMO, despite major advances in therapy [1]. In our center, the mortality rate decreased to 27% using a combination of advanced therapy including pressure limited ventilation with PEEP and permissive hypercapnia, positioning, side differential ventilation, dehydration (if necessary), inhalation of nitric oxide, and extracorporeal lung support when conventional therapy failed to improve pulmonary gas exchange and if the treatment criteria were fulfilled. As described earlier [1], the outcome in our group of patients was associated with the underlying disease (Table 2), ranging from 78% in trauma patients and 58% in patients with pneumonia. These results may be explained partly by the treatment strategy and partly by the criteria for refusal of patients, which are basically the same as used for exclusion for the treatment with extracorporeal lung support. In contrast to the US National ECMO Study, in which the time for a patient on extracorporeal lung support could be limited to 5 days, when no improvement occurred, it is now obvious that some patients require a much longer period of extracorporeal support before successful weaning is possible. In our institution, in which extracorporeal lung assist was started in 1989, mean bypass in the survivor group lasted 23 ± 6 days. Pesenti and coworkers compared mean bypass time of the survivor group treated between 1979 - 1988 and 1988 - 1992 and found an increase of more than 300%, from 153 ± 128 h to 467 ± 321 h, respectively. The bypass time for nonsurvivors did not change significantly [18]. Besides the longer bypass time, using the venovenous perfusion route, keeping the lungs at rest and the technical improvement especially the heparin coated surfaces may have contributed to the reduction in mortality to about 50% in Europe when using extracorporeal lung support (Table 2). However, a historic comparison of actual results and the ECMO study is questionable. Knowledge and experience has been accumulated since then and the insight into the pathophysiology and the mechanisms causing ARDS and promoting the inflammatory process has broadened and influenced therapeutic concepts.

A major criticism of these studies is their uncontrolled, not prospective nature. There is only one study published, which established a prospective randomized study design, comparing conventional therapy with $ECCO_2$-R, showing no significant differences in the survival rate of either group [16]. Again some fundamental shortcomings concerning patient population, bypass technique and ventilator strategy may have finally influenced outcome in this study [5]. Although a prospective randomized study may be desirable, from our point of view, the results in Europe clearly justify the use of extracorporeal respiratory support as a last resort therapy.

After 20 years of accumulated experience with venovenous extracorporeal respiratory support, mortality in more than 400 patients with severe ARDS has been reduced to 49%. These results underline that extracorporeal lung support techniques are an additional and

Table 2: ECMO survival rates for European centers (December 31 1993)

Centers	No. cases	Survival
Milan/Monza	93	41 (44%)
Marburg	150	86 (57%)
Berlin	41	22 (55%)
Paris	64	27 (42%)
Stockholm	26	9 (35%)
Freiburg	19	11 (58%)
Munich	9	7 (77%)
Totals	402	203 (51%)

alternative tool supplementing conventional therapy. The temporary impossibility of supplying sufficient oxygen even using aggressive ventilator therapy with high inspiratory peak pressures, extensive use of PEEP, and high FIO_2 may be overcome. Extracorporeal membrane oxygenation or CO_2 removal allows the possible reduction of iatrogenic factors in the progression of ARDS and for the time to be bought for the restitution of pulmonary gas exchange properties.

References

1. Artigas A, Carlet J, Chastang C, Le Gall JR, Blanch, L and Fernández, R (1992) Adult respiratory distress syndrome: clinical presentation, prognostic factors and outcome In: Artigas A, Lemaire F, Suter PM, Zapol WM (eds.) Adult respiratory distress syndrome. Churchill Livingstone, Edinburgh, pp. 509-523
2. Ashbaugh DG, Bigelow DB, Petty TL, Levine BE (1967) Acute respiratory distress in adults. Lancet 2: 319-323
3. Barber RE, Lee J, Hamilton WK (1970) Oxygen toxicity in man A prospective study in patients with irreversible brain damage. N Engl J Med 283: 1478-1484
4. Bindslev L, Eklund J, Norlander O et al. (1987) Treatment of acute respiratory failure by extracorporeal carbon dioxide elimination performed with a surface heparinized artificial lung. Anesthesiology 67: 117-120
5. Brunet F, Belghith M, Mira J et al. (1993) Extracorporeal carbon dioxide removal and low-frequency positive- pressure ventilation. Chest 104:889-898
6. European ARDS Collaborative Working Group (1988) Adult respiratory distress syndrome (ARDS): clinical predictors, prognostic factors and outcome Intensive Care Med 14 Suppl 1: A300
7. Falke KJ, Thies WR, Lenhsen U, Seifert D, Pesenti A, Schulte HD (1983) Improvement of lung function during clinical extracorporeal CO2 elimination in severe adult respiratory distress syndrome. Thorac Cardiovasc Surg 31: 1-40
8. Gattinoni L, Agostoni A, Pesenti A et al. (1980) Treatment of acute respiratory failure with low-frequency positive-pressure ventilation and extracorporeal removal of CO_2. Lancet 2: 292-294

9. Gattinoni L, Pesenti A, Mascheroni D et al. (1986) Low-frequency positive-pressure ventilation with extracorporeal CO_2 removal in severe acute respiratory failure. JAMA 256: 881-886
10. Gille JP (1974) Respiratory support by extracorporeal circulation with a membrane artificial lung (in French) Bull Physiopathol Respir Nancy 10: 373-410
11. Hill JD, O'Brien TG, Murray JJ et al. (1972) Prolonged extracorporeal oxygenation for acute post-traumatic respiratory failure (shock-lung syndrome) Use of the Bramson membrane lung N Engl J Med 286: 629-634
12. Knoch M, Müller E, Höltermann W, Konder H, Lennartz H (1987) Erfahrungen mit der extrakorporalen CO2-Elimination Anaesthesist 36: 210-216
13. Kolobow T, Spragg RG, Pierce JE, Zapol WM (1971) Extended term (to 16 days) partial extracorporeal blood gas exchange with the spiral membrane lung in unanesthetized lambs. Trans Am Soc Artif Intern Organs 17: 350-354
14. Kolobow T, Gattinoni L, Tomlinson TA, Pierce JE (1977) Control of breathing using an extracorporeal membrane lung. Anesthesiology 46: 138-141
15. Kolobow T, Moretti MP, Fumagalli R et al. (1987) Severe impairment in lung function induced by high peak airway pressure during mechanical ventilation. An experimental study. Am Rev Respir Dis 135: 312-315
16. Morris AH (1993) Evaluation of a new therapy: extracorporeal CO_2 removal, protocol control of intensive care unit care, and the human laboratory. J Crit Care 7(4): 280-286
17. National Heart (1979) Extracorporeal support for respiratory insufficiency. US Department of Health, Education, and Welfare, National Institutes of Health, Bethesda
18. Pesenti A, Gattinoni L, Bombino M (1993) Long term extracorporeal respiratory support: 20 years of progress Intensive Care Crit Care Digest 12(2): 15-17
19. Rossaint R, Slama K, Falke KJ (1991) Therapy of acute pulmonary failure. Dtsch Med Wochenschr 116: 1635-1639
20. Rossaint R, Slama K, Lewandowski K et al. (1992) Extracorporeal lung assist with heparin-coated systems. Int J Artif Organs 15: 29-34
21. Rossaint R, Falke KJ, Lopez F, Slama K, Pison U, Zapol WM (1993) Inhaled nitric oxide in adult respiratory distress syndrome. N Engl J Med 328: 399-405
22. Schulte HD, Bircks W, Dudziak R (1972) Preliminary results with the Bramson membrane lung (Also report of a successful, clinical long-term perfusion). Thoraxchir Vask Chir 20: 54-59
23. Suchyta MR, Clemmer TP, Orme JFJ, Morris AH, Elliott CG (1991) Increased survival of ARDS patients with severe hypoxemia (ECMO criteria). Chest 99: 951-955
25. Tharratt RS, Allen RP, Albertson TE (1988) Pressure controlled inverse ratio ventilation in severe adult respiratory failure. Chest 94: 755-762
26. Uziel L, Cugno M, Fabrizi I, Pesenti A, Gattinoni L, Agostoni A (1990) Physiopathology and management of coagulation during long-term extracorporeal respiratory assistance. Int J Artif Organs 13: 280-287
27. Zapol WM, Snider MT, Hill JD et al. (1979) Extracorporeal membrane oxygenation in severe acute respiratory failure. A randomized prospective study. JAMA 242: 2193-2196

Section 7:

Peritonitis - The Biological Basis for Treatment

Microbial Synergy in Intraabdominal Infections

O.D. Rotstein

The field of infectious diseases has traditionally been dominated by the study of diseases caused by single microorganisms. In order to satisfy Koch's principles, a single organism grown in pure culture was required to initiate infection upon inoculation into an experimental animal. While in a general sense, surgical infections fulfill these criteria, there are several clear differences which make them unique. First, these processes are characterized by the presence of a polymicrobial bacterial flora in the majority of clinical settings (Table 1). For example, the microbial isolates recovered from intraabdominal infections usually consists of a mixture of facultative gram-negative enteric bacili such as *Escherichia coli*, anaerobes such as *Bacteroides fragilis*, and gram-positive bacteria such as *Enterococcus fecalis* [1]. Second, surgical infections frequently occur in a setting of local tissue trauma. While the invading microorganisms are often endowed with their own virulence factors, the coexistent presence of tissue injury renders local host defenses less efficient, thereby promoting the establishment of infection. Finally, surgical infections may be associated with an underlying pathological process. Thus, optimal management usually consists of both directed antimicrobial therapy and surgical intervention to eradicate the source [2]. The purpose of this article is to examine the role of component bacterial species in the pathogenesis of intraabdominal infections and to define some of the mechanisms whereby these microorganisms might interact to augment the virulence of the process, so-called microbial synergy.

E. coli is the most frequently recovered gram-negative enteric microorganism from patients with secondary bacterial peritonitis. While this microbe possesses numerous virulence factors, its surface lipopolysaccharide (LPS) is clearly most responsible for the initiation of the systemic response to intraabdominal infection and hence the associated lethality of this process both in experimental animals and in humans [3-6]. The details of the structure of LPS and the mechanisms whereby it interacts with hosts cells to induce the release of the cytokine cascade are addressed elsewhere in this text. The precise role of anaerobic bacteria such as *B. fragilis* in the pathogenesis of infection is less well defined. Bacteroides LPS is attenuated in terms of its ability to cause death [7]. Neither the intravenous injection of large doses of bacteroides LPS nor the inoculation of high bacterial numbers is able to cause significant mortality in experimental models [8]. Detailed investigations by one group of investigators has revealed that *B. fragilis* plays a central role in the development of intraabdominal abscesses [9-12]. This effect appears to be mediated by a distinct capsular polysaccharide on the cell surface [11, 12]. That bacteroides species contribute to the virulence of intraabdominal infections in humans is best demonstrated by studies evaluating the efficacy of various antimicrobial agents in the treatment of bacterial peritonitis. Regiments containing agents with antianaerobe activity result in an improved clinical outcome compared to those lacking this activity [13].

Microbial synergy is defined as the cooperative interaction of two or more bacterial species that produce a result not achieved by the individual bacteria acting alone [14]. Evidence exists supporting the notion that *E. coli-B. fragilis* synergy occurs with respect to both abscess formation and lethality in experimental intraabdominal infection. For example, while a monomicrobial inoculum of *B. fragilis* caused no deaths in a rat model of intraabdominal infection, the addition of B. fragilis to an inoculum of *E. coli* significantly increased mortality compared to *E. coli* alone (Fig. 1, see [8]). Similarly, each of *E. coli* and *B. fragilis* was able to augment the abscessogenicity of the other microbe when inoculated together into the peritoneal cavity [15].

Table 1: Flora of surgical infections

	Single	Mixed
Abdominal		
Peritoneal cavity	+	+++
Visceral	+++	++
Gynecological	+	+++
Skin and soft tissue	+++, superficial	+++, deep
Head and neck	+	+++
Vascular	+++	+
Bone	+++	+
Brain	+++	++, especially trauma

+++, frequent; ++, occasional; +, rare

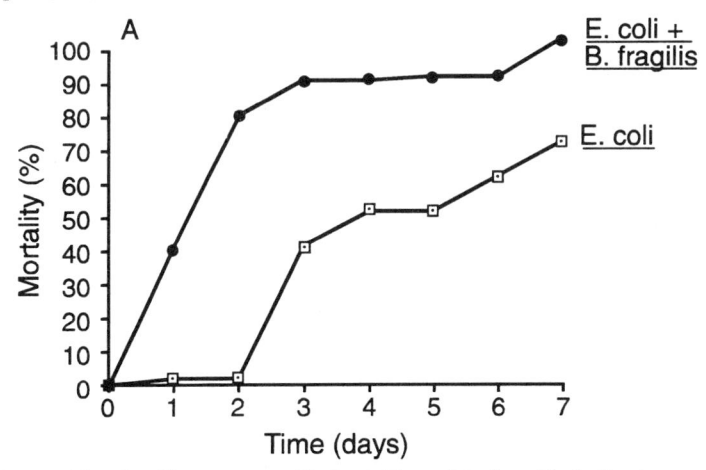

Fig. 1: Bacteroides fragilis augments Escherichia coli-induced lethality in a rat intraabdominal infection model. E. coli and B. fragilis were incorporated alone or in combination into a fibrin clot and inserted into the peritoneal cavity of rats. Mortality was assessed daily. The addition of B. fragilis to E. coli in the fibrin clot augmented lethality compared to E. coli alone. B. fragilis alone caused no deaths (not shown). (Adapted from [24])

Mackowiak [14] defined several possible mechanisms responsible for observed phenomenon of microbial synergy. These include: (1) the ability of one microorganism to provide nutrients for other microbes in a mixed infection; (2) the ability of one bacterial species to impair local host defenses thereby allowing its copathogen to persist and exert its virulence; (3) the alteration of the local milieu by one of the bacterial species resulting in improved survival and/or proliferation by other bacteria within the microenvironment; and (4) transfer of virulence factors between microbes. Within the peritoneal cavity, phagocytic cells including both neutrophils and macrophages play an important role in bacterial clearance and consequent resolution of infection [16]. Based on these observations, several laboratories including our own have examined potential mechanisms whereby anaerobic bacteria such as *B. fragilis* might impair neutrophil function. Data derived from our in vivo synergy studies demonstrated that live but not dead *B. fragilis* were able to augment *E. coli*-induced lethality. This suggested that a product of *B. fragilis* metabolism might be capable of impairing neutrophil function as a possible mechanism contributing to bacterial synergy. Studies examining the effect of *B. fragilis* culture supernatant on neutrophil function demonstrated that neutrophil migration as well as phagocytic killing of *E. coli* was markedly impaired [17, 18]. The inhibitory factor was resistant to heating suggesting it was not a bacterial-derived protease. Further characterization revealed that the factor was low molecular weight and, interestingly, was dependent on low medium pH to exert its effect. The factor was also most active when the supernatant was derived from *B. fragilis* in the late stationary growth phase. Based on these and other considerations, it was speculated that short chain fatty acids (SCFA), known to be normal byproducts of anaerobic bacterial metabolism [19], might be responsible. These molecules were low molecular weight, heat stable and present during stationary phase, thereby complying with the characteristics of the unknown factor. In subsequent studies, SCFA were shown to mimic the pH-dependent inhibition of neutrophil function [20, 21]. Further, when neutrophils were incubated in medium supplemented with concentrations of the various SCFA measured in *B. fragilis* supernatant, the reconstituted medium exerted comparable inhibition of neutrophil function [17]. Similar inhibitory effects of SCFA on neutrophil functions have been reported by other investigators [22-26]. When considered together, these data provided strong evidence for the role of SCFA as the active molecules responsible for the inhibition of neutrophil function by *B. fragilis* filtrate. Figure 2 illustrates a proposed mechanism whereby SCFA (specifically succinate) might exert their effect on neutrophil function. In essence, it was hypothesized that SCFA served as a proton shuttle carrying protons from the extracellular space into the cytoplasmic compartment with resultant intracellular acidification. This notion was attractive since the low pK_a of these weak acids (4.6-4.8) encouraged the formation of an undissociated state, the molecule entered the cytoplasmic compartment and released its proton when exposed to the physiologic intracellular pH. This would lead to progressive acidification of the intracellular space with consequent cellular dysfunction. Three lines of evidence suggested that this mechanism was operative. First, measurements of intracellular pH using fluorescent dye techniques indicated that, at low extracellular pH, succinate-containing medium markedly augmented the magnitude of intracellular acidication compared to control [27]. Second, this effect occurred simultaneously with a significant increase in the uptake of radiolabelled succinate of neutrophils [28]. Finally, the impaired neutrophil function was entirely accounted for by the reduction in intracellular pH, as evidenced by the fact that the inhibition could be reproduced by pharmacological reduction of cytosolic pH in the absence of SCFA [27]. In summary, these studies illustrate a mechanism whereby a normal metabolic product of *B.*

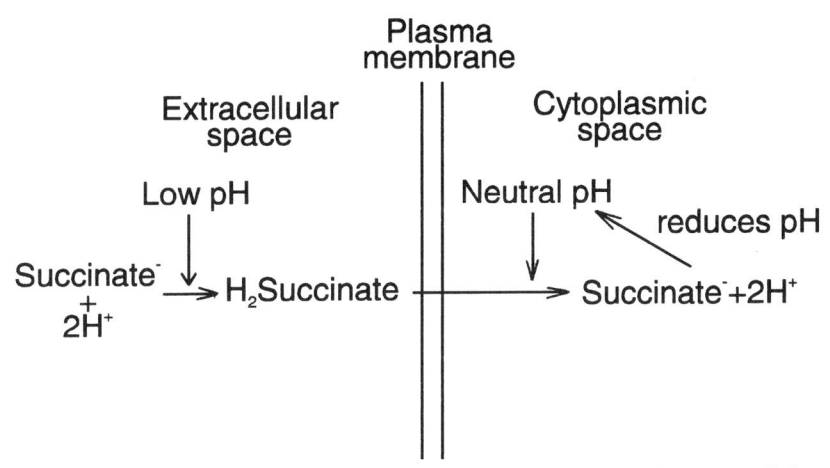

```
                        Plasma
                       membrane
         Extracellular  ║  Cytoplasmic
            space       ║     space
          Low pH        ║   Neutral pH
             │          ║       │      ↖ reduces pH
  Succinate⁻ ↓          ║       ↓
      +     → H₂Succinate → Succinate⁻ + 2H⁺
     2H⁺                ║
                        ║
```

Fig. 2: Mechanism of inhibition of neutrophil function by succinate. At low extracellular pH, the weak acid succinate is protonated and traverses the plasma membrane. Within the cytoplasmic space, the molecule dissociates and releases H^+, thereby causing cytoplasmic acidification. The reduction in intracellular pH accounted for the impaired cellular function induced by succinate. (Adapted from [33])

fragilis might interact with alterations in the local inflammatory microenvironment to effect neutrophil inhibition and thus contribute to synergistic bacterial interactions.

B. fragilis as well as other bacteroides species have been shown to impair phagocytic cell function by other mechanisms (reviewed in [29]). Bacteroides species are able to bind complement components to their cell surface and thus deplete local opsonins [30, 31]. Consequently, opsonin-depleted serum is incapable of serving as a source of opsonins for *E. coli* resulting in impaired phagocytic uptake of these microbes. In addition, the expression and release of various proteases by bacteroides species may serve to degrade the opsonic components of the local milieu and thus cause similar inhibition of *E. coli* uptake and killing [32]. When considered together, these findings suggest that bacteroides species may contribute to synergy both by direct inhibition of neutrophils and also by altering the local conditions which might indirectly retard bacterial clearance.

Bacteroides species may contribute to the pathogenicity of mixed infections by altering other local environmental conditions which may impair the ability of neutrophils to kill bacteria. Fibrin deposition is routinely observed at sites of inflammation including the early stages of peritonitis. Both in vivo and in vitro studies have verified the important contribution of fibrin in the persistence of infection as sites of extravascular infection. During experimental intraabdominal infection, the administration of anticoagulants such as heparin [33] or fibrinolytic agents such as tissue plasminogen activator [34] was shown to augment bacterial clearance and prevent persistent infections such as abscesses (Fig. 3). In vitro studies revealed that fibrin matrices were able to inhibit phagocytic cell function including cell migration and killing capacity. Several mechanisms appear to underlie these effects. The physical structure of the fibrin gel impeded migration of cells through its interstices and thus prevented phagocytic uptake of bacteria [35, 36]. Second, fibrinogen/fibrin degradation products (FDP) have been shown to modify phagocytic cell function. For example, these FDP are able to inhibit phagocytic cell migration and microbicidal functions [37]. Interest-

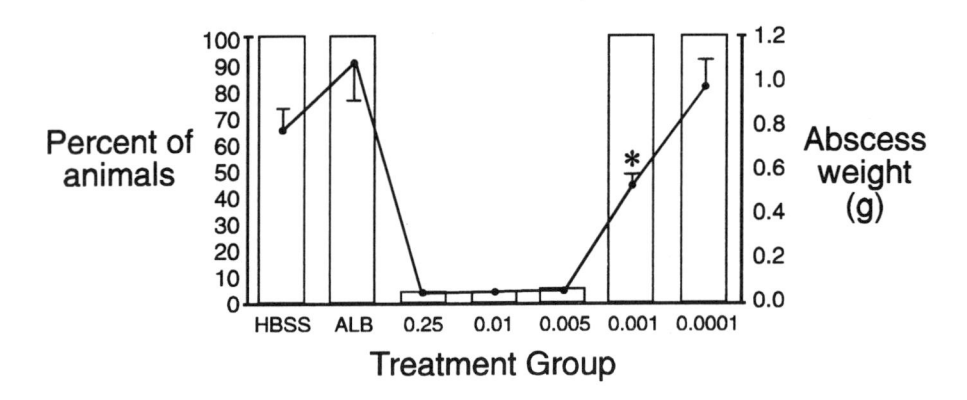

Fig. 3: Fibrinolysis prevents intraabdominal abscess formation. Animals were injected intraperitoneally with salt solution (HBSS), albumin, or various concentrations of recombinant tissue plasminogen activator simultaneous with the inoculation with a Bacteroides fragilis-infected fibrin clot. Tissue plasminogen activator significantly reduced abscess formation. (Adapted from [25])

ingly, FDP as well as fibrinopeptide B have been shown to exhibit chemoattractant properties [38-40]. While this may contribute to neutrophil influx during the early phases of peritonitis, high concentrations of these products may act to desensitize cells and impair their function. Based on the ability of fibrinogen/fibrin and their products to impair resolution of a residual bacterial nidus by phagocytic cells, it was hypothesized that *B. fragilis* might contribute to the virulence of mixed infections by augmenting local fibrin deposition. As noted earlier, bacteroides species possess a large number of proteases, some of which may contribute to the induction of coagulation in the peritoneal cavity [41]. Further, since macrophages are the predominant cell type within the peritoneal cavity during the early hours of peritonitis, it was speculated that *B. fragilis* might initiate fibrin deposition by stimulating macrophages to synthesize procoagulant molecules such as tissue factor on their surface. Incubation of *B. fragilis* with macrophages was shown to induce a dose- and time-dependent increase in their ability to initiate fibrin deposition [42, 43]. Using factor-deficient plasma to perform the assay, the nature of the procoagulant was shown to be consistent with tissue factor-like activity. This stimulatory effect of *B. fragilis* was mediated via a heat-stable surface factor on these microbes and did not require phagocytosis of the microorganism. Subsequent studies indicated that both bacteroides LPS and capsular polysaccharide contributed to the stimulatory effect. Interestingly, very high concentrations of *B. fragilis* ($> 2 \times 10^9$ cfu/ml) prevented the rise in macrophage procoagulant activity in response to *E. coli* LPS. This effect was mediated in part by a soluble *B. fragilis* factor, but not SCFA [44]. Since impaired fibrin sequestration of bacteria in the peritoneal cavity has been shown to augment lethality [34], this observation suggests a mechanism whereby high concentrations of *B. fragilis* might augment *E. coli* lethality, as previously demonstrated using an intraabdominal infection model in rats [8].

In summary, intraabdominal infections are characterized by the presence of a polymicrobial flora consisting predominantly of facultative enteric gram-negative bacteria but also anaerobic bacteria. While each component of the flora exhibits intrinsic virulence, synergistic interactions between bacterial species result in an overall augmentation of the pathogenicity of these infections.

References

1. Lorber B, Swenson RM (1975) The bacteriology of intraabdominal infections. Surg Clin Am 55: 1349-1354
2. Rotstein OD (1992) Peritonitis and intra-abdominal abscesses. In: Care of the surgical patient. Scientific American Publications, New York
3. Raetz CRH, Ulevitch RJ, Wright SD, Sibley CH, Ding A, Nathan CF (1919) Gram-negative endotoxin: an extraordinary lipid with profound effects on eukaryotic signal transduction. FASEB 5: 2652-2660
4. Michie HR, Manogue KR, Spriggs DR, Revhaug A, O'Dwyer S, Dinarello CA, Cerami A, Wolff SM, Wilmore DW (1988) Detection of circulating tumor necrosis factor after endotoxin administration. N Engl J Med 318: 1481-1486
5. Ziegler EJ, McCutchan JA, Fierer J, Glauser MP, Sadoff JC, Douglas H, Braude AI (1982) Treatment of gram negative bacteremia and shock with human antiserum to mutant Escherichia coli. N Engl J Med 307: 1225-1230
6. Dunn DL, Priest BP, Condie RM (1988) Protective capacity of polyclonal and monoclonal antibodies during experimental sepsis. Arch Surg 123: 1389-1393
7. Hofstad T, Kristoffersen T (1970) Chemical characteristics of endotoxin from Bacteroides fragilis NCTC 9343. J Gen Microbiol 61: 15-19
8. Rotstein OD, Kao J (1988) The spectrum of Escherichia coli - Bacteroides fragilis pathogenic synergy in an intraabdominal infection model. Can J Microbiol 34: 352-357
9. Onderdonk AB, Cisneros RL, Crabb JH, Finberg RW, Kasper DL (1989) Intraperitoneal host cellular responses and in vivo killing of Bacteroides fragilis in a bacterial containment chamber. Infect Immun 57: 3030-3037
10. Shapiro ME, Onderdonk AB, Kasper DL, Finberg RW (1982) Cellular immunity to Bacteroides fragilis capsular polysaccharide. J Exp Med 154: 1188-1197
11. Onderdonk AB, Kasper DL, Cisneros RL, Bartlett JG (1977) The capsular polysaccharide of Bacteroides fragilis as a virulence factor: comparison of the pathogenic potential of encapsulated and unencapsulated strains. J Infect Dis 136: 82-89
12. Tzianabos AO, Onderdonk AB, Rosner B, Cisneros RL, Kasper DL (1993) Structural features of polysaccharides that induce intra-abdominal abscesses. Science 262: 416-419
13. Berne TV, Yellin AW, Appleman MD, Heseltine PNR (1982) Antibiotic management of surgically treated gangrenous or perforated appendicitis. Am J Surg 144: 8-13
14. Mackowiak PA (1978) Microbial synergism in human infections (second of two parts). N Engl J Med 298: 83-87
15. Rotstein OD, Kao J, Houston K (1989) Reciprocal synergy between Escherichia coli and Bacteroides fragilis in an intra-abdominal infection model. J Med Microbiol 29: 269-276
16. Dunn DL, Barke RA, Ewald DC, Simmons RL (1987) Macrophages and translymphatic absorption represent the first line of host defense in the peritoneal cavity. Arch Surg 122: 105-110

17. Rotstein OD, Vittorini T, Kao J, McBurney MI, Nasmith PR, Grinstein S (1989) A soluble Bacteroides by-product impairs phagocytic killing of Escherichia coli by neutrophils. Infect Immun 57: 745-753
18. Rotstein OD, Pruett TL, Sorenson JJ, Fiegel VD, Nelson RD, Simmons RL (1986) A Bacteroides by-product inhibits human polymorphonuclear leukocyte function. Arch Surg 121: 82-88
19. Gorbach SL, Mayhew JW, Bartlett JG, Thadepalli H, Onderdonk AB (1976) Rapid diagnosis of anaerobic infections by direct gas-liquid chromatography of clinical specimens. J Clin Invest 57: 478-484
20. Rotstein OD, Pruett TL, Fiegel VD, Nelson RD, Simmons RL (1985) Succinic acid, a metabolic by-product by Bacteroides species, inhibits polymorphonuclear leukocyte function. Infect Immun 48: 402-408
21. Rotstein OD, Wells CL, Pruett TL, Sorenson JJ, Simmons RL (1987) Succinic acid production by Bacteroides fragilis. A potential bacterial virulence factor. Arch Surg 122: 93-98
22. Eftimiadi C, Buzzi E, Tonetti M, Buffa P, van Steenbergen MTJ, de Graaff J, Botta GA (1987) Short-chain fatty acids produced by anaerobic bacteria alter the physiologic responses of human neutrophils to chemotactic peptides. J Infect 14: 43-53
23. Botta GA, Eftimiadi C, Costa A, Tonetti M, van Steenbergen TJM, de Graaff J (1985) Influence of volatile fatty acids on human granulocyte chemotaxis. FEMS Microbiol Lett 27: 39-72
24. Eftimiadi C, Tonetti M, Cavallero A, Sacco O, Rossi GA (1990) Short-chain fatty acids produced by anaerobic bacteria inhibit phagocytosis by human lung phagocytes. J Infect Dis 161: 138-142
25. Topley N, Alobaida HMM, Davies M, Coles GA, Williams JD, Lloyd D (1988) The effect of dialysate on peritoneal phagocyte oxidative metabolism. Kidney Int 34: 404-411
26. Liberek T, Topley N, Jörres A, Petersen MM, Coles GA, Gahl GM, Williams JD (1993) Peritoneal dialysis fluid inhibition of polymorphonuclear leukocyte respiratory burst activation is related to the lowering of intracellular pH. Nephron 65: 260-265
27. Rotstein OD, Nasmith PE, Grinstein S (1987) The Bacteroides by-product succinic acid inhibits neutrophil respiratory burst by reducing intracellular pH. Infect Immun 55: 864-870
28. Rotstein OD, Nasmith PE, Grinstein S (1988) pH-dependent impairment of the neutrophil respiratory burst by the Bacteroides byproduct succinate. Clin Invest Med 11: 259-265
29. Rotstein OD, Pruett TL, Simmons RL (1985) Mechanisms of microbial synergy in polymicrobial surgical infections. Rev Infect Dis 7: 151-170
30. Vel WAC, Namavar F, Verweij-Van Vught AMJJ, Pubben ANB, MacLaren DM (1986) Interactions between polymorphonuclear leukocytes, Bacteroides species, and Escherichia coli: their role in the pathogenesis of mixed infection. J Clin Pathol 39: 376-382
31. Dijkmans BAC, Leijh PCJ, Braat AGP, van Furth R (1985) Effect of bacterial competition on the opsonization, phagocytosis, and intracellular killing of microorganisms by granulocytes. Infect Immun 49: 219-224
32. Bjornson HS (1984) Enzymes associated with the survival and virulence of gram-negative anaerobes. Rev Inf Dis 6: S21-S24
33. Hau T, Simmons RL (1978) Heparin in the treatment of experimental peritonitis. Ann Surg 187: 294-298
34. Rotstein OD, Pruett T, Simmons RL (1986) Fibrin in peritonitis inhibits phagocytic killing of Escherichia coli by human polymorphonuclear leukocytes. Ann Surg 203: 413-419
35. Rotstein OD, Kao J (1988) Prevention of intra-abdominal abscesses by fibrinolysis using recombinant tissue plasminogen activator. J Infect Dis 158: 766-772

36. Ciano PS, Colvin RB, Dvorak AM, McDonagh J, Dvorak HF (1986) Macrophage migration in fibrin gel matrices. Lab Invest 54: 62-70
37. Kazura JW, Wenger JD, Salata RA, Budzynski AZ, Goldsmith GH (1989) Modulation of polymorphonuclear leukocyte microbicidal acitivity and oxidative metabolism by fibrinogen degradation products D and E. J Clin Invest 83: 1916-1924
38. Skogen WF, Senior RM, Griffin GL, Wilner GD (1988) Fibrinogen-derived peptide BB1-42 is a multidomained neutrophil chemoattractant. Blood 71: 1475-1479
39. Senior RM, Skogen WF, Griffin GL, Wilner GD (1986) Effect of fibrinogen derivatives upon the inflammatory response Studies with human fibrinopeptide B. J Clin Invest 77: 1014-1019
40. Stecher VJ, Sorkin E (1972) The chemotactic activity of fibrin lysis products. Intl Arch Allergy 43: 879-886
41. Much H (1908) Uber eine vorstufe des fibrinfermentes in kulturen von Staphylokokkus aureus. Biochem 14: 143-155
42. Rosenthal GA, Levy G, Rotstein OD (1989) Induction of macrophage procoagulant activity by Bacteroides fragilis. Infect Immun 57: 338-343
43. Sinclair SB, Rotstein OD, Levy GA (1990) Disparate mechanisms of induction of procoagulant activity by live and inactive bacteria and viruses. Infect Immun 58: 1821-1827
44. Rotstein OD, Vittorini T (1989) Bacteroides fragilis inhibits macrophage procoagulant activity by E. coli endothelium. Surg Forum 40: 109-111

Host Defenses of the Peritoneal Cavity

D.L. Dunn

Introduction

The mammalian host frequently is subjected to the incursion of microorganisms at a variety of sites within the body. These microorganisms are derived from both the external environment and the endogenous microflora of the host. For example, the integument acts as a barrier to prevent the invasion of microorganisms within the external environment, and a variety of epithelial layers that are colonized by endogenous microflora prohibit the invasion of these epithelial layer-associated, commensal microbes. Among the most heavily colonized regions of the body is the gastrointestinal tract. Although microbes are to be found associated with the mucosal barrier throughout the entire gastrointestinal tract, large numbers and diverse species of autochthonous microbes are present in the proximal (oropharynx) and distal (colorectum) gut. Under normal circumstances, the stomach is virtually sterile due to its high acidity and peristalsis. Few numbers and types of bacteria are found in the proximal small intestine, while progressively increasing numbers of microbes are encountered in an aboral direction in the small intestine and the colon. In addition, increasingly larger numbers of anaerobic bacteria are found in the ileum and colon compared to the more proximal small intestine.

Within the colon facultative and strict anaerobic bacteria predominate with such organisms as *Bacteroides fragilis*, *Bacteroides* sp., *Fusobacterium*, *Peptostreptococcus* sp. and *Peptidostreptococcus* sp. and many others being commonly isolated. These anaerobic organisms outnumber aerobic forms that include *Escherichia coli* and other *Enterobacteriaceae*, and *Enterococcus fecalis* and *fecium* 100-300:1. Microbes comprise as much as one third of the dry weight of feces, with as many as 10^{11}-10^{12} organisms present per gram of feces. Thus, anaerobes are present in extremely large numbers (10^{10}-10^{12} per gram of feces), while 10^8-10^{10} aerobes per gram of feces are isolated [1].

These organisms achieve clinical significance when the barrier function of the gastrointestinal tracts fails, typically due to perforation. In that case, the microorganisms present within that portion of the gastrointestinal tract spill out into the normally sterile peritoneal cavity. The peritoneal cavity is a mesothelium-lined potential space that under normal circumstances contains only a small amount (50 ml) of serous, sterile fluid. Infection of this potential space can occur after exogenous introduction of microorganisms in patients in whom no viscus perforation has occurred (primary microbial peritonitis) or after perforation of a viscus with spillage of the autochthonous flora takes place (secondary microbial peritonitis). The change in microbial flora in patients with initial secondary bacterial peritonitis leading to ongoing infection due to normally low virulence pathogens (e.g., *Staphylococcus epidermidis, Streptococcus fecalis, Candida albicans*) has been termed tertiary microbial or persistent peritonitis.

The introduction of microorganisms into the normally sterile peritoneal environment invokes several potent specialized host antimicrobial defense mechanisms: (1) clearance, (2) phagocytosis and killing, and (3) sequestration. Under most circumstances, host defenses present within the peritoneal cavity act to prevent further microbial invasion either by sequestration or eradication of the invading microorganisms. Thus, the rate of microbial division and presence of a variety of virulence factors that bacteria possess, coupled with the size of the initial inoculum and presence of so-called adjuvant substances that act to foster bacterial growth and bacterial synergistic interactions, are countered by a series of extremely potent local host defense mechanisms. For example, it has become increasingly clear that infections caused by aerobic and anaerobic bacteria together can result in a more serious infection than would be expected from the additive effects of either type of organism alone [2, 3]. The outcome of these opposing forces varies from case to case and consists of a spectrum of events that range from complete eradication of infection, more chronic infection in the form of persistent peritonitis and/or abscess formation, or host lethality due to spread of infection to the systemic level.

Experimental studies conducted in rodents demonstrated clearly that the nature of the interaction of invading microbes with resident and recruited host defenses within the peritoneal cavity is complex. Only very large numbers of bacteria (10^{10} colony forming units, cfu) are capable of saturating clearance, phagocytosis, and sequestration mechanisms and causing mortality in all animals. Introduction of 10^7-10^8 cfu leads to a biphasic curve in which initial diminution of bacterial numbers is observed, following which bacterial growth occurs and 50% mortality occurs. Smaller numbers of bacteria invariably are counteracted effectively, a rapid decrease in the number of microorganisms taking place [4]. Comprehending the nature of the interaction of proliferating bacteria with a series of now well defined host defenses has been the target of a great deal of investigative effort. The purpose of this review is to delineate the host defenses of the peritoneal cavity with regard to their activity and relative importance during microbial peritonitis.

Microbial Clearance via Translymphatic Absorption

Early studies led investigators to the conclusion that particles present within the peritoneal cavity were absorbed through the cytoplasm of mesothelial cells. However, studies by Florey and Allen demonstrated that intracellular uptake did not occur, and the latter investigator's research using frog erythrocytes showed that they became entrapped within the gaps between mesothelial cells (stomata) that led into overlying lymphatic channels (lacunae) [5, 6]. Subsequently, Allen observed that graphite particles injected into the peritoneal cavity of rabbits could be identified in the thoracic duct lymph within 3-5 min, indicating the rapidity with which clearance occurred [7]. Steinberg performed similar studies in dogs but introduced bacteria rather than inert particles or erythrocytes into the peritoneum, noting that microbes were removed largely via this clearance mechanism and only to a small extent by flow into mesenteric and omental venules [8]. The importance of these studies was the finding that large numbers of bacteria were isolated first from the thoracic duct lymph [6-10 min) and subsequently from the bloodstream (30-40 min) after peritoneal bacterial challenge and that no uptake of bacteria into intervening lymph nodes occurred. Movement of the diaphragm during inspiration and expiration appeared to open and close the stomata, facilitating entry of fluid and particulate material into lymphatic lacunae. These lacunae coalesce into larger thoracic lymphatic structures that eventually form the thoracic duct. Higgins demonstrated that omentectomy had no effect upon peritoneal clearance of graphite, while transection of the phrenic nerve leading to diaphragmatic atrophy increased translymphatic absorption of graphite in dogs [9]. Other studies using polystyrene spheres indicated that the maximal size of particulates that could pass through this system was 24 µm, and other confirmatory studies have been performed using both light and scanning electron microscopy [10, 11].

Thus, it is apparent that microbial clearance via translymphatic absorption occurs via specialized structures on the underside of the diaphragm that act as conduits for both fluid and particulate matter. These gaps that are termed stomata (10-16 µm) exist between mesothelial cells that lead into lymphatic structures (lacunae). These lacunae, in turn, lead into lymphatic vessels that coalesce into larger mediastinal lymphatic structures. Subsequently, these lymphatic trunks drain into the thoracic duct, which empties into the venous circulation. Diaphragmatic movement appears to create a pumping action such that fluid and particulates within fluid are forced out of the peritoneal cavity via the aforementioned system. Inert particles, microbes, and even red blood cells are capable of passing out of the peritoneal cavity in this fashion. Large numbers of particulates of all types, including bacteria, are rapidly cleared from the peritoneal cavity into the systemic circulation. For example, inoculation of bacteria into the peritoneum in rodents leads to bacteremia within minutes, and > 50% of an inoculum of 2×10^8 killed radiolabeled *Escherichia coli* are cleared from the peritoneal cavity within 1 h. Radiolabeled bacteria appear in the systemic circulation within 5-10 mins after their introduction into the peritoneal cavity. The potency of this system is such that it is only overloaded by the introduction of huge numbers of microbes ($> 10^{10}$ cfu) [4, 12]. Unfortunately, this potent host defense most probably can exert adverse effects on the host in that removal of bacteria from the peritoneal cavity via this mechanism translates them into the systemic circulation. Although fixed mononuclear cells of the reticuloendothelial system as well as circulating polymorphonuclear leukocytes (PMNs) act to rapidly engulf these microbes, large numbers of microbes are capable of overwhelming these defenses as well. Interaction of gram-negative bacterial endotoxin with systemic host defenses can provoke systemic sepsis and septic shock, a disease process currently associated with 40% mortality.

Microbial Phagocytosis and Killing

Those microbes that are not cleared are rapidly engulfed by resident and recruited phagocytic cells. Few PMNs are present during the initial stages of infection, and resident macrophages act as the first line of peritoneal host defense in concert with clearance to diminish bacterial numbers [4, 12]. Approximately 10^7 macrophages are present within the rodent peritoneal cavity, and these cells exhibit potent phagocytic activity. Immediately after the introduction of microbes into the normally sterile peritoneal cavity, PMNs are recruited, presumably on the basis of chemotactic factors generated by the bacteria themselves as well as by host defense proteins (e.g., C3b, C5a). Within 2-3 h after bacterial challenge, the number of macrophages and PMNs is similar, and thereafter the number of PMNs continues to increase. An influx of leukocytes into the peritoneal cavity continues for 36-48 h. In addition, as few as 10^4 cfu *Escherichia coli* are capable of triggering maximal recruitment of PMNs.

Although PMNs and macrophages exhibit similar activity with regard to phagocytosis and killing, they play somewhat different roles in this system of host defenses. Macrophages are present in relatively low numbers continually and represent a first line, constitutive host defense mechanism. PMNs, however, are not present initially, but serve as an inducible, second-line host defense, being recruited into the peritoneal cavity and serving to prevent proliferation of those bacteria that have escaped the activity of clearance and macrophage phagocytosis.

Microbial Sequestration

Those microorganisms that evade both clearance and phagocytosis are confronted by a final, primitive host defense mechanism [sequestration) that functions to protect the host from the bacterial inoculum. A fibrinogen-rich inflammatory exudate containing plasma opsonins appears during peritoneal infection and fibrin polymerization occurs. Acting in conjunction with the omentum and other mobile viscera, perforations are sealed by fibrin, and as ileus develops contaminated enteric contents are walled off, thereby preventing continued soilage of the peritoneal cavity. The latter mechanism represent a rather crude, albeit effective, way in which infection is contained.

Polymerizing fibrin has the capacity to trap large numbers of bacteria. This process appears to be relatively nonspecific, acting to trap particulates as well as bacteria regardless of external charge or structure characteristics. Thus, either gram negative or gram positive aerobic bacteria or charged or uncharged 5-10 μm polystyrene beads are efficiently trapped in a similar fashion within a fibrin clot as fibrinogen is polymerized by thrombin in vitro. Presumably this same process occurs in vivo within the confines of the peritoneal cavity as one of the initial events in the development of fibrinopurulent peritonitis [13]. Although these host defenses function well within the confines of the peritoneal cavity, adverse systemic effects may occur that are related to these processes (Table 1). Thus, intraabdominal abscess formation is probably promoted both by the fluid influx into the peritoneal cavity which inhibits opsonization and phagocytosis and by the formation of fibrin clots that isolate the bacteria from clearance mechanisms and phagocytic activity. Prevention of overwhelming systemic sepsis via sequestration of infection may be beneficial during the initial stages of infection, but may lead to subsequent intraabdominal abscess formation, chronic infection, and intermittent systemic sepsis.

Summary

Invading microbes encounter a series of local host defenses that are unique to the peritoneal environment. Translymphatic absorption, phagocytosis and killing by macrophages and PMNs, and sequestration by fibrin trapping, omental containment and ileus all serve to interdict microbial proliferation and spread. On balance, peritoneal host defenses function in an extremely efficient fashion, serving to eradicate infection in the vast majority of patients in conjunction with surgical source control, appropriate antimicrobial agent therapy, and intensive care. Unfortunately, large numbers of microbes within the peritoneal cavity may proliferate and overwhelm host defenses initially at the local and thereafter at the systemic level. Not surprisingly, therefore, microbial peritonitis continues to represent a potentially lethal disease process. Further studies are necessary to determine whether or not it may be possible to bolster host defenses at the local and the systemic level to diminish the lethality of this disease process.

Table 1: Host defenses of the peritoneal cavity.

Host defenses	Mechanisms	Constitutive vs. inducible	Potential adverse effect
Clearance	Translymphatic absorption via diaphragmatic stomata and overlying lymphatic lacunae	Constitutive	Systemic sepsis can occur if large numbers of microbes are translated into the systemic circulation.
Phagocytosis	Engulfment and intracellular killing of microbes by: (a) resident macrophage; (b) recruited PMNs	Constitutive Inducible	Release of cytokines, leukocyte enzymes in large quantities could conceivably provoke deleterious effects, although this process probably remains largely confined to the peritoneal cavity.
Sequestration	Several: (a) trapping of microbes by polymerizing fibrin; (b) containment of gross infection by the omentum and ileus	Both Constitutive	Abscess formation with the potential for chronic infection and intermittent systemic sepsis.

References

1. Dunn DL (1990) Autochthonous microflora of the gastrointestinal tract. Perspect Colon Rectal Surg 2: 105-119
2. Dunn DL, Rotstein OD, Simmons RL (1984) Fibrin in peritonitis. IV. Synergistic intraperitoneal infection due to Escherichia coli and Bacteroides fragilis within fibrin clots. Arch Surg 119: 134-144
3. Dunn DL, Barke RA, Ewald DC, Simmons RL (1985) Effects of Escherichia coli and Bacteroides fragilis on peritoneal host defenses. Infect Immun 48: 287-291
4. Dunn DL, Barke RA, Knight NB, Humphrey EW, Simmons RL (1985) Role of resident macrophages, peripheral neutrophils, and translymphatic absorption in bacterial clearance from the peritoneal cavity. Infect Immun 49: 257-264
5. Florey H (1927) Reactions of, and absorption by, lymphatics with special reference to those of the diaphragm. Br J Exp Pathol 28: 479-490
6. Allen L (1936) The peritoneal stomata. Anat Rec 67: 89-99
7. Allen L, Vogt E (1937) A mechanism of lymphatic absorption from serous cavities. Am J Physiol 119: 776-782
8. Steinberg B (1944) Infections of the Peritoneum. Hoeber, New York, p 30.
9. Higgins GM (1930) Phrenic nephrectomy and peritoneal absorption. Am J Pathol 45: 137-157
10. Allen L, Weatherford T (1959) Role of fenestrated basement membrane in lymphatic absorption from peritoneal cavity. Am J Physiol 197: 551-554

11. *Tsilibary EC, Wissig SL (1977) Absorption from the peritoneal cavity: SEM study of the mesothelium covering the peritoneal surface of the muscular portion of the diaphragm. Am J Anat 149: 127-133*
12. *Dunn DL, Barke RA, Ewald DC, Simmons RL (1987) Macrophages and translymphatic absorption represent the first line of host defense of the peritoneal cavity. Arch Surg 122: 105-110*
13. *Dunn DL, Simmons RL (1982) Fibrin in peritonitis. III. The mechanism of bacterial trapping by polymerizing fibrin. Surgery 92: 513-519*

Regulation of Intraabdominal Inflammation: The Cellular Aspect

P. Kinnaert

Peritoneal Structure

The abdominal cavity is lined with a serous membrane, the peritoneum, which also covers the mesentery and the viscera. It normally contains a small amount of fluid (less than 50 ml in humans) and at most 10^7 cells, mainly macrophages (MØs). The peritoneal membrane consists of a single layer of mesothelial cells anchored to a basement membrane which lies on a loose interstitium containing blood microvessels, lymphatics, collagen bundles and a few cells, most of them fibroblasts. However, monocytes and mast cells are also observed usually in the neighborhood of capillaries [1]. It must be remembered that, in the normal state, the abdominal cavity is a virtual space where any intraperitoneal MØ or any contaminant is in close contact with the mesothelial layers of the visceral and parietal peritoneum. Therefore, the inflammatory mediators released by intraperitoneal MØs act immediately on the adjacent mesothelial cells, which in turn are activated and can transmit signals to the cells of the interstitium.Peritonitis induces a classical inflammatory reaction in the interstitium. Moreover, the mesothelial cells no longer form a continuous layer. There are ruptures of the intercellular junctions, with round cells moving into the gaps from the submesothelial layer towards the abdominal cavity. Thus opening of intercellular spaces could facilitate the access of leukocytes from the interstitium to the abdominal cavity [2]. With more severe injury, the mesothelium degenerates and desquamation occurs.

Changes in Peritoneal Cell Populations During Acute Inflammation

The introduction in the peritoneal cavity of an inflammatory stimulus is followed by a rapid influx of polymorphonuclear cells (PMNs), which, in rodents, represent the most important cell type of the exudate already after 4 h. The total number of MØs remains stable for the first 6 h and then starts to increase progressively. However, more precise investigations have demonstrated that there are rapid qualitative changes in this MØ population. Already 1 h after onset of acute inflammation, resident MØs are replaced by recruited MØs [3]. The disappearance of resident MØs from the recoverable cells results from their trapping with PMNs in fibrinous deposits on the peritoneal surface. This observation indicates one of the major limitations of the current studies of intraperitoneal inflammation. Conclusions concerning alterations of the cell population are based on the examination of specimens obtained by peritoneal lavage. These cell suspensions do not represent the whole cell content of the abdomen and we must keep in mind that our present data only concern the recoverable cells.

Production of Chemotactic Factors

Table 1 shows the classical factors usually thought to be responsible for the migration of PMNs towards an infected area. Bacteria release chemotactic peptides. Complement is activated by microbial peptidoglycans or lipopolysaccharides and C5a, a very potent chemoattractant is produced. Intraperitoneal fibrin formation occurs during peritonitis leading to the generation of kinins and fibrin degradation products. MØs release leukotriene B4 (LTB4) within minutes after stimulation while interleukin-8 (IL-8) is produced only after 3 - 5 h [4].

Table 1: Chemotactic factors

Bacterial peptides
Complement derived: C5a
Coagulation related
Lipid mediators, leukotriene B4
Low molecular weight cytokines of the interleukin-8 family

The relative importance of these various mechanisms is not always clear in case of infection. Indeed most of our present knowledge concerning chemotactic factors comes from in vitro studies or experiments in which these agents have been injected subcutaneously or i.p., a rather artificial setting. Kopaniak and Movat demonstrated that complement depletion with cobra venom in rabbits had no effect on subcutaneous PMN accumulation induced by injection of killed *E. coli* [5]. More recently, Mackensie et al. observed that gram-negative organisms were unable to stimulate LTB4 synthesis of human peritoneal MØ although *Staphylococcus aureus* induced a significant increase of the same leukotriene [6]. Finally, there is probably some redundancy of the different chemotactic mechanisms.

Cellular Interactions

In mice, intraabdominal injection of LTB4, a potent chemoattractant, does not increase the number of PMNs in the peritoneal fluid, while IL-1, which is not chemotactic in vitro, induces a rapid influx of PMNs after i.p. administration [7]. This observation indicates that i.p. chemotactic activity is insufficient to provoke the migration of PMNs from the submesothelial microvessels towards the abdominal cavity. However, the effect of IL-1 suggests that more complex mechanisms are needed to transmit information from the peritoneal cavity to the PMNs traveling through the capillaries of the interstitium. It was recently shown that mesothelial cells synthesize and secrete prostaglandins and various interleukins when properly stimulated (Table 2) [8, 9]. Consequently, a cascade of cellular activations progressing from the peritoneal cavity towards the submesothelial microvessels could possibly explain the subsequent migration of the PMNs. In such a model of intraperitoneal inflammation, mesothelial cells are stimulated directly by microorganisms or by tumor necrosis factor (TNF) and IL-1 released by activated intraperitoneal MØs. The latter synthesize and secrete IL-1, which can act on adjacent cells thus quickly amplifying the cellular response. This is facilitated by the close contact of the peritoneal membranes (parietal, visceral, omental) and mobility of abdominal organs, which possibly increases the number of cell interactions. IL-1 from mesothelial origin diffuses into the submesothelial connective tissue where it can induce the production of cytokines by MØs and, finally, activate endothelial cells, thus initiating diapedesis of PMNs. As all these cells also release prostaglandins and chemoattractants (LTB4 and/or IL-8), all the conditions for an inflammatory reaction can be rapidly brought together.

Table 2: Mediators secreted by peritoneal macrophages and mesothelial cells

	Macrophages	Mesothelial cells
TXB2	+	NT
PGE2	+	+
6 Keto PGF1	NT	+
LTB4	+	0
TNF	+	NT
IL-1	+	+
IL-6	+	+
IL-8	+	+

TX, thromboxane; PG, prostaglandin; LT, leukotriene; TNF, tumor necrosis factor; IL, interleukin; NT, not tested.

Few mast cells are present in the peritoneal fluid and in the interstitium, but their number increases during peritonitis. Up to now, mast cells have mainly been implicated in allergic reactions or in defense mechanisms against parasites. However, Qureshi and Jaschik demonstrated, in a mouse model of peritonitis induced by thioglycolate, that mast cells play an important role in the migration of PMNs towards the abdominal cavity [10]. When activated, they release histamine and intraglanular stores of TNF. They also synthesize and secrete cytokines, prostaglandins and leukotrienes [11]. Their role in microbial inflammation remains however to be determined in man.

Adhesion Molecules

Migration of PMNs through the capillary walls is a multistep phenomenon [12]. First, the cells start rolling on the endothelium, a low affinity interaction mediated by selectins. Mel-14, a monoclonal antibody directed against L-selectin, inhibits neutrophil influx at sites of acute inflammation. Firm adhesion of the PMNs to endothelial cells is the next step. Other adhesion molecules are involved in this process: integrins and their ligands from the immunoglobulin super family.

In the case of peritonitis, endothelial cells stimulated by IL-1, TNF or lipopolysaccharide (LPS) express ICAM-1 (intercellular adhesion molecule 1, CD54) which is a ligand for the β_2-integrin CD 11b/CD18 (Mac 1) expressed on PMNs [13, 14]. Activated PMNs increase their surface expression of CD11b/CD18 and the avidity of the molecule for its ligand. This leads to firm adhesion to endothelial cells and, later, transmigration. Antibodies against CD18, the β_2 chain of the integrins, are able to block their activity in vitro. In rabbits, such a monoclonal antibody almost completely inhibited the i.p. inflammatory reactions induced by *E. coli* and *Streptococcus pneumoniae*. However, in situations in which the peritoneal MØs were activated before an i.p. challenge with *Streptococcus pneumoniae*, the PMN infiltrate was only partially reduced by the antibody, indicating that a CD18-independent mechanism of neutrophil emigration exists which could also play a role in postoperative peritonitis [15, 16].

Effects of Previous Contact with Gram-Negative Microorganisms

In mice and rats, previous contact with live or killed *E. coli* increases subsequent i.p. inflammatory reactions induced by the same microorganism. The phenomenon is not mediated by circulating antibodies [17]. It is long-lasting (at least 2 months in rats) and preliminary results with nude mice indicate that it is T cell-independent. These findings are in keeping with the observation of Sawyers et al., that mice pretreated with *E. coli* and *Bacteroides fragilis* developed more intraabdominal abscesses than controls when injected i.p. with a mixture of both microorganisms [18].

Conclusions

Although much progress has been made recently in our understanding of the pathophysiology of intraabdominal inflammatory processes, our knowledge of their regulatory mechanisms still remains incomplete. There is evidence that these mechanisms may differ for various microorganisms. Presently, we can explain the rapid amplification of the inflammatory response by a cascade of cellular activations but we do not know exactly why in most cases it is self-limiting and why in other instances it runs amok and destroys the host. More studies are clearly needed to determine what is beneficial and what is detrimental for the host before we can use immunomodulators intelligently in the clinical setting.

References

1. *Gotloib L, Shostak A (1990) Peritoneal ultrastructure. In: Nolph KD (ed.) Peritoneal dialysis. Kluwer, Dordrecht, pp. 67-95*
2. *Verger C, Luger A, Moore HL, Nolph K (1983) Acute changes in peritoneal morphology and transport properties with infectious peritonitis and mechanical injury. Kidney Int 23: 823-831*
3. *Melnicoff MJ, Horan PK, Morahan PS (1989) Kinetics of changes in peritoneal cell populations following acute inflammation. Cell Immunol 118: 178-191*

4. Rankin JA, Sylvester I, Smith S, Yoshimura T, Leonard EJ (1990) Macrophages cultured in vitro release leukotriene B4 and neutrophil attractant / activation protein (interleukin 8) sequentially in response to stimulation with lipopolysaccharide and zymosan. J Clin Invest 86: 1556-1564
5. Kopaniak MM, Movat HZ (1983) Kinetics of acute inflammation induced by Escherichia coli in rabbits II. The effect of hyperimmunization, complement depletion and depletion of leukocytes. Am J Pathol 110: 13-29
6. Mackenzie RK, Coles GA, Williams JD (1991) The response of human peritoneal macrophages to stimulation with bacteria isolated from episodes of continuous ambulatory peritoneal dialysis-related peritonitis. J Infect Dis 163: 837-842
7. Sayers TJ, Wiltrout TA, Bull CA, Denn AC III, Pilaro AM, Lokesh B (1988) Effect of cytokines on polymorphonuclear neutrophil infiltration in the mouse. Prostaglandin and leukotriene independent induction of infiltration by IL-1 and tumor necrosis factor. J Immunol 141: 1670-1677
8. Rapoport J, Douvdevani A, Conforti A, Zlotnik M, Chaimowitz C (1992) Peritoneal mesothelial cells synthesize IL-1 (abstract) J Am Soc Nephrol 3: 416
9. Topley N, Mackenzie R, Jörres A, Coles GA, Davies M, Williams JD (1993) Cytokine networks in continuous ambulatory peritoneal dialysis: interactions of resident cells during inflammation in the peritoneal cavity. Perit Dial Int 13 (Suppl 2): S283-S285
10. Qureshi R, Jakschik BA (1988) The role of mast cells in thioglycollate induced inflammation. J Immunol 141: 2090-2096
11. Galli SJ (1993) New concepts about the mast cell. N Engl J Med 328: 257-265
12. Laski LA (1992) Selectins: interpreters of cell-specific carbohydrate information during inflammation. Science 258: 964-969
13. Arnaout MA (1990) Structure and function of the leukocyte adhesion molecules CD11/CD18. Blood 75: 1037-1050
14. Diamond MS, Staunton DS, de Fougerolles AR, Stacker SA, Garcia-Aguilar J, Hibbs ML, Springer TA (1990) ICAM-1 (CD54): A counter receptor for Mac 1 (CD11b/CD18). J Cell Biol 111: 3129-3139
15. Doershuk CM, Winn RK, Coxson HO, Harlan JM (1990) CD18-dependent and -independent mechanisms of neutrophil emigration in the pulmonary and systemic microcirculation of rabbits. J Immunol 144: 2327-2333
16. Mileski W, Harlan J, Rice C, Winn R (1990) Streptococcus pneumoniae-stimulated macrophages induce neutrophils to emigrate by a CD18 independent mechanism of adherence. Circ Shock 31: 259-267
17. Kinnaert P, Van Geertruyden N, Bournonville B, Struelens M (1993) Modulation of inflammatory reactions by previous contact with Escherichia coli in rats. Eur J Surg 159: 387-392
18. Sawyer RG, Adams RB, Spengler MD, Pruett TL (1991) Preexposure of the peritoneum to live bacteria increases later mixed intraabdominal abscess formation and delays mortality. J Infect Dis 163: 664-667

Generalized Response in Secondary Peritonitis

E.H. Farthmann, U. Schöffel

Monitoring of the Generalized Response

Intraperitoneal stimuli, directly or through cellular irritation, lead to a local inflammatory response with activation of cellular and plasmatic systems within the peritoneal blood vessels. The resulting vasodilation and leukocyte activation cause an enhancement of microvascular permeability which is common to all forms of peritonitis.
Activating substances as well as products of activation readily reach the systemic circulation and elicit a metabolic response of the organism and a variety of systemic signs which can easily be recorded [1, 2].
If the inflammatory focus persists, or if the inflammatory stimulus leads to a reaction which overwhelms the mechanisms of local confinement, a spillover of the inflammation occurs and leads to a generalized inflammatory response (systemic inflammatory response syndrome, SIRS; whole body inflammation).
Clinically, the differentiation between a state with systemic signs of a local inflammation and the state of a generalized inflammation is difficult to establish. The level of systemic signs might reflect a gradual difference. This, however, is certainly influenced by the degree of the intraabdominal reaction as well as by the general responsiveness of the patient [3]. Since the generalized inflammation invariably leads to organ dysfunction, its detection is essential for the diagnosis of sepsis or SIRS.
For the grading of the severity of peritonitis, several approaches may be useful [1, 2, 4-13]. General scoring systems, such as APACHE II or SSS or MOF, rating the risk and the physiologic response; peritonitis indices which include local aspects (Mannheim peritonitis index, MPI; Peritonitis index Altona, PIA II); and the monitoring of intraperitoneal or systemic signs of intraabdominal inflammation by measuring markers or mediators of the acute inflammatory response. This appears to be the most direct way for grading the severity of any form of peritonitis. As to the monitoring of the clinical course, only the recording of organ function or repeated measurements of systemic inflammatory parameters are useful.
For the monitoring of the inflammatory response a wide variety of plasma parameters might be determined. Basically, most of the known mediators and markers resulting from the activation of plasmatic systems (e.g., complement split products, fibrinopeptides) or from cellular activation (e.g., cytokines, leukocytic enzymes, prostanoids, soluble receptor complexes) as well as hepatic acute phase proteins reflect the degree of the inflammation [1, 2,

14, 15]. This does not seem to be influenced by the biologic activity of the compound nor by its role which may either be activating, modulating, inhibitory or inert.

The Systemic Response, Not Intraabdominal Inflammation, Determines Outcome

In patients with peritonitis we have previously shown that, out of 14 parameters representing the activation state of the different systems as well as inhibitory capacity of the plasma, three parameters showed significantly different levels between survivors and fatalities at the time of admission: C3a, the split-product of complement factor 3 as sign of the activation of the complement cascade; FPA (fibrinopeptide A), the first split-product of fibrinogen marking factor XII activation and elastase-α1-proteinase-inhibitor complex (Eα_1PI) as a marker of leukocyte stimulation [1]. These three parameters have also been useful in detecting postoperative intraabdominal complications [16].
In a recent series of 51 consecutive patients with secondary peritonitis, we evaluated the use of different classification and grading systems at the time of the first surgical intervention. This series included 35 patients with perforation of the gastrointestinal tract. The overall mortality was 27 % and bacteria were found in 74.5 % of peritoneal exudates (Table 1). With the exception of perforated appendicitis and of the two patients with necrotizing pancreatitis, the anatomic origin of the infections did not seem to influence the outcome in this series.

Table 1: Patient population

	n	Died	Age (x)	History (x)(h)	Positive bacteriology
Perforation	35	7	59	36	29
• Stomach/duodenum	15	2	60	26	10
• Small intestine	9	3	51	45	9
• Large intestine	7	2	72	37	6
• Appendix	4	0	53	48	4
Ischemia	5	1	59	28	2
Hepatobiliary system	5	1	63	43	3
Pancreatitis	2	2	65	48	1
Other	4	3	68	36	3
Total	51	14	61	36	38

Comparing the different classification systems (Fig. 1), the line graphs connect the mean scoring values for the different groups of patients. The respective scales are arbitrarily chosen so that the majority of lethal cases should lie in the outer areas.

Indicated in the left upper quarter are two general scoring systems (APACHE II, SSS), in the left lower quarter the two peritonitis indices. On the right side markers of the inflammatory response (systemic on top, local below) with signs of the activation of cellular and plasmatic systems combined to an activation score. We chose three parameters and their respective cut-off points derived from our former studies on the monitoring of the inflammatory response in early peritonitis [1, 16]. The score describes the number of parameters exceeding

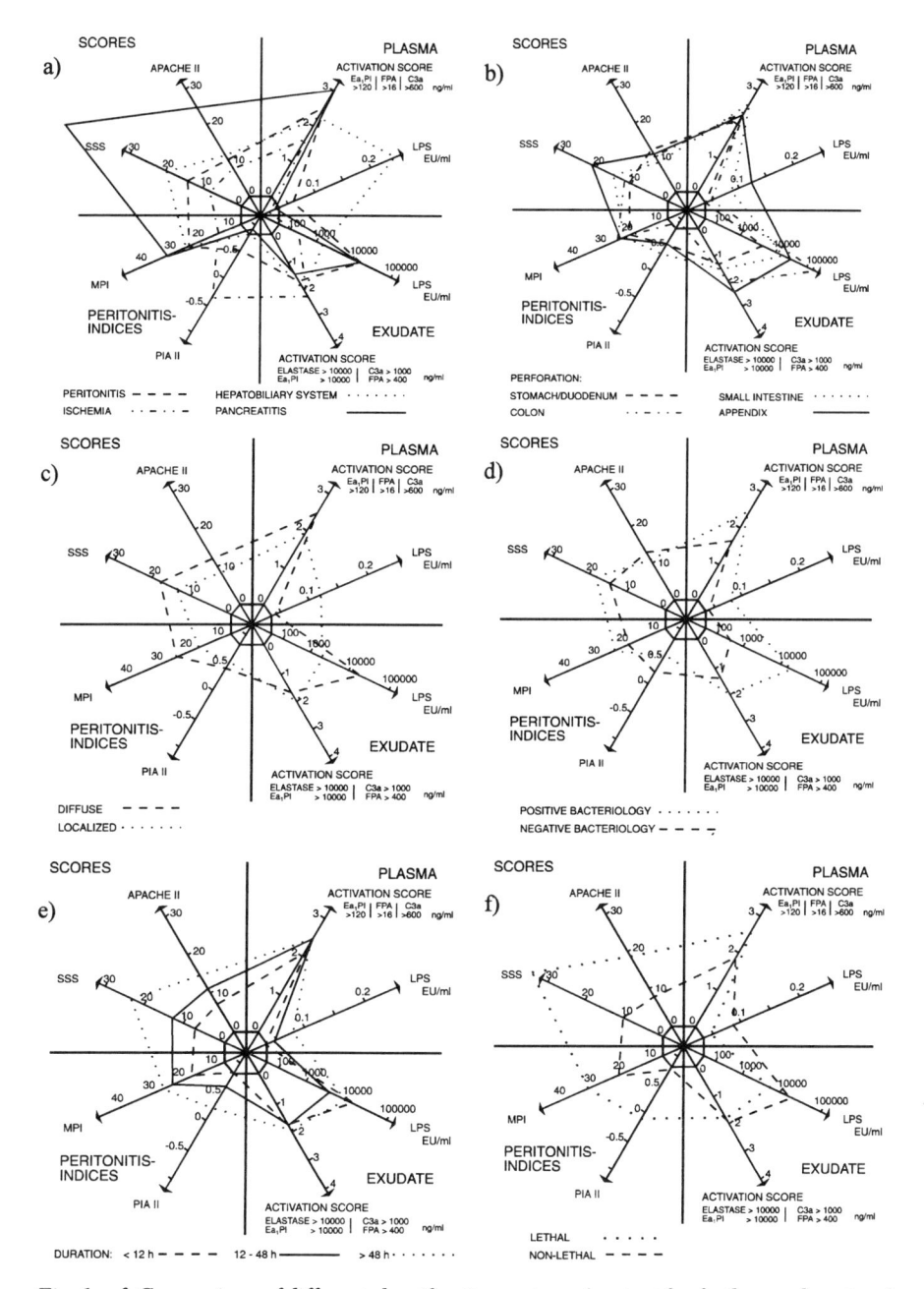

Fig. 1 a-f: Comparison of different classification systems (see text for further explanations). The line graphs connect the mean values obtained for each parameter.
a) Comparison of different etiologies; b) anatomic origin; c) diffuse and localized processes; d) bacteriological findings; e) length of history; f) outcome

their cut-off points and, of course, might be calculated with other constellations of inflammatory parameters too. The local activation score contains free leukocytic elastase as an additional parameter in the peritoneal exudate. Endotoxin levels are additionally indicated in both the plasma and the exudate.

The comparison of different etiologies (Fig. 1a) such as perforation of the intestinal tract, bowel wall ischemia, infectious processes of the hepatobiliary tract, and pancreatitis reveals that necrotizing pancreatitis is a systemic disease rather than an intraperitoneal inflammation, even if organ failure and the typical necrotic exudate raise the MPI value. Mesenteric ischemia has a high loading in PIA. Further differences concern the intraabdominal endotoxin levels, which were highest in the perforation group, systemic endotoxin levels up to a mean of 0.23 in the hepatobiliary group and the highest values in MPI, SSS, APACHE II and systemic activation score in the pancreatitis group.

Within the perforation group, the anatomic origin seems not to be of major importance since the differences mostly concern the intraabdominal endotoxin levels, which of course were highest in the exudates after colon perforation (Fig. 1b).

Comparing localized and diffused processes, these rather small differences are explained by special loadings in both of the indices. The difference in the general activation score reaches significance and correlates to the 11% dying in the group with localized processes (Fig. 1c). Between the groups with and without bacteriologically proven infections, the main differences concern the inflammatory response and, of course, the endotoxin levels (Fig. 1d).

The time from onset of disease to therapy naturally influences the degree of impairment of organ function and thus also the peritonitis indices. The fast increase in the activation score is most important in the postoperative state in which diagnosis may be delayed (Fig. 1e).

Lastly, the socres work best in the comparison of the lethal to the surviving group (Fig. 1f). The important finding is that the intraperitoneal inflammatory response seems not to influence the outcome while the degree of systemic inflammatory response does. For the classification of peritonitis, each of these scores may be useful and each has certain limitations. However, with respect to the necessary monitoring of the postoperative course and of therapeutic effects, we suggest both the recording of organ function and the continuous monitoring of the systemic inflammatory response. Similarly, it has been shown that the systemic rather than the local effects determine the outcome in a series of patients with intraabdominal infection [17].

The missing correlation between the severity of the local inflammation and the severity of the generalized response is difficult to explain. The nature of the intraabdominal stimulus, variations in intraabdominal reactions, the capacity of local defense mechanisms, a distinction between peritoneal and intraabdominal reactions, variable resorptive conditions, or the individual capacity to limit the systemic response may all play a decisive role.

The Systemic Response, Not Intraabdominal Infection, Determines Outcome

The importance of the systemic response as a determinant of outcome is established and thus forms the basis of most of the common grading systems in peritonitis. However, its independence from the presence of intraperitoneal bacteria or of their control is just gaining wider acceptance. It has been shown that sepsis scores are independent of infection control and that these sepsis scores, and not variables related to the infection, are predictive for the further course [18]. Furthermore, infections are not a necessary cause of MOF and their presence does not determine outcome [19]. These authors concluded that many infections occurring in patients with multiorgan failure (MOF) are a consequence, not a cause, of MOF. With intraabdominal infection, experimental results confirm that the quantification of the initial host response has more impact on risk than the quantification of the infection [20]. In our own series, the presence of intraabdominal bacteria influenced the systemic response to a certain extent (Fig. 1e). However, there are no significant differences in severity or outcome variables with respect to bacterial findings (Table 2).

Table 2: Bacterial findings and outcome variables

	n	Mortality (%)	Length of history (h)	APACHE II	SSS	MPI	Endotoxin EU/ml plasma	SSS day 5	Later infectious complications	Positive blood culture
Bacteria + Sensitive[a]	38	28.9	39.7	11.4	17.75	25.6	0.08	16.2	6	7
□ +	13	23.1	34.8	8.3	16.5	23.2	0.082	15.9	1	2
□ ±	16	31.3	47.3	12.7	18.0	29.4	0.081	16.1	5	2
□ −	9	33.3	33.2	14.6	19.2	22.3	0.075	16.4	0	3
Bacteria −	13	23.1	28.0	12.0	14.7	19.8	0.04	15.4	0	0

[a] Sensitive to antibiotic therapy (cefuroxime/metronidazole).

Conclusions

The generalized response in secondary peritonitis combines systemic signs of local inflammation and a generalized inflammation. The severity of any form of peritonitis is determined by this generalized response. This response, and not the intraabdominal infection, and not the intraabdominal inflammation, determines the outcome. For the classification of secondary peritonitis and for the monitoring of the postoperative course, we therefore suggest the recording of organ functions as well as a continuous monitoring of the inflammatory parameters.

References

1. Schöffel U, Zeller T, Lausen M, Ruf G, Farthmann EH (1989a) Monitoring of the inflammatory response in early peritonitis. Am J Surg 157: 567-572
2. Függer R, Zadrobilek E, Götzinger P, Klimann S, Rogy M, Winkler S, Andel H, Mittelböck M, Roth E, Schulz F, Fritsch A (1993) Perioperative TNFα and IL-6 concentrations correlate with septic state, organ function, and APACHE II scores in intraabdominal infection. Eur J Surg 159: 525-529
3. Christou NV (1990) Systemic and peritoneal host defense in peritonitis. World J Surg 14: 184-190
4. Knaus WA, Draper EA, Wagner DP, Zimmermann JE (1985) APACHE II: a severity of disease classification system. Crit Care Med 13: 818-829
5. Stevens LE (1983) Gauging the severity of surgical sepsis. Arch Surg 118: 1190-1192
6. Elebute EA, Stoner HB (1983) The grading of sepsis. Br J Surg 70: 29-31

7. Goris RJA, Boekhorst TPA, Nuytinck JKS, Gimbere JSF (1985) Multiple organ failure. Generalized auto-destructive inflammation. Arch Surg 120: 1109-1115
8. Wittmann DH, Teichmann W, Müller M (1987) Development and validation of the Altona peritonitis index - PIA II. Langenbecks Arch Chir 327: 834-835
9. Wacha H, Linder MM, Feldmann U (1987) Mannheim peritonitis index - prediction of risk of death from peritonitis. Theor Surg 1: 169-175
10. Ohmann C, Wittmann DH, Wacha H, and the Peritonitis Study Group (1993) Prospective evaluation of prognostic scoring systems in peritonitis. Eur J Surg 159: 267-274
11. Poenaru D, Christou NV (1991) Clinical outcome of seriously ill surgical patients with intraabdominal infection depends on both physiologic (APACHE II score) and immunologic (DTH score) alterations. Ann Surg 213: 130-136
12. Nyström, PO, Bax R., Dellinger EP et al. (1990) Proposed definitions for diagnosis, severity scoring, stratification, and outcome for trials on intraabdominal infection. World J Surg 14: 148-158
13. Sawyer RG, Rosenlof LK, Adams RB, May AK, Spenglers MD, Pruett TL (1992) Peritonitis into the 1990s: changing pathogens and changing strategies in the critically ill. Am Surg 58: 82-87
14. Tsukada K, Katoh H, Shiojima M, Suzuki T, Takenoshita S, Nagamachi Y (1993) Concentrations of cytokines in peritoneal fluid after abdominal surgery. Eur J Surg 159: 475-479
15. Schöffel U, Sach M, Burger J et al. (1991) Local inflammatory response and severity of intraabdominal infection. Surg Res Comm 10 (Suppl): 61
16. Schöffel U, Kopp K-H, Lausen M, Ruf G, Farthmann EH (1989b) Monitoring of postoperative intraabdominal septic complications following major abdominal surgery. Surg Res Comm 5: 49-53
17. Ponting GA, Sim AJW, Dudley HAF (1987) Comparison of the local and systemic effects of sepsis in predicting survival. Br J Surg 74: 750-752
18. Marshall J, Sweeney D (1990) Microbial infection and the septic response in critical surgical illness. Arch Surg 125: 17-23
19. Poole GV, Muakkassa FF, Griswold JA (1993) The role of infection in outcome of multiple organ failure. Am Surg 59: 727-732
20. Jönsson B, Berlund J, Skau T, Nyström PO (1993) Outcome of intraabdominal infection in pigs depends more on host responses than on microbiology. Eur J Surg 159: 571-578

Scores in Peritonitis and Their Limitations

H. Wacha, Ch. Ohmann L.M. Reichert, and the SIS-E Peritonitis Study Group

Definition of Scores and Their Design

Scores consist of weighted points derived from single risk factors. Risk factors are prognostic variables such as clinical characteristics and objective findings (e.g., natural risk factors, physiological data, laboratory data). Their values are calculated by mathematical analysis (MPI) [1] or weighted by experts (Apache II) [2]. Some single risk factors, such as organ failure, are strong predictors of death. Scores are sums of risk factors expressed in numbers predicting the probability of dying from a certain disease.

History of Peritonitis Scoring

The desire to compare different collectives with peritonitis dates back to the early 1920s [3]. Early studies of peritonitis compared different age groups, durations of disease, anatomical source of perforation, that is, empirically chosen clinical data and natural risk factors.

Polk [4] recognized remote organ failure as a sign of occult intraabdominal infection. Eiseman et al. [5] believed that a large data base was required to predict the probability of survival given such facts as age, preexisting disease, organ system failure, duration of failure and likelihood of eliminating a source of sepsis. In 1980, Fry concluded that multiple system organ failure (MSOF) remained a principal cause of death and was primarily due to infection.

In 1979 we published our first results using an empirical peritonitis index based on age, natural risk factors, specific risk factors, origin, and spread of peritonitis in 1253 patients.

Prospective validation of this empirical index was done in 1983. Our clinical prognostic prediction for peritonitis was supported by a multivariate mathematical decision model, which enabled us to objectify the selection of prognostic variables and to quantify prognostic statements regarding the outcome of surgical therapy. A total of 37 parameters were tested; 20 were incorporated into a multiple log-logistic discrimination analysis. Only eight proved to be relevant (Table 1).

At about the same time (1981), Knaus [2] constructed an acute physiology score (APS), based on 34 physiological measurements, to classify patients admitted to intensive care units (Table 2).

In 1982 Knaus published the APACHE II, which was composed of three parts: (1) acute physiology score with 12 laboratory values and physical findings, (2) points for age, and (3) points for overall health status (HS).

Table 1: Mannheim peritonitis index: rounded loading of individual risk factors

Risk factors	Loading
Age 50 years	5
Female	5
Organ failure	7
Malignancy	4
Duration of peritonitis 24 h	4
Origin not colon	4
Diffuse peritonitis	6
Exudate	
• clear	0
• cloudy purulent	6
• fecal purulent	12

Index represents total loadings

Table 2: Scores in peritonitis: considered risk factors

Year	Author	Duration	Anatomic origin	Age	Multiorgan failure	Cancer	Spread	Health status	Other
1920	Körte	+	+	+					
1974	Polk				+				
1979	Linder and Wacha	+	+	+	+	+	+		
1981	Knaus					+[a]	+[a]		
1982	Knaus			+		+[b]	+[b]	+	
1982	Le Gall			+	+				
1983	Bohnen et al.				+				
1983	Pine et al.			+	+				Bowel Infarction, malnutrition, alcoholism
1983	Elebute and Stoner				+				pre, intra-and postoperative infection
1983	Stevans				+				Seven organ systems
1983	Wacha	+	+	+	+	+	+		
1984	Meakins		+		APS				

[a]With respect to cancer and spread, 32 laboratory values were considered.
[b]With respect to cancer and spread, 12 laboratory values were considered.

Le Gall [8] added age and previous health status to the primary proposed score of Knaus, the APS. Age < 50, good previous HS and less than two visceral failures were important predictors of late survival (1 year). The sepsis severity score of Stevens [9] defines seven organ systems (lung, kidney, coagulation, cardiovascular, gastrointestinal tract, liver and nervous). Meakins [10] added to the APS of Knaus [2] anatomical and functional classifications.

Bohnen noted, in 1983, that there was no generally available method to predict early organ dysfunction [11]. Organ failure again was found to be a strong predictor of death. A discriminant equation based only on preoperative variables correctly assigned the outcome of death or survival in 92% of patients.

In contrast to the findings of other groups who evaluated preoperative peritonitis, postoperative peritonitis was characterized by lack of the influence of age on outcome, late operation, and more frequent organ failure. However, Pine showed that organ malfunction, shock at any time and age > 65 were the most significant variables for the prediction of death following intraabdominal infection [12]. Alcoholism, malnutrition and intestinal infarction were good predictors as well.

As we are primarily interested in comparing outcomes in different groups and with different treatment regimens, the scoring method of Elebute and Stoner was of minor interest. They incorporated pre-, intra- and postoperative signs of tissue infection, including all kinds of infection, from wound sepsis to peritonitis.

Use in Clinical Practice

In the following years all these scoring systems were tested by statistical means and used in various studies. Some authors tried to ameliorate the prediction of outcome by adding different laboratory data.

The sepsis score of Elebute and Stoner [13], which included platelet count, endotoxin level and AT III correlated well in a study of Grundmann [14] with the severity of the disease, but could not predict final outcome.

Others [15] found platelet count below $0.1 \times 10^{12}/l$ for more than 4 days to be associated with death. Confusing results based on TNF-α levels were reported recently: TNF-α levels did not correlate with the severity of injury score and Glasgow coma scale [16] but did correlate well with the APACHE II score [17]. Although it is well known that, e.g., an elevated level of C-reactive protein (CRP) can indicate postoperatve septic complications [18], the predictive value is only 69% [19].

Acute phase protein did not significantly improve prediction of outcome above that from the septic score of Elebute and Stoner [13].

None of the markers or mediators of systemic or local inflammatory response studied by Schöffel [20] had better predictive values than the scoring systems mentioned above (Fig. 1). So, which score is the best? Dellinger et al. [21] studied the APS score with the anatomical classification system of Meakins [10] in a prospective study of 187 patients. The APS, malnutrition and age were the strongest predictors for survival or death. The authors showed clearly that it is not primarily the location or the type of abscess, but the host response which determines the patients outcome.

Skau compared two indices, the APS and SSS score, and found good interrelations between the methods [22]. The score correlated better with mortality than did age, chronic disease, anatomy or cause of the disease.

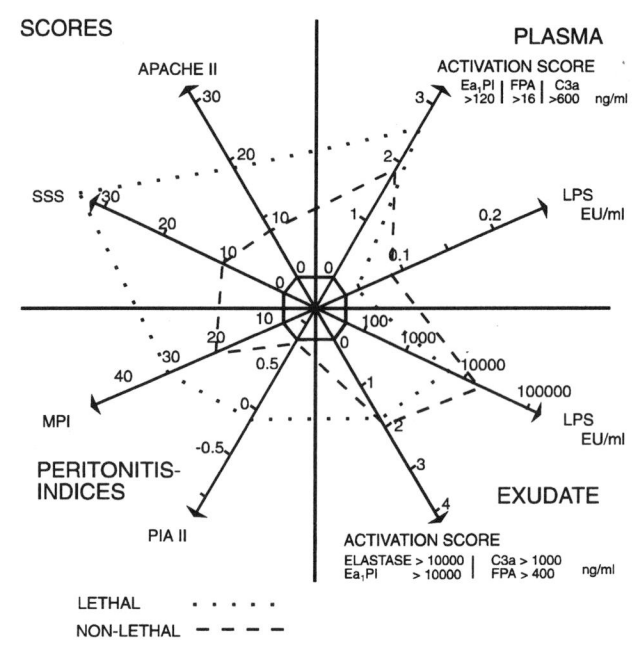

Figure 1: Prediction of mortality

This is astonishing, since age and chronic disease were the two factors Knaus added to the APS to form the much better APACHE II score [7].

Statistical Evaluation

For statistical evaluation three forms of peformance criteria are used: the discriminatory ability, sharpness and reliability.

In a prospective multicenter trial 271 patients from 12 centers in Germany (1987/88) were evaluated for a prognostic scoring system in peritonitis. Data necessary to calculate the Apache II, the MPI (Mannheim peritonitis index) and PIA (peritonitis index Altona) were recorded. The predictive performance of discriminatory ability, sharpness and reliability were investigated.

The Apache II score had a better discriminatory performance than the others. This is surprising because Apache II is not designed to predict risk of death from peritonitis.

Nevertheless, the Apache II does not achieve optimal discrimination. Even with selection of an appropriate cut off point it is not possible to have a false positive or negative result rate of less than 20%! (Fig.2).

The sharpness of prediction is measured by the distribution of score values (Fig 3). Apache II scored 25% of the patients in the lower risk group, and only a few patients (2/271) in the high risk group; 74%, the majority of patients, had a moderate risk of dying.

The distribution of the MPI score is more central and symmetrical, but more than 60% of the patients belonged to the low risk group and in only one third could no sharp prediction be achieved. Thus, the MPI is sharper than the APACHE II.

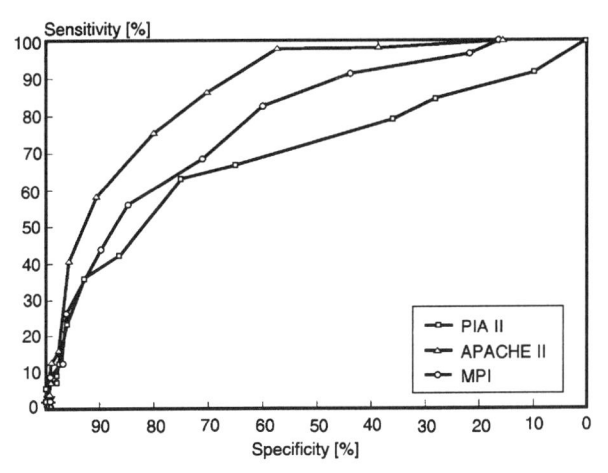

Figure 2: Discriminatory ability of PIA (peritonitis index-Altona), APACHE II, and MPI (Mannheim peritonitis index)

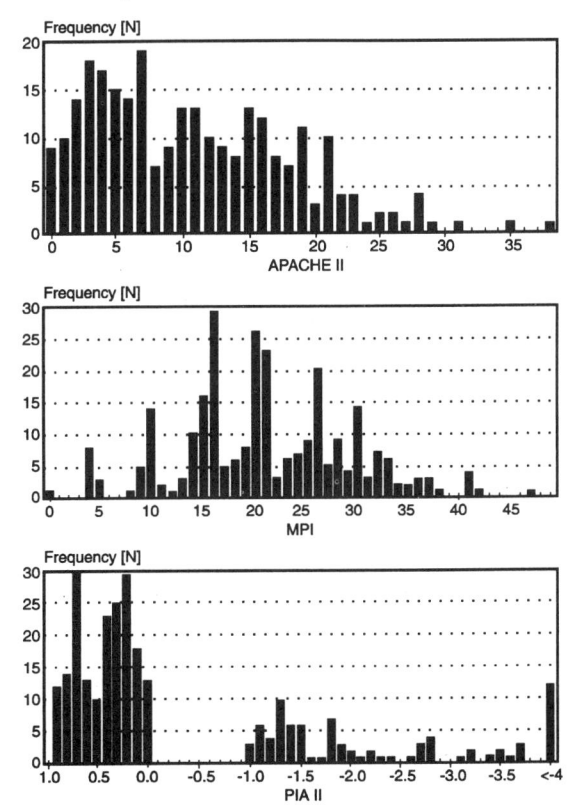

Figure 3: Sharpness of prediction of APACHE II, MPI (Mannheim peritonitis index) and PIA (peritonitis index-Altona) II

Regarding the reliabilty of the scores, Apache II showed no significant differences between observed and predicted death rates, whereas the MPI overestimated the risk of dying in the higher risk groups, and underestimated in the very low risk group (Fig.4).

In summary, Apache II is superior to other scores with respect to discriminatory ability and reliability. Apache II is less effective in terms of sharpness. Nevertheless an individual prediction about the outcome of peritonitis cannot be made.

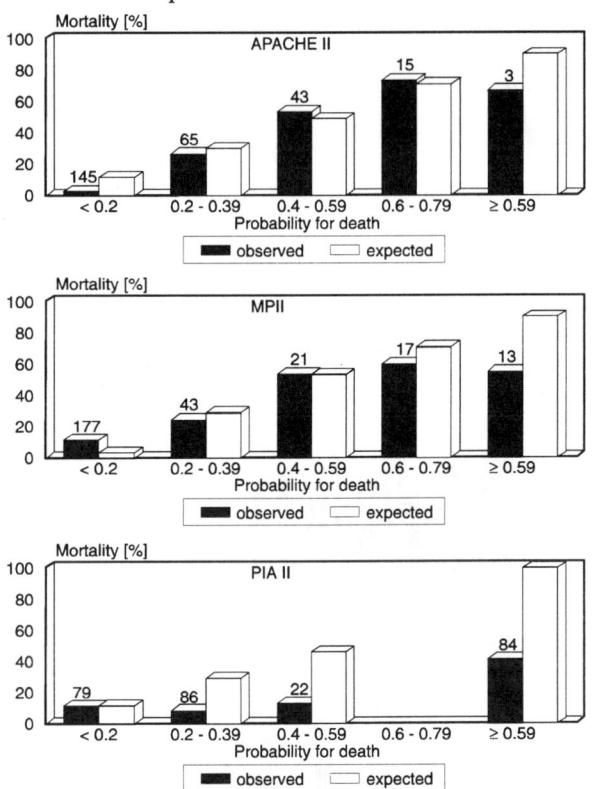

Figure 4: Reliability in predicting the probability of death: APACHE II, MPI (Mannheim peritonitis index) and PIA (peritonitis index-Altona) II

Clinical Results

Our own results from the former peritonitis study group of the Paul Ehrlich Gesellschaft are in contrast to the findings of Rogy et al. [23], who showed that the MPI was superior to the Apache II.

In a paper recently published by Billing et al. [24] more than 2000 cases of peritonitis from seven centers were scored by the MPI. A sensitivity of 86% and an accuracy of 83% were found. Looking at these centers interesting differences could be detected (Figs. 5, 6). In one center with a low average score, all patients suffered from perforated ulcer. In another center 40% of patients had perforated appendicitis with a very low mortality rate. In spite of these great differences in the severity of peritonitis, the MPI correlated well with letality in each center and in the whole study. The authors were able to develop a European therapy standard for treating peritonitis.

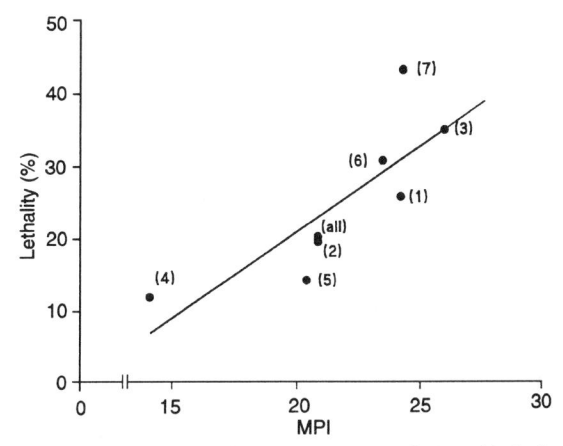

Fig. 5: Correlation between MPI (Mannheim peritonitis index) and lethality in various study centers (numbered). (From [24])

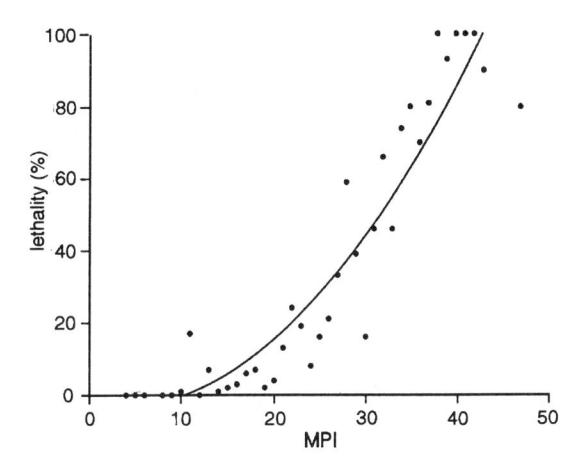

Figure 6: Correlation between MPI (Mannheim peritonitis index) and lethality: all study centers (2003), for each Mannheim peritonitis index (MPI) (From [24])

Much larger trials with the APACHE II have been conducted in France and USA. In one of his first studies Knaus detected differences in death rates for gastrointestinal diseases in France compared to the USA [2]. It is important to mention this because differences in treatment regimens can only be detected if seperate diagnostic groups have been defined. This valuable differentiation is lost by putting all patients together in one analysis. However, neither the MPI nor the APACHE II could always predict well the outcome of specific diseases. Krenzien (1990) could demonstrate superiority of a specific prognostic index of perforated peptic ulcer compared to the MPI [25, 26].

In spite of comparable APACHE II mean values (14, 14, 12), Schein found extremely different mortality rates from postoperative, fecal peritonitis and infected pancreatic necrosis, with death rates 14% to 56% (Table 3). He concluded that the value of planned relaparotomy has yet to be proven in postoperatve peritonitis and necrotizing pancreatitis [27].

Wittman concluded from the fact that the observed mortality was far beyond the predicted mortality that ettapen lavage must have improved therapy [28] (Fig. 7).

In a prospective, open, consecutive, nonrandomized trial using the APACHE II score for comparison, Christou et al. [29] reported no significant differences in mortality between patients treated with a "closed abdomen" technique (mortality 31%) and those treated with variations of the "open abdomen" technique (mortality 44%).

Table 3: APACHE II mean values and mortality in postoperative and fecal peritonitis and infected pancreas

	Postoperative peritonitis	Fecal peritonitis	Infected pancreas
Mortality (%)	55	14	56
Mean APACHE II score	14	14	12

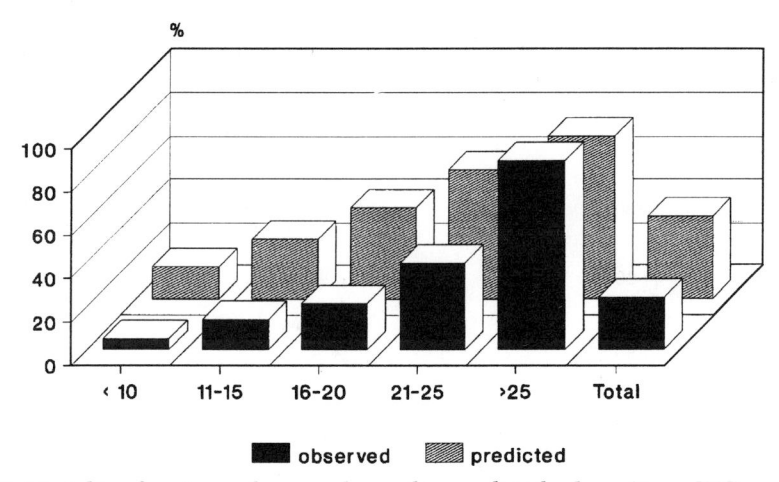

Fig. 7: Mortality after etappenlavage: observed vs. predicted values. (From [28])

Discussion and Conclusions

Scoring systems have been constructed to allow comparison of different patient populations in different institutions. The sum of risk points predicts the outcome of a patient and makes the allocation to a risk group possible. None of the scores is able to predict death for the individual patient. Nevertheless scores have been used in some institutions to decide which therapy to initiate [30]. Some practitioners have thought of excluding patients with extremly high scores from entering the ICU.

Recently, computer software programs have made it possible to collect even more data from the patient than before, and better prediction of survival is reported by the computer than doctors on the ICU. The German magazin "Der Spiegel" reported that the computer believed

80% of the patients would leave the ICU, compared to 75% by the doctors [31]. Is that how we would like to use the scores?

We conclude from the studies above that it is dangerous to use mean values to compare different groups. Mean values can mask specific risk faktors such as occur in ulcer perforation or pancreatitis. Only well defined homogeneous risk groups should be entered in a study.

But how many parameters are necessary to define risk groups? Natural risk factors and organ system failure are the strongest predictors of outcome. Laboratory data and physiological measures reflect the established organ failure, but are not able to predict organ failure itself. Even if they could, they would lose their predictive value since they are manipulated by therapy.

We learned from our last prospective multicenter trial on 350 patients that very few parameters are necessary to allocate patients with peritonitis to a low or high risk group. There were no deaths under the age of 40 years; 69% with no organ failure had a 5% mortality. In 31% with one and more organs failed, the mortality ranged from 17 to 80% (Table 4).

In cases when the source of infection was eradicated, only 14% of 323 patients died; if not, half the patients died.

One operation was performed in 80% of the patients, with a mortality of 14% (Table 5).

The MPI correlated well with the mortality and again the sharpness of prediction of this score was very good. Persistence of organ failure measured by the Goris score [32] on day 1 after the operation was an even better predictor of outcome than the initial score. Intraabdominal complications and bacterial complications were threefold higher if more than two organs failed (Table 6).

Table 4: Prospective multicenter observational study of peritonitis: organ failure and mortality

Organ failure	Number of patients (%)	Mortality (%)
None	176 (69)	5
One organ	23 (9)	17
Two organs	28 (11)	43
Three organs	14 (6)	79
Unknown	3 (1)	0
Total	254	18.5

Table 5: Prospective multicenter observational study of peritonitis: surgical procedure and mortality

Procedure	Patients n (%)	Mortality n (%)
Single operation	204 (80)	29 (14)
planned relaparatomy	17 (7)	5 (29)
Etappen lavage	19 (8)	4 (21)
Controlled closed lavage	5 (2)	2 (40)
Others	9 (4)	7 (78)
Total	254	47 (19)

Table 6: Goris score on the first postoperative day: prediction of future complications (From [32])

Goris score	<2	>2
Patients (n)	215	130
Intraabdominal complications (%)	12	31
• Insufficienci of suture	4	9
• Abscess	5	12
• Rupture of abdomen	3	5
• Fistula	2	7
• Bleeding	1	5
• Other	3	7
Bacterial complications	20	60
• Wound infection	11	20
• Sepsis	5	33
• Pneumonia	7	32
• Infection of soft tissues	2	7
• Other	0	3
Unplanned relaparatomy (%)	9	18

Summary

Scores have been used to compare groups of patients with different diseases and from different institutions. A reduction in mortality from severe peritonitis has yet to be achieved, as there is no decrease in mortality if eradicaton by surgery is not possible [33]. To study this problem will be the aim of our next multicenter trial.

New scores to judge the severity of the peritonitis when entering the hospital are not needed. What we do need are precisely defined entrance criteria; a consensus in the initial therapy; new measurements to characterize the course of the disease; and, as mortality rates come down, new outcome criteria and new treatment regimens.

References

1. *Wacha H, Linder MM, Feldmann U, Wesch G, Gundlach E, Steifensand RA (1987) Mannheimer Peritonitis-Indez - prediction of risk of death from peritonitis - construction of a statistical and validation of an empirically based index. Theor Surg 1: 169-177*
2. *Knaus WA, Wagner DP, Le Gall JR, Draper EA et al. (1982) A comparison of intensive care in USA and France. Lancet 2: 642-646*
3. *Körte W (1927) Die Chirurgie des Peritonaeum. Encke, Stuttgart*
4. *Polk HC, Shields C.L. (1977) Remote organ failure: a valid sign of occult intra-abdominal infection. Surgery 81/3: 310-313*
5. *Eiseman B, Beart R, Norton L (1977) Multiple organ failure. Surg Gynecol Obstet 144/3: 323-326*

6. Fry DE, Pearlstein L, Fulton RL, Polk HC (1980) Multiple system organ failure. The role of uncontrolled infection. Arch Surg 115: 136-140
7. Knaus WA, Zimmermann JE, Wagner DP, Draper EA, Lawrence DE (1981) Apache - acute physiology and chronic health evaluation: a physiologically based classification system APS. Crit Care Med 9/8: 591-597
8. Le Gall J-R, Brun-Bruisson CH, Trunet P, rapin M (1982) Influence of age, previous health status, and severity of acute illness on outcome from intensive care. Crit Care Med 10/9: 575-577
9. Stevens EL (1983) Gauging the severity of surgical sepsis (SSS). Arch Surg 118: 1190-1192
10. Meakins JL, Solomkin JS, Allo MD, Dellinger P, Howard RJ, Simmons RL (1984) A proposed classification of intra-abdominal infection. Arch Surg 119: 1372-1378
11. Bohnen J, Boulanger M, Meakins J, McLean PM (1983) Prognosis in generalized peritonitis. Relation to cause and risk factors. Arch Surg 118: 285-289
12. Pine RW, Wertz M, Lennard St, Dellinger P, Carrico J, Minshew BH (1983) Determinants of organ malfunction and death in patients with intra-abdominal sepsis. Arch Surg 118: 242-249
13. Elebute EA, Stoner HB (1983) The grading of sepsis. Br J Surg 70: 29-31
14. Grundmann R, Hornung M (1988) Verlaufskontrolle septischer Patienten auf den Intensivstation mit Hilfe von "Sepsisscore", Endotoxin - und AT-III - Bestimmung. Langenbecks Arch Chir 373: 166-172
15. Housinger TA, Brinkerhoff C, Warden GD (1993) The relationship between platelet count, sepsis and survival in pediatric burn patients. Arch Surg 128/1: 65-66
16. Rabinovici R, John R, Vernick J, Feuerstein G (1993) Serum tumor necrosis factor-alpha profile in trauma patients. J Trauma 35/5: 698-702
17. Offner F, Philippe J, Vogelaers D, Colardyn F, Baele G, Leroux-Roels G (1990) Serum tumor necrosis factor levels in patients with infectious disease and septic shock. J Lab Clin Med 116(1): 100-105
18. Lohde E, Kraas E (1993) Versorgung von postoperativen Komplikationen nach Eingriffen wegen Peritonitis. In: Haring R (ed.) Peritonitis. Thieme, Stuttgart, pp. 75-81
19. Mustard RA, Bohnen JA, Haseeb S, Kasina R (1987) C-reactive protein levels predict postoperative septic complications. Arch Surg 122: 69-73
20. Schöffel U, Farthmann EH (1990) Classification of intraabdominal infection. Congress on peritonitis. Vienna Nov 1990
21. Dellinger EP, Wertz MJ, Meakins JL (1985) Surgical infection stratification system for intraabdominal infection. Arch Surg 120: 21-29
22. Skau T, Nystrom P-O, Carlson C (1985) Severity of illness in intra-abdominal invection. Arch Surg 120: 152-158
23. Rogy M, Fugger R, Schemper M, Koss G, Schulz (1990) Unterschiedliche Aussagekraft von zwei verschiedenen Prognose - Scores bei Patienten mit Peritonitis. Chirurg 61: 297-300
24. Billing A, Frohlich D, Fugger R, Dau H, Krenzien J, Nitsche D, Schulz F, Thiede A, Wacha H, Schildberg FW (1994) Outcome prediction with the Mannheimer Peritonitis Index in 2003 multicenter patients. Br J Surg 81: 209-213
25. Krenzien J, Roding H (1990) Prognosis of perforated peptic ulcer - stratification of risk factors and validation of scoring systems in predicting the postoperative outcome. Theor Surg 5: 26-32
26. Krenzien J, Lorenz W (1990) Scoring - Systeme für schwere intraabdominale Infektionen. Zentralbl Chir 115/17: 1065-1079
27. Schein M (1990) Planned reoperations and open management in critical intra-abdominal infections: prospective exeperience in 52 cases. World J Surg 15: 537-545
28. Wittmann D, Aprahamian C, Bergstein JM (1990) Ettapen lavage advanced diffuse peritonitis managed by planned multiple laparotomies. World J Surg 14: 218-226

29. Christou NM, Barie PS, Dellinger EP, Waymack JP, Stone HH (1993) Prospective evaluation of management techniques and outcome. Surgical Infection Society intra-abdominal infection study. Arch Surg 128(2): 193-196
30. Dionigi R, Cremaschi RE, Jemos V, Dominioni L, Monico R (1986) Nutritional assessment and severity of illness classification Systems: a critical review on their clinical relevance. World J Surg 10: 2-11
31. Anon (1994) Noten in 20 Fachern. Spiegel 2: 158-159
32. Goris RJA, Boeckhorst TPA, Nuytinck JKS (1985) Multiple organ failure: generalized autodestructive inflammation? Arch Surg 120: 1109
33. Billing A, Frohlich D, Mialkowskyj O, Stockstad P, Schildberg FW (1992) Peritonitisbehandlung mit der Etappenlavage: Prognosekriterien und Behandlungsverlauf. Langenback Arch Chir 377: 305-313
34. Linder MM, Wacha H (1993) Stellenwert von Peritonitis-Indices für die klinisch - prognostische Beurteilung der Peritonitis. In: Haring R (ed.) Peritonitis. Thieme, Stuttgart, pp. 41-47

Correlations Between Endotoxin, Gamma-Interferon, Biopterin and Serum Phospholipase A_2 Activities During Lethal Gram-Negative Sepsis in Rats

A. Hunsicker, W. Kullich, W. Weissenhofer, D. Lorenz, J. Petermann, K. Boden, H. Rokos

Introduction

The purpose of our study was to establish a standardized reproducible animal model of intraperitoneal sepsis, induced by *E. coli*-endotoxemia in LEW.1W rats, to investigate early immunoserological responses in order to find a mediator based system to evaluate peritonitis-sepsis. In the pilot phase of this study we measured the levels of endotoxin, phospholipase A_2 and neopterin (biopterin) as possible markers to predict the outcome of peritonitis.

Approximately 40% of the patients with gram-negative sepsis develop shock, with a mortality of about 90% [1-3]. Endotoxin plays a central part in this process. Redl [4] described endotoxin as the central mediator in the septic process. This potent bacterial antigen has toxic effects on all organ systems, even resulting in multiple organ failure. The process is thought to occur by the systemic activation of cascade reactions involving inflammatory mediators as well as those activating cellular and humoral immune defenses [1, 5, 6]. In this process macrophages produce a broad spectrum of markers, which represents the immune activation [4].

The cytokine interferon-γ (IFN-γ) is released by T lymphocytes and stimulates macrophages to secrete tumor necrosis factor (TNF) and interleukin-1 (IL-1). The macrophage mediated stimulation of eicosanoid metabolism, with activation of phospholipase A_2, (PLA_2), releases lipid mediators [5], and PLA_2 serum concentration correlates with the duration and severity of the septic event [7, 8]. The pteridine derivative neopterin is another sensitive marker of macrophage stimulation [9, 10]. It is produced in the tetrahydrobiopterin (BH_4) cycle after an IFN-γ stimulus [11]. Neopterin could be measured in humans and primates only [12-14], whereas rats produce neopterin only in non detectable concentrations in their complete metabolism of BH_4. Therefore, one can only estimate biopterin concentrations in rats.

Materials and Methods

Diffuse peritonitis was induced by means of an intraperitoneal injection of a mixture of *E. coli* and hemoglobin, in accordance with the methods of Hau and Simmons, Pruett et al. and Kullich and Weissenhofer [15-19].
A total of 42 male LEW.1W rats (weight 318 q 44 g; age: 10.1 q 1.7 weeks) were used. *E. coli* were obtained from a patient suffering from severe diffuse peritonitis. They were characterized as K1:H$^+$, mannose resistant; hemagglutination negative; hemolysine negative; colicin positive; dulcitol fermentation negative. The control group of animals received an intraperitoneal injection of 6.0 ml physiological saline solution. The peritonitis group was injected with 6.0 ml of a mixture containing 0.1 ml of a suspension containing 10^{10} *E. coli*/ml and 2.9 ml of diluted hemolytic autogenous blood (hemoglobin concentration 3%) and 3.0 ml of a 0.9% NaCl solution.
E. coli strain (API 20 E, bio Merieux), was spread thickly with a spatula on Columbia agar (Oxoid), incubated for 18 h at 35C and then rinsed with a sterile 0.9% NaCl solution free of pyrogen (Delta Pharma Co.). The microbial suspension was homogenized and suspended at a density of 1 x 10^{10} organisms-ml (McFarland-Standard; Vitec Systems ATB 1550, bio Merieux. The hemoglobin solution was produced with autogenic rat blood extracted after intraperitoneally anesthetizing the animals with thiopental Nycomed Arzneimittel, Munich, FRG; 40 mg/100 g body weight) by means of cardiac puncture under sterile conditions. The blood was deep frozen three times at -30C under sterile conditions to cause hemolysis. Before use, the hemolysed blood was adjusted to a hemoglobin content of 3% using a 0.9% NaCl solution.
As a consequence of the results of the initial experiments, the duration of the experiment was limited to 6 h. At the end of this period, the animals were subjected to a general intraperitoneal anesthesia (thiopental). All the blood was extracted from the animals within 3 min by means of intracardial puncture under septic conditions. Then the animals were dissected and the organs inspected.
Measurement of endotoxin content in the rat was performed by means of a quantitative, chromogenic, limulus amebocyte lysate test, checked and approved by the FDA (QCL 1000, Whittaker Bioproducts Inc., Walkersville, Md, USA). This genuine, quantitative endotoxin test can identify endotoxin concentrations from 0.01 - 10 EU/ml. The measurement of the staining reaction was carried out by using a microtiter plate of photometer with an extinction at 405 nm (SLT EAR 400 FW, SLT, Austria) [20].
Total biopterin in the serum was determined by means of radioimmunoassay (double antibody method) [21]. Firstly, the acid oxidation of the unstable BH_4 to biopterin was brought about in 15 min using manganese dioxide (6 mg in 20 fl 1 N HCl/100 fl serum). After neutralization with diluted NaOH solution, addition of the specific biopterin antibodies and subsequent centrifugation, the residue was subjected directly to radioimmunoassay.
Phospholipase A_2 in the serum was measured by an enzymatic staining test for free fatty acids (Boehringer Mannheim Biochemica). PLA_2 causes lecithin to split it into lysolecithin and free fatty acids. The fatty acids thus formed were then measured quantitatively. The colored matter was determined with a spectral photometer (SUMAL PE2 Carl Zeiss, Jena) at a wavelength of 450 nm. The activity is calculated by amounts of free fatty acids released per unit of time.
Plasma IFN-γ was measured by means of solid-phase enzyme-linked immunosorbent assay, based on the sandwich principle (ELISA, Cell Biology Products HBT Holland, Biotechnology; supplier for Austria: Biomedica Vienna). The test uses two monoclonal antibodies specific to rat IFN-γ. The enzyme reaction was determined at 405 nm [20].

The statistical calculation (descriptive statistics, Mann-Whitney U test, correlates with Pearson r; linear discriminant analysis) was made on a personal computer using the software package SPSS - PS +, Vers. 4.01 (SPSS Inc., USA).

Results

In contrast to the sham-treated rats, the peritonitis animals showed significant differences in the concentrations of endotoxin, IFN-γ, biopterin and PLA_2 activity. The endotoxin range was from 0.064 EU/l (SD = 0.19) to 102.38 EU/l (SD = 145.40) ($p < 0.0001$)(Fig. 1). IFN-γ levels ranged from 147.9 pg/ml (SD = 141.6) to 4591 pg/ml (SD = 6541) ($p < 0.0001$) (Fig. 2) circulating PLA_2 activities ranged from 116.2 (SD = 45.4) to 185.4 U/l (SD = 105.4) ($p < 0.01$). Biopterin levels ranged from 54.4 nmol/l (SD = 17.2) to 127.8 nmol/l (SD = 76.8) ($p < 0.001$)

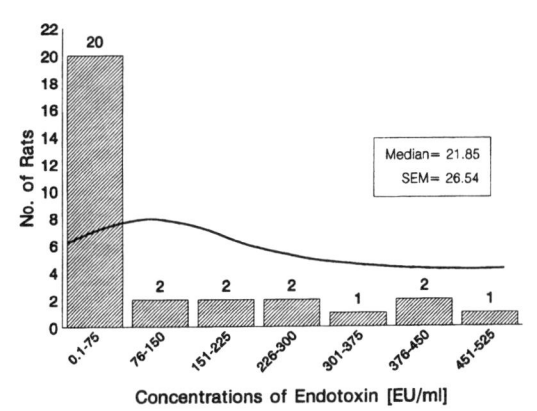

Fig. 1: Distributions of estimated endotoxin levels in the penultimate phase during gram-negative sepsis in LEW.1W rats

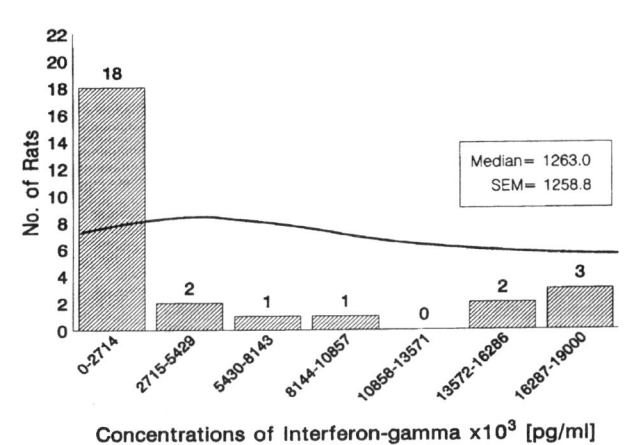

Fig. 2: Distributions of estimated interferon-γ (IFN-γ) expression in the penultimate phase during gram-negative sepsis in LEW.1W rats

For the peritonitis group there were strong correlations between endotoxemia and elevated levels of IFN-γ ($r_p = 0.72; p < 0.0001$)(Fig. 3) and biopterin synthesis ($r_p = 0.82; p < 0.0001$) (Fig. 4). The increase of IFN-γ levels correlated with the regulatory synthesis of the pteridine derivative biopterin ($r_p = 0.73; p < 0.0001$) and with PLA$_2$ activity ($r_p = 0.50; p < 0.005$) (Fig. 5, 6).
Biopterin synthesis correlated slightly with PLA$_2$ activity ($r_p = -0.38; p < 0.05$). In the peritonitis animals, the mean serum PLA$_2$ activity was 62.8% higher than the level in the saline animal group. During the penultimate phase of the septic shock, the difference was slightly significant ($p < 0.01$).
In the animals with peritonitis it was impossible to demonstrate any significant correlations between penultimate serum PLA$_2$ activity and the degree of endotoxemia ($r_p = 0.24$).
Using parameters of endotoxin, IFN-γ levels, biopterin and PLA$_2$ activity, the statistical procedure of the linear discriminant analysis allowed us to distinguish between nonseptic animals and septic animals correctly at a rate of 86.4% (Fig. 7).

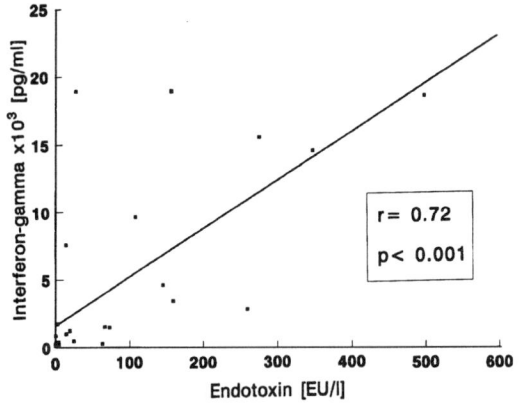

Fig. 3: Correlations between the degree of endotoxemia and the enhanced expression of interferon-γ (IFN-γ) in the prefinal phase of septic shock. The correlation coefficients of linear regression ($r_p = 0.80$) were statistically highly significant ($p < 0.0001$)

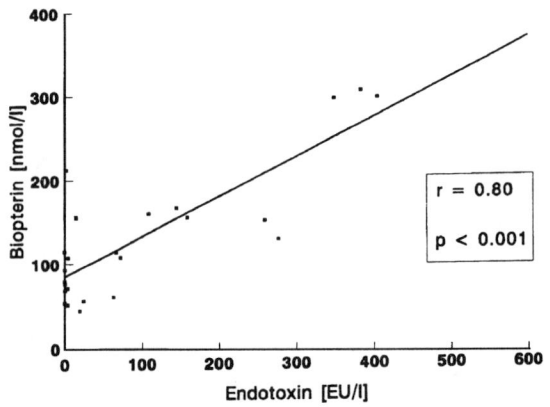

Fig. 4: Correlations between the degree of endotoxemia and the enhanced synthesis of biopterin in the penultimate phase of septic shock. The correlation coefficients of linear regression ($r_p = 0.80$) were statistically highly significant ($p < 0.0001$)

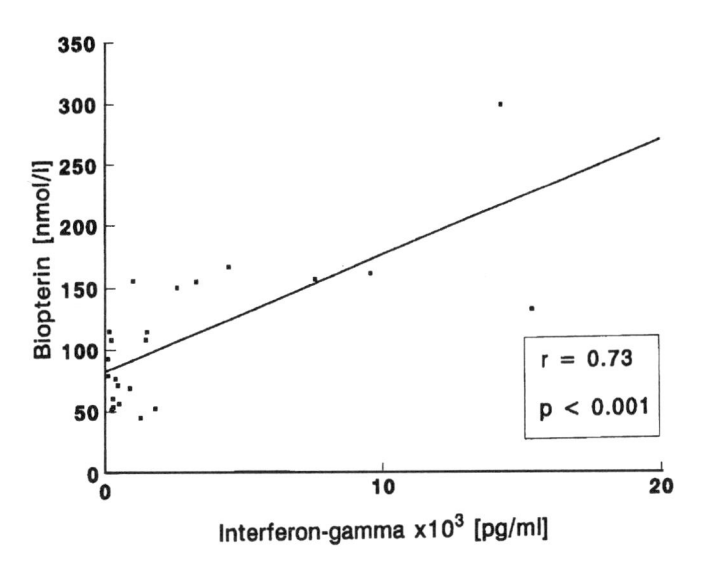

Fig. 5: Correlations between the elevated expression of γ-interferon (IFN-γ) and the enhanced synthesis of the pteridin derivative biopterin in the penultimate phase of septic shock. The correlation coefficients of linear regression ($r_p = 0.73$) were statistically highly significant ($p < 0.0001$)

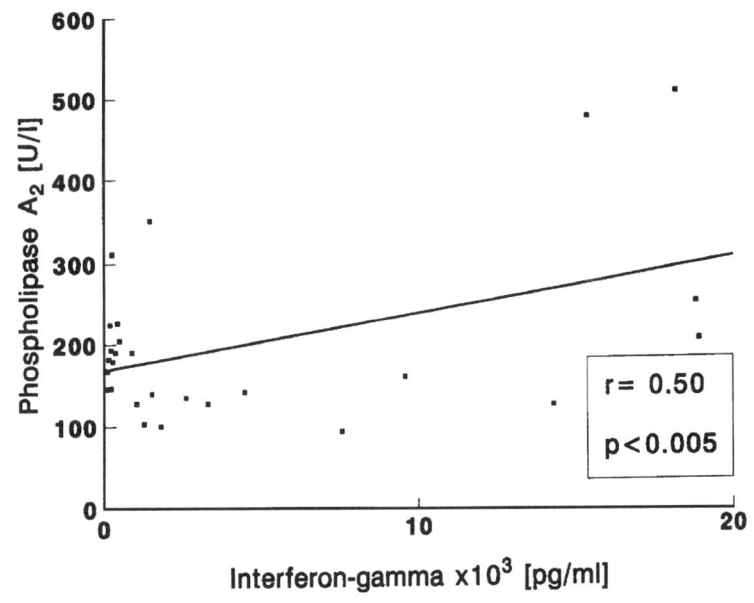

Fig. 6: Correlations between the elevated expression of interferon-γ (IFN-γ) and the enhanced serum phospholipase A_2-activity during the penultimate phase of septic shock. The correlation coefficients of linear regression ($r_p = 0.73$) were statistically highly significant ($p < 0.0001$)

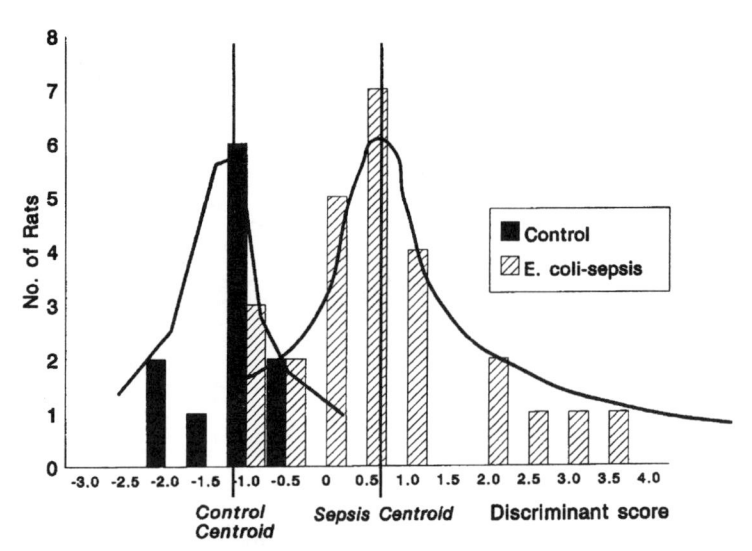

Fig. 7: Canonical discriminant functions and estimated discriminant scores of the linear discriminant analysis between sham-treated and experimental LEW.1W rats during the penultimate phase of E. coli sepsis. At a rate of 86.4% all animals were correctly classified into septic and nonseptic groups; but this procedure, among the septic animals, 19% were scored into the nonseptic group based on the parameters of endotoxin, interferon-γ, biopterin and phospholipase A_2 activity

Discussion

We used LEW.1W rats in a standardized reproducible animal model because of their good immunological responsiveness [22, 23]. Sepsis was induced by a hemoglobin/*E.coli* suspension, which is an accepted and well-tried model. After intraperitoneal injection of this mixture, all animals suffered from a fulminant peritonitis-sepsis and died within 6 h.

Our animal experiments suggest that the course of sepsis correlates with the level of endotoxin. Phospholipases of the A_2 type are released mainly during generalized septic infection in nearly all tissues or circulating cell populations, including monocytes/macrophages [10]. As a result of the formation of arachidonic acid, phospholipases play an important regulatory role in the release of inflammatory mediators [25]. PLA_2 concentrations in humans markedly increased 5-6 h after the beginning of endotoxemia. Maximal enzyme activities were found after 24 h [26]. This increase in serum PLA_2 activities remained 6 h after the induction of gram-negative sepsis in rats. Kellermann et al. [10] found a slight correlation between PLA_2 activities and neopterin concentrations in human sepsis, however, we were not able to demonstrate such relation in the LEW rat model.

In the initial stages of the immune response, a situation comparable to the one in experimental sepsis in this animal model, T-lymphocytes recognize microbial agents and by the release of IFN-γ activate the monocyte/macrophage system [20].

Huber et al. [11] and Bitterlich et al. [27] showed that IFN-γ selectively stimulates mononuclear phagocytes to produce pteridines like neopterin. Since rats do not produce detectable neopterin [12] the related pteridine biopterin was considered as a marker for increased synthesis of pteridines in activated phagocytic cells. Neopterin is suitable for differentiating between patients suffering from sepsis or nonseptic disease, and neopterin is especially helpful in the clinical follow-up of patients with septic disease [9]. It was demonstrated in patients that neopterin is a suitable marker for evaluating monocyte and macrophage stimulation in septic shock and organ failure [28].

The correlation of biopterin with endotoxin levels and with the release of IFN-γ also revealed clearly significant biological connections between them. This result suggests that the secretion of biopterin from activated macrophages is induced by both IFN-γ and directly by endotoxin [20].

Conclusion

Endotoxin, IFN-γ, biopterin and PLA$_2$ measurements are sufficient for early recognition and estimation of the extent of the immunological activation process in peritonitis-sepsis. These explored parameters allow a distinction between septic and nonseptic disorders with high probability.

References

1. DiPiro JT (1990) Pathophysiology and treatment of gram-negative sepsis. Am J Hosp Pharm 47: 6-10
2. Neugebauer 1987
3. Nyträm PO, Bax R, Patchen Dellinger R, Dominioni L, Knaus AW, Meakins JL, Ohmann Ch, Solomkin JS, Wacha H, Wittmann H (1990) Proposed definitions for diagnosis, severity scoring, stratification, and outcome for trials on intraabdominal infections. World J Surg 14: 148-158
4. Redl H, Strohmaier W, Schlag G, Pacher R, Woloszczuk W, Inthorn D, Troppmair J, Huber C (1989) Possible use of monocyte/macrophage activation marker neopterin from clinical monitoring of sepsis-related multiorgan failure. In: Faist E (ed.) Immune consequences of trauma, shock and sepsis. Springer, Berlin, Heidelberg, New York, pp. 109-113
5. Hardid (1990)
6. Philippe JJ, De Buyzere ML (1988) Endotoxin: detection and clinical significance. Acta Clin Belg 43: 429-436
7. Vadas P (1984) Elevated phospholipase A2 levels: correlation with the haemodynamic and pulmonary changes in gram-negative septic shock. J Lab Clin Med 104: 873
8. Vadas P, Pruzanski W, Stefanski E, Sternby B, Mustard R, Bohnen J, Fraser I, Farewell V, Bombardier V, Bombardier C (1988) Pathogenesis of hypotension in septic shock. Crit Care Med 16: 1
9. Hausen A, Fuchs D, Reibnegger G, Werner ER, Wachter H (1989) Neopterin in clinical use. Pteridines 1: 3-10
10. Kellermann W, Frentyel-Beyme R, Welte M, Jochum M (1989) Phospholipase A in acute lung injury after trauma and sepsis: Its relation to the inflammatory mediators PMN-Elastase, C3a and neopterin. Klin Wochenschr 67: 190-195
11. Huber Ch (1984) Immune response-associated production of neopterin. J Exp Med 160: 310

12. Duch S, Browers SW, Woolf JH, Nichol CA (1984) Biopterin cofactor biosynthesis: GTP cyclohydrolase. Neopterin and biopterin in tissues and body fluids of mammalian species. Life Sci 35: 1895-1901
13. Ohlenschlger G, Berger L (1989) Biochemische und klinische Beobachtungen zu den Immunomodulatoren: Interferone (IFN), Interleukin-2 (IL-2), Tumornekrose-Factor (TNF) und dem Immunmarker Neopterin (Teil I). Biolog Medizin 4: 496-508
15. Han (1978)
16. Han (1981)
17. Pruett TL, Rotstein OD, Fiegel VD, Sorenson JJ, Nelson RD, Simmons RL (1984) Mechanism of the adjuvant effect of hemoglobin in experimental peritonitis. VIII Surgery 96: 375-382
18. Pruett TL, Rotstein OD, Wells CL, Sorenson JJ, Simmons RL (1985) Mechanism of the adjuvant effect of hemoglobin in experimental peritonitis. IX Surgery 96: 371-377
19. Kullich W, Weissenhoffer W (1988) Thyroid function and endotoxinemia in experimental peritonitis. Surg Res Comm 3: 159-164
20. Kullich W, Weissenhoffer W, Hunsicker A, Rokos H (1993) Immune stimulation of the interferon-γ and biopterin synthesis with endotoxin in animal-experimental peritonitis. Pteridines, 8/1993
21. Rokos H (1989) Radioimmunoassay for determination of biopterin. Pteridines 1/4: 224
22. Greenhouse DD, Festing MFW, Hasan S, Cohen AL (1990) Catalogue of inbred strains of rats. In: Hedrich HJ (ed.) Genetic monitoring of inbred strains of rats. Fischer, Stuttgart, pp. 433-434
23. Hedrich HJ (1990) List of congenic and segregating inbred strains. In: Hedrich HJ (ed.) Genetic monitoring of inbred strains of rats. Fischer, Stuttgart, pp. 481-486
24. Büchler (1989)
25. Bastian BC, Römisch J, Paques E-P, Burg G (1991) Lipokortine und Phospholipasen: Neue Aspekte in der Physiologie der Glukokortikosteroidwirkung. Hautartz 42: 417-423
26. Vadas P, Pruzanski W, Farewell V (1991) A predictive model for the clearance of soluble phospholipase A_2 during septic shock. J Lab Clin Med 118: 471-475
27. Bitterlich G, Szabo G, Werner ER, Larchner C, Fuchs D, Hausen A, Reibnegger G, Schultz TF, Troppmeier J, Wachter H, Dierich MP (1988) Selective induction of mononuclear phagocytes to produce neopterin by interferon. Immunobiol 176: 228-235
28. Redl H, Schlag G, Bahrami S, Dinges HP, Schade U, Ceska M (1991) Markers of endotoxin related leukocyte activation and injury mechanisms. In: Levin J (ed.) Bacterial endotoxins: cytokine mediators and new therapies for sepsis. Progress in clinical and biological research. New York, pp. 83-100

Granulocyte-Colony-Stimulating Factor Prophylaxis and Treatment in Postoperative Peritonitis: Animal Experiments and a Successful Case Report

K.-P. Reimund, F. Weitzel, W. Lorenz, I. Celik, M. Kurnatowski,
W. Mannheim, A. Heiske, K. Neumann, B. Greger, M. Bartscherer,
M. Rothmund

Introduction

Postoperative peritonitis is still one of the most important complications in abdominal surgery. Despite surgical and antibiotic therapeutic approaches in the clinical routine, mortality rate ranges from 30% to 70% in humans [1]. Recently it was accepted that a developing peritonitis or sepsis is not only caused by the bacterial infection alone but that infection is only one component of a complex network of interactions. This is described as the systemic inflammatory response syndrome (SIRS), an overwhelming systemic inflammatory reaction of the host that is not introduced by bacteria but as a consequence of cytokine release [2]. The modulation of functions of several cytokines, e.g., interleukin 1 (IL-1), interleukin 6 (IL-6), and tumor necrosis factor-a (TNF-α), that have been shown to play an important role in the pathophysiology of sepsis and multiple organ failure [3] is a new strategy of pharmacological interventions. Such interventions (e.g., monoclonal antibodies against cytokines, cytokine receptor antagonists, specific transcription and translation inhibitors and antisense DNA) have been attempted in several animal models [4, 5] and in in vitro experiments in cell cultures. As a consequence of preclinical studies in animal models the effect of some of these new therapeutic agents was investigated in controlled clinical trials. Most of these trials in sepsis, such as the Ziegler study [6], were not successful because of methodological flaws in trial design and the later observation that the animal model did not adequately reflect the clinical situation in humans.

Therefore, before clinical trials in human subjects are started, a need for more clinically relevant animal models was claimed in order to successfully investigate the action of drugs modulating the effects of cytokines.

Design of a Clinically Relevant Animal Model for Postoperative Abdominal Peritonitis

The initial goal of this study was to develop a clinically relevant animal model for postoperative abdominal peritonitis and to investigate the prophylactic effect of the granulocyte-colony stimulating factor (G-CSF) as one of the cytokines modulating the cytokine network. Characteristics of such a clinically relevant model included:
1. Administration of clinically relevant antibiotics, which are also used against contamination and as prophylaxis in human peritonitis, in a dose- and time-dependent manner
2. Development of a common procedure of anesthesia to include the immune suppressive effect of anesthetic drugs
3. A laparotomy as a complete procedure of abdominal surgery and inoculation of a stool suspension into the peritoneal cavity (pelvic region), similar to human postoperative peritonitis
4. The usage of human stool suspensions in order to have human bacteria in the animals which are sensitive to the antibiotics employed in human postoperative sepsis
5. Administration of an opioid analgesic, as in the postoperative situation in humans, to reduce postoperative stress and the metabolic response to injury
6. Administration of G-CSF in the presence of antibiotics in different doses and at different times

The effect of G-CSF, an 18.8 kDa glycoprotein and one of the cytokines modulating the cytokine network, was investigated in this study because the usefulness of G-CSF has been reported in several animal models of sepsis associated with neutropenia [7-10] and in treatment of and protection from neutropenia due to anticancer chemotherapy and bone marrow transplantation [11]. G-CSF can increase granulocyte production in bone marrow, stimulate activation of mature granulocytes [12] and suppress TNF-α release, one of the causal mediators in sepsis and inflammation, from macrophages [13].

Conditions of the Animal Model and Different Settings for the Experiments

Materials

The rats (male Wistar rats, 200 g) were kept under controlled standardized conditions (27°C, 55% humidity, 12 h artificial day/night rhythm in standard cages) for at least 4 days before the experiment started. They were fed with a standard diet (Altromin 1313), water ad libitum and deprived of food 12 h before the experiments.

Human stool was collected from several healthy, adult, male volunteers and prepared separately for each volunteer in the same standardized method under anaerobic conditions. The stool was mixed immediately after collection in a 1:1 ratio with prereduced thioglycolate boullion containing 10% sterile barium sulfate (w/v), 10% glycerine (v/v). Catalase (preparation from bovine liver, 0.19 mg corresponding to 2000-5000 U/mg) was added to 100 ml of this suspension. The mixture was blenderized for 10 min to a macroscopically homogenous suspension and filtered through sterile surgical gauze in an anaerobic chamber. About 200 samples with 10-15 ml aliquots for each of three batches were pipetted into sterile glass tubes and frozen at -80°C for at least six months until needed. This insured that all animals received the same quality of fecal inoculum. Quality control was performed by assessing the mortality rates over the period of the experiment.

All animals, cell lines and chemicals used in the experiment were commercially available. Sources of supply and further details have been previously reported [14].

Methods

Animal Experiment. The time schedule of the animal experiment (Fig. 1a) started with the administration of G-CSF or placebo (Ringer) subcutaneously 12 h before laparotomy. One hour before operation, anesthesia with haloperidol-fentanyl was given intraperitoneally. Additionally, the animals received volume substitution (Ringer) and antibiotic (Augmentan: 10 mg/kg i.v. amoxicillin + 1 mg/kg i.v. clavulanic acid) or placebo (Ringer) intravenously. The stool suspension (1.5 ml/kg) was inoculated by laparotomy, imitating the clinical situation. Administration of antibiotic or placebo was repeated 1 h postoperatively. At the same time, the animals received an analgesic drug (Tramadol) subcutaneously for postoperative pain relief. This was given every 12 h for the whole observation period of 120 h. The main endpoint of the experiment was the 120 h mortality. All animals that survived were killed and pathological and microbiological examinations were performed. The outcome was assessed by two criteria: 120 h mortality rate and - as a biochemical marker - serum TNF-α levels 1 h after operation.

Case Study. Following the successful animal experiments, G-CSF was administered to a 35-year-old patient with polyposis coli who developed postoperative peritonitis 3 days after proctocolomucosectomy, J-pouch and loop ileostomy. Therefore relaparotomy was performed, showing diffuse peritonitis without any indication that leakage had occurred at the anastomosis or in the pouch. A peritoneal lavage was performed and the abdomen was closed. Due to postoperative neutropenia indicating a septic situation, G-CSF (300 %g subcutaneously) was administered once. Two days later an improvement of the abdominal infection during relaparotomy was seen. Fifty-six days after operation, the patient was discharged from the hospital (Fig. 1b).

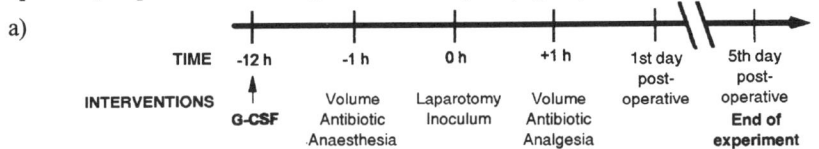

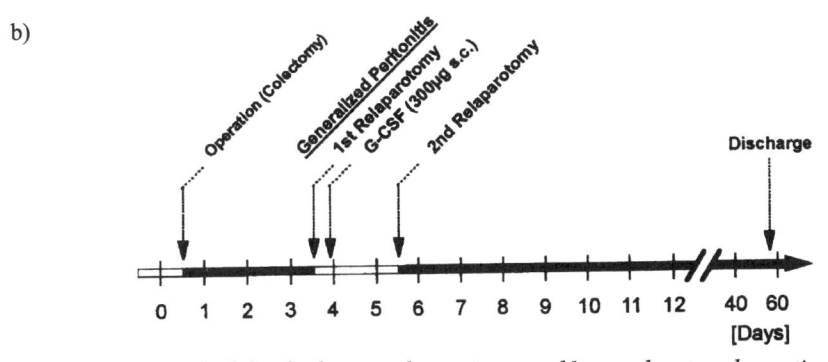

*Fig. 1. a, b: Time schedule of **a** the animal experiment and **b** granulocyte-colony-stimulating factor (G-CSF) administration in a patient with postoperative peritonitis*

G-CSF prophylaxis. In the main experiment four different groups (ten animals/group) were compared with each other concerning mortality and serum TNF-α levels. The latter were measured because TNF-α is an important proinflammatory cytokine and a common denominator of inflammatory reactions. We examined whether a correlation between TNF-α levels, treatment and mortality rate was obtained in this animal model, with the goal of adapting the results to a clinical setting.

The four groups were:

1. Animals treated with sterile heat-inactivated inoculum, to determine whether mortality is caused by toxic effects or is a consequence of the developing peritonitis
2. Control animals receiving the fecal inoculum alone, to generate postoperative peritonitis without any pharmacological interventions
3. Antibiotic treated animals given an antibiotic once before and once after operation with inoculation of stool suspension
4. Animals treated with rhu G-CSF (recombinant human G-CSF, 50 %g/kg s.c., 12 h before inoculation) additional to antibiotic and inoculation of stool suspension

TNF-α assay. Blood for determination of serum TNF-α levels was obtained immediately before and 1 h after operation by puncture of retroorbital vein plexus. TNF-α was determined essentially as described in Espevik and Nissen-Meyer [15]. Briefly, mouse fibrosarcoma cells at a concentration of $1 \times 10^4/200$ %l culture medium consisting of RPMI-1640 supplemented with 2 mM L-glutamine, 4.4 mM sodium hydrogen carbonate and 10% (v/v) fetal calf serum (FCS), were incubated with serially diluted test samples in 96-well, flat-bottomed microtiter plates (37°C, 5% CO_2, 18 h). The dye, methyl-thiazol-tetrazolium salt (MTT; 5mg/ml, 1/10 v/v), was added for determination of cytotoxicity. After incubation for 4 h at 37°C the dye was removed and cells were lysed by addition of 100 %l of 95% isopropanol/5% formic acid. Plates were analyzed on microplate ELISA reader at a test wavelength of 560 nm and a reference wavelength of 690 nm. The titer of TNF-α was calculated in units/ml, defined as the reciprocal of the dilution necessary to cause death of 50% of the cells. Activities in pg/ml are given as equivalents of murine recombinant TNF-α (pg/ml) per 5×10^4 cells. The calculation of units was performed by applying a probit analysis to the data.

Microbiological Analysis. The microorganisms were grown on chocolate agar (tryptic soy-agar supplemented with 10% defibrinated sheep blood, heated for 10 min to 80°C), blood agar (Columbia agar supplemented with 10% defibrinated sheep blood), Endo agar, Mac-Conkey agar and Sabouraud agar in a microaerobic (Anaerocult C) and anaerobic (Anaerocult A) atmosphere. The phenotypical examination of all strains was examined by testing the carbohydrate fermentation reactions according to Kauffmann [16] or by using commercially available enzyme activity and fermentation tests.

Pathology. The animals were killed by extended exposure to carbon dioxide gas in a special chamber. Organs were taken out and fixed in 10% buffered formalin. Embedding of the organs and microtomy of the specimens was performed by using standard procedures. The specimens were stained with haematoxylin/eosin before microscopic assessment.

Statistics. For descriptive analysis mean values, standard errors of the means (SEM), rates and proportions were used. For inferential statistics nominal data were analyzed by chi^2-tests, ordinal data by one step analysis of variance for four groups after logarithmic transformation of the original data.

Evaluation of the Animal Model

Dose-Response Curves

The experimental conditions and dose response curves for fecal inoculum, antibiotic and G-CSF in the presence of antibiotic were developed in a total of 295 rats.

The dose-response curve with fecal inoculum was reproducible for all experiments. A 100% mortality rate was achieved with a concentration range of 1.5 - 2 ml/kg of the 50% suspension (Fig. 2a). By increasing the amount of inoculum, a titration of damage was possible. The mortality did not depend on the kind of inoculum, whether fresh/native or frozen/rethawed stool suspension was used.

The dose-response curve with antibiotic shows a 60% mortality with the clinically recommended dose (Fig. 2b). With very high, not clinically relevant, doses of antibiotic a complete protection of animals was achieved.

With a combination of G-CSF and antibiotic in clinically relevant doses and inoculation of 1.5 ml of stool suspension, the mortality could be reduced remarkably (Fig. 2c). The most effective concentration of G-CSF was in the range of 25 - 75 %g/kg body weight. Here 80% of the animals survived, in contrast to 40% with antibiotic alone. Doses below 25 %g G-CSF were less effective.

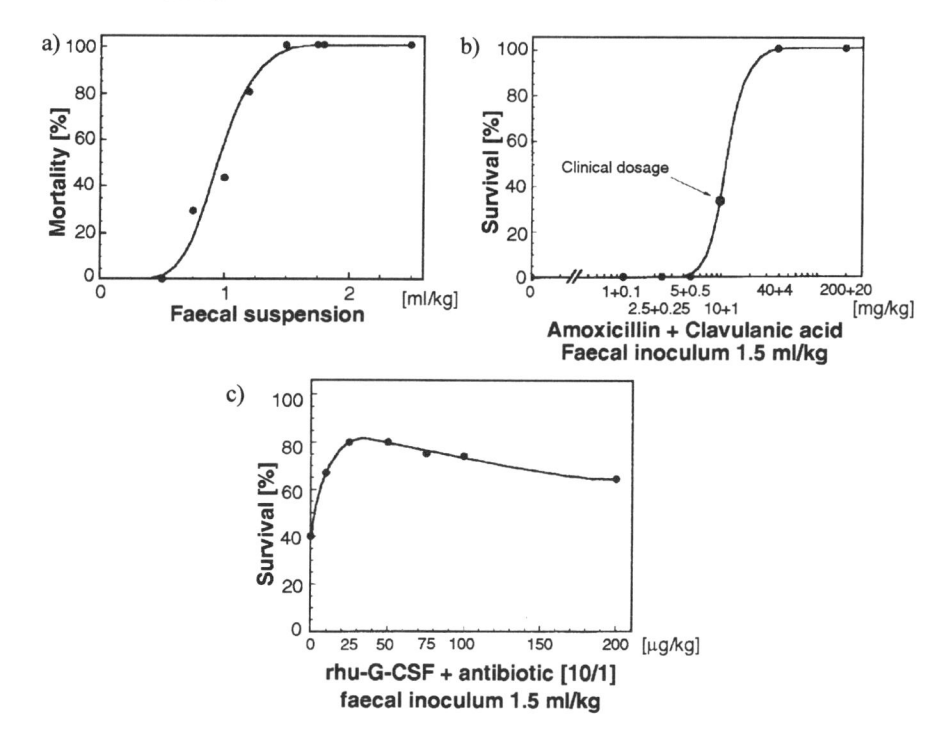

Fig. 2: Dose-response curves for defining the conditions of the animal model; rhu-G-CSF, recombinant human granulocyte-colony-stimulating factor

Microbiological Findings

Microbiologic assays of thawed aliquots sampled during the experiments showed 42 different bacteria (Table 1). Three of the detected bacteria species were antibiotic resistant. A comparison of fresh/native with frozen/rethawed aliquots revealed no change even after 6 months frozen storage. Analysis of abscesses in dead animals showed 19 different bacteria species and an organ specific distribution. Ten of the detected species were not inoculum-related and thus rat-specific germs translocated from the gut during the course of peritonitis. No gram-negative anaerobic bacteria were detectable in these animals. In one animal which died after 48 h, bacteria species were reduced from 42 to three due to antibiotic treatment (Fig. 3). Organ-specific distribution of inoculum bacteria and one rat-specific germ were found, analogous to the control situation in this animal. All bacteria were sensitive to the antibiotic used. Amoxicillin/clavulanic acid-resistant germs in the stool suspension (*Hafnia alvei, Stenotrophomonas maltophilia* and *Bacillus sp.*) were not detectable in antibiotic-treated animals.

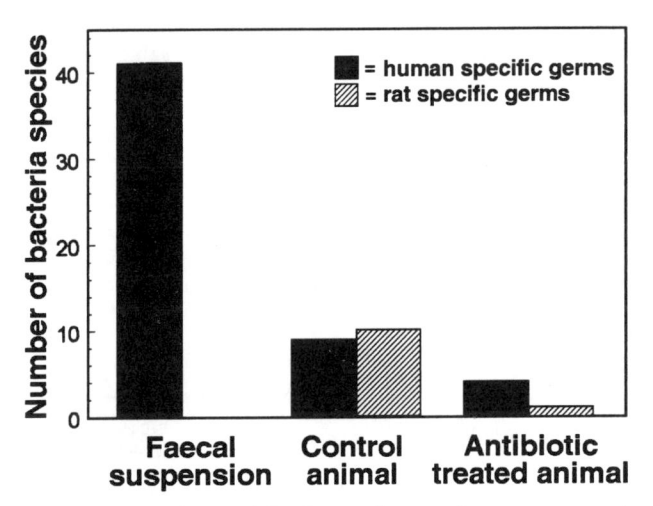

Fig. 3: Microbiological analysis of fecal inoculum and seven organs in control and antibiotic-treated animals

Prophylaxis with G-CSF and Antibiotic: Correlation with serum TNF-α

With sterile inoculum (heat-inactivated), a basal amount of TNF-α (2.6 pg/ml serum) was measurable and no animals died. Animals of the control group receiving only fecal inoculum without any pharmacological intervention had a 14-fold increase of serum TNF-α levels compared to those animals inoculated with sterile stool suspension, thereby indicating that TNF-α was a causal mediator for the developing peritonitis. This resulted in a 100% mortality. In antibiotic-treated animals a reduction of serum TNF-α levels to 17.1 pg/ml and a mortality of 60% was found, whereas in the G-CSF treated group no TNF-α was measurable and mortality was only 20%. The results are summarized in Fig. 4.

Table 1: Qualitative/quantitative microbiological culture of fecal inoculum in treated animals and organ distribution of bacteria

Bacteria	Fecal inoculum	Control (organ)	Antibiotic-treated (organ)
Aerobic gram-negative			
Escherichia coli	$2\text{-}4 \times 10^4$ cfu/ml	+	+(1-7)
Hafnia alvei	+		
Stenotrophomonas maltophilia	+		
Proteus mirabilis a, b			(1-7)
Neisseria sicca a		(5)	
Moraxella phenylpyruvica a		(6)	
Aerobic gram-positive			
Enterococcus faecium	+	+	+(1, 5, 6)
Enterococcus faecalis	5×10^4 cfu/ml	+(5, 6)	
Corynebacterium bovis	$2\text{-}4 \times 10^4$ cfu/ml		
Staphylococcus aureus	+	+(5, 6)	
Staphylococcus cohnii a		(5, 6)	
Staphylococcus warneri	+		
Bacillus sp.	+		
Bacillus sp. 1 a		(5, 6)	
Bacillus sp. 2 a		(5, 6)	
Anaerobic gram-negative			
Bacteroides fragilis	+		
Bacteroides thetaiotamicron	+		
Bacteroides uniformis	+		
Bacteroides distasonis	+		
Bacteroides capillosis	+		
Bacteroides gracilis	+		
Bacteroides eggerthii	+		
Bacteroides levii	+		
Bacteroides vulgatus	+		
Prevotella oralis	+		
Prevotella oris	+		
Prevotella buccae	+		
Prevotella loescheii	+		
Prevotella sp.			+(3, 5)
Porphyromonas gingivalis	+		
Fusobacterium mortiferum	+		
Fusobacterium varium	+		
Wolinella sp.	+		
Anaerobic gram-positive			
Clostridium perfringens	+	+(4, 5, 6)	
Clostridium histolyticum[a]		(5)	
Clostridium clostridiiforme	+	+(3)	
Clostridium innocuum[a]		(1, 6)	
Clostridium difficile	+		
Clostridium ramosum	+		

Clostridium subterminale	+	+(3)	
Clostridium septicum	+		
Clostridium tertium	+		
Eubacterium aerofaciens	+		
Eubacterium lentum	+		
Eubacterium limosum	+		
Listeria minutis	+		
Propionibacterium agnes	+	+(3, 6)	
Propionibacterium granulosum	+		
Lactobacillius acidophilus[a]		(6)	
Bifidobacterium adolescentis	+	+(3, 4, 5, 6)	
Bifidobacterium sp. [a]		(3, 4, 5, 6)	
Not identified gram-labile Bacterium	+		
Fungi			
Candida albicans	5×10^3 cfu/ml		

Due to culture conditions quantitative analysis of bacteria species was possible only in some cases. For germs marked by sp.(species, e.g., *Bacillus sp.* 1 and 2), a detailed characterization was not possible.

The organ distribution of different bacteria species was performed by analyzing abscesses of spleen (1), kidney (2), lung (3), liver (4), gut (5), peritoneum (6), and blood from heart and pleural cavity (7). The presence of a bacteria species in one of the investigated organs is marked in the table by the corresponding numbers.

+, $\leq 10^3$ colony-forming units/ml (cfu/ml).

[a] Rat-specific germs ($\leq 10^3$ colony-forming units /ml) present in control animals.

[b] Rat-specific germs present in antibiotic-treated animals.

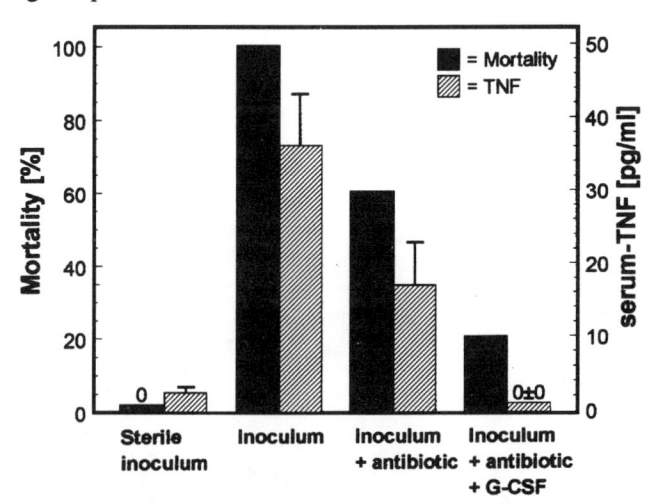

Fig. 4: Mortality at 120 h and serum tumor necrosis factor-a (TNF) levels in the four animal groups: relation to use of antibiotics, granulocyte-colony-stimulating factor (G-CSF), and inoculum, n = 5 for all groups except antibiotic + inoculum (n = 10); mortality, $p < 0.01$ (chi^2 test); TNF (ANOVA after log transformation): $p < 0.02$ (a/b) and $p < 0.05$ (b/c). TNF data are mean ± SEM from all animals in one group. TNF value of each animal is the mean value of a triple measurement

Administration of G-CSF for Treatment of a Patient with Postoperative Peritonitis

Starting with the administration of G-CSF, clinical and inflammatory parameters were continuously monitored. IL-1, IL-6, TNF-a, and the soluble TNF receptors were also measured, as was leukocyte count, C-reactive protein (CRP), and elastase. The neutrophil count increased progressively after a single dose of G-CSF to more than 30 000/%l in a 12 day period (Fig. 5). At the day of discharge, a normal leukocyte count was observed.

During the entire observation period no TNF-a or IL-1 was detectable. In contrast, enormous levels of IL-6 (26 000 pg/ml) and high levels of CRP (216 mg/l, normal value: < 5 mg/l) and elastase (240 %g/l, normal value: < 40 %g/l) were measured before G-CSF administration. These parameters declined in the postadministration period to normal levels at day of discharge. IL-6 declined within 2 days to normal levels. The amount of the soluble 75 kDa TNF receptor in serum was slightly increased (5156 pg/ml) and did not change during the observation period. In contrast, tenfold higher serum levels of the 55 kDa TNF receptor (7165 pg/ml) were found before G-CSF administration. These levels declined to normal values at day of discharge (Fig. 5).

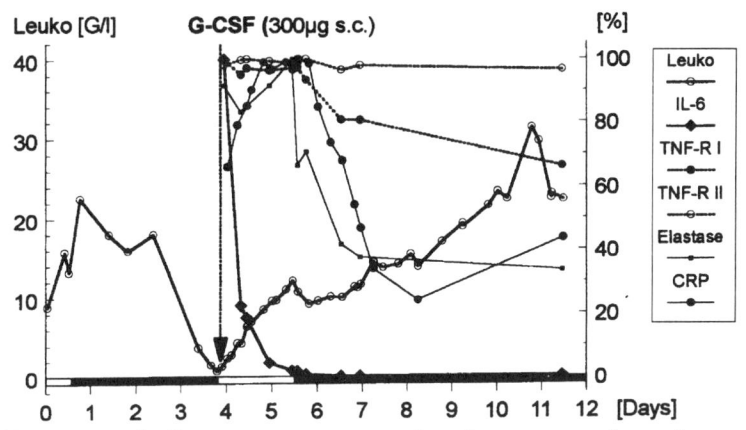

Fig. 5: Time course of inflammatory parameters after administration of granulocyte-colony-stimulating factor to a patient with postoperative peritonitis. Thick line, filled circles, leukocytes; thick lines, diamonds, interleuki-6 (IL-6); dotted line, filled circles, tumor necrosis factor (TNF) receptor I; dotted line, open circles, TNF receptor II; thin line, filled squares, elastase; thin line, filled circles, C-reactive protein (CRP)

Discussion

Cytokines are an important component in the pathophysiology of sepsis. Studies (Ziegler [6], Wenzel [1], Lorenz [17], Zanetti [18]) published so far have not given final answers concerning the therapeutic use of both cytokines and agents that attack cytokine activities such as anti-endotoxin antibodies or cytokine receptor antagonists. The reasons have been the different effects of new treatment strategies in subgroups, especially in those with gram-positive sepsis, in whom detrimental effects appeared.

Therefore more clinically relevant models are necessary to determine the therapeutic impact of cytokines. The model of postoperative peritonitis presented here is suitable to accomplish this goal. The use of human stool suspension caused a peritonitis with pus and abscesses in the abdomen; almost all other clinical aspects can be adjusted according to the situation in humans. Comparing the microbiological analysis of stool suspension and control animals a reduction of bacteria species was found in the latter, demonstrating that there was no totally immunocompromised state and that defense against infection occurred. In contrast to other models [19], animals did not die within the first 6 h, but 24-30 h after operation. This indicates a causal connection of death and the developing peritonitis. Also the translocation of bacteria, which means finding germs not present in the stool suspension, showed a similarity to the situation in human peritonitis.

With a clinically relevant and recommended dose of antibiotic, mortality was 60%, representing the clinical situation. Addition of G-CSF to the antibiotics reduced mortality to 20%, thereby suggesting a new concept of prophylaxis. TNF-a, an important contributor to inflammatory conditions [20-22], was suppressed by G-CSF. Suppression of TNF-a release from macrophages is one possible mechanism of G-CSF protection in this model.

The usefulness of the drug was demonstrated in treatment of and protection from neutropenia due to anticancer chemotherapy and bone marrow transplantation [11]. In our experience G-CSF treatment in a patient with postoperative peritonitis and leukopenia resulted in increased leukocyte count, decreased of inflammatory parameters, and recovery from disease. These promising data can now be studied further in new clinical trials.

Acknowledgement

We thank Armin Demant and Ingeborg Muttschall for support in performing the animal experiments. This work was supported by cooperative grants of Deutsche Forschungsgemeinschaft (Grant We 1807/1-1) and Amgen, Inc. (Europe).

References

1. Wenzel RP (1992) Anti-endotoxin monoclonal antibodies: a second look. N Eng J Med 326: 1151-1153
2. Bone RC and the members of the American College of Chest Physicians/Society of Critical Care Medicine, Consensus Conference Committee. Members of the American College of Chest Physicians/Society of Critical Care Medicine, Consensus Conference (1992) Definitions for sepsis and organ failure and guidelines for the use of innovative therapies in sepsis. Crit Care Med 20: 864-874
3. Ertel W, Morrison MH, Wang P, Ba ZF, Ayala A, Chaudry IH (1991) The complex pattern of cytokines in sepsis: association between prostaglandins, cachectin and interleukins. Ann Surg 214: 185-195
4. Roilides E, Pizzo PA (1992) Modulation of host defenses by cytokines: evolving adjuncts in prevention and treatment of serious infections in immunocompromised hosts. Clin Infect Dis 15: 508-524
5. Christman JW (1992) Potential treatment of sepsis syndrome with cytokine-specific agents. Chest 102: 613-617

6. Ziegler EJ, Fisher CJ, Sprung CL, Straube RC, Sadoff JC, Foulke GE, Wortel CH, Fink MP, Dellinger RP, Teng NNH, Allen IE, Berger HJ, Knatterud GL, LoBuglio AF, Smith CR, HA-1A Sepsis Study Group (1991) Treatment of gram negative bacteremia and septic shock with HA-1A human monoclonal antibody against endotoxin. N Engl J Med 324: 429-436
7. Hebert JC, Oreilly M, Gamelli RL (1990) Protective effect of recombinant human granulocyte colony-stimulating factor against pneumococcal infections in splenectomized mice. Arch Surg 125: 1075-1078
8. Iida J, Saiki I, Ishihara C, Azuma I (1988) Protective activity of recombinant cytokines against sendai virus and herpes simplex virus (HSV) infections in mice. Vaccine 7: 229-233
9. Silver GM, Gamelli RL, O'Reilly M (1989) The beneficial effect of granulocyte colony-stimulating factor (G-CSF) in combination with gentamicin on survival after pseudomonas burn wound infection. Surgery 106: 452-456
10. Tanaka N, Kumamoto Y, Hiros T, Yokoo A (1989) Study of the prophylactic and therapeutic effect of human granulocyte-colony stimulating factor (G-CSF) on experimental pyelonephritis induced by Pseudomonas aeruginosa in neutropenic mice. Kansenshogaku Zasshi 63: 145-155
11. Metcalf D (1991) The colony-stimulating factors: discovery to clinical use. Philos Trans R Soc Lond [Biol] 333: 147-173
12. Demetri GD, Griffin JD (1991) Granulocyte colony-stimulating factor and its receptor. Blood 78: 2791-2808
13. Görgen I, Hartung T, Leist M, Niehörster M, Tiegs G, Uhlig S, Weitzel F, Wendel A (1991) Granulocyte colony-stimulating factor treatment protects rodents against lipopolysaccharide-induced toxicity via suppression of systemic tumor necrosis factor a. J Immunol 149: 918-924
14. Lorenz W, Reimund K-P, Weitzel F, Celik I, Kurnatowski M, Schneider C, Mannheim W, Heiske A, Neumann K, Rothmund M (1994) G-CSF prophylaxis before operation protects against lethal consequences of postoperative peritonitis. Surgery 116: 925-934
15. Espevik T, Nissen-Meyer J (1986) A highly sensitive cell line WEHI 164 clone 13, for measuring cytotoxic factor/tumor necrosis factor from human monocytes. J Immunol 95: 99-105
16. Kauffmann S (ed.) (1954) Enterobacteriaceae. 2nd ed. Ejnar Munksgaard, Copenhagen
17. Lorenz W (1993) Clinical trials in sepsis and septic shock: a scrutiny of methodology. Theor Surg 8: 59-60
18. Zanetti G, Glauser M-P, Baumgartner JD (1993) Anti-endotoxin antibodies and other inhibitors of endotoxin. New Horizons 1: 110-119
19. Wichterman KA, Baue AE, Chaudry IH (1980) Sepsis and septic shock - a review of laboratory models and a proposal. J Surg Res 29: 189-201
20. Tiegs G, Wolter M, Wendel A (1984) Tumor necrosis factor is a terminal mediator in galactosamine/endotoxin-induced hepatitis in mice. Biochem Pharmacol 38: 627-631
21. Beutler B, Mislark IW, Cerami AC (1985) Passive immunization against cachectin/tumor necrosis factor protects mice from the lethal effect of endotoxin. Science 229: 869-871.
22. Lehmann V, Freudenberg MA, Galanos C (1987) Lethal toxicity of lipopolysaccharide and tumor necrosis factor in normal and D-galactosamine-treated mice. J Exp Med 165: 657-663

Protective Effects of Hydroxyethyl Starch-Deferoxamine in Early Sepsis

D. Moch, B. Schröppel, M.H. Schoenberg, H.-J. Schulz, B.-E. Hedlund U.B. Brückner

Reactive oxygen metabolites (ROM) are an important factor in the pathogenesis of endotoxin-induced sepsis. Endotoxin primes the PMN-leukocytes, leading to an enhanced oxygen radical generation. These species induce lipid peroxidation of cell membranes and cause cell membrane disintegration and ultimately tissue damage. On the other hand, lipid peroxidation prompts further accumulation of PMNs. The most toxic radical in this context, the hydroxyl radical, is generated from superoxide and hydrogen peroxide by the iron-driven Haber-Weiss and Fenton reactions. The iron chelator deferoxamine (DFO) is able to suppress these iron-catalyzed reactions [12]. When, however, applied intravenously DFO acts as a cardiodepressant. In order to avoid these negative circulatory side-effects we used a DFO conjugated to hydroxyethyl starch (HES-DFO) [8].

The aim of our study was: (1) to quantitate the injury to the lung and the kidney as primary shock organs in the very early phase of sepsis and to elucidate (2) whether the generation of oxygen radicals is involved in this pathophysiology and (3) whether the conjugate HES-DFO could prevent these tissue damages.

Materials and Methods

The study was performed on 70 male Sprague-Dawley rats weighing 360 ± 60 g. The animals were randomly separated into two groups treated immediately prior to sepsis, receiving either 3 ml (representing a dose of 45 mg DFO/animal intravenously) of the conjugate (Biomedical Frontiers, Minneapolis, USA) or only 3 ml of the carrier starch solution. During halothane anesthesia the left carotid artery and external jugular vein were cannulated. After a small mid-abdominal laparotomy, sepsis was induced via cecal ligation and puncture (CLP) [15]. The mean arterial pressure (MAP) was measured immediately prior to as well as 30, 60, 120, and 240 min following induction of sepsis. At these time points, 2 ml of blood were also withdrawn for quantitative analysis of the plasma concentration of endotoxin by means of a specific chromogenic LAL test [2].

At each timepoint 5 or 10 animals were put to death. The kidneys and the lungs were rapidly harvested and instantaneously frozen in liquid nitrogen. In addition, ten rats were immediately put to death for evaluation of baseline values. In the tissue specimen the contents of PMN myeloperoxidase (MPO) [13], reduced and oxidized glutathione (GSH/GSSG) [6], malondialdehyde (MDA) [14], and conjugated dienes (CD) [5] were determinedusing modifications of published procedures. Five animals that had been operated on but without CLP sepsis served as controls to exclude methodological bias.

A two-way analysis of variance for repeated measures was used to determine differences between groups or over time. Statistical significance was accepted at the 95% confidence level ($p < 0.05$).

Results

Thirty minutes after sepsis induction the plasma endotoxin concentration exceeded 6.8 EU/ml in both groups, indicating severe sepsis, regardless of treatment. MAP decreased slightly but significantly in all animals during sepsis. In the lungs (Table 1) MPO concentration was increased in the starch group as soon as 30 min after induction of sepsis. Concomitantly, the GSH level in the tissue decreased and lipid peroxidation occurred as shown by the elevated MDA and CD levels. The pretreatment with HES-DFO diminished the PMN accumulation in lung tissue and, consequently, the MPO concentration was reduced. Moreover, lung MDA and CD levels were significantly lower in the conjugate-treated animals at nearly all time points.

Table 1: Content of PMN-myeloperoxidase (MPO), reduced (GSH) and oxidized (GSSG) glutathione, as well as the lipid peroxidation products malondialdehyde (MDA) and conjugated dienes (CD) in lung tissue in CLP sepsis in rats.

Time (min) Group (n)		Basis (10)	30 HES (5)	30 HES-DFO (8)	60 HES (5)	60 HES-DFO (8)	120 HES (5)	120 HES-DFO (9)	240 HES (5)	240 HES-DFO (7)
MPO (U/g protein)	Median	484	1165	1050	1385	1443	1618	995	1719	1064
	Minimum	231	291	256	645	703	843	334	1172	464
	Maximum	564	3000	1463	2301	2237	2205	2058	2276	2021
GSH (μmol/g protein)	Median	39.1	27.9	27.5	23.5	28.9	26.9	28.9	20.8	26.3
	Minimum	22.6	17.7	17.6	19.8	22.9	22.4	20.9	18.7	18.4
	Maximum	54.3	45.7	38.9	29.3	43.2	31.2	43.4	26.1	32.4
GSSG (μmol/b protein)	Median	0.74	0.59	0.88	0.53	0.46	0.58	1.18	0.77	0.58
	Minimum	0.34	0.34	0.48	0.19	0.22	0.19	0.16	0.31	0.16
	Maximum	0.98	0.94	1.40	1.38	1.45	0.94	1.94	1.41	1.30
MDA (mol/g protein)	Median	230	326	174*	388	164*	463	160*	437	178*
	Minimum	150	282	161	225	76	338	74	288	28
	Maximum	335	456	220	636	465	590	389	774	321
CD (nmol/g protein)	Median	9.1	14.5	10.3	9.2	6.2*	14.4	8.8*	9.6	9.0
	Minimum	2.5	7.5	8.8	7.7	3.3	11.6	4.3	6.7	1.5
	Maximum	18.3	22.1	22.9	19.0	10.6	29.0	10.9	13.2	11.1

*$p < 0.05$ starch (HES) vs. starch-deferoxamine (HES-DFO).

Histomorphological examinations revealed marked microatelectases associated with destruction of the alveolar septa and splicing of the basal membranes in the HES-treated rats. In contrast, the anti-oxidative prophylaxis resulted in nearly normal and well-ventilated alveoli, and only some enlarged reticular fibers without splicing were observed.

In the kidneys (Table 2) almost similar results were found. The tissue MPO levels differed neither within nor between groups. The slight decrease in the GSH content seen after 60 min in the HES-DFO group revealed oxidative stress but to a less pronounced degree. The most impressive effect of iron chelation, however, was demonstrated by the so-called lipid peroxidation products. At each timepoint MDA and CD levels were markedly lower than in the rat streated only with HES. The pathohistological micrographs of the starch group demonstrated tubulotoxic and mitochondrial damage, whereas HES-DFO treatment attenuated these alterations.

Table 2: Content of PMN myeloperoxidase (MPO), reduced (GSH) and oxidized (GSSG) glutathione, as well as the lipid peroxidation products malondialdehyde (MDA) and conjugated dienes (CD) in kidney tissue in CLP sepsis in rat.

Time (min)		0	30		60		120		240	
Group (n)		Basis	HES	HES-DFO	HES	HES-DFO	HES	HES-DFO	HES	HES-DFO
		(10)	(5)	(8)	(5)	(8)	(5)	(9)	(5)	(7)
MPO	Median	19	11	12	10	7	11	7	9	8
(U/g protein)	Minimum	3	5	4	90	1	7	2	6	4
	Maximum	36	18	36	13	19	15	27	12	15
GSH	Median	33.7	23.7	21.5	19.0	21.4	24.8	19.5	18.1	24.6
(μmol/g protein)	Minimum	21.4	16.9	16.0	15.1	12.2	18.9	11.9	15.6	12.9
	Maximum	53.0	35.6	33.7	20.8	32.5	34.7	39.8	33.5	29.8
GSSG	Median	0.88	0.78	0.82	0.57	0.73	0.59	0.67	1.29	0.27
(μmol/b protein)	Minimum	0.23	0.67	1.18	0.16	0.12	0.15	0.15	0.14	0.17
	Maximum	1.94	1.01	1.50	1.62	1.08	1.95	1.76	2.60	1.12
MDA	Median	994	793	235*	691	201*	1158	273*	861	340*
(mol/g protein)	Minimum	564	145	119	345	137	732	147	552	143
	Maximum	1005	1107	485	1121	349	1213	348	1509	409
CD	Median	11.6	20.9	14.5	21.5	12.7*	27.2	13.6*	14.5	15.7
(nmol/g protein)	Minimum	6.7	15.4	4.1	12.1	8.2	18.5	3.4	13.1	2.9
	Maximum	22.1	27.3	25.4	25.3	16.7	29.5	24.5	21.1	17.8

*$p < 0.05$ starch (HES) vs. starch-deferoxamine (HES-DFO).

Discussion and Conclusion

Endotoxin obviously triggers the generation of ROM during gram-negative sepsis. In in vivo-systems PMN leukocytes [7], vascular and alveolar endothelial cells [4], alveolar macrophages [9, and mesangial and tubular cells [1] are given as the source of these ROM. Our results confirm the suggestions that there are different sources of ROM in both the lungs and kidneys. The high molecular weight ofthe conjugate HES-DFO [8] prevents any membrane penetration and hence intracellular accumulation. Therefore, the prevention of the iron-driven catalysis of hydroxyl radicals must occur in the extracellular space.

The concentration of myeloperoxidase, as an indirect measure of PMN accumulation, was significantly increased in lung tissue. This result is in accordance with the histological findings of a marked interstitial PMN permeation. Other studies [11] also reported a pulmonary PMN infiltration after an endotoxin challenge. Accumulated PMNs, on the other hand, are most likely responsible for the enhanced ROM generation in sepsis. After activation these cells release highly aggressive oxygen species that react with many biological substances, particularly with polyunsaturated fatty acids (PUFA). This reaction is called lipid peroxidation (LPO). Since all cell membranes abound in PUFA, the peroxidation of these molecules leads to a disintegration of cell membrane structures, resulting ultimately in cell death and hence tissue damage.

Lipid peroxidation leads to two primary breakdown products, low molecular weight lipid-derived aldehydes and alcohols, often referred to as thiobarbituric acid reactive substances (TBARS), of which malondialdehyde (MDA) is a major component, and low molecular weight lipids, conjugated dienes (CD). Both MDA/TBARS and CD, when measured in plasma and/or tissue, are considered as indirect markers of LPO in vivo [5]. In the present study HES-DFO significantly reduced the extent of LPO in the lungs. This is documented by lower MDA and CD levels. The pathohistological findings also reflect this biochemical benefit of HES-DFO.

The data of the kidneys reveal a different pathway. In fact, the anti-oxidative therapy with HES-DFO attenuated renal LPO and the histological findings are consistent with the observed membrane protection. However, the stimulus for generation of ROM in renal tissue is governed by activation other than that by PMN since the MPO concentration never exceeded physiological values.

Because the macromolecule HES-DFO is not glomerularly filtered [10] and there are no relevant concentrations of HES-DFO in the urine within the first 2 h, the observed protective effects of the conjugate suggest ROM production probably in the vascular endothelial or mesangial cells [1].

On the basis of our results we conclude: (1) There is an early generation of oxygen radicals in peritonitis-induced sepsis. (2) These oxygen radicals appear to be important mediators inducing kidney and lung damage. (3) Iron-driven reactions seem to be pivotal for the development of these alterations. (4) In the kidneys the generation of the O_2 species is apparently endothelium or mesangium derived, whereas (5) in the lungs its release is governed by PMN leukocytes. (6) This is proven by the fact that the iron chelator HES-DFO was able to markedly attenuate LPO of cell membranes and (7) hence reduce the morphological injury. (8) This substance might therefore be an additional and efficient tool in treating early sepsis and septic shock. Further studies are required to further establish the exact mechanism of protection.

References

1. *Baud L, Ardaillou R (1986) Reactive oxygen species: production and role in the kidney. Am J Physiol 251: F765-F776*
2. *Berger D, Marzinzig E, Marzinzig M, Beger HG (1988) Quantitative endotoxin determination in blood - chromogenic modification of the limulus amebocyte lysate test. Eur Surg Res 20: 128-136*

3. Braughler IM, Duncan LA, Chase RL (1986) The involvement of iron in lipid peroxidation. Importance of ferric to ferrous ratios in initiation. J Biol Chem 22: 10282-10289
4. Brigham (1987) Antioxidants protect cultured bovine lung endothelial cells from injury by endotoxin. J Appl Physiol 63: 840-850
5. Buege IA, Aust SD (1978) Microsomal lipid peroxidation. Methods Enzymol 52: 302-306
6. Griffith OW (1980) Determination of glutathione and glutathione disulfide using glutathione reductase and 2-vinylpyridine. Anal Biochem 106: 207-212
7. Grisham MB, Everse J, Janssen F (1988) Endotoxemia and neutrophil activation in vivo. Am J Physiol 254: H1017-H1022
8. Hallaway PE, Eaton JW, Panter SS, Hedlund BE (1989) Modulation of deferoxamine toxicity and clearance by covalent attachment to biocompatible polymers. Proc Natl Acad Sci USA 86: 10108-10112
9. Johnson KJ, Ward PA, Kunkel RC, Wilson BS (1986) Mediation of IgA-induced lung injury in the rat - role of macrophages and reactive oxygen products. Lab Invest 54: 499-506
10. Paller MS, Hedlund BE (1988) Role of iron in postischemic renal injury in the rat. Kidney Int 34: 474-480
11. Repine IR (1992) Scientific perspectives on adult respiratory distress syndrome. Lancet 339: 466-469
12. Summers MR, Jacobs A, Tudway D, Perera P, Ricketts C (1979) Studies in deferoxamine and feroxamine metabolism in normal and iron-overloaded subjects. Br J Haematol 42: 547-555
13. Suzuki K, Ota H, Sasagawa S, Sakatani T, Fujikura T (1987) Assay method for myeloperoxidase in human polymorphonuclear leukocytes. Analyt Biochem 132: 345-352
14. Yagi S (1976) A simple fluorometric assay for lipoperoxide in blood. Biochem Med 15: 212-216
15. Yelich MR (1990) Glucoregulatory, hormonal, and metabolic responses to endotoxicosis or cecal ligation and puncture sepsis in the rat: a direct comparison. Circ Shock 31: 351-363

Section 8:

Acute Pancreatitis - Biology and Therapeutic Consequences

Biochemical Pattern, Systemic Complications, and Outcome in Acute Pancreatitis

C. Niederau, R. Lüthen, J.W. Heise, H. Becker

Introduction

The diagnosis of acute pancreatitis is based on clinical symptoms and signs and on increases in serum concentrations of amylase or lipase. Major increases of serum pancreatic enzymes (more than three- to fivefold of the upper normal limit) virtually confirm the diagnosis of acute pancreatitis, in particular when the patient presents with a typical clinical picture. The diagnosis may be further supported by imaging procedures such as ultrasound and computed tomography (CT). However, neither these imaging techniques nor all the further laboratory and technical measurements are needed to confirm the diagnosis but are carried out to assess the severity of pancreatitis and its prognosis.

The severity of pancreatitis varies from a mild, continuously healing edematous form to a severe necrotizing disease with complications at distant extrapancreatic organs and a mortality rate which may exceed 50% [7, 86, 98]. Although there is still no specific therapy for acute pancreatitis, the improvements in supportive care may help to decrease the high mortality in necrotizing pancreatitis. Therefore it is important to identify patients with necrotizing pancreatitis at the earliest possible stage in order to assure adequate supportive treatment. It is well known that hypovolemic shock due to sequestration of fluid into the retroperitonaeum and other third spaces is a major life-threatening condition during the first 24 - 48 h [98]. During the early stage of necrotizing pancreatitis a variety of vasoactive and toxic compounds are released into the systemic circulation. These substances are thought to cause the pulmonary, cardiovascular, and renal complications which determine the clinical course during the first 2 weeks. The mortality seen later in the course of necrotizing pancreatitis is usually due to septic complications. Assessment of the prognosis should therefore indicate the severity of the disease and should help to identify which of the various possible complications may occur.

CT is generally regarded as the gold standard for differentiation between edematous and necrotizing pancreatitis [6, 15]. Ultrasound is less helpful for this purpose [102]. Although CT is the most reliable imaging technique to identify necrosis, up to 20% of necrotizing forms may be falsely diagnosed as edematous pancreatitis by CT early after the onset of the disease. Also, edematous pancreatitis may be falsely diagnosed as necrotizing pancreatitis in a considerable percentage of patients during the early stage of the disease [15]. Therefore, additional information based on clinical observations and laboratory measurements are needed to determine the severity, complications, and prognosis of acute pancreatitis.

Multifactorial Systems of Grading the Severity of Pancreatitis

The first widely accepted multifactorial system of grading the severity of pancreatitis was described and applied by Ranson et al. [95, 96]. This scoring system includes 11 prognostic factors, six of which are determined directly after admission. A further five laboratory and clinical factors are assessed within 24 h after admission. Thus, Ranson's score cannot be fully obtained during the first two days of the disease. Imrie et al. [52] have introduced a scoring system slightly modified from Ranson's grading; and later modified their own scoring system to better evaluate the prognosis in biliary pancreatitis [90]. Neither modification of Imrie's score (also called the Glasgow score) allows assessment of the prognosis during the first 2 days after admission. This delay in characterizing the severity of pancreatitis is therefore a drawback of all the major standard scoring systems. Recently, the APACHE illness grading system (acute physiology and chronic health evaluation) [65, 75] was used to predict the outcome in acute pancreatitis [72, 118]. The original APACHE system is very complex and difficult to use in the clinical routine [65, 75]. A simplified modification, the APACHE II system, utilizes 12 routinely available physiological and laboratory measurements with an additional weighing for age and preadmission health status [66]. The major drawback of the APACHE II system is the need to assess the score on multiple occasions during the course of the disease. Furthermore, the APACHE II system is still more complex and difficult to use than Imrie's or Ranson's system in clinical practice. It has been shown that only the peak of the APACHE II scores during the first 3 days after admission is superior to the older standard scoring systems [72]. Thus, the diagnostic delay using the APACHE II system is even greater than that of the older systems. The APACHE system may, however, be useful to accurately assess the prognosis of patients with a very severe course treated on intensive care units [118].

Biochemical Pattern

The serum activities of all pancreatic digestive enzymes rise sharply within the first 24 h of acute pancreatitis. Part of these enzymes may leave the pancreatic acinar cell via the basolateral site due to a blockade in regular luminal secretion [2]. Probably a major part of the pancreatic enzymes in serum originates from necrotic exocrine tissue. In the usual course of acute pancreatitis serum concentrations of digestive enzymes decline steadily over the initial 3-6 days after the beginning of the disease. When determining the initial increase in serum enzymes as a diagnostic test for acute pancreatitis, the sensitivity and specificity are similar for different types of digestive enzymes, including amylase, trypsin, lipase, and elastase. Minor serum increases of these enzymes (< 2-3 times the upper normal limit) can be seen in a variety of nonpancreatic diseases such as ulcus perforation, cholecystitis, intestinal obstruction and ischemia, renal failure, and gynecological diseases. Major serum increases of pancreatic digestive enzymes (> 3 times the upper normal limit) have, however, a good specificity for acute pancreatitis and are only rarely seen in nonpancreatic diseases [18, 32, 107]. Thus, in the case of a typical clinical picture determination of serum (or urinary) amylase is usually sufficient to confirm the diagnosis provided that the increase in serum amylase is marked, and that the measurement is made during the first 24 h of the attack. The serum elevations of most pancreatic enzymes decline so rapidly that the diagnostic value is already markedly reduced 48-72 h after the beginning of pancreatitis [119]. The decrease in serum enzyme levels is more rapid for amylase than for lipase. Therefore serum measurements of enzymes other than amylase may be of some additional value later in the course of pancreatitis. The height of the increase in serum pancreatic enzymes is not of prognostic importance [13, 119].

Acute Phase Reactants and Other Biochemical Markers of the Severity of Pancreatitis

Despite the combination of CT and one of the scoring systems about 10 - 15% of fatal or complicated cases of necrotizing pancreatitis cannot correctly be predicted early in the course of the disease. Therefore investigators have sought for additional and better laboratory markers to predict a severe and complicated course of pancreatitis [18-20, 38, 43, 70, 79, 93, 95]. These laboratory signs include lactic dehydrogenase (also included in the scoring systems), phospholipase A2 [20, 93], C-reactive protein (CRP) [18, 20, 79], α_1-antitrypsin, a2-macroglobulin [43], serum methemalbumin [38, 81], granulocyte elastase [43] and trypsinogen-activating peptide (TAP) [45]. Many of the markers represent acute-phase reactants. The sensitivity of these laboratory signs for detecting pancreatic necrosis varies between 50% and 93% depending on the cutoff level used for these parameters. As yet only the measurement of lactic dehydrogenase and to some degree also that of CRP are used for this purpose in clinical practice. The other laboratory methods are not standardized and not available to most clinicians. It also remains to be evaluated whether one of these parameters offers significant information in addition to that obtained by the combined use of CT, clinical scoring, and CRP.

Mediators of Systemic Complications in Acute Pancreatitis

The recent advances in immunological research have enabled us to measure a great number of cytokines and other substances which mediate damage to tissues remote to the organ where the original disease began. Release of the mediators, on the one hand, mirrors a consequence of the disease but, on the other hand, also represents a factor which may determine the final outcome. Some of these mediators can be used both as diagnostic and as prognostic tools. Many alterations in cytokines in acute pancreatitis resemble those seen in sepsis. Therefore, the definition of systemic inflammatory response syndrome (SIRS) [16] can be used equally in sepsis and in pancreatitis:
- Body temperature > 38C or < 36C
- Pulse rate > 90/min
- Respiratory rate > 20/min or $PaCO_2$ < 32 mmHg
- Leukocytes > 12.000 µl or 4000µl
  or > 10 % nonsegmented leukocytes

The term SIRS is used to indicate that septic, bacterial infections as well as severe, primarily abacteremic diseases such as trauma and acute pancreatitis have common characteristics of activation of the cascades of inflammatory mediators and cytokinines. The initial events which lead to SIRS, are however, different in the various diseases in which a SIRS may occur. In acute pancreatitis activated pancreatic digestive enzymes are probably the primary factors which further stimulate the release and formation of substances such as interleukins 1, 4, 6 and 8 [44, 76], tumor necrosis factor-α, intercellular adhesion molecule 1 and platelet-activating factor [25], NO-related compound, bradykinin, kallikrein, histamine, prostaglandins, inflammatory cells [61], and free radicals [41] (for review on inflammatory mediators and cytokines see [44]). It is still a matter of debate as to which of the pancreatic digestive enzymes is most important for the activation and release of other mediators and thus for the pathogenesis of the systemic complications. Trypsin is probably very important because it triggers the activation of other proteolytic enzymes. Various proteases are known to act at multiple sites in the activation cascade of the coagulation, fibrinolysis, and complement systems. Lipase and phospholipase may via release of free fatty acids and lysolecithin cause membrane damage.

Release of proteases from damaged cells may accelerate the formation of xanthine oxidase from xanthine dehydrogenase and may thereby contribute to oxidative damage [26, 77]. Many of the cytokines and mediators released in acute pancreatitis also act on the microcirculation of extrapancreatic tissue both by directly altering the vascular tone and by inducing a prethrombotic state due to coagulopathic changes. Despite the enormous increase in knowledge about mediators and cytokines, their interaction and contribution to systemic complications in the extremely complex situation of acute pancreatitis are still unclear.

Hemodynamic and Cardiovascular Complications

Hypovolemic shock has been the major cause of early death in acute pancreatitis [60, 98, 109, 112]. There is a massive plasma volume deficit during the initial hours of a severe attack of acute pancreatitis mainly due to sequestration into the retroperitoneum. The deficit in intravascular volume may reach 25%-40% already during the first 6 h of pancreatitis [4, 22]. In addition to the more local sequestration of fluid into the retroperitoneal space there is a systemic damage to capillaries with a subsequent loss of fluid into nonpancreatic tissues and "third spaces" including lungs, subcutaneous tissue, pleural space, peritoneal space, and intestine [34, 110, 111] (Fig. 1). In patients with severe pancreatitis 10-12 l fluid may need to be replaced during the initial 24 h.

The cause of the systemic capillary leak of fluid is probably multifactorial, due to a release of a variety of cytokines, inflammatory mediators, proteases, phospholipases, and free radicals [110, 111] (Fig. 1). The value of adequate volume replacement is so evident that it has never been studied in controlled clinical trials. Randomized experimental studies have, however, clearly shown that volume replacement dramatically reduced the mortality in acute hemorrhagic pancreatitis [87]. Volume replacement also proved to be more important for the outcome than prophylactic inhibition of proteases or hyperoxygenation [87].

More than 20 years ago it was first suggested that a special small molecular weight peptide (800 - 1000 Da) in the circulation reduces the volume output of the left cardiac ventricle. Because of this negative inotropic effect the putative peptide was termed myocardial depressant factor (MDF) [73, 74, 78]. Initial studies also showed a reduction in the left verticular function [27, 59]. Later studies, however, demonstrated that the hemodynamic situation in severe necrotizing pancreatitis is characterized predominantly by a decrease in the peripheral and pulmonary resistance [9, 17, 59] similar to the situation in sepsis [104].

The later studies even reported that the overall cardiac output is increased. Probably due to the MDF-mediated depression the cardiac output cannot compensate for the marked reduction in the peripheral resistance [23]. The final result, the marked reduction in peripheral pulmonary vascular tone and the potentially depressed myocardial function, is a shock situation with an increase in pulse rate and a decrease in arterial tension. In this context it is also noteworthy that as yet the MDF peptide has not been identified in its molecular structure. Furthermore, substances which have been shown to inhibit the depressant action of MDF in experimental situations, such as protease inhibitors, prostaglandins, thromboxane antagonists, and flucocorticoids [73, 74] are unable to improve the outcome of patients with severe pancreatitis.

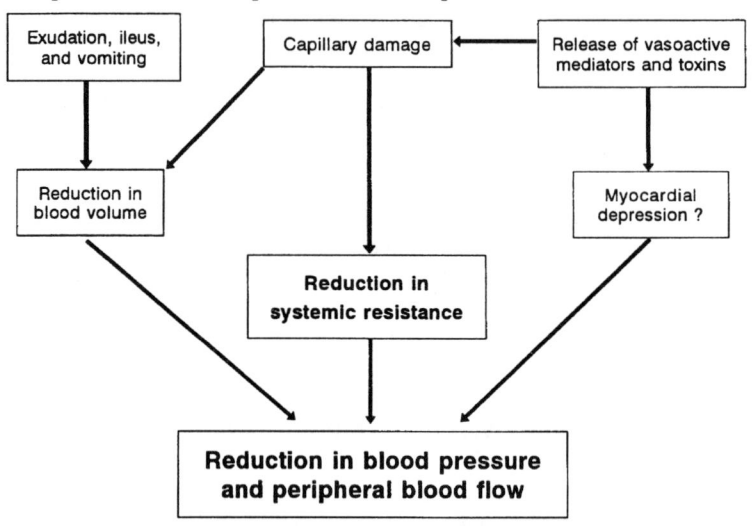

Fig. 1: Pathophysiology of hemodynamic complications in acute pancreatitis

Renal Failure

Alterations in renal function are observed in 15%-35% of patients with acute pancreatitis [5, 53, 89, 91]. The full clinical picture of acute renal failure occurs in 10%-20% of patients, who usually have a severe form of pancreatitis. Histologically, acute renal failure due to acute pancreatitis is characterized by tubular necrosis in most cases [36, 91]. Clinically the hypovolemic shock is usually the major cause of renal dysfunction (Fig. 2). Thus a close monitoring of hemodynamic alterations and an adequate volume replacement have not only reduced the early mortality due to a hypovolemic shock but also the incidence of renal failure [53, 56]. Consequently, the mortality associated with acute renal failure has been markedly reduced from 60%-100% [5, 12, 53] to values considerably smaller than 50% [3, 89]. Nevertheless, renal failure which requires dialysis treatment is still associated with high mortality in patients with acute pancreatitis. Although hypovolemia is a major factor for the pathogenesis of acute renal failure, other mechanisms may contribute to this systemic complication. This assumption is further supported by the observation that despite the decrease in early mortality due to hypovolemic shock a considerable percentage of patients have still developed renal failure in our present series. Indeed, further studies have shown fibrin deposits in glomerular capillaries in patients with acute renal failure and pancreatitis potentially caused by a prethrombotic state due to a release of substances which activate the coagulation cascade and increase renal vascular resistance [40, 47, 116]. Other studies have suggested that pancreatitis leads to a marked activation of the renin-angiotensin system and in this way contributes to renal failure [41].

```
┌──────────────┐      ┌──────────────┐      ┌──────────────────────┐
│ Hypovolemic  │─────▶│ Reduction in │◀─────│ Release of vasoactive│
│    shock     │      │  blood flow  │      │ toxins and free radicals│
└──────────────┘      └──────────────┘      └──────────────────────┘
                              │                        │
                              ▼                        ▼
┌──────────────┐          ╱───────╲            ┌──────────────────────┐
│Acute tubular │─────────▶│ RENAL │            │ Avtivation of leuco- │
│  necrosis    │          │FAILURE│            │ and thrombocytes     │
└──────────────┘          ╲───────╱            └──────────────────────┘
                           ▲    ▲                        │
                           │    │                        │
┌──────────────────┐       │    │          ┌──────────────────────┐
│ Hyperactivation of│──────┘    └──────────│ Fibrin deposits in   │
│ renin/angiotensin │                      │ glomerular capillaries│
└──────────────────┘                      └──────────────────────┘
```

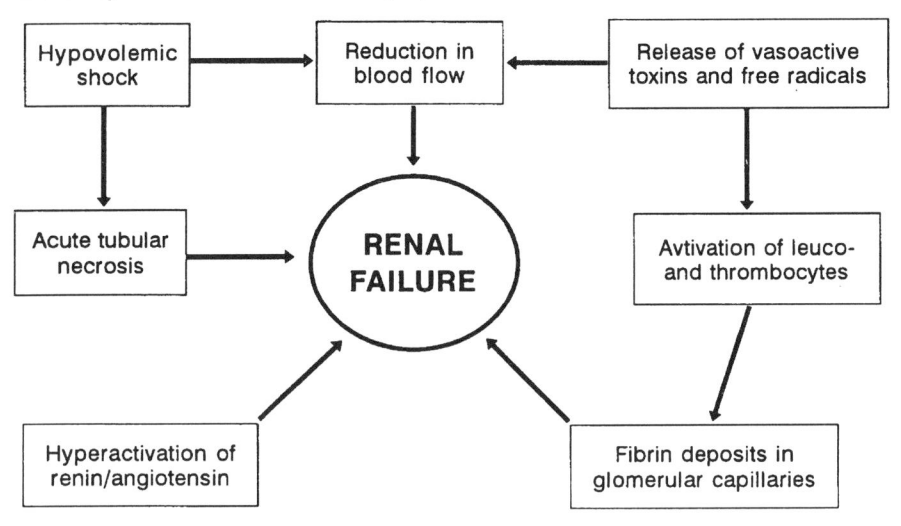

Fig. 2: Pathophysiology of renal complications in acute pancreatitis

Pulmonary Failure

Evidence of functional alteration in respiration is still common in patients with acute pancreatitis. In older series, 45%-69% of patients with acute pancreatitis showed hypoxemia [55, 76] while in the present series this percentage is still 38%. Hypoxemia is marked in most published series that approximately 50% of hypoxemic patients need mechanical ventilation. Hypoxemia and the need for mechanical ventilation are still associated with considerable mortality in patients with acute pancreatitis [98]. The close monitoring of arterial pO_2 is necessary because many hypoxemic patients initially do not show clinical or radiographic evidence for pulmonary failure [55, 76].

Morphologically, hyperemia and congestion in alveolar capillaries can be seen early in acute pulmonary failure due to pancreatitis. Later pulmonary edema and infiltrates occur and may finally lead to hyaline membranes and classical morphological picture of the adult respiration distress syndrome [71, 108]. Damage to pulmonary membranes due to a variety of factors is probably the most important mechanism which leads to respiratory failure in acute pancreatitis (Fig. 3). In addition, pleural effusions, fluid overload, hypalbuminemia, capillary damage, cardiac failure, and an increase in abdominal pressure may contribute to respiratory alterations (Fig. 4). The pathophysiological mechanisms which cause pulmonary membrane damage in acute pancreatitis are still a matter of debate. It is likely that proteases, phospholipase A_2, free fatty acids, and lysolecithin released by the latter enzymes are involved in the damage to pulmonary and capillary membranes in the lung [115].

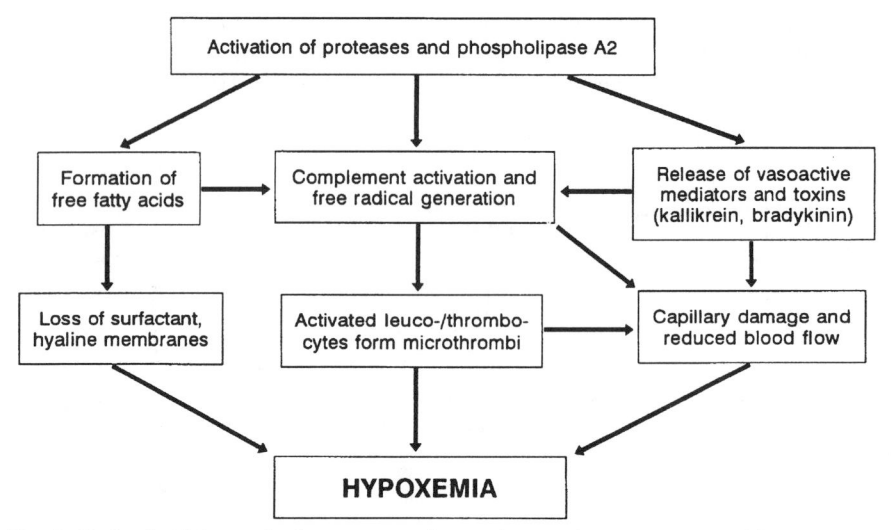

Fig. 3: Pathophysiology of pulmonary membrane damage in acute pancreatitis

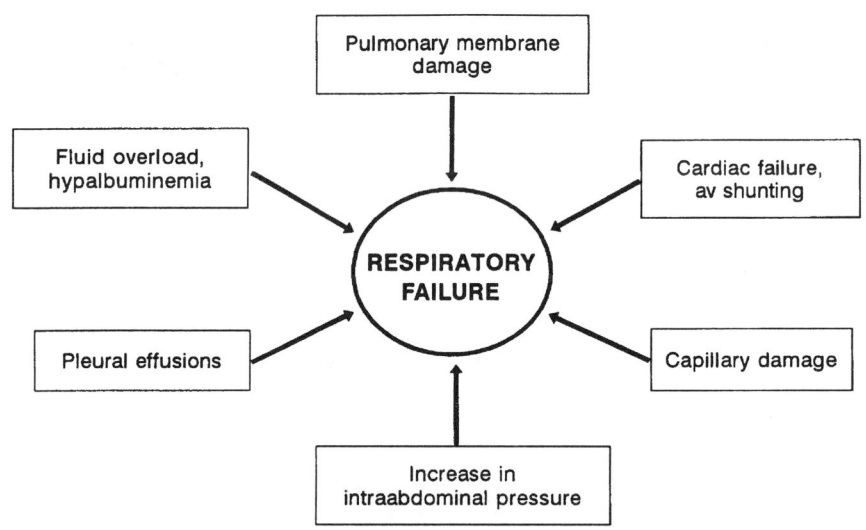

Fig. 4: Pathophysiology of respiratory failure in acute pancreatitis

Phospholipase A_2 may via the release of lysolecithin lead to a destruction of the surfacant factor [50] and may thereby contribute to the development of hyaline membranes [58, 71, 103, 113]. Activated inflammatory cells and thrombocytes may on the one hand lead to intravascular microthrombi [80], and on the other hand, cause damage due to release of free radicals and various toxic mediators [69, 92]. Other studies have shown that complement activation and resulting breakdown products in concert with the release of kinins lead to an increase in the capillary permeability in the lung [80, 92]. Depletion of neutrophils and administration of radical scavengers reduced pulmonary complications in experimental pancreatitis [46]. Other recent studies have suggested that an increase of platelet-activating factor may contribute to respiratory failure in acute pancreatitis [25].

Septic Complications

Today septic complications associated with multiorgan failure (MOF) or multiple organ dysfunction syndrome (MODS) are the most frequent causes of death in patients with acute pancreatitis [89]. Although sepsis may occur early in particular due to cholangitis in the biliary forms of pancreatitis [85], the septic complications which contribute to the death of patients are usually seen 2 - 3 weeks after the onset of pancreatitis [8, 21, 39] (Fig. 5). The spectrum of germs detected in infected pancreatic necrotics is similar to that seen in the transverse colon [8, 21, 39]. A meta-analysis of three studies [8, 21, 39] shows the following frequency of different bacteria in pancreatic necrosis in 280 patients with acute pancreatitis: *Escherichia coli*, 25.9%; *Pseudomonas species*, 15.9%; *Staphylococcus aureus*, 15.3%; *Klebsiella species*, 10.1%; *Proteus species*, 10.1%; *Streptococcus faecalis*, 4.4%; *Enterobacter species*, 2.5%; *Various anaerobic germs*, 15.6%. Thus, there may be a local transmission of bacteria from the colon to the pancreas due to an increase in permeability of the intestinal wall and a decrease in the immune defense due to blockade of the reticuloendothelial system in patients with severe pancreatitis (Fig. 6). Other causes of sepsis in severely ill patients with pancreatitis may originate from surgery, intravenous lines, dialysis, mechanical ventilation, urinary catheters, respiratory infections, and nosocomial germs in intensive care units. The use of antibiotics is again the object of controlled clinical trials since the antibiotics which proved ineffective in previous studies [24, 37, 51] have later been shown not to penetrate even into the normal pancreas [8, 21, 67].

The definition of sepsis has recently been changed from the mere detection of bacteria in blood cultures to the syndrome called SIRS [16]. As yet there is no early prognostic parameter to indicate the development of sepsis in pancreatitis although the severity of the disease and the degree of necrosis are in general correlated with the likelihood of sepsis [11].

Cutaneous, Subcutaneous, and Skeletal Complications

Cutaneous alterations in body wall ecchymosis are well known in patients with acute pancreatitis. These include the Grey-Turner sign at the lateral parts of the abdomen, Cullen's sign in the periumbilical region and Fox' sign near the inguinal ligaments. The latter cutaneous signs of pancreatitis are thought to represent tracking of blood-stained pancreatic exudate through preformed fascia in combination with signs of ischemia, local hemorrhage, and potentially also subcutaneous fat necrosis. The cutaneous signs are seen in approximately 2%-3% of patients with acute pancreatitis and are usually associated with a complicated course of acute pancreatitis [82, 114]. Recent studies have shown that they do not have a prognostic importance in young patients [28]. In older patients the occurrence of the cutaneous signs are associated with a mortality of 30%-40%. The rare subcutaneous or osteolytic fat necrosis is thought to be caused by lipolytic enzymes release in acute pancreatitis [1, 14, 62, 83, 101].

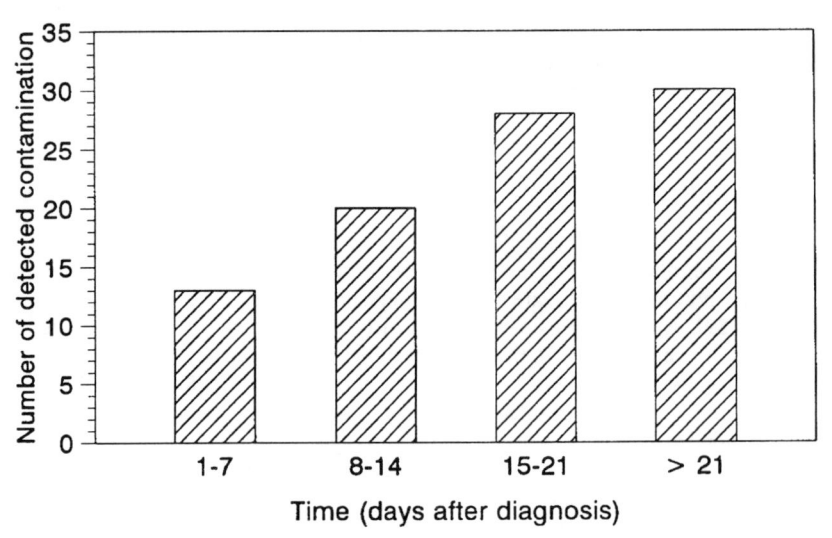

Fig. 5: Time interval between diagnosis of acute pancreatitis and detection of bacterial contamination of pancreatic necrosis (from Gerzof et al. [39], Bassi et al. [8], Büchler et al. [21])

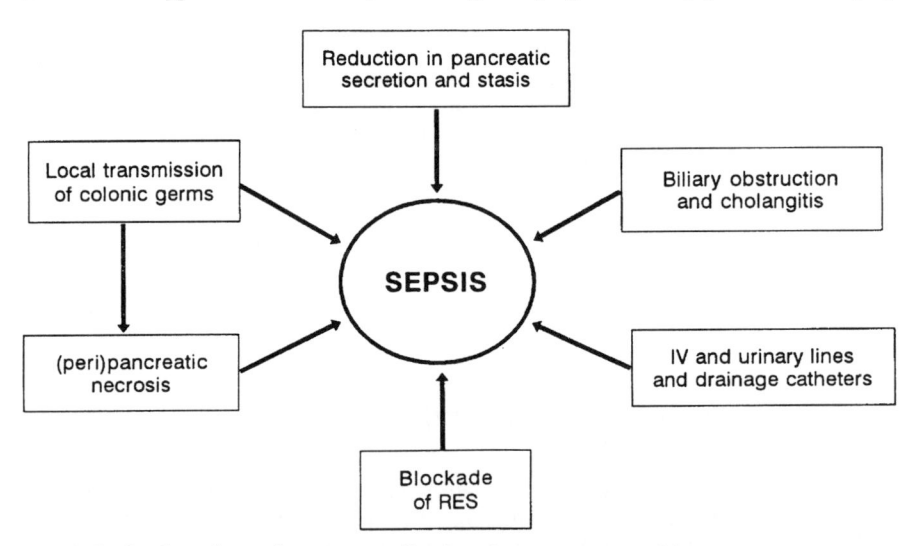

Fig. 6: Pathophysiology of septic complications in acute pancreatitis

Pancreatic Encephalopathy

Some patients with acute pancreatitis develop severe psychotic and neurological disturbances which may be independent of prior alcohol abuse [31, 35]. The clinical syndrome of confusion, hallucinations, aphasia, and sometimes coma has been termed pancreatic encephalopathy [190]. The pathogenesis of the rare pancreatic encephalopathy is unclear.

Metabolic Complications

Many of the great number of metabolic complications in acute pancreatitis are included in the clinical scores which assess the severity of the disease.

Hypocalcemia. Although one of the most frequent metabolic alteration seen in acute pancreatitis, hypocalcemia rarely leads to tetanic symptoms. The lack of clinical consequence of hypocalcemia in pancreatitis is explained by the fact that there is only little change in ionized calcium because of a large reduction in serum albumin [54]. Initially the reduction in calcium has been suggested to be due to loss of calcium in lipolytic fat necrosis [33]. Other factors contributing to hypocalcemia include reduction in serum albumin [54], pH changes, a shift of extracellular calcium into intracellular stores, an inadequate response of parathormone release [30, 99] nd calcium binding in complexes formed by free fatty acids and albumin [115] (Fig. 7).

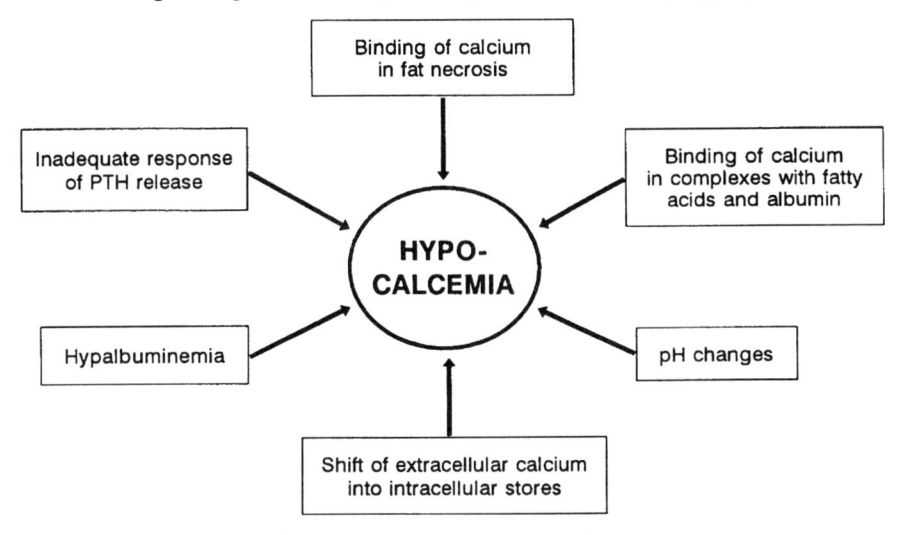

Fig. 7: Pathophysiology of hypocalcemia in acute pancreatitis

Hypertriglyceridemia. A common abnormality in patients with acute pancreatitis is hypertriglyceridemia, which can be either the cause or the consequence of the disease. Increased serum triglycerides occur in approximately 25% of patients. In particular, large increases in serum triglycerides (> 1000 mg%) have been attributed with the pathogenesis of acute pancreatitis. On the other hand, a reduction in lipoprotein lipase may cause or aggravate hypertriglyceridemia in pancreatitis [64].

Hyperglycemia. Acute pancreatitis is often associated with hyperglycemia. Large increases in serum glucose is a bad prognostic sign according to Ranson's score [97]. The factors which contribute to pancreatitis-associated hyperglycemia and diabetes include decrease in the insulin release due to alterations in beta cell function, peripheral insulin resistance, hyperglucagonemia and increases in circulating concentration of cortisol and norepinephrine [29, 105] (Fig. 8).

Coagulopathy. Severe acute pancreatitis often results in a hypercoagulable or prethrombotic state [57, 84, 117] although the classical feature of disseminated intravascular coagulation is only a rare complication in patients with acute pancreatitis [42, 68, 84]. The cause of the pancreatitis-associated coagulophathy is probably the action of activated proteases on the cascade systems of coagulation, fibrinolysis, and complement. The exact sites of action of proteases in the complex mutually interacting systems are as yet unclear. In any case, the prethrombotic and hypercoagulable state may in particular be responsible for the formation of microthrombi in renal and pulmonary microcirculation.

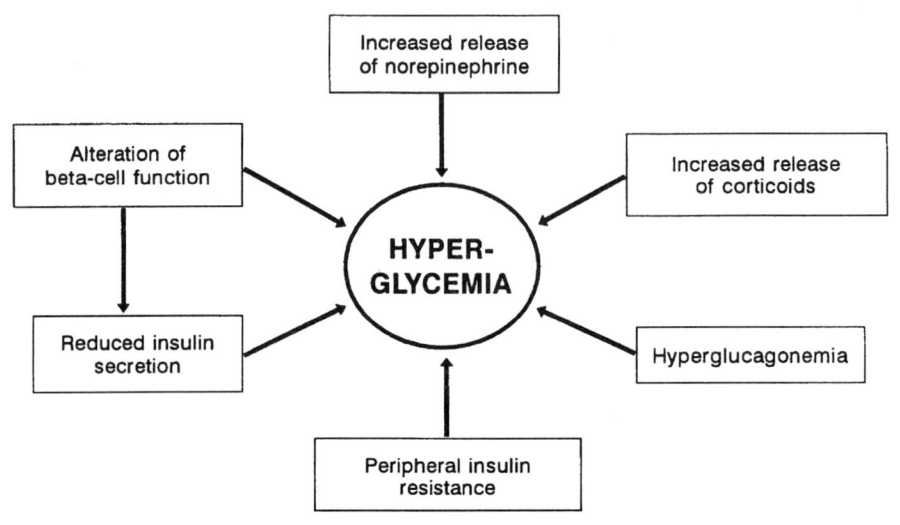

Fig. 8: Pathophysiology of hyperglycemia acute pancreatitis

Multiorgan Failure or Multiple Organ Dysfunction Syndrome

MOF or MODS [16] is associated with a very high mortality in acute pancreatitis as well as in other diseases. Since the systemic complications due to pancreatitis are thought to be mediated by similar factors and mechanisms for a variety of organs, it is to be expected that severe pancreatitis is often associated with MODS such as respiratory, pulmonary and hemodynamic failure. In the present series of patients mortality increased to 59% in those who had more than three systemic complications. Future studies must aim at early intervention in the cascade of immunological and inflammatory events which initiate the systemic damage.

Complications and Outcome in the Recent Series of Patients

The present study analyzes the outcome systemic complications in all 193 patients admitted with acute pancreatitis to the Departments of Medicine and Surgery of the University of Düsseldorf from 1987 to 1992. In both the surgical and the medical patients alcohol was the leading cause of pancreatitis and accounted for about one-third of cases. The biliary cause of pancreatitis was slightly more frequent in the medical patients (30%) than in the surgical patients (21%). In both the Departments of Medicine and Surgery between 6% and 8% of the pancreatitis cases occurred following ERCP. The etiology could not be determined in about 25%-30% of cases in the medical and surgical groups.

In addition, the systemic complications were analyzed for the 152 patients admitted with acute pancreatitis to the Departments of Medicine ($n = 93$) and Surgery ($n = 59$) from 1986 to 1991 (data for 1992 not yet included). Respiratory insufficiency was the most frequent systemic complication, followed by sepsis and renal insufficiency (Table 1). Initial signs of hypovolemic shock developed in only 27% of patients and was associated only with 7% mortality. Respiratory and renal insufficiency in addition to sepsis were, however, associated with high mortalities, from 25 to 38%. Severe respiratory and renal insufficiency requiring mechanical ventilation and dialysis, respectively, were associated with an even higher mortality of 34% and 46%, respectively. The mortality increased to 59% in the presence of at least three systemic complications; such MODS was seen in 22% of all patients.

Table 1: Frequency of systemic complications and associated mortality in 152 patients with acute pancreatitis

	n	Percentage of total	Percentage mortality
All patients	152	100	5
CT without necrosis	66	44	0
<1/3 necrosis	53	34	8
> 1/3 necrosis	33	22	30
initial shock situation	27	18	30
Initial insufficiency[a]	57	38	25
Mechanical ventilation	29	19	34
Renal insufficiency[b]	29	19	38
Dialysis	13	9	46
Sepsis	31	20	26
≥ 3 systemic complications	22	14	59

[a] $pO_2 < 80$ mmHg.
[b] Serum creatinine > 2 mg/%.

Etiology of pancreatitis and initial serum increase in pancreatic enzymes predicted neither complications nor outcome. There were 14 deaths in the 193 patients, 9 surgical and 5 medical patients. Only 2 of 14 deaths occurred during the 1st week, and all other deaths occurred later (after 4-12 weeks) (Figs. 9, 10), generally as the consequence of septic complications and MOF. The two patients who died early in the course of pancreatitis both suffered from untreatable cardiovascular and pulmonary failure. Thus, only 15% of deaths occured early in the course of the disease, whereas this percentage varied between 40% and 70% just 10 years ago. In the literature, the majority of deaths from acute pancreatitis have occurred at two different stages of the disease [98]. A significant proportion of deaths is seen in the early phase of the disease, and a considerable number of deaths occur even during the first 24 h. A high percentage of the early deaths is caused by hypovolemic shock or untreatable cardiovascular failure. The other major proportion of fatalities is seen during the late stages of the disease, often caused by septic complications [10, 98]. This picture, which has been described by several previous reports, has apparently changed during recent years. In the present series only a few deaths were seen in the early phase of the acute pancreatitis. The great majority of fatalities occurred at late stages, i.e., between 4 and 12 weeks after admission. Almost all late deaths were associated with MOF caused by septic complications.

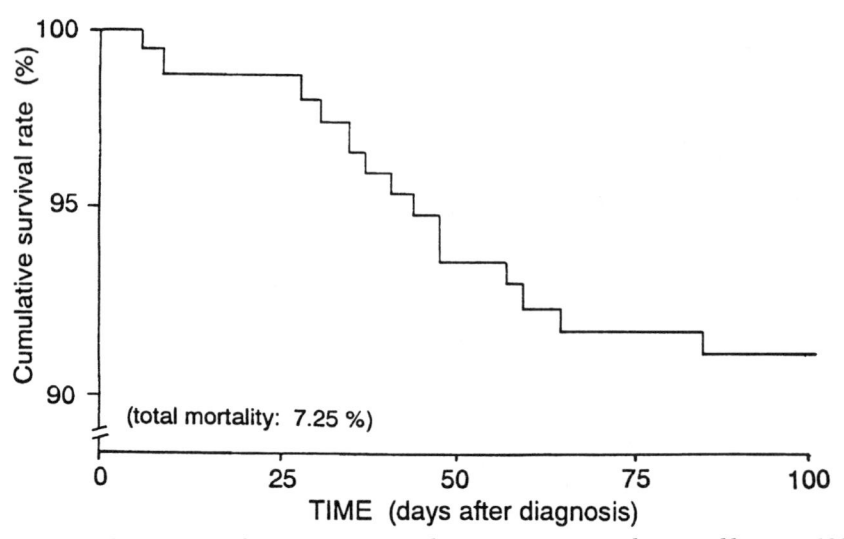

Fig. 9: Cumulative survival in 193 patients with acute pancreatitis diagnosed between 1986 and 1992 in the Departments of Medicine and Surgery of the University of Düsseldorf

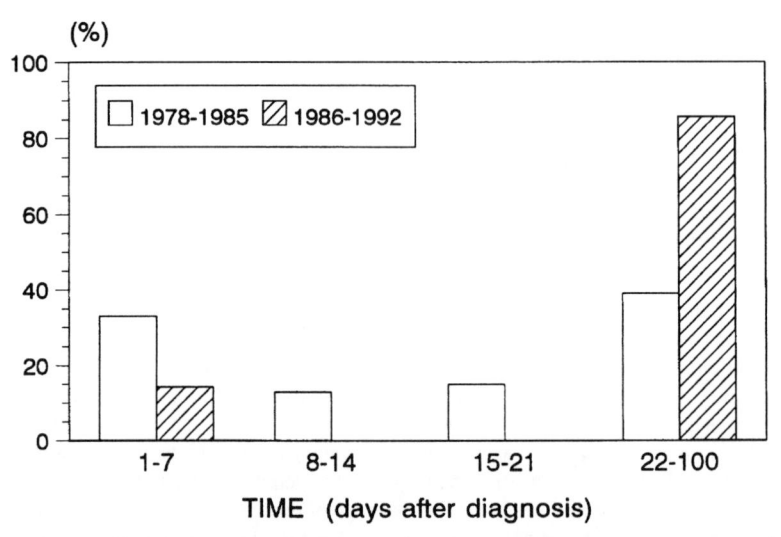

Fig. 10: Percentage of patients dying from acute pancreatitis in the time intervals from 1978-1985 and from 1986-1992 in the Departments of Medicine and Surgery of the University of Düsseldorf

The decrease in the percentage of early deaths might be due to improvements in supportive care, particularly to the advancements in intensive care medicine.

High levels of CRP are correlated with a complicated course and a fatal outcome. Although some cytokines (e.g., interleukin 6) have been found increased in severe disease, the predictive value of these markers is not better than the combination of clinical scores (Ranson, Imrie, APACHE II) with CT or CRP. Ranson and CT scores as well as serum CRP reliably predicted a course with systemic complications; they were less helpful for prediction of sepsis and late mortality. It appears doubtful whether measurements of cytokines will help to better predict the late outcome.

In light of the present series, the advancements in intensive care medicine are probably responsible for the relatively low incidence of manifest hypovolemic shock and for the low early mortality in severe pancreatitis. Most deaths today are caused by late septic complications and MOF. As yet only careful and continuous monitoring of patients (e.g. by APACHE scores) may help to early identify those who develop septic complications and MOF.

The majority of medical patients showed an edemateous form of pancreatitis without major necrosis on CT. In contrast, the majority of the surgical patients presented with necrosis as assessed by CT and had a severe course as indicated by a high Ranson's score (> 3 positive signs). Correspondingly, the mortality of 15% seen in the surgical group was significantly greater than the 5% mortality observed for the medical patients. However, regarding the relationship between mortality and the severity of pancreatitis there was no major difference between surgical and medical patients. In neither groups was there mortality in the absence of necrosis; mortality ranged between 5% and 10% in the presence of minor to moderate necrosis, and increased to more than 20% in patients with major necrosis (Fig. 4). Mortality from biliary causes were only slightly higher than that caused by other factors including alcohol both in the medical and surgical patients and Ranson's score, and CT gradings were not significantly different between the various etiological groups of patients.

The additional measurements of CRP offered only slight advantages compared to the clinical grading and CT. Nevertheless, CRP values were significantly higher in patients with pancreatic necrosis than in those with edema. Similarly, CRP values were significantly higher in patients who died during the course of pancreatitis than in those who survived. In the present series the age of the patients did not help to predict a fatal outcome or a complicated course when used as a single clinical characteristic. The age of the patients who died from pancreatitis was only slightly higher than that of patients who survived the disease. The use of other clinical scores such as Imrie's score or the APACHE II system did not offer major advantages in predicting fatal outcome and complications. The one late death and a number of complications not predicted by CT or Ranson's signs were due to late septic complications in patients with moderate necrosis on CT and two or three positive Ranson's signs. Thus, none of the deaths and only a small number of complications not predicted by CT or Ranson's signs would have been picked up by applying other scoring systems. Additional measurements of CRP also failed to predict the one fatal outcome and the majority of complications not predicted by CT or Ranson's score.

The kind of treatment did not appear as a major prognostic factor. All patients in the present series received maximal supportive care, and only those underwent surgery in whom severe septic complications occurred or a MOF threatened to kill the patient. Accordingly, patients who underwent surgery had the most severe disease (mean Ranson's score = 5.2 ± 1.3). Patients who were treated conservatively in the Surgical Department had virtually the same mortality as those treated (conservatively) in the Department of Medicine.

The occurrence of pulmonary and renal failure were two other major factors which determined the outcome in acute pancreatitis. In the present series these complications were often caused by septic complications which generally occurred at later stages of the disease. The other individual clinical characteristics including age were prognostic factors of only minor importance. The clinical scoring system defined by Ranson [97] still proved helpful to determine a complicated course of pancreatitis (Fig. 11). In our patients scoring systems other than that described by Ranson offered no major advantages. The number of positive Ranson's signs was less helpful for predicting a fatal outcome. The additional use of CRP or one of the various acute-phase reactants and cytokines might slightly increase the prognostic ability of clinical grading. As yet there is no early prognostic parameter to indicate the development of sepsis in pancreatitis although the severity of the disease and the degree of necrosis in general correlate with the likelihood of sepsis [11]. The APACHE system may help to monitor a severe course of acute pancreatitis in patients treated on intensive care units [118].

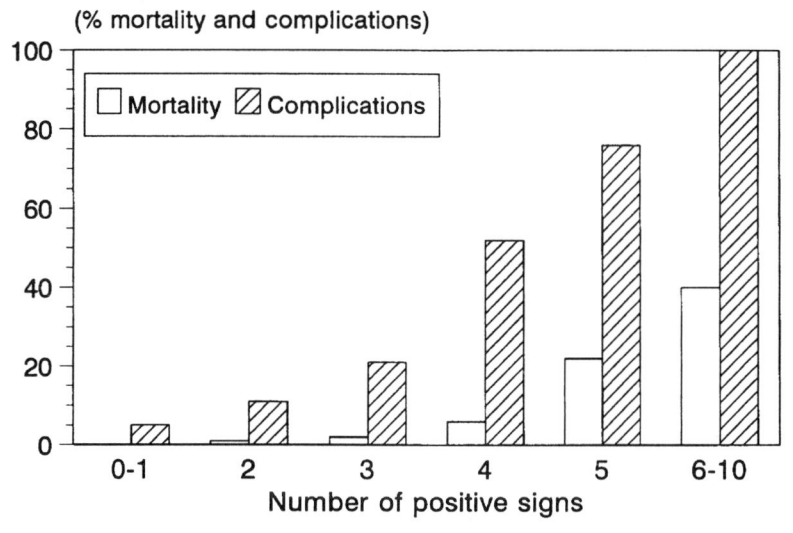

Fig. 11: Mortality and complications according to Ranson's score in 193 patients with acute pancreatitis diagnosed between 1986 and 1992 in the Departments of Medicine and Surgery of the University of Düsseldorf

Acknowledgement

C.N. was supported by the Pinguin Stiftung.

References

1. *Achord JL, Gerle RD (1966) Bone lesions in pancreatitis. Am J Dig Dis 11: 453-460*
2. *Adler G, Rohr G, Kern HF (1982) Alteration of membrane fusion as a cause of acute pancreatitis in the rat. Dig Dis Sci 27: 993-1002*
3. *Agarwal N, Pitchumoni CS (1986) Simplified prognostic criteria in acute pancreatitis. Pancreas 1: 69-73*
4. *Anderson MC, Schoenfeld FB, Iams WB, Suwa M (1967) Circulatory changes in acute pancreatitis. Surg Clin North Am 47: 127-140*
5. *Balsov JT, Jorgensen HE, Nielsen R (1962) Acute renal failure complicating severe acute pancreatitis. Acta Chir Scand 124: 348-354*

6. Balthazar EJ, Robinson DL, Megibow AJ, Ranson JHC (1990) Acute pancreatitis: values of CT in establishing prognosis. Radiology 174: 331-336
7. Barkin JS, Garrido (1986) Acute pancreatitis and its complications: diagnostic and therapeutic strategies. Postgrad Med 79: 241
8. Bassi C, Falconi M, Girelli R, Nifosi F, Elio A, Martini N, Pederzoli P (1989) Microbiological findings in severe pancreatitis. Surg Res Commum 5: 1-4
9. Beger HG, Büchler M, Bittner R, Hess W, Schmitz JE (1986) Hemodynamic data pattern in patients with acute pancreatitis. Gastroenterology 90: 74-79
10. Beger HG, Krautzberger W, Bittner R, Büchler M, Block S (1986) Bacterial contamination of pancreatic necrosis. A prospective clinical study. Gastroenterology 91: 433-438
11. Beger HG, Büchler M, Bittner R (1988) Necrosectomy and postoperative local lavage in necrotizing pancreatitis. Br J Surg 75: 207-212
12. Beisel WR, Herndon Eg, Myers JE, Stones L (1959) Acute renal failure as a complication of acute pancreatitis. Arch Intern Med 104: 539-543
13. Blamey SL, Imrie CW, O'Neill J, Gilmour WH, Carter DC (1984) Prognostic factors in acute pancreatitis. Am J Gastroenterol 77: 1340-1346
14. Blauvelt H (1946) A case of acute pancreatitis with subcutaneous fat necrosis. Br J Surg 34: 207-208
15. Block S, Maier W, Bittner R, Büchler M, Malfertheiner P, Beger HG (1986) Identification of pancreas necrosis in severe acute pancreatitis: imaging procedures versus clinical staging. Gut 27: 1035-1042
16. Bone RC, Balk RA, Cerra FB, Dellinger RP, Fein AM, Knaus WA, Schein RMH, Sibbald WJ (1992) The ACCP/SCCM Consensus Conference Committee: definitions for sepsis and organ failure and guidelines for the use of innovative therapies in sepsis. Chest 101: 1644-1655
17. Bradley EL, Hall JR, Lutz J, Hammer L, Lattouf O (1983) Hemodynamic consequences of severe pancreatitis. Ann Surg 198: 130-133
18. Büchler M, Malfertheiner P, Schoetensack C, Uhl W, Beger HG (1986) Sensitivity of antiproteases, complement factors and C-reactive protein in detecting pancreatic necrosis. Results of a prospective clinical study. Int J Pancreatol 1: 227-235
19. Büchler M, Malfertheiner P, Uhl W, Beger HG (1987) C-reaktives Protein als Entzündungs- und Nekrosemarker in der Gastroenterologie. Med Klin 82: 180-185
20. Büchler M, Malfertheiner P, Schädlich H, Nevalainen TJ, Friess H, Beger HG (1989) Role of phospholipase A2 in human acute pancreatitis. Gastroenterology 97: 1521-1526
21. Büchler M, Malfertheiner P, Friess H, Isenmann R, Vanek E, Grimm H, Schlegel P, Frieß T, Beger HG (1992) Human pancreatic tissue concentration of bactericidal antibiotics. Gastroenterology 103: 1902-1908
22. Carey LC (1979) Extra-abdominal manifestations of acute pancreatitis. Surgery 86: 337-342
23. Cobo JC, Abraham E, Bland RD, Shoemaker WC (1984) Sequential hemodynamic and oxygen transport abnormalities in patients with acute pancreatitis. Surgery 95: 324-330
24. Craig RM, Dordal E, Myles L (1975) The use of ampicillin in acute pancreatitis. Ann Intern Med 83: 831
25. Dabrowski A, Gabryelewicz A, Chyczewski L (1991) The effect of platelet activating factor antagonist (BN 52021) on cerulein-induced acute pancreatitis with reference to oxygen radicals. Int J Pancreatol 8: 1-11
26. DeGroot H, Littauer A (1989) Hypoxia, reactive oxygen, and cell injury. Free Radic Biol Med 6: 541-551
27. Di Carlo V, Nespoli A, Chiesa R (1981) Hemodynamic and metabolic impairment in acute pancreatitis. World J Surg 5: 329-339

28. Dixon AP, Imrie SW (1984) The incidence and prognosis of body wall ecchymosis in acute pancreatitis. Surg Gynecol Obstet 159: 343-347
29. Donowitz M, Hendler R, Spiro HM (1975) Glucagon secretion in acute and chronic pancreatitis. Ann Intern Med 83: 778-781
30. Drew SI, Joffe B, Vinik A (1978) The first 24-hours of pancreatitis. Changes in biochemical and endocrine homeostasis in patients with pancreatitis compared with those in control subjects undergoing stress for reasons other than pancreatitis. Am J Med 69: 795-803
31. Dürr GHK (1979) Acute pancreatitis. In: Howat HT, Sarles H (eds.) The exocrine pancreas. Saunders, London, pp. 352-401
32. Eckfeldt JH, Kolar JC, Elson MK, Shafer RB, Levitt MD (1985) Serum tests for pancreatitis in patients with abdominal pain. Arch Pathol Lab Med 109: 316
33. Edmondson HA, Fields IA (1942) Relation of calcium and lipids to acute pancreatic necrosis: Report of fifteen cases, in one of which fat embolism occurred. Arch Intern Med 69: 177-190
34. Ellison EC, Pappas TN, Johnson JA, Fabri PJ, Carey LC (1981) Demonstration and characterization of the hemoconcentrating effect of ascitic fluid that accumulates during hemorrhagic pancreatitis. J Surg Res 30: 241-48
35. Estrada RV, Moreno J, Martinez E (1979) Pancreatic encephalopathy. Acta Neurol Scand 59: 135-139
36. Frey CF, Brody GL (1966) Relationship of azotemia and survival in bile pancreatitis in the dog. Arch Surg 93: 295-300
37. Finch WT, Sawyers JL, Schenkers S (1976) A prospective study to determine the efficacy of antibiotic in acute pancreatitis. Ann Surg 183: 667
38. Geokas MC, Rinderknecht H, Walberg CB, Weissmann R (1974) Methemalbumin in the diagnosis of acute hemorrhagic pancreatitis. Ann Intern Med 81: 483-486
39. Gerzof SG, Banks PA, Robbins AH, Johnson WC, Spechler SJ, Wetzner SM, Snider JM, Langewin RE, Jay ME (1987) Early diagnosis of pancreatic infection by computed tomography-guided aspiration. Gastroenterology 93: 1315-1320
40. Giacobino JP, Simom GT (1971) Experimental glomerulonephritis induced by minimal doses of trypsin. Arch Pathol 91: 193-200
41. Greenstein RJ, Krakoff LR, Felton K (1987) Activation of the renin system in acute pancreatitis. Am J Med 82: 401-404
42. Greipp PR, Brown JA, Gralnick HR (1972) Defibrination in acute pancreatitis. Ann Intern Med 76: 73-76
43. Gross V, Schvlmerich J, Leser HG, Salm R, Lausen M, Rnckauer K, Schöffel U, Lay L, Heinisch A, Farthmann EH, Gerok W (1990) Granulocyte elastase in assessment of severity of acute pancreatitis. Comparison with acute phase proteins C-reactive protein, alpha$_1$-antitrypsin, and protease inhibitor alpha$_2$-macroglobulin. Dig Dis Sci 35: 97-105
44. Gross V, Leser HG, Heinisch A, Schölmerich J (1993) Inflammatory mediators and cytokines-new aspects of the pathophysiology and assessment of severity of acute pancreatitis. Hepatogastroenterology 40: 522-530
45. Gudgeon AM, Hurley P, Patel G, Shenkin A, Imrie CW, Heath DI, Jehanli A, Wilson C, Austen BM, Hermon-Taylor J (1990) Trypsinogen activating peptides assay in the early prediction of severity of acute pancreatitis. Lancet 335: 4-8
46. Guice KS, Oldham KT, Caty MG, Johnson KJ, Ward PA (1989) Neutrophil-dependent, oxygen-radical mediated lung injury associated with acute pancreatitis. Ann Surg 210: 740-747
47. Gupta RK (1971) Immunohistochemical study of glomerular lesions in acute pancreatitis. Arch Pathol 92: 267-272

48. Hermon-Taylor J, Majee AI, Grant DAW (1981) Cleavage of peptide hormones by beta 2-macroglobulin-trypsin complex and its relation to the pathogenesis and chemotherapy of acute pancreatitis. Clin Chim Acta 109: 203-209
49. Hjelmqvist B, Wattsgard C, Borgström A, Lasson A, Nyman U, Aspelin P, Ohlsson K (1989) Early diagnosis and classification in acute pancreatitis. Digestion 44: 177-183
50. Holm BA, Keicher L, Mingyao L, Sokolowski J, Enhorning G (1991) Inhibition of pulmonary surfactant function. J Appl Physiol 71: 317-321
51. Howes R, Zuidema GD, Cameron JL (1975) Evaluation of prophylactic antibiotics in acute pancreatitis. J Surg Res 18: 197: 203
52. Imrie CW (1974) Observations on acute pancreatitis. Br J Surg 61: 539-544
53. Imrie CW, Blumgart LH (1975) Acute pancreatitis: a prospective study on some factors in mortality. Bull Soc Int Chir 6: 601-603
54. Imrie CW, Allam BF, Ferguson JC (1976) Hypocalcaemia of acute pancreatitis: the effect of hypoalbuminaemia. Curr Med Res Opin 4: 101-116
55. Imrie CW, Ferguson JC, Murphy D, Blumgart LH (1977) Arterial hypoxia in acute pancreatitis. Br J Surg 64: 185-188
56. Imrie CW, Benjamin IS, Ferguson JC et al. (1978) A single-centre double-blind trial of Trasylol therapy in primary acute pancreatitis. Br J Surg 65: 337-341
57. Imrie CW, Shearer MG, Wilson C (1988) Glycoproteins as markers of pancreatic damage in acute pancreatitis. Int J Pancreatol 3: 43-52
58. Interiano B, Stuard ID, Hyde Rw (1972) Acute respiratory distress syndrom in pancreatitis. Ann Intern Med 77: 923-926
59. Ito K, Ramirez-Schon G, Shah PM (1981) Myocardial function in acute pancreatitis. Ann Surg 194: 85-88
60. Jacobs ML, Dagget WM, Civetta JM (1977) Acute pancreatitis: analysis of factors influencing survival. Ann Surg 185: 43-51
61. Karges W, Willemer S, Feddersen ChO, Adler G (1991) Cerulein-induzierte Pankreatitis der Ratte: Einfluß experimenteller Granulozytopenie. Z Gastroenterol 29: 469
62. Keating JP, Shackleford GD, Shackleford PG, Ternberg JL (1972) Pancreatitis and osteolytic lesions. J Pediatr 81: 350-353
63. Kellum JM, De Meester TM, Elkins R, Zuidema G (1972) Respiratory insufficiency secondary to acute pancreatitis. Ann Surg 175: 657-662
64. Kessler JI, Kniffen JC, Janowitz HD (1963) Lipoprotein inhibition in the hyperlipemia of acute alcoholic pancreatitis. N Engl J Med 269: 943-948
65. Knaus WA, Zimmermann JE, Wagner DP, Draper EA, Lawrence DE (1981) APACHE - acute physiology and chronic health evaluation: a physiologically based classification system. Crit Care Med 9: 591-599
66. Knaus WA, Draper EA, Wagner DP, Zimmermann JE (1985) APACHE II: a severity of disease classification system. Crit Care Med 13: 818-829
67. Koch K, Drewelow B, Liebe S, Reding R, Riethling AK (1991) Die Pankreasgängigkeit von Antibiotika. Chirurg 62:
68. Kwaan HC, Anderson MC, Gramatica L (1971) A study of pancreatic enzymes as a factor in the pathogenesis of disseminated intravascular coagulation during acute pancreatitis. Surgery 69: 663-672

69. Lamy M, Dupont-Deby G, Pincemail J, Braun M, Duchateau J, Deby C, Van Erck J, Bodson L, Damas P, Franchimont P (1985) Biochemical pathways of acute lung injury. Bull Eur Physiopathol Respir 21: 221-229
70. Lankisch PG, Schirren CA (1990) Increased body weight as a prognostic parameter for complications in the course of acute pancreatitis. Pancreas 5: 626-629
71. Lankisch PG, Rahlf G, Koop H (1983) Pulmonary complications in fatal acute hemorrhagic pancreatitis. Dig Dis Sci 28: 11-116
72. Larvin M, McMahaon MJ (1989) APACHE-II score for assessment and monitoring of acute pancreatitis. Lancet 2: 201-204
73. Lefer AM (1982) The myocardial depressant factor as a mediator of circulatory shock. Klin Wschr 60: 713-716
74. Lefer AM, Glenn TM, O'Neill TJ, Lovett WL (1971) Inotropic influence of endogenous peptides in experimental hemorrhagic pancreatitis. Surgery 69: 220-228
75. Le Gall JR, Loirat P, Alperovitch A (1984) A simplified acute physiology score for ICU patients. Crit Care Med 12: 975-977
76. Leser HG, Gross V, Scheibenbogen C, Heinisch A, Sal R, Lausen M, Rückauer K, Andreesen R, Farthmann EH, Schölmerich J (1991) Elevation of serum interleukin-6 concentration precedes acute-phase response and reflects severity in acute pancreatitis. Gastroenterology 101: 782-785
77. Littauer A, DeGroot H (1992) Release of reactive oxygen by hepatocytes on reoxygenation: three phases and role of mitochondria. Am J Physiol G1015-G1020
78. Lovett WL, Wangensteen SL, Glenn TM, Lefer AM (1971) Presence of a myocardial depressive factor in patients in circulatory stock. Surgery 70: 223-231
79. Mayer AD, McMahon MJ, Bowen M, Cooper EH (1984) C-reactive protein: an aid to assessment and monitoring of acute pancreatitis. J Clin Pathol 27: 207-211
80. McKenna JM, Craig RM, Chandrasekhar AJ, Cugell DW, Skorton D (1977) The pleuropulmonary complications of pancreatitis. Chest 71: 197-204
81. McMahon MJ, Playforth MJ, Pickford IR (1980) A comparative study of methods for the prediction of severity of attacks of acute pancreatitis. Br J Surg 67: 22-25
82. Meyers MA, Feldberg MAM, Oliphant M (1989) Grey-Turner's sign and cullen's sign in acute pancreatitis. Gastrointest Radiol 14: 30-37
83. Mullin GT, Caperton EM, Crespin EM (1968) Arthritis and skin lesions resembling erythema nodosum in pancreatic disease. Ann Intern Med 68: 75-87
84. Murphy D, Imrie CW, Davidson JF (1977) Haematological alterations in acute pancreatitis. Postgrad Med 53: 310-314
85. Neoptolemos JP, Carr-Locke DL, Leese T, James D (1987) Acute cholangitis in association with acute pancreatitis: incidence, clinical features, outcome and the role of ERCP and endoscopic sphincterotomy. Br J Surg 74: 1103-1106
86. Niederau C, Schulz HU (1993) Current conservative treatment of acute pancreatitis: evidence from animal and human studies. Hepatogastroenterology 40: 538-549
87. Niederau C, Crass RA, Silver J, Ferrell LD, Grendell JH (1988) Effects of hydration, oxygenation, peritoneal lavage, and a new protease inhibitor on experimental acute pancreatitis. Gastroenterology 95: 1648-1657
88. Niederau C, Lüthen R, Niederau M, Strohmeyer G, Ferrell LD, Grendell JH (1990) Pancreatic exocrine secretion in acute experimental pancreatitis. Gastroenterology 90: 1120-1127
89. Niederau C, Lüthen R, Heise JW, Becker H (1992) Prognosis of acute pancreatitis. In: Beger HG, Büchler M, Malfertheiner P (eds.) Standards in pancreatic surgery. Springer, Berlin, Heidelberg, New York, pp. 76-91

90. Osborne DH, Imrie CW, Carter DC (1981) Biliary surgery in the same admission for gallstone-associated acute pancreatitis. Br J Surg 68: 758-761
91. Otto H (1965) Nephropathia pancreatica. Med Klin 60: 1848-1852
92. Perez DH, Horn JK, Ong R (1983) Complement derived chemotactic activity in serum from patients with pancreatitis. Lab Clin Med 101: 123-129
93. Poulakkainen P, Valtonen V, Paananen A, Schröder T (1987) C-reactive protein (CRP) and serum phospholipase A2 in the assessment of the severity of acute pancreatitis. Gut 28: 764-771
94. Ranson JHC, Turner JW, Roses DF, Rifkind KM, Spencer FC (1974) Respiratory complication in acute pancreatitis. Ann Surg 179: 557-566
95. Ranson JHC (1982) Etiologic and prognostic factors in human acute pancreatitis: a review. Am J Gastroenterol 77: 633-638
96. Ranson JHC, Spencer FC (1978) The role of peritoneal lavage in severe acute pancreatitis. Ann Surg 187: 565-575
97. Ranson JHC, Rifkind KM, Roses DF (1974) Prognostic signs and the role of operative management in acute pancreatitis. Surg Gynecol Obstet 139: 69-81
98. Renner IG, Savage WT, Pantoja JL, Renner VJ (1985) Death due to acute pancreatitis. A retrospective analysis of 405 autopsy cases. Dig Dis Sci 30: 1005-1018
99. Robertson GM, Moore EW, Switz DM (1976) Inadequate parathyroid response in acute pancreatitis. N Engl J Med 294: 512-516
100. Rothermich NO, Von Hamm E (1941) Pancreatic encephalopathy. J Clin Endocrinol 1: 873-881
101. Scarpelli DG (1956) Fat necrosis of bone marrows in acute pancreatitis. Am J Pathol 31: 1077-1087
102. Schölmerich J, Johannesson T, Brobmann G, Wimmer B, Thiedemann B, Groß V, Gerok W, Farthmann EH (1989) Die Sonographie bei akuter Pankreatitis-Diagnose, Ätiologieklärung und Prognoseabschätzung. Ultraschall 10: 290-294
103. Schroder T, Lempinen M, Kivilaakso E (1982) Serum phospholipase A2 and pulmonary changes in acute fulminant pancreatitis. Resuscitation 10: 79-87
104. Siegel JH, Greenspan M, Del Guernico LRM (1967) Abnormal vascular tone, defective oxygen transport and myocardial failure in human septic shock. Ann Surg 165: 504-505
105. Soloman SS, Duckworth WC, Jallepalli P (1980) The glucose intolerance of acute pancreatitis. Hormonal response to arginine. Diabetes 29: 22-26
106. Steer ML, Saluja AK (1993) Etiology and pathogenesis of acute pancreatitis. In: Beger HG, Büchler M, Malfertheiner P (eds.) Standards in pancreatic surgery. Springer, Berlin, Heidelberg, New York, pp. 13-24
107. Steinberg WM, Schlesselmann SE (1987) Treatment of acute pancreatitis. Comparison of animal and human studies. Gastroenterology 93: 1420-1428
108. Stömmer P (1984) Lungenschäden durch akute tryptische Pankreatitis. Dtsch Med Wochenschr 109: 454-460
109. Storck G, Pettersson G, Edlund Y (1976) A study of autopsies upon 116 patients with acute pancreatitis. Surg Gynecol Obstet 143: 241-245
110. Tahamont MV, Barie PS, Blumenstock FA, Hussain MH, Malik AB (1982) Increased lung vascular permeability after pancreatitis and trypsin infusion. Am J Pathol 109: 15-26
111. Takada Y, Appert HE, Howard JM (1976) Vascular permeabilitiy induced by pancreatic exudate formed during acute pancreatitis in dogs. Surg Gynecol Obstet 143: 779-783
112. Trapnell JE (1992) The natural history and prognosis of acute pancreatitis. Ann R Coll Surg Engl 38: 265-287

113. Vadas P, Pruzanski W (1986) Biology of disease: role of secretory phospholipases A2 in the pathobiology of disease. Lab Invest 55: 391-399
114. Vigholt-Sorensen E (1989) Subcutaneous fat necrosis in pancreatic disease. A review and two new case reports. J Clin Gastroenterol 10: 741-745
115. Warshaw AL, Lee KH, Napier TW (1985) Depression of serum calcium by increased plasma free fatty acids in the rat: a mechanism for hypocalcemia in acute pancreatitis. Gastroenterology 89: 814-820
116. Werner MH, Hayes DF, Lucas CE, Rosenberg IK (1974) Renal vasoconstriction in association with acute pancreatitis. Am J Surg 127: 185-190
117. Wilson C, Imrie CW (1991) Systemic effects of acute pancreatitis. In: Johnson CD, Imrie CW (eds.) Pancreatic diseases. Springer, Berlin, Heidelberg, New York, pp. 287-297
118. Wilson C, Heath DI, Imrie CW (1990) Prediction of outcome in acute pancreatitis: a comparative study of APACHE-II, clinical assessment and multiple factor scoring systems. Br J Surg 77: 1260-1264
119. Winslet M (1992) Relation of diagnostic serum amylase levels to aetiology and severity of acute pancreatitis. Gut 33: 982-986

Oxygen Free Radicals and Acute Pancreatitis

D. Closa, L. Fernández-Cruz, J. Roselló-Catafau, M. Bardaj, E. Gelpí

Introduction

Acute pancreatitis is a necrotic and inflammatory process characterized by sudden onset in and around the pancreas. With the exception of infectious pancreatitis resulting from direct injury by micro-organisms, other forms of acute pancreatitis irrespective of their etiology are related to autodigestion of the organ by pancreatic enzymes [23]. This disease of the pancreas leads to acinar cell damage, epithelial necrosis, interstitial edema, and migration and activation of granulocytes into the pancreatic tissue [27]. In spite of the great number of studies on the pathogenesis of acute pancreatitis the initial reactions remain poorly known. It is thought that intrapancreatic activation of hydrolytic enzymes induces the rapid autodigestion of the gland. Particularly, intrapancreatic activation of trypsinogen to trypsin could be a key step that initiates a release of pancreatic enzymes from their inactive zymogens [30]. A colocalization of lysosomal hydrolases and pancreatic zymogens into the organelles in acinar cells has also been observed [43]. These cell organelles present increased membrane fragility and could release their content into the cytoplasm. It has been suggested that although many clinical situations are known to initiate acute pancreatitis, oxygen free radicals (OFR) can act as a molecular trigger for some of the effects of pancreas inflammation, such as tissue damage, edema, and inflammatory cells (granulocyte) activation [33].

Oxygen Free Radicals

A free radical can be defined as any species capable of independent existence that contains one or more unpaired electrons [21]. The presence of one or more unpaired electrons sometimes makes the species highly reactive. Molecular oxygen is the major source of biological free radicals. The superoxide radical (O_2-) is the 1-electron reduction product of molecular oxygen. It can be originated in vivo as a chemical accident when some of the electrons passing through the respiratory chain leak from the electron carriers and pass directly onto oxygen, reducing it to superoxide [16]. There are also a functional in vivo formation of superoxide. Activated neutrophils, eosinophils and macrophages can produce

O_2^- as a mechanism to kill microorganisms. This superoxide is generated by a membrane-bound NADPH oxidase system present in these cells [9]. Another important source of superoxide is the enzyme xanthine oxidase. This enzyme is present in two forms: a NADH-dependent form (D-form, or xanthine dehydrogenase) and an O_2-dependent form (O-form, or xanthine oxidase) [40]. Transformation from the D-form to the O-form can be, irreversibly, due to proteolytic cleavage, or, reversibly through -SH group oxidation [13]. This enzyme oxidizes xanthine or hypoxanthine to uric acid, and transfers electrons to NAD^+ (in the D-form) generating NADH, or to O_2 (in the O-form) generating O_2^-.

The superoxide anion can be dismutated to hydrogen peroxide (H_2O_2) nonenzymatically, but in vivo this reaction is catalyzed by superoxide dismutase (SOD) at a rate four orders of magnitude greater [22]. H_2O_2 has no unpaired electron and consequently cannot be described as a radical. (The term "reactive oxygen species" has been introduced to englobe O_2^-, H_2O_2, and OH) [20]. H_2O_2 can be removed by two enzymes: catalase and glutation peroxidase. On the other hand, hydrogen peroxide, in the presence of transition metals, can be easily decomposed generating the hydroxyl radical (OH) which is the most reactive free radical known [21].

The toxicity of OFR is due to their great reactivity in attacking proteins and DNA and initiating the free radical chain reaction known as lipid peroxidation. This reaction occurs when a free radical (specially OH) is generated close to biological membranes [15]. Under these conditions OH attacks the fatty acid chains of the membrane phospholipids. The problem is that when a radical gives or takes an electron to a nonradical this nonradical becomes a radical. This fact explains why the reaction between OH and a membrane fatty acid proceeds as a chain reaction leading to membrane destruction [20].

In vivo there are some defense mechanism against the oxygen free radical production. SOD, catalase, and gluthatione peroxidase are the major intracellular antioxidants. Cell membranes contains α-tocopherol, a lipid-soluble molecule with antioxidant activity [41]. Extracellular defenses from OFR are the α-tocopherol present in lipoproteins, ascorbic acid, and an extracellular isoenzyme of SOD [20]. Nevertheless, the major extracellular antioxidant defense is to prevent the generation of OH by binding the transition metal ions [37]. These ions bound to transferrins, hemoglobin, ceruloplasmin, albumin, etc. do not participate in OH formation.

Acute Pancreatitis

In 1984 Sanfey et al. [34] evaluated the possible role of oxygen free radicals in three models of experimental acute pancreatitis in isolated canine pancreas. Alcoholic pancreatitis was simulated by free fatty acid (FFA) infusion, ischemic pancreatitis was performed by subjecting the pancreas preparation to 2 h of ischemia, and gallstone pancreatitis was simulated by partial duct obstruction and simultaneous secretin stimulation. Pancreatitis was measured by increased pancreatic weight gain, hyperamilasemia and tissular edema. They showed that pretreatment with scavengers (superoxide dismutase and catalase) and/or an inhibitor of xanthine oxidase (allopurinol) significantly ameliorated all three parameters in each model [36]. Consequently they concluded that OFR are mediators involved in the pathogenesis of acute pancreatitis. The fact that allopurinol was effective in prevent pancreatic damage indicates that xanthine oxidase may be the source of these toxic species. The pancreas tissue is rich in hydrolytic enzymes such as chymotrypsin or trypsin. When these zymogens are activated, as a consequence of free fatty acids or pancreatic ischemia, proteolytic activation of xanthine oxidase may easily occur [33]. The subsequent generation of OFR can affect the cell and organelle membranes by lipoperoxidative mechanisms, and enhance zymogen activation, initiating a chain of events which lead to cell death.

An impressive amount of experimental data was generated after the initial work of Sanfey et al. Although in general these data support that OFR may play a role in acute pancreatitis, reported differences in the effectivity of OFR scavengers make difficult the suggestion of a precise role for OFR in this pathology. Obviously differences in experimental designs, models of pancreatitis, dose, time, and route of drug administration can partially explain these differences.

Administration of supramaximal doses of cerulein, a cholecistokinin analogue, induces an edematous acute pancreatitis [18]. In this experimental model, initial workers evaluated the effect of scavenger administration in the amelioration of the structural and biochemical injury associated to acute pancreatitis. It has been reported that treatment with SOD and catalase significantly prevents edema formation, granulocyte accumulation, tissue necrosis, lipid peroxidation, and DNA and RNA increases [19, 38, 39]. Administration of lactoferrin also shows a protective effect in this experimental model of pancreatitis [24]. Lactoferrin can act as an iron chelator, preventing the iron-dependent generation of hydroxyl radicals. During the evolution of this model of pancreatitis changes in sulfhydryl compounds and decreased tissue SOD activity has been reported [10, 11]. Continuous infusion of allopurinol reduced pancreatic weight gain and serum amylase concentration [44]. This ameliorating effect of allopurinol administration suggests that xanthine oxidase activation can also be the source of OFR in this model of edematous acute pancreatitis. Nevertheless there are reports that found no effect of allopurinol administration [32]. In addition, direct measurements of xanthine oxidase in pancreas tissue under cerulein stimulation failed to detect activation of this enzyme [7, 14] (Fig. 1). The usual methods for the determination of xanthine oxidase activity only measure the O-form of this enzyme once it is irreversibly converted from the D-form, since the buffer employed in these determinations contains agents (such as dithiothreitol, DTT) that reduces the -SH groups. These agents are added in the buffer in order to prevent artifactual reversible activation of the enzyme during the process of extraction and determination [13]. In this sense it could be speculated that perhaps in the cerulein induced acute pancreatitis, xanthine oxidase might be reversibly activated to the O-form. Nevertheless, Nordback and Cameron [29] using other models of acute pancreatitis induction, demonstrated that direct DTT administration prevents the OFR-induced damage, but that the protective effect is not impressive in the cerulein induced pancreatitis.

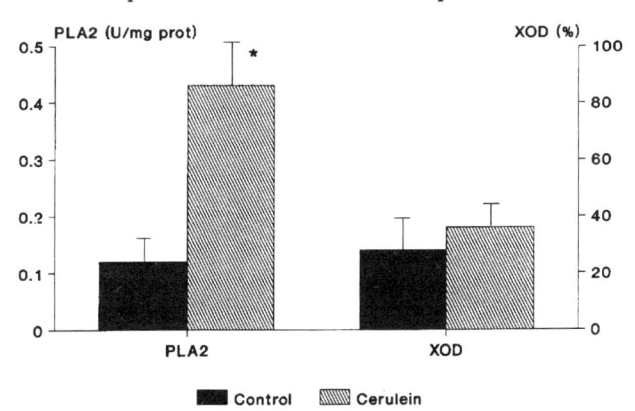

Fig. 1: Phospholipase A_2 (PLA$_2$) and xanthine oxidase (XOD) levels in cerulein-induced acute pancreatitis

It has been suggested that cell damage and oxidation products act as chemoattractants and can activate inflammatory cells, which generates more oxygen free radicals and proteolytic enzymes [2]. Sarr et al. [36] evaluated the role of leukocytes in the production of OFR induced by FFA infusion. Nevertheless, they found that depletion of circulating neutrophils had no effect in edema, weight gain, or hyperamylasemia developed in this model of acute pancreatitis. Despite these observations they could not completely exclude the possibility that resident phagocytes could serve as the source of OFR, and concluded that circulating leukocytes are not essential in the development of pancreatitis Concerning edematous pancreatitis, xanthine oxidase seems to be the source of OFR in some experimental models, but recent reports indicate that other sources could be responsible in cerulein-induced pancreatitis.

Studies in the hemorrhagic pancreatitis suggest that OFR play little if any role in the progression to hemorrhagic pancreatitis. Therefore the administration of free radical scavengers offers controversial results. It has been reported that SOD and catalase administration prevents some of the features of these models [1, 8, 25]. Nevertheless, it has also been reported that the denaturalized enzymes also present a protective effect, suggesting that protection is not conferred by their catalytic activity [31]. Allopurinol administration has also been evaluated in these experimental models. This xanthine oxidase inhibitor shows a small or no effect in the development of the inflammatory process (determined as mortality rate, hyperamylasemia, edema, and vacuolization) [25, 26, 31]. In contrast, there are also reports in the sense that allopurinol exerts a protective effect in the evolution of pancreatitis. Daily allopurinol treatment appears to be effective in order to reduce the initial increases of serum amylase associated to ischemic pancreatitis [3]. In addition, increased levels of xanthine oxidase activity have been measured in experimental necrohemorrhagic pancreatitis induced by bile salt administration in the pancreatic duct [6] or by a coline deficient, ethionine supplemented diet [28]. Furthermore, a great amount of inflammatory mediators was generated during this process, including prostaglandins and lipoxygenase arachidonic acid metabolites [4] (Fig. 2). The presence of leukotriene B_4 in pancreas tissue one hour after pancreatitis induction has been also demonstrated [5]. Leukotriene B_4 has been implicated as a mediator of neutrophil infiltration and appears to play a role as a chemotactic agent amplifying the inflammatory response and resulting in a secondary source of OFR.

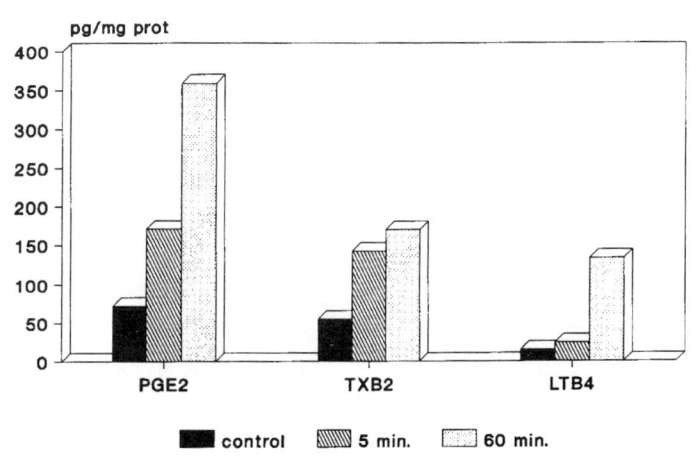

Fig. 2: Arachidonic acid metabolites in taurocholate-induced acute pancreatitis. PGE2, Prostaglandin E_2; TXB2, thromboxane B_2; LTB4, leukotriene B_4

It has been shown that xanthine oxidase activation can occur after cell death in hepatocytes [12]. In pancreas acinar cells, where the concentration of hydrolytic enzymes is greater than in hepatocytes, a great level of enzyme conversion could be expected after cell death in different models of necrohemorrhagic pancreatitis. When the acinar cell dies, endogenous trypsin and other proteolytic enzymes are able to catalyze the xanthine dehydrogenase to xanthine oxidase conversion. Under these conditions, xanthine oxidase could be an important source of OFR which can damage plasmatic membranes of colindant cells. Activated proteases and phospholipases can easily enhance the digestion of oxidant-damaged membranes or denatured membrane components [17]. A significant activation of phospholipase A_2 has been shown after taurocholate induction, but this increase was significantly attenuated with the use of scavengers (SOD) or membrane stabilizers (16,16 dimethyl prostaglandin E_2; Fig. 3). These results reinforce our suggestion that tissue damage could be the result of joint OFR and hydrolytic enzyme activation (Fig. 4), and possibly neutralized using substances that prevents lysosomal and digestive enzyme compartments coalesce. Thus the simultaneous presence of a source of OFR and proteolytic enzymes can initiate a chain of events leading to cell death which is extended to the complete pancreatic lobule [6] (Fig. 4). In this regard, it has been reported that administration of hydrogen peroxide or xanthine plus xanthine oxidase in the pancreas generates increases in amylase and lipase concentrations, hemorrhages, and edema. These features can be prevented by SOD administration, but also by a trypsin inhibitor (gabexate mesilate) [42]. This fact suggests that proteolytic enzymes are mediators in the OFR-induced damage and points to the importance of synergism among hydrolytic enzymes and OFR in the pathogenesis of pancreatitis. It is possible that antioxidant drugs, protease inhibitors, phospholipase A_2 inhibitors, and immunoneutralization of leukocyte and/or endothelial cell adhesion (Fig. 5) could offer a combined valid therapeutic approach in severe pancreatitis.

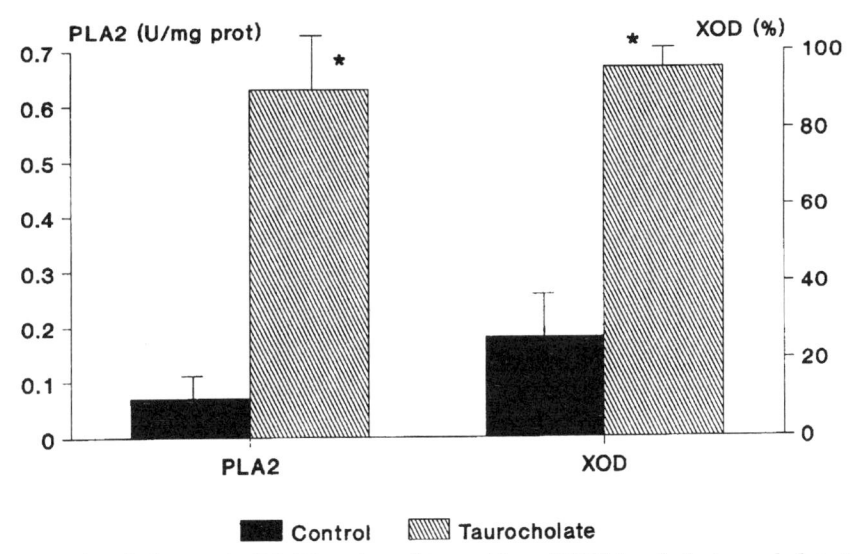

Fig. 3: Phospholipase A_2 (PLA2) and xanthine oxidase (XOD) levels in taurocholate-induced acute pancreatitis

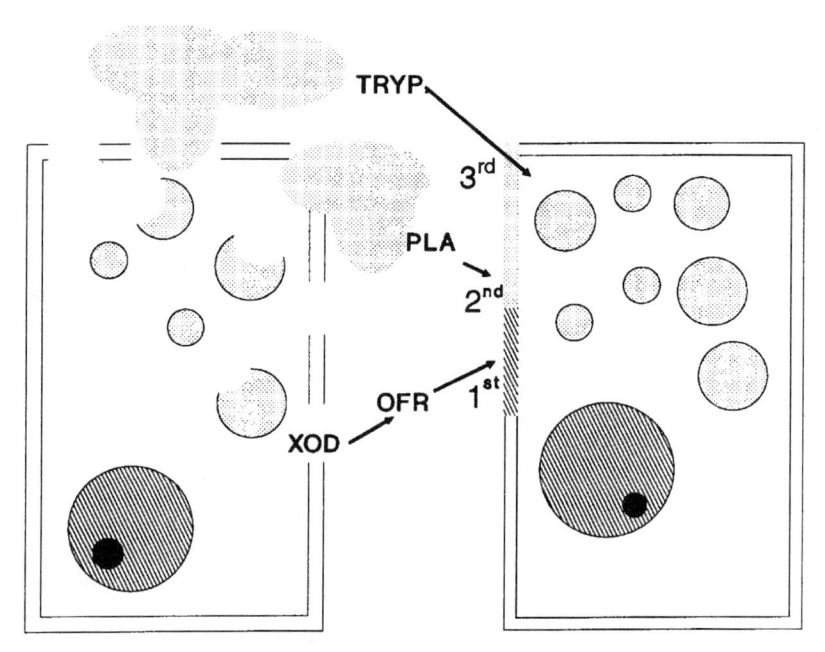

Fig. 4: Sequence of extended acinar damage 1; OFR-mediated membrane disruption; 2, phospholipase digestion of oxidant-damaged membrane; 3, proteolytic cleavage of cell components

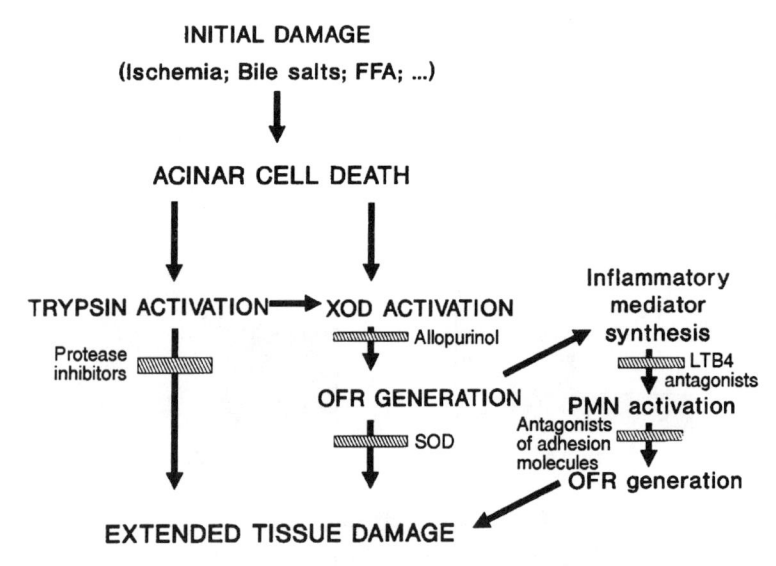

Fig. 5: Sequence of events associated to acute pancreatitis, and possible points of therapeutic action

References

1. Bank S, Sandberg A, Aaron J, Greenwald R, Lendval S (1985) The effect of oxygen free radical scavengers on ethionine induced pancreatitis in mice. Dig Dis Sci 30: 962
2. Braganza JM, Rinderknecht H (1988) Free radicals and acute pancreatitis. Gastroenterology 94: 1111-1112
3. Cassone E, Maneschi EMT, Faccas JG (1991) Effects of allopurinol on ischemic experimental pancreatitis. Int J Pancreatol 8: 227-234
4. Closa D, Roselló-Catafau J, Martrat A, Hotter G, Bulbena O, Fernández-Cruz L, Gelpí E (1993) Changes of systemic prostacyclin and thromboxane A_2 in sodium taurocholate and cerulein induced acute pancreatitis in rats. Dig Dis Sci 38: 33-38
5. Closa D, Roselló-Catafau J, Hotter G, Bulbena O, Fernández-Cruz L, Gelpí E (1993 Cyclooxygenase and lipoxygenase arachidonate metabolism in necrohemorrhagic acute pancreatitis induced in rats by sodium taurocholate. Prostaglandins 45: 315-322
6. Closa D, Bulbena O, Roselló-Catafau J, Fernández-Cruz L, Gelpí E (1993) Effects of prostaglandins and superoxide dismutase administration on oxygen free radical production in experimental acute pancreatitis. Inflammation 17: 563-571
7. Closa D, Bulbena O, Hotter O, Roselló-Catafau J, Fernández-Cruz L, Gelpí E (1994) Xanthine oxidase activation in cerulein- and taurocholate-induced acute pancreatitis in rats. Arch Int Physiol Bioch Biophys 102: 167-170
8. Closa D, Hotter G, Roselló-Catafau J, Bulbena O, Fernández-Cruz L, Gelpí E (1994) Prostanoids and oxygen free radicals in early stages of experimental acute pancreatitis. Dig Dis Sci 39: 1537-1543
9. Curnutte JT, Babior BM (1987) Chronic granulomatous disease. Adv Hum Genet 16: 229-245
10. Dabrowski A, Chwiecko M (1990) Oxygen radicals mediate depletion of pancreatic sulfhydryl compounds in rats with cerulein-induced acute pancreatitis Digestion 47: 15-19
11. Dabrowski A, Gabryelewicz U, Wereszczynska S, Chyczewski L (1989) Oxygen-derived free radicals in caerulein-induced acute pancreatitis. Scand J Gastroenterol 24: 1245-1249
12. DeGroot H, Littauer A (1988) Reoxygenation injury in isolated hepatocytes: cell death precedes conversion of xanthine dehydrogenase to xanthine oxidase. Biochem Biophys Res Commun 155: 278-282
13. DellaCorte E, Stirpe F (1972) The regulation of rat liver xanthine oxidase. Involvement of thiol groups in the conversion of the enzyme activity from dehydrogenase (type D) into oxidase (type O) and purification of the enzyme. Biochem J 126: 739-745
14. Devenyi ZJ, Orchard JL, Powers RE (1987) Xanthine oxidase activity in mouse pancreas: effects of caerulein-induced acute pancreatitis. Biochem Biophys Res Commun 149: 841-845
15. Dix TA, Aikens J (1993) Mechanisms and biological relevance of lipid peroxidation initiation. Chem Rev Toxicol 6: 2-18
16. Fridovich I (1983) Superoxide radical: an endogenous toxicant. Ann Rev Pharmacol Toxicol 23: 239-257
17. Ginsburg I, Misgav R, Pinson A, Varani J, Ward PA, Kohen R (1992) Synergism among oxidants, proteinases, phospholipases, microbial hemolysins, cationic proteins, and cytokines. Inflammation 16: 519-538
18. Grönroos JM, Aho HJ, Hietaranta AJ, Nevalainen TJ (1991) Early acinar cell changes in caerulein-induced interstitial acute pancreatitis in the rat. Exp Pathol 41: 21-30
19. Guice KS, Miller DE, Oldham KT, Townsend CM, Thompson JC (1986) Superoxide dismutase and catalase: a possible role in established pancreatitis. Am J Surg 151: 163-169
20. Halliwell B (1991) Drug antioxidant effect A basis for drug selection? Drugs 42: 569-605

21. Halliwell B, Gutteridge JMC (1989) Free radicals in biology and medicine. Clarendon, Oxford
22. Hassan HM, Schellhorn HE (1988) Superoxide dismutase: an antioxidant defense enzyme. In: Oxy-radicals in molecular biology and pathology. Liss, New York, pp. 183-193
23. Klöppel G, Maillet B (1993) Pathology of acute and chronic pancreatitis. Pancreas 8: 659-679
24. Koike D, Makino I (1993) Protective effect of lactoferrin on caerulein-induced acute pancreatitis in rats. Digestion 54: 84-90
25. Koiwai T, Oguchi H, Kawa S, Yanagisawa Y, Kobayashi T, Homma T (1989) The role of oxygen free radicals in experimental acute pancreatitis in the rat. Int J Pancreatol 5: 135-143
26. Lankisch PG, Pohl U, Otto J, Wereszczynska U, Gröne HJ (1989) Xanthine oxidase inhibitor in acute experimental pancreatitis in rats and mice. Pancreas 4: 436-440
27. Martin E, Bedossa P (1991) Classification des pancréatites. Ann Pathol 11: 4-17
28. Nonaka A, Manabe T, Tamura K, Asano N, Imanishi K, Tobe T (1989) Changes of xanthine oxidase, lipid peroxide and superoxide dismutase in mouse acute pancreatitis. Digestion 43: 41-46
29. Nordback IH, Cameron JL (1993) The mechanism of conversion of xanthine dehydrogenase to xanthine oxidase in acute pancreatitis in the canine isolated pancreas preparation. Surgery 113: 90-97
30. Rinderknecht H (1991) Activation of pancreatic zimogens. Dig Dis Sci 31: 314-320
31. Rutledge PL, Saluja AK, Powers RE, Steer ML (1987) Role of oxygen derived free radicals in diet induced haemorrhagic pancreatitis in mice. Gastroenterology 93: 41-47
32. Saluja A, Powers RE, Saluja M, Rutledge P, Steer ML (1986) The role of oxygen-derived free radicals in caerulein-induced pancreatitis. Gastroenterology 90: 1613
33. Sanfey H (1991) Oxygen free radicals in experimental acute pancreatitis In: Braganza JM (ed.) The pathogenesis of pancreatitis. Manchester University Press, Manchester, pp. 53-65
34. Sanfey H, Bulkley GB, Cameron JL (1984) The role of oxygen derived free radicals in the pathogenesis of acute pancreatitis. Ann Surg 200: 405-413
35. Sanfey H, Bulkley GB, Cameron JL (1985) The pathogenesis of acute pancreatitis: the source and role of oxygen derived free radicals in three different experimental models. Ann Surg 201, 633-639
36. Sarr MG, Bulkley GB, Cameron JL (1986) The role of leukocytes in the production of oxygen-derived free radicals in acute experimental pancreatitis. Surgery 101: 292-296
37. Sato M, Bremner I (1993) Oxygen free radicals and metallothionein. Free Radic Biol Med 14: 325-337
38. Schoenberg MH, Büchler M, Schädlich H, Younes M, Bültmann B, Beger HG (1989) Involvement of oxygen radicals and phospholipase A_2 in acute pancreatitis of the rat. Klin Wochenschr 67: 166-170
39. Schoenberg MH, Büchler M, Gaspar M, Stinner A, Younes M, Melzner I, Bültmann B, Beger HG (1990) Oxygen free radicals in acute pancreatitis of the rat. Gut 31: 1138-1143
40. Stirpe F and DellaCorte E (1969) The regulation of rat liver xanthine oxidase Conversion in vitro of the enzyme activity from dehydrogenase (Type D) to oxidase (Type O). J Biol Chem 244: 3855-3863
41. Sukalski KA, Pinto KA, Berntson JL (1993) Decreased susceptibility of liver mitochondria from diabetic rats to oxidative damage and associated increase in α-tocopherol. Free Radic Biol Med 14: 57-65
42. Tamura K, Manabe T, Andoh K, Kyogoku T, Oshio G, Tobe T (1992) Effect of intraarterial active oxygen species on the rat pancreas. Hepatogastroenterology 39: 152-157
43. Watanabe O, Baccino FM, Sterr ML, Meldonesi J (1984) Supramaximal caerulein stimulation and ultrastructure of rat pancreatic acinar cells: early morphological changes during development of experimental pancreatitis. Am J Physiol 246: G457-467
44. Wisner JR, adn Renner IG (1988) Allopurinol attenuates caerulein induced acute pancreatitis in the rat. Gut 29: 926-929

The Effect of Biliary Obstruction on the Phagocytic Function of the Reticuloendothelial System in the Opossum Model

J. Baas, N. Senninger, H. Elser, F. Willeke, R. Langer, C. Herfarth

Introduction

Extrahepatic biliary obstruction has been shown to cause a depression of the reticuloendothelial system in both man [1-3] and animals [4-6]. In the opossum model, obstruction of the pancreatic and the hepatic duct together is also an important factor in the pathogenesis of biliary pancreatitis [7]. There is a consensus that extrahepatic biliary obstruction causes a depression of the reticuloendothelial system (RES) in the long-term effect (after 3-5 weeks) [8-10], but there are also studies that show an even increased function of the RES during the first days after biliary obstruction [11]. The goal of this study was to clarify the functions of the liver RES in the first week after different biliary obstructions.

Materials and Methods

Animals. We used 18 North American opossums weighing 2700-3200 g. The animals were housed one per cache, maintained on an artificial day-and-night cycle, and fed laboratory food and water ad libitum.
Experimental Groups and Surgical Procedures. All 18 opossums were operated on under intraperitoneal (i.p.) Na-pentobarbital anesthesia (25 mg/kg) using sterile techniques. After placement of a central venous line in the jugular vein, the abdomen was entered via a midline incision. The gallbladder was evacuated and the cystic duct ligated to exclude a possible vent function. Then a specially designed tourniquet was placed around the common hepatic duct above its junction with the pancreatic duct (group II), around the pancreatic duct (group I), or around both ducts (group III). The tourniquet was exteriorized to the back of the animal but not yet closed.
Method of Determination of RES Function. As a test substance we used Nanocoll, a ^{99m}Tc-labeled albumin colloid with a diameter of 25-50 nm. Under Na-pentobarbital anesthesia the animals were fixed on a computerized gamma camera, and about 20 MBq in

a volume of 2 ml Nanocoll colloid was injected rapidly via the central venous line over 2-3 s. During 30 min sequential frames were taken at intervals of 4 s for the first 480 s and at intervals of 30 s for the rest of the time. In the image two regions of interest (ROI) were selected, one containing the liver and the other marking an area in the lower abdomen to measure the background radiation. Time-activity curves were generated for both ROIs and the resulting net liver uptake was calculated using a computer (Fig. 1). As a parameter for this uptake curve we calculated the parameters R and S of the natural logarithmic regression for the net liver curve during the first 1200 s after injection of Nanocoll (Fig. 1) using the formula: count rate = R x LN(time) + S. In all cases the correlation coefficient for the natural log regression was higher than 0.93, thus showing R and S to be very good parameters for the shape of the net liver uptake curve. For the function of the whole RES we took blood samples before and 1, 2, 3, 5, 7, 10, 20, and 30 min after the injection of Nanocoll. The clearance of the test substance was determined, and the corrected phagocytic index a was calculated. Results are expressed as mean ± standard deviation. Significance was tested using Student's t test. A p value below 0.05 was considered significant and one below 0.005 highly significant.

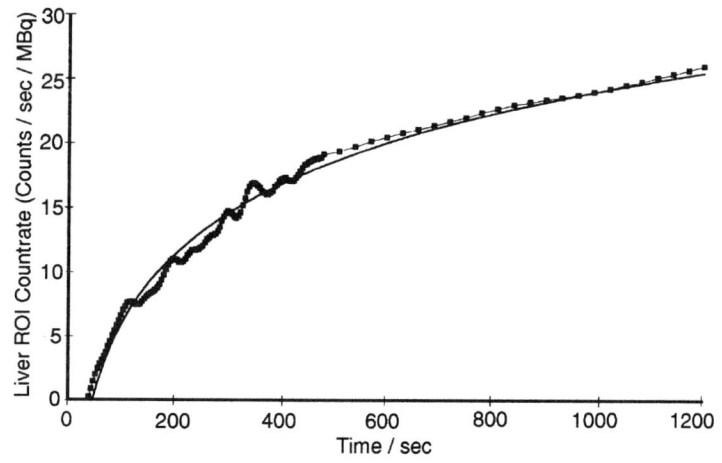

Fig. 1: Liver uptake of Nanocoll and logarithmic regression

Results

In group I there was a slightly diminished function of the whole and the liver RES, starting to be significant on day 5 (Fig. 2). In group II (Fig. 2b) the decrease in parameter a became significant on day 2 and highly significant on day 5. Parameter R became highly significant from day 2 on. The worst RES function occurred in group III (Fig. 2c). From the first day after obstruction, both parameters changed significantly to the worse. Starting on day 2, the change in parameter R was highly significant, as was the change in the phagocytic index on day 6. Comparison of the parameters R and a in each group showed a more diminished function of the liver RES than on the whole RES. From day 5, there were highly significant differences between the groups, with group I having the best and group II the worst RES function (Fig. 3).

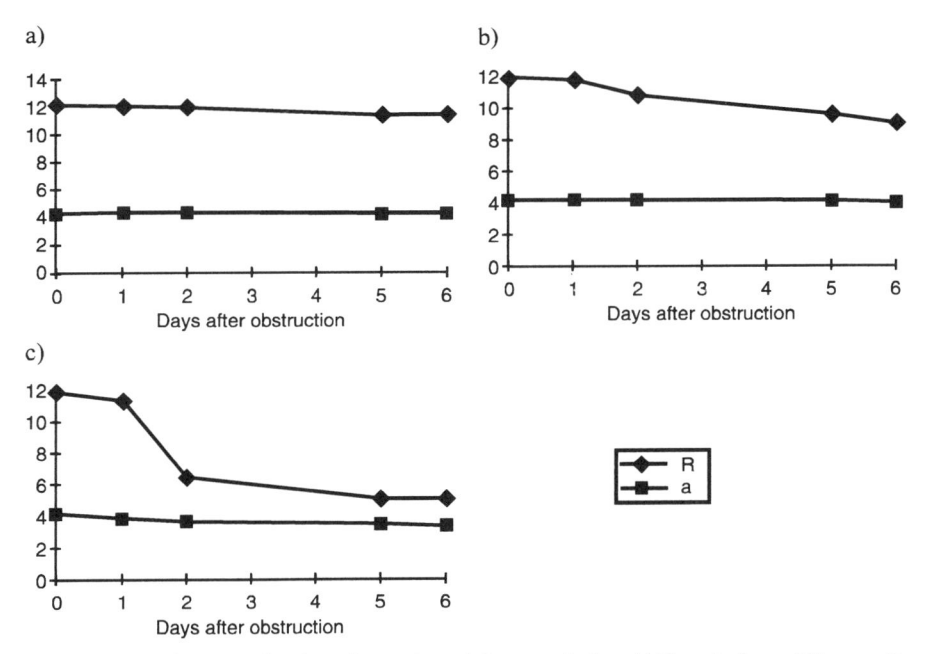

Fig. 2a-c: RES function after duct obstruction. a) Pancreatic duct. b) Hepatic duct. c) Pancreatic and hepatic ducts

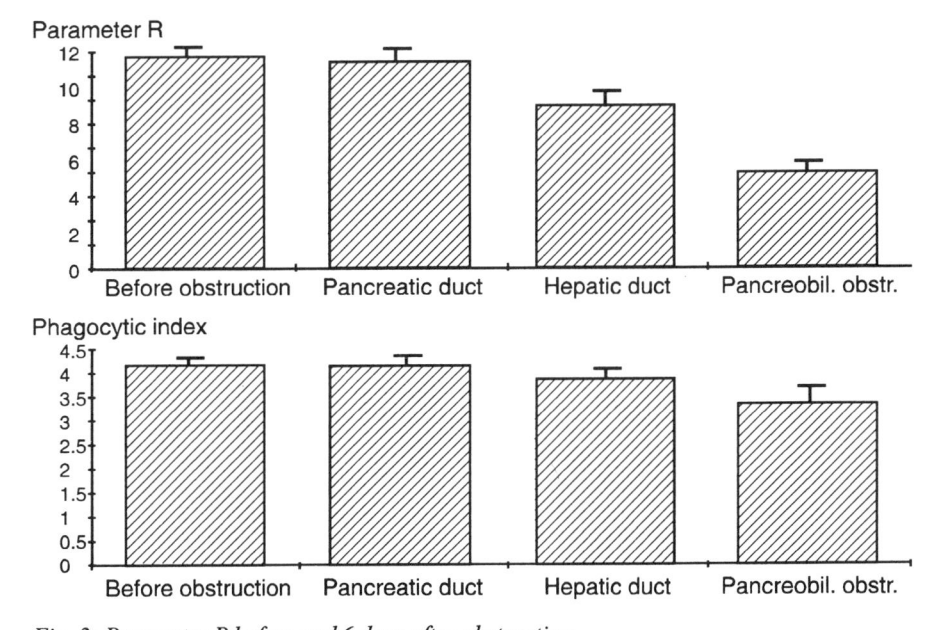

Fig. 3: Parameter R before and 6 days after obstruction

Discussion

In an animal with a single obstruction of the pancreatic duct there is only a small change in the function of the RES that could be related to a temporary load of the phagocytic capacity by the operative procedure and the central lines. But in an animal with an obstructed hepatic duct, the function of the RES, especially in the liver, is strongly impaired. By an additional obstruction of the pancreatic duct, this effect can be even more significant, although no bile reflux is possible. This change in RES function is correlated with the effect on the pancreas. Obstruction of the pancreatic duct alone leads only to mild pancreatic swelling, while obstruction of the pancreatic and hepatic duct together results in a severe hemorrhagic pancreatitis [7].

This effect if well known and has been explained by a bile reflux into the pancreas. In our experiment, however, there was no reflux possible, and despite this a severe pancreatitis occurred. A possible explanation is a diminished function of the RES. A number of mechanisms might account for this effect. Absorption of intestinal endotoxins is increased in obstructive jaundice, and an impaired RES might be unable to clear the postal venous blood of the endotoxins so they could damage the pancreas. Enzymes from the pancreas are set free and could further damage the organ. Their clearance by the RES is also impaired. A damaged RES could leak hydrolases that are toxic to various tissues and could damage cells in the pancreas.

We conclude that single pancreatic duct obstruction in the opossum model is not followed by a strong RES dysfunction, while single or additional obstruction of the hepatic duct leads to a strong impairment of the phagocytic capacity. These misfunctions could be important factors in the pathogenesis of biliary pancreatitis.

References

1. Drivas G, James O, Wardle N (1976) Study of reticuloendothelial phagocytic capacity in patients with cholestasis. Br Med J 1:1568-1569
2. Athlin L, Holmberg SB, Hafstrom L (1991) A clinical review with special reference to phagocytosis. Eur J Surg 157: 163-170
3. O'Conner MJ (1985) Mechanical biliary obstruction, a review of the multisystemic consequences of obstructive jaundice and their impact on perioperative morbidity and mortality. Am Surg 51: 254-251
4. Holman JM, Rikkers LF (1982) Biliary obstruction and host defense failure. J Surg Res 32: 208-213
5. Collier DSJ, Pain JA, Wight DGD, Lovat P, Bailey ME (1986) The Kupffer cell in experimental extrahepatic cholestasis in the rat - a light microscopy, immunohistochemical and electron microscopy study. J Pathol 150: 187-194
6. Katz S, Grosfeld JL, Gross K, Plager DA, Ross D, Rosenthal RS, Hull M (1984) Impaired bacterial clearance and trapping in obstructive jaundice. Ann Surg 199: 14-20
7. Senninger N, Moody FG, Coelho JCU, Van Buren DH (1986) The role of biliary obstruction in the pathogenesis of acute pancreatitis in the opossum. Surgery 99: 688-693
8. Ball SK, Grogan JB, Collier BJ, Scott-Conner CE (1991) Bacterial phagocytosis in obstructive jaundice. A microbiologic and electron microscopic analysis. Am Surg 57: 67-72
9. Pain JA (1987) Reticulo-endothelial function in obstructive jaundice. Br J Surg 74: 1091-1094
10. Vane DW, Redlich P, Weber T, Leapman S, Siddiqui AR, Grosfeld JL (1988) Impaired immune function in obstructive jaundice. J Surg Res 45: 287-293
11. Halpern BN, Biozzi G, Nicol T (1957) Effect of experimental biliary obstruction on the phagocytic activity of the reticuloendothelial system. Nature 180: 503-504

Effect of Sodium Selenite in Combination with Aprotinin on Inflammatory Plasma Markers During Acute Pancreatitis

S. Kopprasch, H. Kühne, T. Zimmermann, A. Dörfler, H.-E. Schröder, K. Ludwig

Introduction

Extensive experimental studies and clinical trials have revealed the preferential role of three biochemical events in the pathogenesis of acute pancreatitis: heightened free radical activity, activation of proteolytic pancreatic enzymes and release of inflammatory mediators. All these processes are involved in damage to the pancreas and, moreover, may contribute to systemic complications such as cardiopulmonary changes, renal failure, sepsis, and coagulation deficiency. The present study assessed the efficacy of the antioxidant selenium in the adjuvant therapy of acute necrotizing pancreatitis (ANP) and acute edematous pancreatitis (AEP). The effects of selenium were evaluated by monitoring the time course of different inflammatory plasma markers during therapy.

Methods

A total of 21 patients with ANP and 20 with AEP were entered into the study protocol. All patients with ANP and 12 with AEP randomized previously in a double-blind fashion received sodium selenite (Selenase, GN Pharm Arzneimittel, Stuttgart). On the first day of therapy 1000 μg was given as a bolus. Thereafter the patients received 600 μg sodium selenite daily by infusion until normalization of serum amylase levels. During the first 6 days of therapy all patients received Trasylol (days 1-3, 500 000 U; days 4-6, 300 000 U). Blood samples were obtained just before the onset of therapy and then daily until patients improved or died. In the present study three patients with ANP died. The following plasma parameters were measured: activity of glutathione peroxidase [6], reduced glutathione [2], kallikreinogen, kallikrein inhibitor capacity, [3] and PMN elastase proteinase inhibitor complex (EL-PI complex; IMAC, Merck, Darmstadt).

Results

During selenium therapy glutathione peroxidase activity increased in patients with ANP (from 1.43 ± 0.78 µkat/l on day 1 to 2.37 ± 0.98 µkat/l on day 20). There was an even more pronounced rise in selenium-treated AEP patients (Fig.1). AEP patients without selenium supplementation revealed only minor changes in plasma glutathione peroxidase activity (slight increase from 1.58 ± 0.63 µkat/l on day 1 to 1.72 ± 0.38 µkat/l on day 5). The time course of plasma malondialdehyde levels depended on the severity of pancreatitis (Fig. 2). Patients with ANP showed a gradual rise until day 8 which was followed by a continuous decrease until day 20. The malondialdehyde level was constantly lower in selenium-treated AEP patients than in AEP patients without selenium supplementation. In contrast to the glutathione peroxidase activity the concentrations of reduced glutathione remained within the range of their initial levels in all patients with acute pancreatitis (data not shown). Obviously the selenium supplementation had no effect on the plasma levels of reduced glutathione.

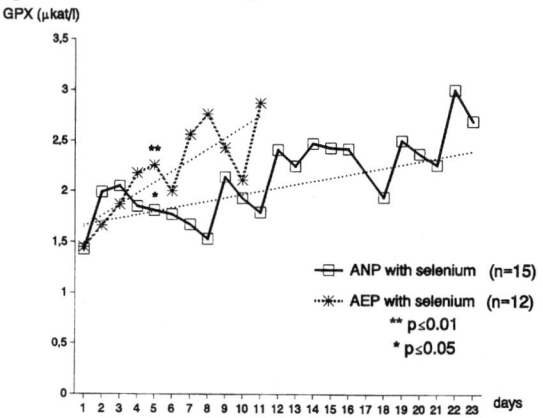

Fig. 1: Activity of plasma glutathione peroxidase (GPX) in patients with mild (AEP) and severe (ANP) acute pancreatitis (means; asteriks, significant difference vs. day 1)

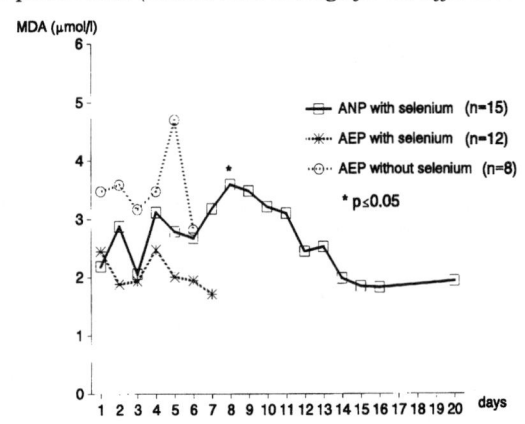

Fig. 2: Changes of plasma malonedialdehyde (MDA) levels during acute pancreatitis (means; *$p \leq 0.05$ vs day 1)

Acute pancreatitis resulted in high initial levels of the plasma EL-PI complex (ANP patients, 336.5 ± 129.9 µg/l; AEP patients, 142.4 ± 113.7 µg/l; reference values, 22.6 ± 18.6 µg/l). During selenium treatment a marked decrease in EL-PI complex was found, with a slight delay in AEP patients (Fig. 3). In contrast, EL-PI complex in AEP patients without selenium increased further after hospitalization, reaching maximum values on day 4 and then falling. The initial decrease in plasma kallikreinogen levels showed a pronounced dependence on the severity of pancreatitis (Fig. 4). Only in AEP patients with selenium administration was a tendency toward normal levels observed. The extent of the kallikreinogen activation correlated with the changes in kallikrein inhibitor capacity (Fig. 5).

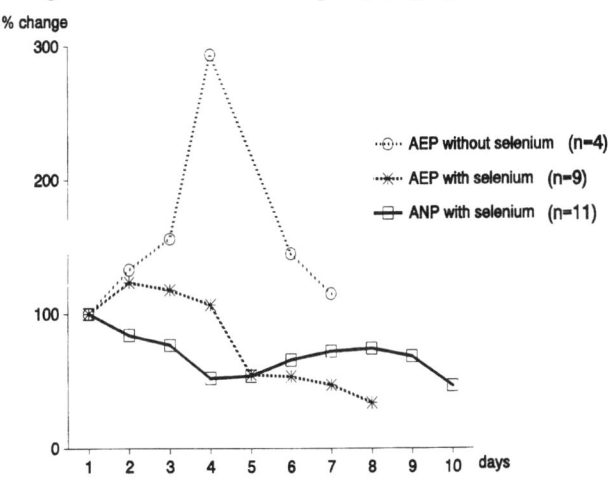

Fig. 3: Time course of EL-PI complex during acute pancreatitis (means; percal changes of our own controls)

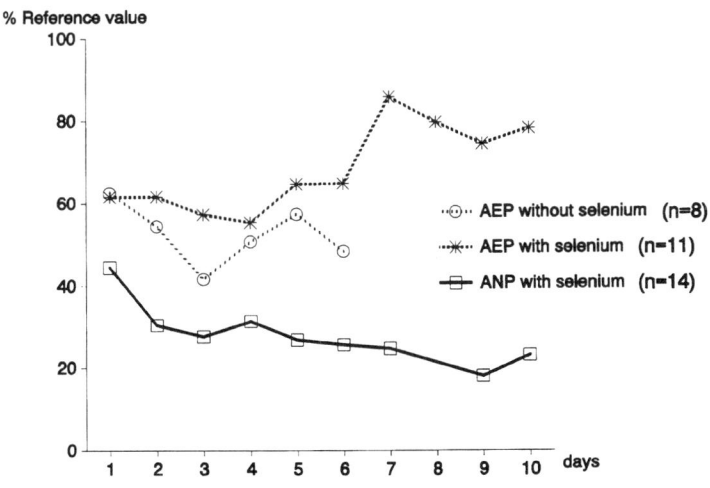

Fig. 4: Changes of plasma kallikreinogen levels in patients with acute pancreatitis (means; percentage of the kallikreinogen reference value: 11.29 ± 1.74 µkat/l)

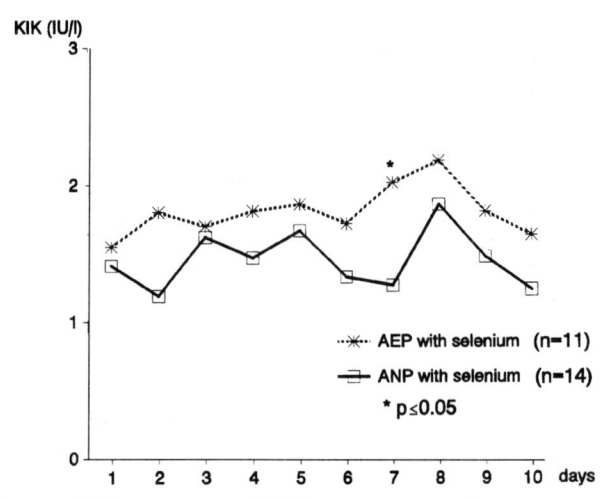

*Fig. 5: Kallikrein inhibitor capacity (KIK) in patients with acute pancreatitis during selenium therapy (means; *p ≤ 0.05 vs day 1)*

Discussion

The benefits of antioxidant therapy in acute pancreatitis have been documented in various animal models [1, 4, 7]. The antioxidant properties of the trace element selenium are based on ist ability to scavenge free radicals directly and to prevent radical formation indirectly by selenium-containing glutathione peroxidases. Plasma glutathione peroxidase is an integral part of the human defense system agianst free radicals. There exists a close correlation between selenium intake and plasma glutathione peroxidase levels [5].
The present study found that selenium supplementation ameliorates the systemic manifestations in patients with acute mild and severe pancreatitis, as reflected by the time course of different plasma inflammatory parameters. It was shown that selenium treatment results in the expected elevation in plasma glutathione peroxidase activity and a decrease in plasma malondialdehyde levels, at least in later stages of pancreatitis. Furthermore, selenium supplementation substantially influenced the time course of PMN elastase release into systemic circulation. The effects on PMN elastase release and the kallikrein-kinin system are possibly triggered indirectly by selenium by stabilization of cellular and subcellular integrity.

References

1. Giuce KS, Miller DE, Oldham KT, Townsend CM, Thompson JC (1986) Superoxide dismutase and catalase: a possible role in established pancreatitis. Am J Surg 151: 163-168
2. Hissin PJ, Hilf R (1976) A fluorometric method for determination of oxidized and reduced glutathione in tissues.Anal Biochem 74: 214-226
3. Lehmann B, Kühne H, Scheuch DW (1981) Zur Kallikreinogenbestimmung in Plasmen unterschiedlicher Spezies.Z Med Lab Diagn 22: 354-355

4. Sanfey H, Bulkley GB, Cameron JL (1984) The role of oxygen-derived free radicals in the pathogenesis of acute pancreatitis. Ann Surg 200: 405-413
5. Steiner G, Menzel H, Lombeck I, Ohnesorge FK, Bremer HJ (1982) Plasma glutathione peroxidase after selenium supplementation in patients with reduced selenium state. Eur J Pediatr 138: 138-140
6. Thomson CD, Rea HM, Doesburg VM, Robinson MF (1977) Selenium concentrations and glutathione peroxidase activities in whole blood of New Zealand residents. Br J Nutr 37: 457-460
7. Zimmermann T, Schuster R, Lauschke G, Trausch M, Albrecht S, Kopprasch S, Kühne H (1991) Chemiluminescence response of whole blood and separated blood cells in cases of experimentally induced pancreatitis and MDTQ-DA-Trasylol-ascorbic acid therapy. Anal Chim Acta 255: 373-381

The Effects of Toxemia on the Cascade Systems of Patients with Acute Pancreatitis

S. Pierrakakis, P. Karydakis, N. Economou, A. Ninos, G. Antsaklis

Introduction

Acute pancreatitis may present as a fulminant disease that results in the systemic inflammatory response syndrome and multiple organ failure syndrome, a state with a particularly unfavorable prognosis. It has been demonstrated previously that with progress of the disease complement is activated and consumed [2]. This process is clearly associated with the pathogenesis of pancreatitis complications [6]. The complement system can be activated by circulating pancreatic enzymes, toxins, or other cascade systems such as coagulation fibrinolysis or kinins. This cascade system activation is clearly related to increased mortality and morbidity. Toxemia, since 1952 an assumed phenomenon, can be now demonstrated and documented. If we can establish toxemia, we can search for and treat any infectious focuses before the development of any serious complications.

The purpose of this study was to evaluate the prevalence of toxemia in patients with acute pancreatitis and to relate this condition to the activation of cascade systems that are encountered in the subsequent complications of the disease. To accomplish this we used the limulus amebocyte lysate test that is based in the coagulation of a special protein of the arthropod *Limulus polephemus*. This is a reliable method and can detect even amounts of toxin of 0.2 ng [4]. We evaluated 45 patients (15 men and 30 women) with a mean age of 59 years (21 - 87 years); most (70%) were between 51 and 80 years old. We considered as severe pancreatitis any case with more than three of Ranson's or Imrie's signs and with one or more positive Agarwal parameter. Two or more consecutive positive limulus tests in the same day were considered as indicative of toxemia.

Results

Sixteen (35.55%) of our patients had toxemia, but in only two cases there was a urinary gram-negative infection. Toxemia detected in these patients is probably the result of bacterial and toxin translocation from the intestinal tract in the portal system. Gallstone pancreatitis accounted for 84% of all cases of acute pancreatitis in the 45 patients of our series. Other causes were alcoholic pancreatitis (6.6%) and duodenal diverticulum (2.2%); the etiology was unknown in 6.6% of cases.

Toxemia is closely related to the activation of cascade systems involved in the systemic inflammatory response syndrome and the final systemic complications of the disease. Toxemia was discovered in 100% of coagulation disorders, 100% of complement C3 consumption cases, 65% of cases of kinin activation, and 50% of those of fibrinolysis activation. Toxemia is clearly linked to both complement consumption and a high number of complications. Among the 35 patients (77.77%) with Ranson score of 2 or less, six (17.1%) had toxemia and nine with low C3; there were three complications. By contrast, all of the ten patients (22.22%) with two or more Ranson points had both toxemia and low C3; among these there were nine complications. Patients who had toxemia and a low C3 level without serious complications were hospitalized for longer periods. The mean value of C4 was elevated in patients with pancreatitis of moderate severity. In the first 24 h the mean value of C3 is reduced in patients with severe pancreatitis. C3 is also further reduced in patients who eventually die, while in those who survive C3 gradually normalizes during recovery. Using Pearson's correlation coefficient and Fisher's method we found a strong correlation between Ranson's criteria, toxemia, low C3, and the rate of complications ($r = 0.72$, $p < 0.001$).

Discussion

A very significant positive correlation was found between Ranson's criteria and toxemia. The way in which toxemia increases morbidity and mortality remains obscure. According to our results toxemia is perhaps the initiating factor of the activation and subsequent consumption of the complement. Toxemia may also be closely related to the activation of other cascade systems. The cascade system activation is responsible for the systemic inflammatory response syndrome and the multiple organ failure syndrome that eventually results. During the bacteremia that precedes septic shock, complement is activated by the alternative pathway. The same procedure has been observed in patients with severe acute pancreatitis [1].

A positive correlation was also observed between Ranson's criteria and C3. Complement's components C3 and C4 act as acute-phase compounds and their levels increase during the inflammatory diseases due to their increased production. The same components are reduced during the process of severe acute pancreatitis [3]. Serial blood samples must be evaluated to ascertain the actual levels of C3 and C4. During the course of severe acute pancreatitis these components seem to be consumed more rapidly than they can be produced, whilst in milder cases of pancreatitis production of C3 and C4 is greater than their consumption. This is reflected in the detected elevated values. The opposite is the case in severe acute pancreatitis.

We furthermore observed a positive correlation between Ranson's criteria and the rate of complications, but found that the presence of toxemia cannot predict the development of any specific complication. Chemical peritonitis that is the result of acute pancreatitis liberates toxins from the gut to the systemic circulation. The toxemia that ensues is probably the main causative role for the complications of the disease. Treating this peritonitis can be decisive for the survival of the patient [5].

References

1. Foulis AK, Murray WR, Galloway D et al. (1982) Endotoxemia and complement activation in acute pancreatitis in man. Gut 23: 656-661
2. Goldstein I, Cola D, Radin A et al. (1978) Evidence of complement catabolism in acute pancreatitis. Am J Med Sci 275: 257-264
3. Horn JK, Ranson J, Ong R et al. (1980) Evidence of complement catabolism in experimental acute pancreatitis. Am J Pathol 101: 205-216
4. Levin J (1987) The limulus amebocyte lysate test: perspectives and problems. In: Detection of bacterial endotoxins with the limulus amebocyte lysate test. Liss, New York, pp. 1-23
5. Ranson J, Spencer F (1987) The role of peritoneal lavage in severe acute pancreatitis. Ann Surg 187: 565-573
6. Pierrakakis S (1986) Complement's activation in acute pancreatitis. Thesis, University of Athens

ICU Treatment of Patients with Acute Necrotizing Pancreatitis

R. Függer, P. Götzinger, T. Sautner, H. Andel, G. Huemer

Introduction

Despite rigorous efforts to improve the survival of patients suffering from acute necrotizing pancreatitis, mortality rates in the reported series remain in the range between 10% and 30%, depending on individual risk factors [1, 4, 6]. The main cause of death is multiple organ failure, either as a consequence of acute pancreatitis or of infectious and septic complications occurring in the course of the disease. Although acute necrotizing pancreatitis is a sterile inflammation at the onset, the development of systemic inflammatory response syndrome and multiple organ failure dysfunction as a consequence of pancreatic insult per se is well known [7]. However, bacterial contamination of pancreatic necrosis had been documented to occur as early as during the first week of the disease [1]. Therefore infection as the cause of systemic inflammatory response syndrome and multiple organ failure is of significant importance in the course of acute necrotizing pancreatitis and the most frequent cause of death. The removal of pancreatic necrosis is seen as the therapeutic goal in the treatment of acute necrotizing pancreatitis. Therefore intensive care therapy and surgery are forced to cooperate closely. Surgical procedures must eliminate necrotic tissue, abscesses, and other septic intra-abdominal foci. Intensive care therapy must prevent organ failures or, in the case of established organ dysfunction, to treat or support insufficient function. Beyond these two aspects, monitoring of organ functions in the intensive care unit and the interpretation of the course of organ function/dysfunction plays a key role in the indication for surgical revision.

Scoring Systems

Several scoring systems are applied to determine the severity of acute necrotizing pancreatitis. The Ranson score [8] is a specific score designed to assess the severity of pancreatitis by means of several selected parameters (serum calcium, blood urea nitrogen, hematocrit fall, base deficit, arterial pO_2, and fluid sequestration) in the first 48 h of pancreatitis. The Ranson score is widely accepted and shows a good correlation with prognostic outcome. However, in recent years other commonly used ICU scores, especially APACHE II [5], have been introduced for severity scoring and prognostic stratification in patients with acute necrotizing pancreatitis. Wilson and Larvin demonstrated that the APACHE II score most accurately predicts outcome and response to therapy [6, 13]. Another advantage of the APACHE II is the immediate availability at the time of admission. In addition, scores are absolutely necessary to compare reported patient series of various centers and with differing surgical strategies.

Organ Dysfunction

At the time of admission to the ICU patients may have established organ dysfunction or infectious complications of acute necrotizing pancreatitis. Previous operations of pancreatic necrosis before allocation to a specialized ICU and surgical center impair the outcome significantly because of a high incidence of organ dysfunctions and infected pancreatic necrosis. Of 125 patients with acute necrotizing pancreatitis 49 (39.2%) were transferred to our unit for further treatment after initial operations of pancreatic necrosis in other departments [4]. The incidence of organ dysfunction and infection at admission were: 18% cardiovascular failure (defined as need for norepinephrine or dobutamine for adequate perfusion), 34% pulmonary dysfunction (need for mechanical ventilation), 15% renal failure (need for continuous hemofiltration), 10% hepatic dysfunction (serum bilirubin > 3 gm/% or normotest < 50%), and 85% bacterial infection of pancreatic necrosis. The median APACHE II score was 15 (range 4 - 30).

Cardiovascular Dysfunction

Cardiovascular function is of crucial importance in acute necrotizing pancreatitis because failure reveals consecutive dysfunction of other organ systems. As generally known from sepsis or severe injury, a hyperdynamic cardiovascular state can be identified in the early phase of pancreatitis, even in absence of infectious complications. The major function of the circulatory system is the delivery of oxygen to the periphery. If oxygen delivery is insufficient, metabolic acidosis and dysfunction of other organs occur.

Therefore the two goals of circulatory support are to maintain a hyperdynamic cardiovascular state and to keep oxygen delivery sufficient [9]. Although there is controversy over whether oxygen delivery should be normal or supranormal, most intensivists try to achieve supranormal values. Therefore, the two goals of circulatory support are to maintain a hyperdynamic state and to keep oxygen delivery in a supranormal level. A cardiac index of more than 4.5 is the aim of therapeutic measures such as fluid support (cristalloids and/or colloids) and inotropics (norepinephrine, dobutamine, dopamine). Although there are differing opinions about the choice of fluid and inotropics, the importance of maintaining a hyperdynamic cardiovascular function is not disputed.

Except for the cardiac index, oxygen delivery depends on the arterial oxygen saturation and the oxygen-carrying capacity. Regarding a sufficient DO_2, arterial oxygen saturation should be more than 90% and hemoglobin between 10 and 12 mg/dl.

Overall, desired values of hemodynamic parameters in cardiovascular support of patients with acute necrotizing pancreatitis correspond to ranges known from the therapy of severe septic conditions.

These are:
Heart rate: < 120/min
Cardiac index: > 4.5 l min^{-1} m^{-2}
Mean arterial pressure: > 70 mmHg (normal)
Mean pulmonary artery pressure: < 20 mmHg
Pulmonary artery wedge pressure: 12 - 16 mmHg
Oxygen delivery: > 600 ml min^{-1} m^{-2}
Oxygen consumption: > 170 ml min^{-1} m^{-2}
Mixed venous oxygen saturation: > 70%

As a basic measure continuous arterial monitoring by an arterial catheter (a. radialis) is obligatory. In the case of an unsteady state, advanced cardiovascular monitoring by pulmonary artery catheter is indicated. Transesophageal echocardiography and recent technologies such as continuous cardiac output measurement extend the spectrum of cardiovascular monitoring.

Pulmonary Dysfunction

Pulmonary insufficiency, usually presenting as fully developed adult respiratory distress syndrome, is a frequent organ failure in acute necrotizing pancreatitis. Of the patients admitted to our unit 34% presented respiratory failure, defined as the necessity for mechanical ventilation. Although there are many different definitions of pulmonary dysfunction, this may simply be summarized as evidence of tachypnea (> 20/min) and an increase in arterial oxygen saturation (<90%) and paO$_2$ (< 50 mmHg). The therapy of pulmonary failure is mechanical ventilation (intermittent positive pressure ventilation). Some centers apply airway pressure release ventilation (biphasic positive airway pressure) in selected patients. For severe adult respiratory distress syndrome several therapeutical measures such as NO or extracorporal oxygenation are being studied and may play a role in future therapeutic concepts.

Renal Dysfunction

Renal failure may present as oliguric or nonoliguric. The causes are generally prerenal or renal; decreased plasma volume and impaired cardiac output are typical factors in renal dysfunction in acute necrotizing pancreatitis. This mechanism is well known from other conditions associated with a high frequency of renal failure, such as shock, severe trauma, and sepsis. However, toxic lesions of the parenchyma, for example due to nephrotoxic antibiotics or other drugs, may also play a role in renal dysfunction. To prevent dysfunction, low-dose dopamine bypass (2 µg kg^{-1} min^{-1} is generally administered. Furthermore, a steady circulatory state with a cardiac index above 4.5 and a mean arterial pressure higher than 70 mmHg is essential to avoid nephrotoxic drug effects. Nevertheless, the frequency of renal failure is high. In our patients 15% needed hemofiltration at the time of admission. Continuous pump driven veno-venous hemofiltration is the therapy of choice in established renal failure and generally preferred to hemodialysis. The indication of hemofiltration depends on the level of blood urea nitrogen, hyperpotassemia, and fluid balance; the possibility of positive effects with respect to toxin elimination are controversial [10].

Hepatic Dysfunction and Coagulation

Walvatne and Cerra define hepatic dysfunction as serum bilirubin above 3 mg/dl without biliary obstruction, evidence of hematoma, or transfusion reaction [11]. The frequency in our patients at admission was 10%, mostly affecting the synthetic function of the liver. As alcohol abuse, often associated with chronic hepatic failure or even cirrhosis, is a frequent cause of acute necrotizing pancreatitis, preexisting liver dysfunction must be noted. Therefore, substitution of components of blood coagulation may be necessary. In our ICU we substitute a normotest lowed than 30% and angiotensin III lower than 60%. For prevention of treatment of disseminated intravascular coagulation, heparin and aprotinin are administered according to laboratory coagulation test results.

Additional ICU Treatment

There are several other intensive care measures that are not specific to acute necrotizing pancreatitis. Some of these are subject of controversial debate. We use sucralfate for prophylaxis of ulcer stress bleeding in all our patients with pancreatic necrosis. Furthermore, every patient receives a nasogastric tube for continuous evacuation of the stomach. However, we do not use enteral nutrition in the early period of acute pancreatitis and provide complete parenteral nutrition. Frequent operative revisions, paralysis and elevated gastrointestinal, and biliary and pancreatic secretion are the reason for our restricting enteral feeding to the phase of recovery. Selective oral gut decontamination is another controversy among intensivists and surgeons. Although some report decreased bronchial infection in decontaminated patients, no positive effect with respect to survival has been shown. Based on these results we use oral decontamination only in immunosuppressed patients but not generally in all our pancreatitis patients.

Importance of Infection

Bacterial infection of pancreatic necrosis significantly worsens outcome. This has been shown in several studies [1, 2, 12] and in our own series [4]. However, not only infected necrotic tissue affects prognosis negatively. Survival is significantly decreased in cases of diffuse peritonitis, possibly due to intestinal fistulas, bacteremia, and bronchopulmonary infection (Table 1). Generalized infection with consecutive multiple organ failure is the leading cause of death in acute necrotizing pancreatitis. Beyond surgical elimination of septic intra-abdominal foci, adequate antibiotic therapy directed to germs found in bacteriological specimen is of essential importance.

Indication of Surgical Revision

Monitoring of organ functions in the intensive dare unit is of great help in surgical decision making. Organ dysfunction caused by persistent abdominal infection such as abscesses, peritonitis, or infected necrosis, has been known since the 1970s [3]. In cases of impaired organ function or failure to improve despite adequate ICU treatment an intraperitoneal focus should be suspected. In the absence of any extrapancreatic od extra-abdominal origin of organ dysfunction, deterioration in organ function is an indication for reoperation. The decision for operative revision may be supported by computed tomography controls in the case of organ dysfunction. On our unit, a surgical regimen of necrosectomy, open drainage by laparotomies and consecutive reoperations for the elimination of pancreatic necrosis is established [4]. In the period 1985-1988 most reoperations were performed in preplanned intervals, resulting in a high incidence of intestinal fistulas associated with this aggressive surgical regimen. A more individual, less aggressive concept with planned revision in the beginning and restriction of further reoperation to impending organ failure detected by intensive care monitoring ("on demand") decreased the rate of fistulas and mortality (Table 2).

Table 1: Effect of infection on mortality

	n	Mortality	
		n	%
Necrotic tissue (n=125)			
Noninfected	19	2	10
Infected	106	38	36
Blood culture (n=119)			
Negative	80	15	19
Positive	39	25	64
Bronchial infection (n=119)			
Negative	49	12	25
Positive	70	28	40

Negative, no bacterial infection; Positive, bacteriologically confirmed infection.

Table 2: Indication to revision in acute necrotizing pancreatitis

	APACHE II (median)	Revision		Mortality
1985/1988	15	Clinical	10%	28%
		Planned	80%	
		On demand	10%	
Since 1989	15	Planned	36%	17%
		On demand	64%	

References

1. Beger HG, Bittner R, Block S, Büchler M (1986) Bacterial contamination of pancreatic necrosis. Gastroenterology 91: 433-438
2. D'Egidio A, Schein M (1991) Surgical strategies in the treatment of pancreatic necrosis and infection. Br J Surg 78: 133-137
3. Fry DE, Pearlstein L, Fulton RL, Polk HC (1980) Multiple organ failure, the role of uncontrolled infection. Arch Surg 115: 136-140
4. Függer R, Schulz F, Rogy M, Herbst F, Mirza D, Fritsch A (1991) Open approach in pancreatic and infected pancreatic necrosis: laparotomies and preplanned revisions. World J Surg 15: 516-521
5. Knaus WA, Draper EA, Wagner DP, Zimmerman JE (1985) APACHE II: a severity of disease classification system. Crit Care Med 13: 818-829
6. Larvin M, McMahon MJ (1989) APACHE II score for assessment and monitoring of acute pancreatitis. Lancet 2: 201-204
7. Members of the American College of Chest Physicians/Society of Critical Care Medicine Consensus Conference Committee (1992) Definition for sepsis and organ failure and guidelines for the use of innovative therapies in sepsis. Crit Care Med 20: 864-874
8. Ranson JHC, Rifkind KM, Roses DF, Fink SD, Eng K, Spencer FC (1974) Prognostic signs and the role of operative management in acute pancreatitis. Surg Gynecol Obstet 139: 69-80
9. Shoemaker WC (1986) Hemodynamic and oxygen transport patterns in septic shock: physiologic mechanisms and therapeutic implications. In: Sibbald WC, Sprung CL (eds.) Perspectives on sepsis and septic shock. Society of Critical Care Medicine, Fullerton
10. Sporn P (1992) Hämofiltrations- und Dialysemethoden in der operativen Intensivmedizin. Chirurg 63: 993-998
11. Walvatne C, Cerra FB (1990) Hepatic dysfunction in multiple organ failure. In: Deitch E (ed.) Multiple organ failure. Thieme, Stuttgart
12. Widdison AL, Karanjia ND (1993) Pancreatic infection complication acute pancreatitis. Br J Surg 80: 148-154
13. Wilson C, Heath DI, Imrie CW (1990) Prediction of outcome in acute pancreatitis: a comparative study of APACHE II, clinical assessment and multiple factor scoring systems. Br J Surg 77: 1260-1264

Surgical Treatment of Necrotizing Pancreatitis

W. Uhl, M.W. Büchler

Introduction

Clinical management of acute pancreatitis is based on the observation that most patients have a mild, self-limiting disease [1-3]. However, there are uncertainties with regard to the therapeutic schedule since a specific and effective pharmacotherapy is not available, and the effectiveness of a surgical therapy of necrotizing pancreatitis has not been substantiated by controlled prospective clinical data up to now. In patients with acute pancreatitis and local septic complications following a bacterial infection of the necrotic material surgical therapy was proved undoubtedly superior to the conservative treatment protocol in the past [4-6].

The goals of surgical management of necrotizing pancreatitis are: removal of necrotic peri- and intrapancreatic tissue, emptying of pancreatogenic ascites in the peritoneal cavity and the lesser sac, and blocking of the inflammatory and necrotizing process to prevent systemic release of vasoactive and toxic substances. A further very important step in operative therapy is preserving vital intact pancreatic tissue. This is based on the experience that from a morphological point of view the necrotizing process is often represented mainly by fatty tissue necroses in and around the vital exocrine and endocrine pancreatic parenchyma [7, 8].

In the past, a variety of surgical treatment modalities have been propagated, including pancreatic resection [9-11], peritoneal dialysis [12-14], multiple tube drainage [15], surgical débridement and suction drainage [5, 16], necrosectomy with postoperative continuous local lavage of necrotic cavities [17], various forms of open packing [18-21], and nonoperative drainage using percutaneous techniques [22-24]. However, the results of an operative therapy for necrotizing pancreatitis depend not only on the surgical technique used but also on the patient series, severity of concomitant morbidity factors, timing of surgical intervention, extent of the necrotizing process, and - most important - on bacterial infection of the necroses [6, 25].

Indication for Surgical Management

The development of pancreatic parenchymal and/or extrapancreatic necroses are undoubtedly the critical feature determining the prognosis of acute pancreatitis. For the early assessment of the severity of acute pancreatitis single, simple to determine, and reliable blood parameters, such as C-reactive protein, PMN elastase, and phospholipase A_2 catalytic activity have been shown to have high accuracy rates for detecting pancreatic necroses in morphological well-defined patient populations with acute pancreatitis [26-28]. Therefore, today contrast-enhanced computed tomography can be restricted to those cases with high values of these necroses-indicating parameters in dealing with special questions such as the evaluation of the intra- and extrapancreatic extent of necroses (Fig. 1).

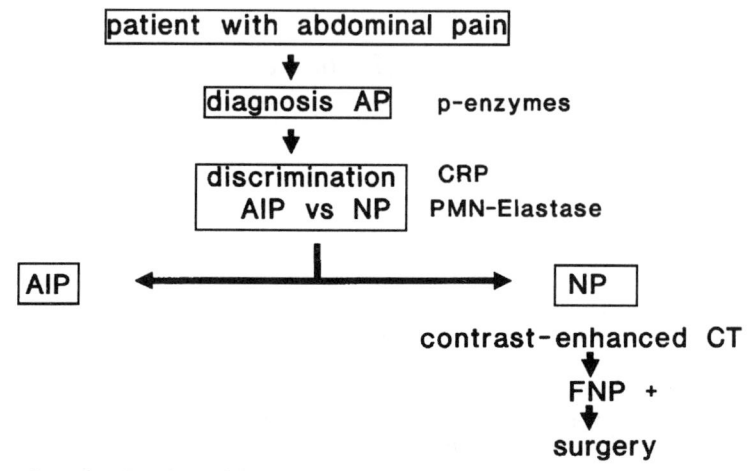

```
        patient with abdominal pain
                     ↓
              diagnosis AP       p-enzymes
                     ↓
             discrimination     CRP
              AIP  vs  NP       PMN-Elastase
   AIP  ←──────────┴──────────→   NP
                                contrast-enhanced CT
                                       ↓
                                      FNP +
                                       ↓
                                     surgery
```

Fig. 1: Algorithm for clinical decision-making in acute pancreatitis. AIP, acute edematous pancreatitis; NP, acute necrotizing pancreatitis; FNP, fine needle puncture

There is no question that patients with proven severe necrotizing pancreatitis should be treated in an intensive care unit, as the early phase of the disease is characterized by organ complications such as shock, lung and kidney failure caused by the release of vasoactive and toxic substances [29]. A certain percentage of patients with necrotizing pancreatitis and organ complications can be treated successfully by intensive care measures alone, and thus an operation can be avoided [30]. Intensive care measures involve specific therapy forms against pulmonary, renal and cardiocirculatory dysfunctions.

Surgical management is indicated in patients who:

- exhibit infected necroses
- do not respond to maximal ICU treatment within 3-5 days

Specifically, from a clinical point of view, surgical management is indicated in patients who develop signs of a surgical acute abdomen and septic complications caused by a bacterial infection of necroses, primarily by gram-negative germs from the intestinal flora such as *Escherichia coli*, *Pseudomonas* and/or *Streptococcus faecalis*. The overall contamination rate of the necrotic material is approximately 40% in the first week of the disease [6]. Persisting organ failure such as pulmonary and/or renal insufficiency, severe cardiovascular insufficiency, and metabolic disorders are further indications for surgical therapy if these complications worsen over a period of at least 3 - 5 days of maximum intensive care treatment. The assessment of nonresponse of the local and systemic organ complications to conservative therapy is a very important interdisciplinary step and the basis of the decision for surgery.

According to morphological and bacteriological criteria found by contrast-enhanced computed tomography [31] for the evaluation of intra- and extrapancreatic necroses and fine needle aspiration [32], with Gram staining and cultures of the exudate and/or necroses patients with proven infected necroses are clear candidates for surgical intervention. Patients with focal or minor necroses present a moderate clinical picture and therefore respond mostly to conservative therapy [30].

A total of 170 patients suffering from necrotizing pancreatitis were surgical treated at the Department of General Surgery, University of Ulm, between May 1982 and December 1992. An acute surgical abdomen developed in about 8% and sepsis in about 39%; 48% had to be operated on for systemic organ complications which had not responded to intensive care therapy (Table 1).

Table 1: Indications for surgical management of patients with proven necrotizing pancreatitis ($n = 170$)

	n	%
Acute surgical abdomen	14	8.0
Sepsis	67	39.0
Multiorgan systemic failure (despite ICU treatment 3-5 days)	82	48.0
Shock	34	20.0
Pulmonary insufficiency	94	55.0
Renal failure	14	8.0
Severe metabolic disorders	9	5.0

Timing of Surgery

The operative therapy of necrotizing pancreatitis is based on an exhaustive application of conservative intensive care measures. The timing of surgical intervention in severe acute pancreatitis is still under discussion today. The intervention can be performed early, that is in the acute phase, if complications arise which make an early operation absolutely necessary [33, 34], or if the diagnosis is still uncertain [35], but the intervention can also be delayed [24]. The rationale for delaying surgical therapy is to wait until demarcation of the necroses has occurred. However, the problem is that the demarcation process cannot be evaluated objectively. Furthermore, there are no sufficiently objective data about the response to conservative therapy and the efficiency of maximum intensive care treatment protocols (e.g., long-term artificial respiration or hemofiltration). However, a minimum period of intensive care therapy should be observed. In our series surgery was carried out on the ninth day on average (range 1 - 64 days) after the onset of acute abdominal symptoms, and on the fifth day (on average) of ICU treatment (range 0 - 56 days). Early operative intervention in the first week of the disease is indicated only in the small group of patients with fulminant necrotizing pancreatitis (subtotal to total necroses of the pancreatic gland) and in proven early bacterial infection of the necroses.

Techniques of Surgical Treatment

Surgical treatment of necrotizing pancreatitis centers on the removal of the necroses and the continuous evacuation of pancreatic fluids, which may contain bacterial and biologically active compounds. Thus, peritoneal dialysis [13, 14] alone cannot be considered an adequate therapy for acute pancreatitis, as has been demonstrated by Mayer et al. [14]. In this study hospital mortality was the same in the control group and in the group treated with peritoneal dialysis (27% and 28%, respectively). According to current clinical studies, a significant reduction in organ complications and mortality rate cannot be achieved, nor is it to be expected, as the effects of peritoneal lavage are restricted to the abdominal cavity and have no influence on the persisting necrotizing process in the retroperitoneal spaces. This therapeutic approach does not provide for an evacuation of necrotic or bacterially infected tissue.

The exclusive operative implantation of several thick drainage tubes into the omental bursa, combined with a bile duct drainage (cholecystectomy plus T-drainage), gastrostomy, and jejunostomy is only partly successful, as necrostomy is missing. This treatment form, known as triple-tube drainage [15] and applied mostly in United States clinics in the 1970s, aims at draining ascitic fluid from the lesser sac and inhibiting exocrine pancreatic secretion. Application of this surgical procedure has shown, however, that it does not lead to a substantial reduction of morbidity and mortality. As necroses and bacterially infected intra- and retropancreatic inflammatory process are not removed, it is not surprising that pancreatic abscesses grow up to 40% after application of this tripple-tube drainage [36].

Surgical treatment of necrotizing pancreatitis with the classical resection techniques - hemipancreatectomy, partial or total pancreaticoduodenectomy - aims at the total removal of the diseased pancreatic tissue or the whole organ [9-11]. Partial or total pancreaticoduodenectomy also requires removal of otherwise healthy organs (duodenum, parts of the stomach, etc.) and this imposes additional stress on the severely ill patient. Furthermore, surgeons must be aware that in quite a number of cases with necrotizing pancreatitis only the external parts of the pancreas are necrotic, the pancreatic parenchyma around the pancreatic duct being intact. This type, known as superficial necrotizing pancreatitis, can easily be mistaken by the surgeon as a total necroses of the gland and lead to a wrong kind of treatment [7], if he does not know the overall morphology, which might be seen from contrast-enhanced computed tomography of the pancreas. Except for the very rare case of total pancreatic necrosis, pancreatic resection involves the risk of overtreatment and increases in late morbidity and mortality which are caused mainly by endo- and exocrine insufficiency.

As the exclusive lavage or drainage of the retroperitoneum is not able to reduce the high morbidity and mortality rates in necrotizing pancreatitis, other surgical principles, combined with débridement of necroses, have been introduced. In the Mayo series published by Becker et al. [37] hospital mortality of patients with pancreatic abscess was 40% and the reoperation rate 31% (Table 2). The authors were dissatisfied with these results, feeling that surgical necrosectomy with drainage alone was insufficient for a significant reduction in mortality. Therefore, additional treatment protocols following surgical débridement were developed. These surgical modalities comprise the application of open packing with multiple redressing, multiple stump drainage with lavage or planned frequent reoperations with or without a zipper [11, 18, 20, 21]. Multiple redressings and frequent reoperations remove the necroses and are carried out in combination with intraoperative lavage. The Boston series reported by Warshaw and Jin [5] showed a significant decrease in hospital mortality of patients with necrotizing pancreatitis or pancreatic abscess (Table 2). The overall hospital mortality in the Boston series was 24%; in a later period only 1 of 19 patients died. In Atlanta the open packing technique is applied exclusively [21]. Multiple redressings, however, entail many reoperations, a prolonged intensive care phase, and an enormous additional stress for the patient. Multiple reoperations are also the cause of an increased occurrence of intestinal fistula, stomach outlet stenosis, mechanical ileus, incisional hernia, and complications with local severe bleeding (Table 2).

Table 2: Results of surgical débridement/necrosectomy in necrotizing pancreatitis/pancreatic abscess

Reference	n	Hospital mortality % n	Hospitalization days	Postop. complications[a] (%)	Reoperations (%)	Additional surgical technique
Becker el al. [37]	62	40 (25/62)		80	31	Drainage
Warshaw and Jin [5]	45	24 (11/45)	49	84	27	Multiple suction
Bradley [21]	28	11 (3/28)	46	4-36	100	drainage Open packing

[a]Pancreatic fistula, enteric fistula, gastric obstruction, incisional hernia, retroperitoneal hemorrhage.

More recently, interventional techniques for the nonoperative management of necrotizing pancreatitis were introduced. Good results have been reported with large draining tubes placed percutaneously in the necrotic areas [22, 23], using imaging procedures and avoiding surgical intervention completely. So far the experience with this new treatment protocol is limited, however, and obviously this method cannot guarantee the complete removal of necrotic areas. Every second patient in the van Sonnenberg [23] series had to be operated on after drainage, since the removal of necrotic tissue and the bacterially infected necroses was not efficient enough.

Necrosectomy and Closed Continuous Local Lavage

For the treatment of pancreatic necroses we strongly advocate surgical débridement - necrosectomy - supplemented by intraoperative and postoperative closed continuous local lavage of the lesser sac and of the necrotic cavities in the retroperitoneum involved [2]. This provides an atraumatic and continuous evacuation of devitalized necrotic tissue as well as removal of bacterially infected dead tissue and biologically active substances from the ongoing necrotizing process after necrosectomy.

After opening of the abdominal cavity, using an upper abdominal midline incision in most patients, the gastrocolic and duodenocolic ligaments are divided, and the pancreas is exposed. The extent of necroses in the head, body and tail of the gland can easily be assessed and measured. Débridement of necrosectomy, either digitally or by the careful use of instruments, permits the exclusive elimination of all demarcated devitalized tissue, preserving the vital pancreatic parenchymal tissue. After surgical débridement, a thorough hemostasis with transfixion stitches, using monofilament suture material, is mandatory. It has become increasingly clear that it is not necessary to remove every gram of devitalized tissue because any tissue being or becoming necrotic is rinsed out by the lavage fluid. After the surgical débridement and suturing of bleeding vessels, an extensive intraoperative lavage is performed using 3 - 6 l of normal saline to clear the surface of the pancreatic and peripancreatic tissues. For the postoperative closed continuous local lavage (the necrotizing process is of course still going on) two or more large (28 - 34 F) double-lumen silicon rubber tubes are inserted so that a regionally restricted lavage is effected at least. The gastrocolic and duodenocolic ligaments are sutured to create a closed retroperitoneal lesser sac compartment for the postoperative continuous lavage. In the first postoperative days the amount of lavage fluids is 20-40 l per tube, a fast reduction taking place during the following days, depending on the clinical course and the appearance of the outflowing liquid. For the lavage a slightly hyperosmotic fluid is used, generally the normal solution for continuous ambulatory peritoneal dialysis. Lavage can be stopped as soon as there are no more signs of acute pancreatitis, and after the necrotic cavities have been completely cleansed. This is confirmed by the measurement of pancreatic enzyme levels in the return fluid, and by assessing its sterility. Finally, the drainage tubes are removed.

170 patients with necrotizing pancreatitis have been treated by this protocol (Table 3). The patients had a severe type of pancreatitis with 4.7 Ranson points (mean) and an infection rate of 43%. The mean postoperative lavage duration was 39 days, and the amount of lavage fluid was 8 l per day (median). In the postoperative period after necrosectomy and during closed local lavage treatment systemic organ complications were rare and occurred mainly in connection with local complications. There were 64 patients (37.6%) who had to be reoperated on, mostly for an abscess or an ongoing necrotizing process forming in the area of the original necrotic cavity which was not drained by the tubes. In these patients with the severe type of necrotizing pancreatitis hospital mortality was 14% (24/170). Death was mostly related to the extent of necroses and the presence of bacterial infection of the necroses. The mortality rate of patients with infected necroses was approximately twice as high as that of patients with sterile pancreatic necroses (20% vs. 11%).

Table 3: Results of necrosectomy and continuous local lavage in necrotizing pancreatitis ($n=170$)

Preoperatively	Severity of disease; Infected necroses	4.7 Ranson points (median) 43%
Postoperatively	Hospitalization	61 days (median among survivors)
	Lavage duration	39 days (mean)
	Lavage fluid	8l/24 h (median)
	Reoperation	37.6% (64/170)
	Hospital mortality	14.1% (24/170)

References

1. Warshaw AL (1980) A guide to pancreatitis. Compr Ther 6: 49-55
2. Beger HG, Büchler M (1986) Decision-making in surgical treatment of acute pancreatitis: operative or conservative management of necrotizing pancreatitis? Theor Surg 1: 61-68
3. Büchler M (1991) Objectification of the severity of acute pancreatitis. Hepatogastroenterology 38: 101-108
4. Beger HG, Krautzberger W, Bittner R, Block S, Büchler M (1985) Results of surgical treatment of necrotizing pancreatitis. World J Surg 90: 927-979

5. Warshaw AL, Jin G (1985) Improved survival in 45 patients with pancreatic abscess. Ann Surg 202: 408-417
6. Beger HG, Krautzberger W, Bittner R, Büchler M, Block S (1986) Bacterial contamination of pancreatic necrosis. A prospective clinical study. Gastroenterology 91: 433-438
7. Leger L, Chiche B, Ghouti A, Lovel A (1978) Pancreatitis aigues necrose capsulaire superficielle et atteinte aprenchsmateuse. J Chir (Paris) 115: 65-70
8. Becker W (1981) Pathological anatomy and pathogenesis of acute pancreatitis. World J Surg 5: 303-313
9. Edelmann G, Boutelier P (1974) Le traitement des pancréatites aigues nécrosantes par l'ablation chirurgicale précoce des portions nécrosées. Chirurgie 100: 155-167
10. Alexandre JH, Guerreri MT (1981) Role of total pancreatectomy in the treatment of necrotizing pancreatitis. World J Surg 5: 369-377
11. Hollender LF, Meyer C, Marrie A, daCosta SE, Castellanos JG (1981) Role of surgery in the management of acute pancreatitis. World J Surg 5: 361-368
12. Wall AJ (1965) Peritoneal dialysis in the treatment of severe acute pancreatitis. Med J Aust 2: 281-287
13. Lasson A, Balldin G, Genell S, Ohlsson K (1984) Peritoneal lavage in severe acute pancreatitis. Acta Chir Scand 150: 479-484
14. Mayer AD, McMahon MJ, Corfield AP, Cooper MJ, Williamson RCN, Chir M (1985) Controlled clinical trial of peritoneal lavage for the treatment of sever acute pancreatitis. N Engl J Med 312: 399-404
15. McCarthy MC, Dickermann RM (1982) Surgical management of severe acute pancreatitis. Arch Surg 117: 476-480
16. Watermann NG, Walsky RS, Kasdan ML (1968) The treatment of acute hemorrhagic pancreatitis by sump drainage. Surg Gynecol Obstet 126: 963-974
17. Beger HG, Büchler M, Bittner R, Block S, Nevalainen T, Roscher R (1988) Necrosectomy and postoperative local lavage in necrotizing pancreatitis. Br J Surg 75: 207-221
18. Knol JA, Eckhauser FE, Strodel WE (1984) Surgical treatment of necrotizing pancreatitis by marsupialization. Am Surg 50: 340-345
19. Stone HH, Strom PR, Mullins RJ (1984) Pancreatic abscess management by subtotal resection and packing. World J Surg 8: 340-345
20. Wertheimer MD, Norris CS (1986) Surgical management of necrotizing pancreatitis. Arch Surg 121: 484-487
21. Bradley EL III (1987) Management of infected pancreatic necrosis by open drainage. Ann Surg 206: 542-550
22. Gerzof SG, Robbins AJ, Johnson WC, Birkett DH, Nabseth DC (1981) Percutaneous catether drainage of abdominal abscess: a five-year experience. N Engl J Med 305: 643-657
23. Van Sonnenberg E, Wing VW, Casola G, Nakamoto SK, Mueller PR, Ferruci JT, Halasz NA, Simeone JF (1984) Temporizing effect of percutaneous drainage of complicated abscess in critically ill patients. Am J Roentgenol 142: 821-826
24. Larvin M, Chlamers AG, Robinson PJ, McMahon MJ (1989) Debridement and closed cavity irrigation for the treatment of pancreatic necrosis. Br J Surg 76: 465-471
25. Büchler M, Malfertheiner P, Friess H, Bittner R, Vanek E, Schlegel P, Beger HG (1989) The penetration of antibiotics into human pancreas. Infection 17: 20-25
26. Büchler M, Malfertheiner P, Schoetensack C, Uhl W, Beger HG (1986) Sensitivity of antiproteases, complement factors and C-reactive protein in detecting pancreatic necrosis. Results of a prospective clinical study. Int J Pancreatol 1: 227-235

27. Büchler M, Malfertheiner P, Schädlich H, Nevalainen TJ, Friess H, Beger HG (1989) Role of phospholipase A2 in human acute pancreatitis. Gastroenterology 97: 1521-1526
28. Uhl W, Büchler M, Malfertheiner P, Martini M, Beger HG (1991) PMN-elastase in comparison with CRP, antiproteases, and LDH as indicators of necrosis in human acute pancreatitis. Pancreas 6: 253-259
29. Beger UH, Bittner R, Büchler M, Hess M, Schmitz JE (1986) Hemodynamic data pattern in patients with acute pancreatitis. Gastroenterology 90: 74-79
30. Büchler M, Malfertheiner P, Uhl W, Beger HG (1988) Conservative treatment of necrotizing pancreatitis in patients with minor pancreatic necrosis. Pancreas 3: 592
31. Block S, Maier W, Clausen C, Bittner R, Büchler M, Malfertheiner P, Beger HG (1986) Identification of pancreas necrosis in severe acute pancreatitis. Gut 27: 1035-1042
32. Gerzof SG, Banks PA, Robbins AH (1984) Role of guided percutaneous aspiration in early diagnosis of pancreatic sepsis. Dig Dis Sci 29: 950
33. Kivilaakso E, Frøki O, Nikki P, Lempinen M (1981) Resection of the pancreas for acute fulminant pancreatitis. Surg Gynecol Obstet 152: 493-498
34. Poston GJ, Williamson RCN (1990) Surgical management of acute pancreatitis. Br J Surg 77: 5-12
35. Ranson JHC, Rifkind KM, Roses DF, Fink SD, Eng K, Spencer FC (1974) Prognostic signs and the role of operative management in acute pancreatitis. Surg Gynecol Obstet 139: 69-81
36. Warshaw AL (1974) Inflammatory masses following acute pancreatitis. Surg Clin North Am 54: 620-637
37. Becker JM, Pamberton JH, DiMagno EP, Jestrup DM (1984) Prognostic factors in pancreatic abscess. Surgery 96: 455-460

Section 9:

Infections in Transplantation: Epidemiology, Prevention and Treatment

Epidemiology of Infections After Bone Marrow Transplantation

H. Einsele, H. Hebart, U. Schumacher

Introduction

Even after the introduction of new antibacterial, antifungal, and antiviral agents in the treatment and prophylaxis of patients after bone marrow transplantation infections remain a major cause of morbidity and mortality after allogeneic marrow transplantation [1]. The incidence and the type of infectious complications depend largely on the source of the transplant and the transplantation modality. Recipients of an autologous marrow transplant develop fewer infectious complications than patients who undergo allogeneic bone marrow transplantation due to more rapid immune reconstitution and the lack of graft-versus-host disease (GvHD) and the consequent immunosuppressive therapy [2]. GvHD is one of the major risk factors for the development of infection [3]. Patients suffering from GvHD are specifically at risk of developing infectious complications due to the markedly disturbed immune reconstitution affected by the graft-versus-host reaction and its immunosuppressive treatment. Patients with acute GvHD usually do not die of target organ failure but rather of the complications of associated infections.

Following bone marrow transplantation - independent of the source of the transplant - there is an early phase of severe neutropenia and disturbance of a variety of granulocyte functions which renders these patients particularly sensitive to bacterial and fungal infections. In the later posttransplant period, especially in recipients of an allogeneic bone marrow transplant a severe combined disturbance of T- and B-lymphocyte function mainly determines the spectrum of infectious complications observed in these patients.

A distinct and very predictable pattern of infectious complications can be observed due to these different phases of disturbance of host defense which characterize the changing balance between the recovery of normal granulocyte and lymphocyte function and the ongoing immunosuppressive influence of GvHD and its treatment. Bacterial, viral, and fungal infections thus occur in a very predictable manner over the months following marrow transplant.

Bacterial Infections

The risk of bacterial infections is highest immediately following transplant during the period of neutropenia. The neutropenic period generally lasts for 3 - 4 weeks following marrow infusion until the neutrophil count rises above 500/µl. The bacteria causing infectious complications in this early posttransplant period originate mainly from the gastrointestinal tract, mouth and skin. Therefore apart from the effectiveness of the protective environment most of these patients are kept in laminar air-flow units, principally the mode of decontamination determines the incidence of bacterial infections in the marrow transplant recipient.

Due to alterations in the decontamination protocols - particularly the increased use of cotrimoxazol and of chinolones for enteral decontamination - the rate of gram-negative infections has been markedly decreased since the early 1970s. At that time gram-negative organisms (the three predominant being *Pseudomonas aeruginosa*, *Klebsiella pneumoniae*, and *Escherichia coli*) accounted for 71% of bacteremia [1]. A high rate of septic shock and death in untreated or inadequately treated granulocytopenic patients occurred during the course of a septicemia with these pathogens [1]. Gram-positive organisms, including both coagulase-positive and -negative staphylococci, have recently accounted for 61% of bloodborne infections after marrow transplant. The most frequently documented gram-positive organisms causing bacteremia are *Staphylococcus epidermidis* and *S. aureus*, as well as *Streptococcus viridans* and *pneumoniae*. While these organisms are generally less pathogenic than gram-negative organisms in granulocytic patients, there are exceptions. *Streptococcus mitis* (a subspecies of *S. viridans*) sepsis has been associated with fulminant, mostly fatal, shock. A common feature in patients with this complication is the presence of severe mucositis.

Fungal Infections

The incidence of fungal infections following allogenic bone marrow transplantation ranges from 9.5% [4] to 20% in some recent studies. Fungal infections are inherent, with a high mortality due to both diagnostic and therapeutic difficulties. The ability to distinguish patients at risk would therefore be of great value for early therapeutic intervention. Well-known risk factors for the development of invasive fungal infection in marrow transplant recipients are long-term and intensive application of broad-spectrum antibiotic therapy, a prolonged neutropenic period following marrow transplantation, the use of a central venous access, acute and chronic GvHD, and steroid treatment for GvHD.

Using bivariate logistic regression analysis at the time of bone marrow transplantation high recipient age, low bone marrow cell-dose, recipient cytomegalovirus (CMV) seropositivity, and splenectomy were significant risk factors for deep fungal infection [5]. In a multivariate analysis, only splenectomy, recipient CMV seropositivity, and low marrow cell dose were held significant [5]. On day 30 after bone marrow transplantation antithymocyte globulin treatment and GvHD grades II-IV were significant risk variables in bivariate regression and probability tests.

Candida is the most frequent nosocomial fungal pathogen in the marrow transplant recipient. Clinical syndromes in these patients include superficial colonization, superficial or invasive cutaneous infections, mucous membrane infection, deep organ infection or disseminating infection [6]. The term invasive fungal infection refers to the penetration of *Candida* species into tissue below the epithelial surface and/or infection of viscera. *Candida* infections are mostly endogenous infections. This means that infection starts by colonization, and *Candida* may be a part of the normal oral, vaginal, and gastrointestinal flora of the adult. In infants, additionally, cutaneous colonization is a common event. During hospitalization it has been reported that more than 50% of patients become colonized with *Candida* species [7]. *C. albicans* is the most commonly isolated species causing disseminating infections, followed by *C. tropicalis* in immunosuppressed populations [8]. Organs most often infected are the kidneys, brain, heart, lungs, eyes, skin, skeletal muscle, liver, spleen, bone, and joints [9]. In an affected organ, multiple small micro- or macroabscesses develop, but these seldom become large enough, except in neutropenic patients, for detection by contrast radiography or ultrasonography. *Candida* can overcome the epithelial barrier and reach the blood stream through catheters; thus systemic infection can occur via intact mucosa, for example, intestinal manipulation, chemotherapy, and irradiation to the gut mucosa further increases the possibility for the fungi to gain access into the vascular system. If the infection is disseminated, many *Candida* organisms are removed by Kupffer cells in the liver or trapped by capillars of the lung. Therefore only few yeast cells reach the systemic circulation resulting in the low sensitivity of blood cultures.

Whereas about 80% of transplant recipients are colonized by *C. albicans*, only 5% of these patients develop disseminated infection. In contrast, only 30% of patients are colonized by *C. tropicalis*, but 56% of these patients with long-term granulocytopenia develop disseminated infection.

Aspergillus species are soil-dwelling fungi, which in contrast to *Candida* can be often isolated from air samples, dust, food, and plants within hospitals. The most pathogenic species of *Aspergillus* are *A. fumigatus*, *A. flavus*, and *A. niger*. The infection is nosocomial and usually acquired by airborne transmission by direct inoculation from occlusive bandages. Furthermore, outbreaks of *Aspergillus* infections have occurred when construction work has been carried out in the hospital or nearby. Clinical syndromes include allergic aspergillosis, pulmonary infection with cavitation, and hemorrhage, which can be fatal. The upper respiratory tract and sinuses are the main parts of entrance of *Aspergillus* species for dissemination to other organs such as the kidneys, heart with myocardial infarction, and brain infection with or with out hemorrhages and infarction.

Cytomegalovirus

CMV infection remains the major cause of infectious morbidity and mortality during the first 100 days after allogeneic bone marrow transplantation but may also occur after autologous bone marrow transplantation. The incidence of CMV infection has been found to be much lower following autologous bone marrow transplantation than allogeneic bone marrow transplantation, but severe clinical manifestations, such as CMV-induced interstitial pneumonia may also occur [10, 11]. The median time of onset of CMV disease at our institution is 56 days after transplant [12]. The use of CMV-seronegative blood products can prevent CMV infection at least in CMV-seronegative patients receiving a transplant from a CMV-seronegative donor.

CMV infections occur at a high frequency in CMV-seropositive patients and those receiving a transplant from a CMV-seropositive donor (up to 80%) [13]. Clinical manifestations of CMV infection include interstitial pneumonia, enteritis, hepatitis, encephalitis, and rarely retinitis and adrenalitis as commonly seen in AIDS patients. The most threatening manifestation of CMV disease is CMV-induced interstitial pneumonia. Even when receiving the most effective therapy, a combination of ganciclovir and CMV-hyperimmunoglobulin - after an initial good response [14, 15] - only 31% of allogeneic marrow transplant recipients developing CMV-induced interstitial pneumonia survive the first 3 months following the onset of the disease. CMV-enteritis and hepatitis is also associated with high morbidity and mortality in marrow transplant recipients. New therapeutic strategies have therefore been developed for these patients: preemptive therapy and prophylaxis with antiviral agents.

Two studies [16, 17] have demonstrated significant reduction in the incidence of CMV disease by preemptive therapy with ganciclovir introduced at the time of first detection of the virus by culture technique. Due to the fact that culture assays have failed to detect CMV prior to the onset of CMV disease in 13% - 23% of patients, placebo-controlled studies [18] were performed to evaluate the prophylactic ganciclovir in the CMV-seropositive patient. In spite of a marked reduction in CMV infection and disease the survival rate is not better than in the placebo group, possibly due to an increase in the incidence of other infectious complications. New techniques such as polymerase chain reaction (PCR) and antigenemia assay are therefore applied to diagnose CMV infection in these patients earlier and thus to introduce antiviral therapy earlier [12]. PCR assays seem to be suitable even for a preemptive approach, due to the fact that they have been shown to provide a negative predictive value of 100% [19].

Herpes Simplex Virus Infection

Herpes simplex virus (HSV) infection develops primarily from reactivation of latent virus in patients who are seropositive for HSV at the time of transplant [20]. HSV infection occurs early after transplant, with a median time of onset of 9 days in patients not receiving prophylactic acyclovir and 78 days in patients routinely receiving prophylaxis from the time of conditioning until day 30 after transplant. Due to the fact that GvHD and its treatment markedly reduce the cell-mediated immunity which is essential for the control of virus infections, at least at our institution patients with chronic GvHD receive antiviral prophylaxis with acyclovir at least until day 180 after marrow transplantation.

Late Infections After Bone Marrow Transplantation

Most long-term survivors after bone marrow transplantation are healthy and need no further immunosuppression. However, 30% have mild to severe chronic GvHD characterized by immunodeficiency, frequent bacterial infections, and clinical lesions resembling those seen in autoimmune collagen vascular disease [21, 22]. Patients with chronic GvHD have persistent problems with host defense barriers due to mucosal atrophy and decreased lubrication of mucosal surfaces (sicca syndrome) and to decreased or absent secretory IgA, decreased opsonizing antibody, and functional neutrophil defects [23]. Therefore patients with chronic GvHD continue to have problems with bacterial infections; in fact, they are a major cause of death in these patients.

Most often patients with chronic GvHD affected by infections of the upper and lower respiratory tracts, skin infections, and septicemia [24]. Due to the markedly disturbed B cell function - especially the production of opsonizing antibodies - the most common cause of bacterial infections is encapsulated bacteria, such as *Streptococcus pneumoniae* and *Haemophilus influenzae*. In patients with chronic GvHD sinusitis, otitis media, and bacterial pharyngitis are the most common sites of bacterial infections, often caused by gram-negative bacteria, staphylococci and pneumococci. Pneumonia and bronchitis - other common infections in the patient with chronic GvHD - are caused mainly by *S. pneumoniae* or *Staphylococcus aureus*. Further manifestation of bacterial infections in these patients are purulent conjunctivitis and cystitis. Apart from bacterial infections, fungal infections may also occur, mainly with Candida species confined to the oral mucosa but also *Aspergillus* and *Nocardia* infections have also been described in these patients.

Prophylaxis with daily cotrimoxazol for the duration of treatment of chronic GvHD has been successful in reducing bacterial infections from 66% among patients not taking prophylaxis to 47% in patients receiving prophylaxis. Alternatively, oral penicillin has been used for prophylaxis of bacterial infections in patients receiving therapy for chronic GvHD.

Due to markedly disturbed T-B cell interaction during chronic GvHD patients affected by this complication often have subnormal levels of circulating immunoglobulin, which may predispose them to recurrent sinopulmonary infections. We are therefore currently evaluating weekly adjuvant immunoglobulin replacement with intravenous immunoglobulin (200 mg/kg body weight) in patients with severe chronic GvHD to determine whether this approach by immunomodulation cannot only ameliorate the GvHD but also reduce the incidence of infections and pulmonary complications in these patients.

References

1. Bowden RA, Meyers JD (1985) Infectious complication following marrow transplantation. In: Plasma therapy and transfusion technology, vol 6, no 2, pp. 285-302
2. Shiobara S, Harada M, Tori T et al. (1982) Difference in posttransplant recovery of immune reactivity between allogeneic and autologous bone marrow transplantation. Transplant Proc 2: 429-433
3. Paulin T, Ringden O, Nilsson B, Lönnqvist B, Gahrton G (1987) Variables predicting bacterial and fungal infections after allogeneic marrow engraftment. Transplantation 43: 393-398
4. Tollemar J, Homberg K, Ringden O, Lönnqvist B (1989) Surveillance tests for the diagnosis of invasive fungal infections in bone marrow transplant recipients. Scand J Infect Dis 21: 205-212
5. Tollemar J, Ringden O, Boström L, Nillson B, Sundberg B (1989) Variables predicting deep fungal infections in bone marrow transplant recipients. Bone Marrow Transplant 4: 635-641
6. Meunier F (1988) Fungal infections in the compromised host. In: Rubin RH, Young LS (eds.) Clinical approach to infection in the compromised host. Plenum, New York, p 193
7. Weber DJ, Rutala WA (1989) Epidemiology of hospital-acquired fungal infections. In: Holmberg K, Meyer R (eds.) Diagnosis and therapy of systemic fungal infections. Raven, New York, p 1
8. Wingard JR, Merz WG, Saral R (1979) Candida tropicalis: a major pathogen in immunocompromised patients. Ann Intern Med 91: 539
9. Edwards JE Jr (1989) Candidemia and Candida catheter-associated sepsis. In: Holmberg K, Meyers R (eds.) Diagnosis and therapy of systemic fungal infections. Raven, New York, p 39
10. Jules-Elysee K, Stover DE, Yahalom J, White DA, Gulati SC (1992) Pulmonary complications in lymphoma patients treated with high-dose therapy and autologous bone marrow transplantation. Am Rev Resp Dis 146: 485-491
11. Wingard JR, Chen DY, Burns WH et al. (1988) Cytomegalovirus infection after autologous bone marrow transplantation with comparison to infection after allogeneic bone marrow transplantation. Blood 71: 1432-1437
12. Einsele H, Ehninger G, Steidle M et al. (1991) Polymerase chain reaction to evaluate antiviral therapy for cytomegalovirus disease. Lancet 338: 1170

13. Petersen FB, Bowden RA, Thornquist M, Meyers JD, Buckner CD, Counts GW, Nelson MT, Newton BA, Sullivan KM, McIver J, Thomas ED (1987) The effect of prophylactic immune globulin on the incidence of septicemia in marrow transplant recipients. Bone Marrow Transplant 2: 141-148
14. Emanuel D, Cunningham I, Jules-Elysee K, Brochstein JA, Kernan NA, Laver J et al. (1988) Cytomegalovirus pneumonia after BMT successfully treated with the combination of ganciclovir and high-dose intraneous immunoglobulin. Ann Intern Med 109: 777-782
15. Reed EC, Bowden RA, Dandlike PS, Lillebay KE, Meyers JD (1988) Treatment of cytomegalovirus immunoglobulin in patients with bone marrow transplants. Ann Intern Med 109: 783-788
16. Goodrich JM, Moi M, Gleaves CA, Dumond C, Cays M, Ebeling DF et al. (1991) Early treatment with ganciclovir to prevent cytomegalovirus disease after allogeneic BMT. N Engl J Med 325: 1601-1607
17. Schmidt GM, Horak DA, Niland JC, Duncan SR, Forman SJ, Zaia JA (1991) A randomized controlled trial of prophylactic ganciclovir for CMV pulmonary infection in recipients of allogeneic bone marrow transplants. N Engl J Med 324: 1005-1011
18. Goodrich JM, Bowden RA, Fisher L, Keller C, Schoch G, Meyers JD (1993) Ganciclovir prophylaxis to prevent cytomegalovirus disease after allogeneic BMT. Ann Intern Med 118: 173-178
19. Einsele H, Ehninger G, Steidle M, Fischer I, Bihler S, Garneth A, Valbracht A, Schmidt H, Waller HD, Müller CA (1993) Lymphocytopenia as an unfavorable prognostic factor in patients with cytomegalovirus infection after BMT. Blood 82: 1672-1678
20. Wade JC, Newton B, Flournoy N, Meyers JD (1984) Oral acyclovir for prevention of herpes simplex virus reactivation after marrow transplantation. Ann Intern Med 100: 823-828
21. Noel DR, Witherspoon RP, Storb R, Atkinson K, Doney K, Mickelson EM, Ochs HD, Warren RP, Weiden PL, Thomas ED (1987) Does graft-versus-host disease influence the tempo of immunologic recovery after allogeneic human marrow transplantation? An observation on 56 long-term survivors. Blood 51: 1087-1105
22. Atkinson K, Storb R, Prentice RL, Weiden PL, Witherspoon RP, Sullivan K, Noel D, Thomas ED (1979) Analysis of late infections in 89 long-term survivors of bone marrow transplantation. Blood 53: 720-731
23. Sullivan KM, Deeg HJ, Sanders JE, Shulman HE, Witherspoon RP, Doney K, Appelbaum FR, Schubert MM, Stewart P, Springmeyer S, McDonald GB, Storb R, Thomas ED (1984) Late complications after marrow transplantation. Semin Hematol 21: 53-63
24. Atkinson K, Farewell V, Storb R, Tsoi M-S, Sullivan KM, Witherspoon RP, Fefer A, Clift R, Goodell B, Thomas ED (1982) Analysis of late infectious after human bone marrow transplantation: role of genotypic nonidentity between marrow donor and recipient and of nonspecific suppressor cells in patients with chronic graft-versus-host disease. Blood 60: 714-720

Infections in Lung - Transplant Recipients

A. Michalopoulos, V. Kadas, A. Anthi, E. Papadakis, J. Kriaras, G. Tzelepis, S. Geroulanos

Introduction

Over the past decade single lung transplantation has become a well-established therapeutic modality for many types of end-stage lung disease and chronic pulmonary hypertension [1, 2]. Because of several advantages over double lung or heart-lung transplantation, single lung transplantation continues to increase at an exponential rate [3].
Despite substantial progress in the postoperative care of pulmonary graft recipients pulmonary infections remain a significant cause of morbidity and mortality and a major determinant of early patient mortality [4]. Indeed, patients after lung transplantation have far more infectious complications than recipients of other solid organ transplants. The increased susceptibility to infection is attributed to several factors, including pulmonary hilar stripping, ischemic lung injury, immunosuppressive agents, mechanical ventilation, and exposure of both donor and recipient to ICU bacteria [5]. In addition, impaired mucociliary clearance due to alterations in ciliary action of respiratory epithelium and impaired phagocytosis of alveolar macrophages has been reported as another contributing factor [6, 7].

Bacterial Infection

The transplanted lung is particularly vulnerable to bacterial infection. It has been reported that bacterial pneumonia occurs in up to 60% of patients following lung transplantation. Although it can occur at any time after transplantation, it is most common in the early postoperative period [8]. Bacteria are the most frequent caus of pneumonia in the first postoperative month. Horvath et al. [9] reported that 12 of 15 recipients of single lung transplants had a significant infectious episode. Overall, 24 infections occurred in the first year after transplantation. Twenty of the infections were considered to be severe, and 19 involved the respiratory system. Ten cases were bacterial pneumonias. An infection rate of 38% of bacterial pneumonia was reported by Deusch et al. [10] in 29 lung transplant recipients within 2 weeks after lung transplantation.

Contributing factors in the development of bacterial post-transplant pneumonia include immunosuppressive therapy with corticosteroids, azathioprine, and cyclosporin A due to different mechanisms and alterations in the natural lung defence mechanisms induced by transplantation. Early infection is more likely in the setting of prolonged mechanical ventilation and reduced host response in the allogenic and immunosuppressed environment. Transfer of bacteria from the donor lung to the recipient is another local predisposing factor for the development of early postoperative pneumonia. In the late postoperative period (occurring after 100 days) the major predisposing factors appear to be the presence of chronic rejection and diseased airways [7], while bacterial airway colonisation and obliterative bronchiolitis may contribute to the development of infection.

During the early postoperative period *Staphylococcus aureus*, *Enterobacter spp.*, *Pseudomonas spp.*, *Haemophilus influenzae*, and *S. pneumonia* are the most common pathogens [3]. *Mycoplasma hominis*, *Legionella pneumophila*, and typical and atypical *Mycobacteria* can sometimes be isolated. Maurer et al. [11] and Deusch et al. [10] reported as more frequent bacterial organisms isolated gram-negative bacilli (*Klebsiella*, *Escherichia Coli* and *Pseudomonas*).

Patients with pulmonary infection are usually symptomatic. The most common symptoms are fever, shortness of breath and coughing.

The diagnosis of early bacterial pulmonary infection is usually difficult because of the similarity of symptoms with allograft rejection. The pathogen is revealed by means of sputum and blood cultures. When the cultures fail to help, bronchoalveolar lavage (BAL) is performed. The value of bronchoscopy for the diagnosis of infections or rejection in lung transplant recipients is controversial. Cultures are usually more sensitive for detection of bacterial infection [12]. Simbley et al. [13] studied the role of transbronchial biopsies in the management of lung transplant recipients and found histological evidence of infection in 17% of clinically stable or asymptomatic patients. Persistently high serum levels of interleukin 6 (IL-6) indicate the presence of infection, while a spiked elevation of IL-6 could have a predictive value in diagnosing rejection [14].

Intravenous antibiotics and chest physiotherapy are the mainstay of therapy.

Another factor to be considered is cross-infection, which clearly demonstrates the significance of early identification and treatment of any organisms colonising the trancheobronchial tree of donors. Zenati et al. [15] found culture-positive tracheal specimens in up to 76% of donors. The Pittsburgh transplant group recommends antibiotic treatment of all donors to lower the prevalence of subsequent infection in transplant recipients [16]. The organisms isolated from the recipient infections from the Pittsburgh series, however, were different from those initially identified in the donor tracheobronchial tree except in three patients who had systemic *Candida* infections.

The role of anti microbial prophylaxis in lung transplantation has not been fully determined. A study from the University of Pittsburgh [17] shows that the routine postoperative antibiotic administration significantly decreases the incidence of early pneumonia from 50% to 9%. The antibiotics used were a combination of ceftazidime, clindamycin, and an amino glycoside. Although these results appear extremely encouraging, further studies are needed before this approach becomes a widely acceptable form of therapy.

Bacterial pneumonia is one of the most common causes of early morbidity and mortality, especially in the first 2 weeks after transplantation. It is the first life-threatening infection that the recipient faces in the early postoperative period [18]. An evaluation of early causes of death at the University of Pittsburgh showed that infection is responsible for the majority of deaths (35%) [3]. Snell et al. [19] found that younger lung recipients tend to die from graft rejection while older patients (over the age of 50 years) die from infection.

Viral Infections

Cytomegalovirus (CMV) infection remains a substantial cause of morbidity in pulmonary allograft recipients. CMV is a common infectious agent and the most common pathogen in the period between 4th and 8th weeks after transplantation. The overall prevalence of CMV infection is about 50% in this period. The precise frequency of infection depends on a number of factors, such as the degree and type of immunosuppression and the immune status of the recipient. It is also largely determined by the transmission of CMV from the latently infected donor or the previous presence of virus in transplant recipient [20]. The use of immunosuppressive agents to prevent graft rejection is the most important factor responsible for reactivating latent infection and contributes to the occurrence of primary infection. Recurrence of infectious virus from the latent viral genomes is the initiating event in the pathogenesis of CMV infection after lung transplantation [21]. In a group of 46 lung transplant recipients who survived more than 1 month after operation, Ettinger et al. [22] documented a CMV infection rate of 92% in the patients who were donor negative/recipient positive, donor positive/recipient positive or donor positive/recipient negative. The incidence of CMV pneumonitis was 75%. Interestingly, no donor negative/recipient negative patient in this study experienced CMV infection.

From a clinical standpoint CMV infection is usually referred to as symptomatic or not, with or without lung involvement [23]. The CMV infection usually occurs at a median of about 50 days after transplantation [24]. Fever, myalgias, malaise, abdominal discomfort, pneumonitis, interstitial pneumonia, and/or hepatitis, leukopenia and thrombocytopenia are the common manifestations of CMV infection, which is usually mild. Infection with this virus may be chronic or recurrent. Lungs are the most common site for CMV recurrence.

CMV infection can be diagnosed serologically by means of the complement fixation test, enzyme-linked immunosorbent assay, and the detection of specific antibody to CMV (IgM and IgG) [25]. Isolation of virus from blood, urine, saliva, or BAL culture is extremely important in establishing the diagnosis. Fluorescent monoclonal antibodies against the early CMV antigen have been developed to ensure a rapid and reliable method of CMV detection [26]. The diagnosis of CMV pneumonitis is based on BAL and transbronchial lung biopsy [27, 28]. Differential cell counts and measurement of lymphocyte proliferation using specimens of BAL may be valuable in the diagnosis of CMV infection in lung transplant recipients [29]. Buffone et al. [30] found that polymerase chain reaction amplification of CMV DNA recovered from BAL and peripheral blood samples provides a powerful means of monitoring allowing detection of viral replication earlier than tissue culture after lung transplantation. The early diagnosis of CMV infection remains a keystone for patient after lung transplantation.

The current treatment of CMV infection is ganciclovir. A combination of ganciglovir and CMV immune globulin has also been suggested to treat severe CMV infections and CMV pneumonitis [31]. The most common adverse reaction of ganciglovir is neutropenia, while the CMV immune globulin has rare side effects [32, 33].

CMV prophylaxis remains controversial. Duncan et al. [34] treated 13 recipients at risk for CMV infection with 3 weeks of ganciclovir (IV 5 mg/kg twice a day for 14 days, starting 5 days after the transplantation, followed by 1 week of the drug at a dose of 5 mg/kg per day), followed by oral acyclovir (800 mg three times a day for an additional 2 months). CMV infection developed in 38% of recipients, which represents a decline in the incidence of CMV infection [34]. In contrast, Bailey et al. [35] reported no benefits with prophylactic use of ganciclovir along with polyvalent immune globulin in seven seronegative recipients of seropositive organs. The value of high dose acyclovir for CMV in this population is also not clear. Bolman et al. [36] reported higher than 50% incidence of CMV infection but no death in 44 lung recipients using 3200 mg/day oral acyclovir. Controlled trials of anti viral prophylaxis will be important in lung transplantation but require multicenter studies.

CMV infection has also been linked to both bronchiolitis and rejection. Although several studies in heart-lung recipients found a strong correlation between CMV infection and bronchiolitis the whole issue is controversial [37, 38]. Also the correlation between CMV infection and rejection is not fully verified.

Herpes simplex virus (HSV) and Epstein-Barr virus are found more frequently in lung transplant recipients than in other forms of transplantation. Maurer et al. [39] found 51 infection episodes in 40 lung recipients. Twelve of these episodes were viral (six disseminated zoster, four, HSV pneumonia, and two CMV pneumonia). Clinical manifestations include mucocutaneous lesions of the mouth, throat, and nose. Useful tools for the diagnosis of viral infection are serology, viral cultures, BAL, and transbronchial biopsy. Acyclovir is the treatment of choice. Antiviral prophylaxis (acyclovir 200 mg d.i.d.) is used mainly for HSV and CMV, especially during the first 3 months after transplantation. De Hoyos et al. [40] noted a reduction in HSV pneumonitis after the introduction of acyclovir prophylaxis.

Protozoal Infections

Apart from viral infections, a high incidence of *Pneumocystis carinii* pneumonia (PCP) has been reported in lung transplant recipients. The incidence of PCP in the absence of prophylaxis in transplant recipients ranges between 3% and 15%, while in heart-lung recipients a prevalence of 43% has been found [41]. PCP usually occurs after the third post transplantation month. Main symptoms are fever, cough and shortness of breath. Sometimes the patients are asymptomatic. Chest X-ray usually reveals diffuse infiltrates. PCP diagnosis is established quickly by means of BAL or transbronchial biopsy. Prophylaxis with oral administration of trimethoprim-sulfamethoxazole has proven effective in preventing PCP in heart-lung or lung transplant recipients [42]. Nathan et al. [43] suggest that inhaled pentamidine (300 mg on a monthly basis) is an effective and well-tolerated form of PCP prophylaxis in post-lung transplantation patients. In addition to morbidity and mortality, PCP has a potential for precipitating late rejection.

Fungal Infections

Because of increased frequency of airway colonisation *Candida albicans* commonly invades the lung tissue and causes life-threatening infection in lung transplant recipients throughout the intermediate postoperative period. The spectrum of clinical manifestations is wide. Sometimes *Candida* is found in association with *Aspergillus*. Treatment of choice is fluconazole because of its low toxicity. Antifungal prophylaxis remains controversial. Fluconazole is often used. The combination of low-dose amphotericin and itraconazole has a wider antifungal spectrum and remains a good alternative [44]. Although these agents have been used in lung transplant recipients, more studies and further experience is necessary before their routine prophylactic use [9].

References

1. Cooper JD (1991) Current status of lung transplantation. Transplant Proc 23: 2107-2114
2. Haydock DA, Trulock EP, Kaiser LR, Ettinger NA, Triantafillou AN, Ochoa LL (1992) Lung transplantation. J Thorac Cardiovasc Surg 103: 329-340
3. Heritier F, Madden B, Hodson ME, Yacoub M (1992) Lung allograft transplantation: indications, preoperative assessment and postoperative management. Eur Respir J 5: 1262-1278
4. American Thoracic Society (1993) Report of the ATS workshop on lung transplantation. Amer Rev Respir Dis 147: 772-776
5. Aeba R, Stout J, Francalancia N, Keenan R, Duncan A, Yousem S, Burckart G, Yu V, Griffith B (1993) Aspects of lung transplantation that contribute to increased severity of pneumonia. J Thorac Cardiovasc Surg 106: 449-457
6. Read RC, Shankar S, Rutman A, Feldman C, Yacoub M, Cole PJ (1991) Ciliary beat frequency and structure of recipient and donor epithelia following lung transplantation. Eur Respir J 4: 796-801
7. Shankar S, Fulsham L, Read RC, Theodoropoulos S, Cole PJ, Madden B (1991) Mucociliary function after lung transplantation. Transplant Proc 23: 1222-1223
8. Dauber JH, Paradis IL, Dummer JS (1990) Infectious complications in pulmonary allograft recipients. Clin Chest Med 11: 291-308
9. Horvath J, Dummer S, Loyd J, Walker B, Merrill W, Frist W (1993) Infection in the transplanted and native lung after single lung transplantation. Chest 104(3): 681-685
10. Deusch E, End A, Grimm M, Graninger W, Klepetko W, Wolner E (1993) Early bacterial infections in lung transplant recipients. Chest 104(5): 1412-1416
11. Maurer JR, Tullis DE, Grossman RF, Vellend H, Winton TL, Patterson GA (1992) Infectious complications following isolated lung transplantation. Chest 101(4): 1056-1059
12. Walts AE, Marchevsky AM, Morgan M. Pulmonary cytology in lung transplant recipients: recent trends in laboratory utilisation. Diagn-Cytopathol 7(4): 353-358
13. Simbley RK, Berry GJ, Tazelaar HD, Kraemer MR, Theodore J, Marshall SE, Billingham ME, Starnes VA (1993) The role of transbronchial biopsies in the management of lung transplant recipients. J Heart Lung Transplant 12(2): 308-324
14. Yoshida Y, Iwaki Y, Pham S, Dauber JH, Yousem SA, Zeevi A, Morita S, Griffith BP (1993) Benefits of posttransplantation monitoring of IL-6 in lung transplantation. Ann Thorac Surg 55(1): 89-93
15. Zenati M, Dowling RD, Armitage JM, Kormos RL, Dummer JS, Hardesty RL, Griffith BP (1989) Organ procurement for pulmonary transplantation. Ann Thorac Surg 48(1): 882-886
16. Dowling RD, Zenati M, Yousem SA, Pasculle AW, Kormos RL, Armitage JM, Griffith BP, Hardesty RL (1992) Donor transmitted pneumonia in experimental lung autografts. Successful prevention with donor antibiotic therapy. J Thorac Cardiovasc Surg 103: 767-772
17. Girffith BP, Hardesty RL, Armitage JM, Hattler BG, Pham SM, Keenan RJ, Paradis I (1993) A decade of lung transplantation. Ann Surg 218: 310-320
18. Low DE, Kaiser LR, Haydock DA, Trulock E, Cooper JD (1993) The donor lung: infectious and pathologic factors affecting outcome in lung transplantation. J Thorac Cardiovasc Surg 106: 614-621
19. Snell GI, De-Hoyos A, Winton T, Maurer JR (1993) Lung transplantation in patients over the age of 50. Transplantation 55(3): 562-566
20. Ho M. Cytomegalovirus infection and indirect sequelae in the immunocompromised transplant patient. Transpl Proc 23(2S): 2-7

21. Balthesen M, Messerle M, Reddehase MJ (1993) Lungs are a major organ site of Cytomegalovirus latency and recurrence. J Virol 67(9): 5360-5366
22. Ettinger NA, Bailey C, Trulock EP, Storch GA, Anderson D, Raab S, Spitznagel EL, Dresler C, Cooper JD (1993) Cytomegalovirus infection and pneumonitis. Impact after isolated lung transplantation. Washington University Lung Transplant Group. Am Rev Respir Dis 147(4): 1017-1023
23. Dummer JS, White LT, Ho M, Griffith BP, Hardesty RL, Bahnson HT (1985) Morbidity of CMV infection in recipients of heart-lung transplants who received cyclosporine. J Infect Dis 152: 1182-1191
24. Schmuth M, End A, Grimm M, Ringel, Wiser W, Wieselthaler G, Wollenek G, Klepetko W (1993) Cytomegalovirus infection following lung transplantation. Dtsch Med Wochenschr 118(11): 365-370
25. Wreghitt T (1989) Cytomegalovirus infections in heart and lung transplant recipients. J Antimicrob Chemother 23S: 49-60
26. Emanuel D, Peppard J, Stover D, Gold J, Armstrong D, Hammerling U (1986) Rapid immunodiagnosis of CMV pneumonia by bronchoalveolar lavage using human and murine monoclonal antibodies. Ann Intern Med 104: 476-481
27. Paradis IL, Grgurich WF, Dummer JS, Dekker JS, Dekker A, Dauber JH (1988) Rapid detection of CMV pneumonia from lung lavage cells. Am Rev Respir Dis 138: 697-702
28. Higenbottam T, Stewart S, Wallwork J (1988) Transbronchial lung biopsy to diagnose lung rejection and infection of heart-lung transplants. Transplant Proc 20S: 767-769
29. Maurer R, Gough E, Chamberlain D, Patterson G, Grossman RF (1989) Sequential bronchoalveolar lavage studies from patients undergoing double lung and heart-lung transplant. Transpl Proc 21(1): 2585-2587
30. Buffone GJ, Frost A, Samo T, Demmler GJ, Cagle PT, Laurence EC (1993) The diagnosis of CMV pneumonitis in lung and heart-lung transplant patients by CPR compared with traditional laboratory criteria. Transplantation 56(2): 342-347
31. Hutter JA, Scott J, Wreghitt T, Higenbottam T, Wallwork J (1993) The importance of Cytomegalovirus in heart-lung transplant recipients. Chest 95: 627-631
32. Watson FS, O' Connell JB, Amber IJ, Renlund DG, Classen D, Johnston JM, Smith CB, Bristow MR (1988) Treatment of CMV pneumonia in heart transplant recipients with DHPG. J Heart Transplant 7: 102-105
33. Metselaar HJ, Velzing J, Rothbarth PH, Bakl AH, Mochtar B, Weimar W (1989) Prophylactic use of anti-CMV immunoglobulins in heart transplant recipients: a study of safety. Transpl Proc 21: 2504-2505
34. Duncan SR, Paradis IL, Dauber JH, Yousem SA, Hardesty RL, Griffith BP (1992) Ganciclovir prophylaxis for CMV infections in pulmonary allograft recipients. Am Rev Respir Dis 146: 1213-1215
35. Bailey TC, Trulock EP, Ettinger NA, Storch GA, Cooper JD, Powderly WG (1992) Failure of prophylactic ganciclovir to prevent Cytomegalovirus disease in recipients of lung transplants. J Infect Dis 165: 548-552
36. Bolman RM, Shunqay SJ, Estrin JA, Hertz MI (1991) Lung and heart-lung transplantation. Ann Surg 214: 456-470
37. Keenan RJ, Lega ME, Dummer JS, Paradis IL, Dauber JH, Rabinowich H, Yousem SA et al. (1991) Cytomegalovirus serologic status and postoperative infection correlated with risk of developing chronic rejection after pulmonary transplantation. Transplantation 51: 533-538

38. Scott JP, Higenbottam TW, Sharples L, Clelland CA, Smyth RL, Stewart S, Willwork A (1991) Risk factors for obliterative bronchiolitis in heart-lung transplant recipients. Transplantation 51: 813-817
39. Maurer JR, Tullis DE, Grossman RF, Vellend H, Winton I, Patterson GA (1992) Infectious complications following isolated lung transplantation. Chest 101: 1056-1059
40. De Hoyos AL, Patterson GA, Maurer JR, Ramirez JC, Miller JD, Winton TL (1992) Pulmonary transplantation. J Thorac Cardiovasc Surg 103: 295-306
41. Gryzan S, Paradis IL, Zeevi A, Duquesnoy RJ, Dummer JS, Griffith BP (1988) Unexpectedly high incidence of Pneumocystis Carinii infection after lung-heart transplantation. Am Rev Respir Dis 137: 1268-1274
42. Kramer KR, Stoehr C, Lewiston NJ, Starnes V, Theodore J (1992) Trimethoprim-sulfamethoxazole prophylaxis for Pneumocystis carinii infections in heart-lung and lung transplantation - how effective and for how long? Transplantation 53: 586-589
43. Nathan S, Ross D, Zakowski D, Kass R, Koerner S (1994) Utility of inhaled pentamidine prophylaxis in lung transplant recipients. Chest 105: 417-420
44. Denning DD, Tucker RM, Hanson LH, Stevens DA (1989) Treatment of invasive aspergillosis with itraconazole. Am J Med 86: 791-800

Fungal Infections Following Solid-Organ Transplantation

E.E. Etheredge, L.M. Flint

Introduction

Infections continue to be major causes of morbidity and mortality in recipients of solid-organ transplants (SOT). Bacteria, viruses, fungi, and protozoa plague the immunosuppressed host, for whom any infection has an exaggerated potential for severity. The unfortunate suppression of host defenses by the nonspecific effects of routine immunosuppressive medications is the major predisposing factor, but others include: diabetes mellitus, hepatitis, leukopenia, postsplenectomy status, uremic state, cadaver allograft transplantation, repeated treatment of persistent or recurrent rejection [1], concurrent infection such as cytomegalovirus (CMV) [2] and recipient female gender [3].
Fungi are ubiquitous organisms that find expression as pathogens in a bewildering array of clinical conditions that range from a simple superficial mucosal vaginitis in a normal host to a disseminated, lethal infection that spares virtually no organ in the immunocompromised host. The compromised host is the setting for malignant infections by many fungi, including ones not previously recognized as potential pathogens. *Candida* and *Aspergillus* species cause more than 80% of fungal infections after SOT [4], but *Cryptococcus, Coccidioides, Histoplasma, Mucor, Rhizopus, Tinea, Torulopsis,* and others are pathogens [5].
Fungal infections following SOT are third in frequency, following viral and bacterial infections, but among severe infections following SOT fungal infections entail the greatest mortality [4]. This high mortality is attributed to (a) difficulty of early diagnosis in the face of a low index of suspicion, (b) lack of effective therapy, especially for *Aspergillus*, (c) toxicity and drug-interactions of antifungal antibiotics and (d) limited data on effective antifungal prophylaxis [4]. It is important to emphasize that most fungal infections occur in association with other pathogens. In a large series of kidney and kidney-pancreas recipients [3] fungus was reported as the sole pathogen in 5.6% of the patients but as a copathogen with bacteria in 10.3%, with virus in 3.3%, with virus and bacteria in 10.6%, and with virus, bacteria and parasite in 1.8%. It has been noted that 90% of opportunistic infections occur in recipients of SOT who have viral infections [2]. Dunn [5] makes an important observation that fungal infections have associated copathogens especially during

periods of intense immunosuppression but present frequently as the sole infectious agent during periods of maintenance immunosuppression.

In considering epidemiological factors Rubin [6] has put forth the community and hospital exposures model. For the former he notes that the major focus should be recent or remote exposures to the geographically restricted, systemic mycoses such as *Blastomyces dermatitidis, Coccidioides immitis and Histoplasma capsulatum*, and that reactivation, or primary infection or superinfection, with dissemination can occur. For the latter he describes two hazards: domiciliary and nondomiciliary. The domiciliary hazard is exposure in the room or ward where the patient is housed. Domiciliary epidemics feature a clustering of cases in time and space. Nondomiciliary exposures, such as those in the radiology departments, are thought to be the more frequent nosocomial problem, but its epidemic is difficult to identify and investigate. The diagnosis of fungal infection may be difficult, but it is facilitated by the mandatory consideration of fungus as a pathogen in the differential diagnosis at any time following SOT. Many writers suggested that it is useful to consider fungal infections within three time frames: 1 month post-SOT, 1-6 months, and over 6 months. Within the first month following SOT, all things "surgical" are potential factors. Preexisting conditions, the type of transplant, wound contamination, urinary stents and catheters, central venous lines, wound reentry, and anastomotic leak are but a few examples. The potential of a contaminated graft must also be considered. Immunosuppression is routinely the most intense during this period. Paya [4] states that 80% of fungal infections occur within the first 2 months following SOT. Within the second time frame (1-6 months following SOT) one may see the emergence of the aggressive, opportunistic fungal infections such as *Aspergillus*. This is also true for the third time frame, when sporadic or epidemic fungal infections continue to emerge, especially in SOT recipients with poorly functioning allografts and cumulative high dose immunosuppression. Rubin [6] emphasizes the point that fungal infections that present outside the time frame may reflect an unusual epidemiologic hazard and should be investigated.

The mainstay of diagnosis of fungal infections is the history and physical examination. Serious infections, such as with *Cryptococcus neoformans*, may present with a vague history of malaise, low-grade fever and cough. Subtle findings on physical examination, especially skin lesions, may identify major disseminated disease, as with *Candida folliculitis* and *cryptococcal* and *Aspergillus* skin lesions. Skin biopsy should be used aggressively. Even in the absence of focal or localizing neurological findings, symptoms of headache or vague neurological dysfunction should prompt computed tomography of the head and, if not contraindicated, lumbar puncture for spinal fluid analysis. In addition to the routine tests and cultures for spinal fluid analysis, one should order india ink preparation and cryptococcal antigen.

Routine chest and flat and erect abdominal roentgenograms and cultures of blood, urine, sputum, and drainage from any site are standard. Computed tomography and/or ultrasonography are first-line diagnostic tests if an intraabdominal or retroperitoneal infection is suspected, and guided needle aspiration may be employed to sample suspect fluid collections. Pulmonary lesions must be diagnosed aggressively. Bronchoscopy is indicated for bronchoalveolar lavage, brushings or biopsy for stains and cultures. Occasionally, open lung biopsy is required for definitive diagnosis.

Rhinolaryngoscopic examination may be required for the rhinocerebral infections caused by *Mucor* and *Rhizopus* species. Esophagoscopy is indicated to evaluate dysphagia or odynophagia, commonly caused by *Candida* esophagitis. Biopsy may be required to distinguish *Candida* lesions from those of CMV.

Fungal Infections Following Renal Transplantation

Fungal infections following renal SOT account for only about 5% of all infections in this group, the lowest rate for any SOT. The most common presentations are fungemia associated with urinary tract infection, catheter-related sepsis, and esophagitis [7]. *Candida* is the most common fungal pathogen. We routinely transplant without the use of central venous catheter, and in our experience fungemia from any cause is rare. We also find that candiduria is uncommon (1.6% of patients) and is usually detected in a surveillance culture. *Candida* urinary tract infection is commonly related to prolonged urinary catheter drainage. A very rare complication of *Candida* urinary tract infection is obstruction of the kidney by a fungal ball [8, 9]. Esophagitis appears to be more common in patients treated for rejection with OKT_3, but our overall incidence is too low to prove an association statistically. *C. vulvovaginitis* is not uncommon, especially in the diabetic recipient.

Candidemia in the transplant patient carries a risk of late visceral complications in over 50% [2] *Candida* pneumonia is very uncommon and probably occurs from aspiration or bloodstream seeding. While *C. albicans* is the most common *Candida* species causing pneumonia, *C. tropicalis* appears to be more pathogenic for the neutropenic patient, and *C. parapsilosis* appears to be associated chiefly with total parenteral nutrition [10].

Aspergillus is a virulent fungus with great invasive potential, entering the host via the lungs, sinuses, and areas of skin breakdown. *Aspergillus* infections appear sporadically, frequently in association with allograft dysfunction and intensified antirejection therapy or in near-epidemic numbers from intense aerosol exposure, especially associated with construction and even that at the hospital. Aspergillosis is the most frequent and most serious of the pulmonary mycoses [11] and most cases occur within the first 4 months following SOT. *A. fumigatus* accounts for most of the cases while *A. flavus* and *A. niger* account for most of the rest. The condition presents as an acute pneumonia with high fever, cough, and pleuritic pain [10], but Rubin [12] notes that *aspergillus* infection may present with fever alone, fever and a nonproductive cough or chest discomfort, or fever and evidence of disseminated infection. The pulmonary infection is a necrotizing, hemorrhagic bronchopneumonia with fungal invasion of the blood vessels. This special characteristic accounts for the tendency to disseminate: dissemination to vital organs occurs in 50% of patients before the diagnosis of invasive aspergillosis [13].

C. neoformans is the most common pathogen of central nervous system infection following renal SOT, but it enters the host via the lungs. Isolated cryptococcal lung disease, however, accounts for only about 19% of infections with *C. neoformans* [10]. The disease may be identified on a routine chest radiograph as multiple pulmonary nodules [13], but Wolensky [10] notes that it has a wide spectrum, ranging from a subacute illness with systemic signs of fever and weight loss and symptoms of cough and pleuritic pain to an acute, febrile pneumonia or disseminated disease. The history of a pulmonary component may be lacking and the patient presents with a meningitis and a history of headaches and fever, sometimes of some weeks' duration. Rubin [12] notes that about one-third of meningitis patients have a history of cough that identifies the pulmonary component. As noted above, skin lesions of *C. neoformans* occur in 20%-30% of patients [13]. Cryptococcosis is almost exclusively a late disease, occurring after 6 months or more following SOT.

Rhinocerebral mucormycosis is a rare, invasive, locally destructive disease caused by genera of the *Mucoraceae*, namely *Mucor* and *Rhizopus*. Rubin [12] notes that any prolonged acidosis and iron-mobilizing treatment with deferoxamine are predisposing factors for mucormycosis [14].

Infection from the geographically restricted mycoses (*Histoplasma capsulatum, Coccidioides immitis, and Blastomyces dermatitidis*) are uncommon but not rare. These mycoses have similar characteristics, including the fact that dormant infections may be reactivated, even to dissemination, or primary infection with dissemination or even superinfection can occur [6]. Again, the spectrum of presentation mimics others described. The chest radiograph may be compelling, while skin lesions or neurologic findings may narrow the focus. Tolkoff-Rubin and Rubin [13] note that *histoplasmosis* in the renal transplant recipient is an exogenous infection, usually presenting in the disseminated stage and showing central nervous system involvement in about 20% of patients. Similarly, coccidioidal mycosis is characterized by dissemination in two-thirds of patients, of whom 90% of patients have pulmonary disease, 50%-60% skin disease, and 33%-50% central nervous system disease. Blastomycosis is very uncommon but a few cases have been reported [15].

Fungal Infections Following Liver SOT

The incidence of fungal infections following orthotopic liver transplants (OLT) is somewhat higher than that for renal transplants, ranging from about 13% to 35% [16]. The spectrum of fungal diseases after OLT closely mimics that for kidney transplantation but includes peritonitis and intraabdominal abscesses that reflect the surgical conditions of OLT. In a large series of 303 patients with OLT a 24% incidence of fungal infections was reported of which 84% were caused by *Candida* species. Of special note is the finding of *Candida* species in 10/17 patients with disseminated disease and *Aspergillus flavus* in 6/17 [17]. It has been noted from Castaldo's data that 62% of *aspergillus* infections were disseminated but only 16% of candida infections. Observed clinical complexes were: disseminated infection (26%), peritonitis (24%), pneumonitis (21%), multiple sites of colonization (18%), fungemia (15%) and other sites (22%). Overall, fungal infections account for 23.6% of the deaths following OLT, and the actuarial 1-year patient survival of adult recipients with fungal infections was only 44%, compared to 88.5% of those recipients with no fungal infections. Discriminant analysis identified the variables most predictive of fungal infection: retransplantation, reintubation, bacterial infections, intraoperative blood transfusions, urgent status before transplantation, number of steroid boluses, vascular complications, prolonged antibiotic use, method of biliary reconstruction, and risk score. The aggressive behavior of this fungus is underscored by the observation of local surgical wound infection caused by *A. fumigatus* in recipients of OLT [18].

Fungal Infections Following Heart Transplantation

The most common fungal pathogen following heart SOT is *Candida*, with *C. albicans* predominating [19] although Paya [4] cites *Aspergillus* as the most common and calls this a distinguishing feature of fungal infections in cardiac transplantation. Certainly the dominance of *Aspergillus* species in pulmonary and disseminated forms is universally accepted, as is its lethality. Oropharyngeal colonization with *Candida* is very common and superficial to moderate candida infection of the mouth and esophagus are prevalent. An important clinical point is that there was a 44% presence of histologically confirmed CMV in patients who die of *Aspergillus* infection [20]. Blood-borne *Candida* from catheter sepsis and disseminated *Candida* can be fatal, but the disseminated type of infection rarely involves the lungs [21]. These infections peak within the first 2 months following transplantation. Both *Candida* species [22] and *Aspergillus* [23] may cause mediastinitis and devastating surgical complications including ruptured aortic pseudoaneurysm. The diagnostic approach to these infections is standard, but the efficacy of fine needle aspiration of the lung for the rapid diagnosis of pulmonary aspergillosis has been reported [24]. The established heart transplant recipient is subject to the complete array of geographically restricted and sporadic, opportunistic mycoses.

Fungal Infections Following Lung and Heart-Lung Transplantation

Fungal infections following pulmonary and heart-lung SOT are fairly common, and *Candida* species account for more than 60% of the infections, with *Aspergillus* being the next most common [25]. In a series of isolated single and double lung transplants, Maurer et al. [26] reported only two pulmonary fungal infections of 35 total pulmonary infections and three fungal septicemias. Kramer et al. [27] have described a form of invasive aspergillosis, ulcerative tracheobronchitis, in a series of heart-lung and single lung recipients. The disease is characterized by deep mucosal ulceration, initially limited to the anastomosis site and large airways, and two of six patients died of disseminated aspergillosis. Both *Candida* and *Aspergillus* species have been reported in association with surgical complications such as anastomotic dehiscence with resulting mediastinitis, empyema, and pseudoaneurysm.

Fungal Infections Following Kidney-Pancreas Transplants

Fungal infections following kidney-pancreas transplantation are more common than fungal infections after kidney transplant alone. The diabetic condition, bicarbonate wastage, and acidosis associated with urinary drainage, gastrointestinal contamination of the donor and technical complications of this intra-abdominal operation are factors for fungal infection, especially peritonitis and intra-abdominal abscess formation. *Candida* is the dominant fungal pathogen. Reporting a series of combined kidney pancreas transplants in patients before and after dialysis is required, Stratta et al. [28] noted a remarkably low incidence of major fungal infection overall (3.3%), but details were lacking. Another overview reporting a contemporary series of kidney-pancreas and pancreas transplants reported an overall 7.4% graft loss from infection (pathogens not enumerated) [29]. Sollinger et al. [30] reported an experience with 100 consecutive simultaneous kidney-pancreas transplants (with bladder drainage) in which there was but one cryptococcal infection and one *Candida esophagitis*. Intra-abdominal fungal infections or abscesses require aggressive drainage and often multiple operations (Tesi, 1994, personal communication).

Prophylaxis Against Fungal Infections

The oral administration of the antifungal nystatin is widely used to prevent oral and esophageal *Candida* infection. The minimal use of central venous lines and avoidance of prolonged bladder drainage are keys to prevent fungal line sepsis and fungal urinary tract infections. Low-dose trimethoprim-sulfamethoxazole has been shown to reduce markedly the incidence of urinary tract infections after renal transplant [31] and others using the same regimen have noted a reduction of infections by pathogens sensitive to these drugs (*Pneumocystis carinii, Nocardia asteroides, Listeria monocytogenes and Toxoplasmosis gondii*). This may be germane to antifungal prophylaxis since the trimethoprim-sulfamethoxazole regimen is also associated with a reduction in colonization by *Candida* [32].

There is a uniform call for antifungal prophylaxis in liver transplantation, but meaningful data, especially from randomized, prospective studies, are lacking. A recent report notes that selective bowel decontamination with quinolones and nystatin reduced gram-negative and fungal infections in 17 consecutive patients receiving OLT, compared to historic controls [33]. Similar reductions in fungal infection by use of nystatin was reported [34] in another nonrandomized study. Another group [35] reported that the selective use of intravenous amphotericin B in high-risk patients was associated with a low incidence and mortality rate, compared to other published series. However, their study was not randomized, and their data were not presented to show efficacy even in their treated group. A small, randomized, prospective study of selective decontamination in pediatric liver transplants used enterally administered nonabsorbable antibiotics including amphotericin B. While the treatment regimen was associated with a statistically significant reduction in gram-negative infections, it did not significantly reduce the incidence of fungal infections [36].

Treatment of Fungal Infections Following SOT

It is beyond the scope of this chapter to detail the treatment regimens for the myriad of fungal infections following SOT. However, a number of observations are worth summarizing.

Fungal infections resulting from surgical complications require *surgical* therapy. Intense antifungal antibiotic therapy will be required but is inadequate until foreign bodies are removed, abscesses completely drained, devitalized tissue débrided, and sources of contamination such as anastomic leaks controlled. These principles apply to virtually every organ or anatomic region infected by fungi.

Serious infection by any pathogen, including fungi following SOT requires a consideration of reduction of immunosuppressive therapy. This consideration is especially problematic since opportunistic infections frequently cluster in association with periods of most intense immunosuppression, especially the treatment of rejection. There are no algorithms of clinical certainty to guide these critical decisions.

Amphotericin B continues to be the benchmark antibiotic for serious fungal infections. However, its multiple side effects such as nephrotoxicity make its use difficult, especially given the near-universal use of cyclosporine and the potential for synergistic toxicity. Liposomal amphotericin-B seems to have therapeutic potential.

Itraconazole and fluconazole appear to have an important, if incompletely defined, role in the treatment of fungal disease following SOT. Ketoconazole, known to raise cyclosporine levels, has little efficacy. The clinical applications of these azole agents have been well reviewed [4].

As emphasized by many authors, the development of effective prophylaxis against invasive fungal infections following SOT is mandatory and should be grounded on the risk factors identified. The efficacy and safety of the prophylactic measures must be verified by randomized, prospective trials. Given the overall compromise of host defense attendant contemporary immunosuppression, it appears that the development of effective prophylaxis offers far more immediate promise than new therapeutic agents or regimens in combating the impact of fungal infections following SOT.

References

1. Dunn DL, Najarian JS (1990) Infectious complications in transplant surgery. In: Shires CT, Davis J (eds.) Principles and management of surgical infection. Lippincott, Philadelphia, pp. 425-464
2. Rubin RH (1988) Infection in the renal and liver transplant patient. In: Rubin RH, Young LS (eds.) Clinical approach to infection in the compromised host. Plenum, New York, p 557
3. Brayman KL, Stephanian E, Matas AJ et al. (1992) Analysis of infectious complications occurring after solid-organ transplantation. Arch Surg 127: 38
4. Paya CN. (1993) Fungal infections in solid-organ transplantation. Clin Infect Dis 16: 677
5. Dunn DL (1990) Problems related to immunosuppression. Infections and malignancy occurring after solid organ transplantation. Crit Care Clin 6(4): 955-977
6. Rubin RH. (1993) Fungal and bacterial infections in the immunocompromised host. Eur J Clin Microbiol Infect Dis 12 Suppl 1: S42
7. Cohen J, Hopkin J, Kurtz J (1988) Infectious complications after renal transplantation. In: Morris PJ (ed.) Kidney transplantation. Principles and practice. 3rd edn. Saunders, Philadelphia, pp. 533-573
8. Walzer Y, Bear RA (1983) Ureteral obstruction of renal transplant due to ureteral candidiasis. Urology 21: 295
9. Ratner LE, Clayman RN, Hanto DW (1990) Obstructive uropathy due to ureteral candidiasis in a renal allograft. Clin Transplant 4: 202
10. Wolensky E (1994) Mycotic, actinomycotic and nocardial pneumonia. In: Baum GL, Wolensky E (eds.) Texbook of pulmonary diseases, 5th edn. Little, Brown, Boston, pp. 503-520
11. Brinkman RJ Jr (1994) Hospital acquired pneumonia. In: In: Baum GL, Wolensky E (eds.) Texbook of pulmonary diseases, 5th edn. Little, Brown, Boston, pp. 457-479
12. Rubin RK (1993) Infectious complications of renal transplantation. Kidney Int 44: 221
13. Tolkoff-Rubin NE, Rubin RH (1992) Clinical approach to viral and fungal infections in the renal transplant patient. Semin Nephrol 12: 364
14. Sauve A, Manzi S, Perfect J et al. (1989) Deferoxamine treatment as a risk factor for zygomycete infection. J Infect Dis 159: 151
15. Serody JS, Mill MR, Detterbeck FC et al. (1993) Blastomycoses in transplant recipients: report of a case and review. Clin Infect Dis 16: 54
16. Arnow PM (1991) Infections following orthotopic liver transplantation. HPB Surg 3: 221
17. Castaldo P, Stratta, RJ, Wood RP et al. (1991) Clinical spectrum of fungal infections after orthotopic liver transplantation. Arch Surg 126: 149
18. Pla' MP, Berenguer J, Arzuaga JA et al. (1992) Surgical wound infections by Aspergillus fumigatus in liver transplant recipients. Diagn Microbial Infect Dis 15: 703
19. Hummel M, Thalmann V, Jautzke G et al. (1992) Fungal infections following heart transplantation. Mycoses 35: 23
20. Thalmann V, Kehrein B, Jautzke G et al. (1990) Pilzinfektionen in Autopsiegut nach Herztransplantation. Wiss Sitz Berl Ges Pathol 262: 11-12
21. Hofflin JM, Potasman I, Baldwin JC et al. (1987) Infectious complications in heart transplant recipients receiving cyclosporine and corticosteroids. Ann Intern Med 106: 209
22. Glower DD, Douglas JM, Gaynor JW et al. (1990) Candida mediastinitis after a cardiac operation. Ann Thorac Surg 49: 157
23. Byl B, Jacobs F, Antoine M et al. (1993) Mediastinitis caused by Aspergillus fumigatus with ruptured aortic pseudoaneurysm in a heart transplant recipient: case study. Heart Lung 22: 145
24. McCalmont TH, Silverman JF, Geisinger KR (1991) Cytologic diagnosis of aspergillosis in cardiac transplantation. Arch Surg 126: 394

25. Dauber JH, Paradis IL, Dummer JS (1990) Infectious complications in pulmonary allograft recipients. Clin Chest Med 11: 291
26. Maurer JR, Tullis E, Grossman RF et al. (1992) Infectious complications following isolated lung transplantation. Chest 101: 1059
27. Kramer MR, Denning DW, Marshall SE, Ross DJ et al. (1991) Ulcerative tracheobronchitis after lung transplantation. A new form of invasive aspergillosis. Am Rev Respir Dis 144: 552
28. Stratta RJ, Taylor RJ, Ozaki CF et al. (1993) A comparative analysis of results and morbidity in type I diabetics undergoing preemptive versus postdialysis combined pancreas-kidney transplantation. Transplantation 55: 1097
29. Sutherland DER, Dunn DL, Goetz FC et al. (1989) A 10-year experience with 290 pancreas transplants at a single institution. Ann Surg 210: 274
30. Sollinger HW, Knechtle SJ, Reed A et al. (1991) Experience with 100 consecutive simultaneous kidney-pancreas transplants with bladder drainage. Ann Surg 214: 703
31. Tolkoff-Rubin NE, Cosimi AB, Russel PS et al. (1982) A controlled study of trimethoprim-sulfamethoxazole prophylaxis of urinary tract infection in renal transplant recipients. Rev Infect Dis 4: 614
32. Fox BC, Sollinger HW, Belzer FO, Maki DG. (1990) A prospective, randomized, double-blind study of trimethoprim-sulfamethoxazole for prophylaxis of infection in renal transplantation: clinical efficacy, absorption of trimethoprim-sulfamethoxazole, effects on the microflora and the cost benefit of prophylaxis. Am J Med 89: 255
33. Gorensek MJ, Carey WD, Washington II JH et al. (1993) Selective bowel decontamination with quinolones and nystatin reduces gram-negative and fungal infections in orthotopic liver transplant recipients. Cleve Clin J Med 60: 139
34. Weisner RH, Hermans PE, Rahela J et al. (1988) Selective bowel decontamination to decrease gram-negative aerobic bacterial and Candida colonization and prevent infection after orthotopic liver transplantation. Transplantation 45: 570
35. Mora NP, Cofer JB, Solomon H et al. (1991) Analysis of severe infections (INF) after 180 consecutive liver transplants: the impact of amphotericin-B prophylaxis for reducing the incidence and severity of fungal infections. Transplant Proc 23: 1528
36. Smith SD, Jackson RJ, Hannakan CJ et al. (1993) Selective decontamination in pediatric liver transplants. A randomized, prospective study. Transplantation 55: 1306

Cytomegalovirus Prophylaxis by Passive Immunization in High-Risk Kidney and Heart Transplant Recipients

W. Weimar, H.J. Metselaar, A.H.M.M. Balk

Introduction

Cytomegalovirus (CMV) infections remain a major clinical problem after bone marrow and solid-organ transplantation. Especially CMV-seronegative recipients of an allograft from a CMV seropositive donor are at risk to develop life-threatening CMV disease as primary infections may run a fulminant course under circumstances of immunosuppression. Also, serious CMV-related morbidity can be expected in patients treated with mono- or polyclonal anti-T-cell preparations, for example, OKT3 and antilymphocyte serum or antithymocyte globulin (ATG) for the prevention or therapy of acute rejection episodes. CMV prophylaxis with immunoglobulins, both selected and notselected for anti-CMV antibody titers, is often used. However, despite a number of randomized controlled trials and numerous uncontrolled observations, controversy remains over the efficacy of passive immunization against CMV in clinical transplantation. Other factors adding to the confusion include differences among the various reports in study design, inclusion criteria for high-risk groups, immunosuppressive regimens and the variability of total antibody content, specific neutralizing titers, and administration schedules of the globulin preparations used.

We here report on our experience with a standardized anti-CMV hyperimmunoglobulin preparation given to solid-organ transplant recipients at high risk to develop CMV disease. We performed a double-blind placebo-controlled trial study in kidney transplant recipients treated with rabbit ATG for biopsy-confirmed rejection. We also describe our analysis of routine administration of anti-CMV immunoglobulin to CMV-seronegative heart transplant recipients. In the latter study we compared the incidence of CMV infection and disease in these passively immunized patients with the same parameters in untreated heart transplant recipients with naturally acquired CMV seropositivity.

Material and Methods

Immunoglobulin Preparation

The anti-CMV immunoglobulin preparation was produced from cold ethanol precipitated large plasma pools with high titers of antibody against CMV (Cytotect, Biotest Pharma, Dreieich, Germany). Cold sterilization was performed with β-propionolactone treatment [1]. The final preparation contained 100 mg protein/ml (95% IgG). It had an anti-CMV IgG titer of 40 000 enzyme-linked immunosorbent assay (ELISA) U/ml (50 U/ml ELISA against the Paul Ehrlich standard) and a CMV neutralizing titer of 1:3000/ml. During and after transplantation only buffy-coat depleted blood transfusions were given. Blood-donors were not regularly screened for CMV IgG antibodies.

Virology

Initially the CMV serological status of the transplant recipients was screened for anti-CMV IgG by an ELISA developed in our own laboratory. From March 1989 a commercial kit was used (ETI-Cytok G, Sorin Biomedics Saluggia, Italy). Recipients with pretransplant IgG titers of less than 1:100 U or less than 1:500 U were considered seronegative. Until March 1989 IgM antibodies were determined by an indirect immunofluorescence assay and subsequently by ELISA (ETI-Cytok M reverse, Sorin). Similarly serum of the allograft donor was screened for CMV antibodies. Monitoring for CMV infection after transplantation involved testing urine, throat-wash, and blood for isolation of the virus and antibody determinations on days 7, 14, 28, 56, and 72 and every 3 months thereafter. Additional specimens were obtained when CMV disease was suspected. Isolation of CMV was performed by a low-speed centrifugation assay in combination with immunofluorescence using monoclonal antibodies against early antigen (EA) of CMV. Buffy-coat samples were cultured on human embryonic lung fibroblasts and screened for cytopathic changes. From 1991 monoclonal antibodies against CMV pp65 antigen were used to detect virus antigen in peripheral blood leukocytes. CMV infection was defined as any appearance of IgM, any isolation of CMV from urine, throat-wash, or blood, or any demonstration of the antigen. CMV disease was presumed when infection coexisted with two of the following symptoms: otherwise unexplained fever over 38°C for at least 2 consecutive days: gastrointestinal, lung, retina or central nervous system involvement; leucocytopenia ($< 2.5 \times 10^9$/l); thrombocytopenia ($< 100 \times 10^9$/l); elevation in serum alanine or aspartate aminotransferase ($> 2 \times$ normal). Lung, central nervous system or gastrointestinal tract involvement was confirmed by biopsy or culture. Depending on the severity of symptoms, either no specific measures were taken, or patients were treated by decrease/interruption of immunosuppressive medication and/or by administration of ganciclovir.

Patients

In the kidney transplant study 152 patients treated with cyclosporine and low-dose steroids were potentially eligible for a prophylactic study in patients given ATG. In 110 cases (72%) no rejection was diagnosed while in 42 patients biopsy-confirmed rejection necessitated therapy with rabbit ATG in which circulating T cells were kept below 150 mm^3 for 14 days. Forty patients agreed to participate and were randomized to receive either globulin ($n = 20$)

or a 20% albumin preparation (Merieux, Lyon, France). Both preparations were dissolved in 250 ml saline and given intravenously over a period of 1 h at a dose of 100 µg/kg body weight. Globulin/albumin infusion was administered on the day of ATG treatment and on days 7, 14, 35, 56, and 77 thereafter.

In the heart transplant study we analyzed 146 consecutive patients. There were 65 CMV sero-negative heart recipients, and each received immunoglobulin starting at the day of operation. A first dose of 150 mg/kg body weight was administered shortly before the end of extracorporeal circulation. Thereafter doses of 100 µg/kg were given on days 2, 7, 14, 28, 42, 56, and 72. This regimen resulted in geometrical mean preinfusion IgG titers of 1700-2100 ELISA units during the first 2 weeks and remained at a median of 1050 U during the following 3 months, decreasing rapidly thereafter.

Results

The incidence of symptomatic CMV disease in the 110/152 kidney transplant patients who were not treated for rejection was low. Only seven patients showed signs of CMV morbidity, which was significantly ($p < 0.05$, χ^2 test) lower than in the patients who became eligible for the double-blind study.

Table 1 summarizes the results of this study in kidney transplant recipients treated with rabbit ATG for rejection. We analyzed 39 patients, as one patient died within 14 days of the study. Of these 39 patients 8 belonged to a CMV-seronegative donor/recipient pair. In these 8 combinations the virus was not involved, no virus was isolated, patients were consequently not at risk for CMV disease. In the remaining 31 high-risk kidney transplant recipients we found no statistically significant difference between globulin and placebo-treated patients as to virus isolation, viremia, CMV disease, or lung involvement. CMV-related disease was more frequently observed in the 9 seronegative recipients at risk than in the 22 seropositive patients (78% vs. 27%, $p < 0.02$), and lung involvement was observed only in seronegative recipients ($p < 0.01$). None of the 16 globulin-treated patients died from CMV infection, in contrast to 4/15 placebo treated patients (difference 27%, 95% CI, 3%-50%, n.s.). However, in patients with virus isolation, or viremic or viral disease the difference in CMV-related mortality between treated and placebo was statistically significant ($p < 0.05$; Fig. 1).

Table 1: The incidence of CMV isolation and disease in globulin/placebo-treated kidney transplant recipients stratified for CMV serostatus of the donor/recipient combination (all patients received ATG for biopsy-confirmed acute rejection)

CMV serostatus donor / recipient	Globulin treatment				Placebo treatment			
	-/-	+/-	±/+	Total	-/-	+/-	±/+	Total
No status	3	5	11	19	5	4	11	20
Virus isolation	0	5	10	15	0	3	8	11
Viremia	0	5	6	11	0	3	5	8
Disease	0	4	3	7	0	3	3	6
Lung involvment	0	2	0	2	0	3	0	3
CMV-related death	0	0	0	0	0	3	1	4

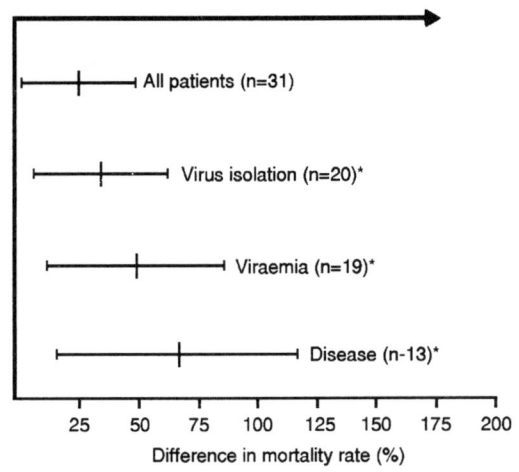

*Fig. 1: Anti-CMV immunoglobulin therapy versus placebo treatment in kidney transplant recipients treated with ATG for rejection. Effect on CMV-related mortality in all patients at risk, those with virus isolation, those with viraemia, and those with CMV disease. Approximate 95 confidence intervals for difference in mortality rates. *$p < 0.05$*

Table 2 shows the incidence of CMV infection and disease in 146 heart transplant recipients, including 65 seronegative recipients treated with passive immunisation. Of these 65 patients 29 received a heart from a seropositive donor. CMV infection occurred in 21/65 seronegative and in 40/81 seropositive recipients (n.s.). The incidence of CMV infection in seronegative recipients of a CMV-matched donor heart (3/34) was significantly lower than in seronegative recipients of a positive donor heart and lower than in seropositive recipients, but no significant difference in infection was found between the two latter groups (18/29 vs. 40/81). Although primary infection more frequently resulted in CMV disease than secondary infection (11/21 vs. 10/40), no difference in incidence of disease was noted between seronegative and seropositive patients (11/65 vs. 10/81), nor was there a difference in the severity of symptoms following primary or secondary infection. There was a higher incidence of CMV disease in all patients who received a heart from a seropositive donor versus a seronegative donor. However, after transplantation of a heart from a seropositive donor a comparable incidence of CMV disease was observed in our passively immunized seronegative patients versus our seropositive patients.

Table 2: The incidence of CMV infection and disease in heart transplant recipients [seronegative recipients ($n = 65$) had globulin treatment]

CMV serostatus donor/recipient	-/-	+/-	±/+
No status	35	30	81
Virus isolation	3	14	30
Virus serology	3	14	33
Viremia	3	18	40
Disease	3	8	10
Lung involvment	0	2	4
CMV-related death	0	0	0

Discussion

The present report summarizes the data from our previously published studies [2, 3]. We concluded that passive immunization with anti-CMV globulin during 3 months in high-risk kidney and heart transplant recipients affords partial protection against the more serious consequences of CMV infection. However, it does not prevent CMV replication, nor does it reduce the overall incidence of CMV disease. The partial protection is reflected by the ability of the globulin preparation to attenuate the severity of CMV disease, thus preventing overwhelming organ involvement and CMV-related death. Our analysis in heart transplant recipients it suggests that this partial protection against CMV closely resembles the natural acquired immunity associated with pretransplant seropositivity for CMV.

Our study in kidney transplant recipients also points in that same direction as, in our hand, the efficacy of the globulin preparation was mainly the result of preventing CMV-related mortality in the seronegative recipients of kidneys from seropositive donors. When the literature is searched on the subject of passive immunization against CMV in transplantation, only 18 properly controlled randomized trials are evaluable for evaluation. In their recently published meta-analysis of these studies Glowacki and Smaill [4] concluded that prophylactic immunoglobulin has a clinically significant beneficial effect on symptomatic CMV disease and CMV-related death with common odds ratio of approximately 0.58. Our observations are in line with this, and we feel there is a place for anti-CMV hyperimmunoglobulin prophylaxis, especially in high-risk solid-organ transplant recipients.

References

1. Prince AM, Stephan W, Brotman B (1983) Beta-propiolactone/ultraviolet irradiation: a review of its effectiveness for inactivation of viruses in blood derivates. Rev Infect Dis 5: 92-107
2. Metselaar HJ, Rothbarth PhH, Brouwer ML, Wenting GJ, Jeekel J, Weimar W (1989) Prevention of cytomegalovirus related death by passive immunization. A double blind placebo controlled study in kidney transplant recipients treated for rejection. Transplantation 48: 264-266
3. Balk AHMM, Weimar W, Rothbarth PH, Metselaar HJ, Meeter K, Mochtar B, Simoons ML (1993) Passive immunization against Cytomegalovirus in allograft recipients. The Rotterdam Heart Transplant Program experience. Infection 21: 1-6
4. Glowacki LS, Smaill FM (1993) Meta-analysis of immune globulin prophylaxis in transplant recipients for the prevention of symptomatic cytomegalovirus disease. Transplant Proc 25: 1408-1410

Posttransplant Lymphoproliferative Disorders: Pathogenesis Presentation, and Approaches to Therapy

V.A. Morrison, B.A. Peterson, D.L. Dunn

Introduction

In the late 1960s it was first recognized that renal allograft recipients have an increased incidence of de novo malignancies following transplantation [1, 2]. The risk of malignancies in this population is 6%, which is 100 times the risk in the general population matched for age. The most common malignancies occurring in these patients are tumors of the skin or lip, followed by lymphoproliferative disorders. The risk of posttransplant lymphoproliferative disorders (PTLD) arising in the renal allograft recipient is 40 times that of the general population. Although initially described in renal transplant patients, PTLD have also been found in liver, heart, heart-lung, and bone marrow transplant recipients [3-5] and in patients with congenital immunodeficiency disorders [6, 7]. A morphologic spectrum of these disorders was seen, with histologic lesions varying from a reactive polyclonal hyperplasia to a monoclonal malignant lymphoma. Hypotheses for the occurrence of these disorders include impaired immune surveillance related to the chronic immunosuppressive therapy, chronic antigen stimulation from the allograft, direct oncogenic effects of the immunosuppressive therapy, Epstein-Barr virus (EBV) induced lymphoproliferation, and combinations of these factors [8]. Further investigation has implicated EBV as having a significant role in the etiology of the PTLD.

Pathogenesis

Epstein-Barr virus is a DNA virus which is a member of the Herpes family of viruses. This virus selectively infects and transforms human B-lymphocytes which express surface immunoglobulin and have EBV membrane receptors. Two types of cellular infections may be caused by EBV [9]. The first type of infection is productive, replicative (or lytic) infection in which mature infectious virus particles are assembled and released, resulting in cell death. Initially in the cycle of viral particle assembly, Epstein-Barr nuclear antigen (EBNA) and lymphocyte-determined membrane antigen (LYDMA) are expressed. This is followed by expression of early membrane antigen (EMA) and early antigen (EA), the latter of which inhibits cellular RNA, DNA, and protein synthesis. The synthesis of viral DNA subsequently occurs, followed by the production of viral capsid antigen (VCA) and late membrane antigen (LMA). Subsequent assembly and release of the viral particles occur, resulting in the death of the B-lymphocyte. The time from initial cell infection to viral particle release ranges from 10 to 14 days.

The second type of EBV infection is a nonreproductive infection in which the virus is incorporated into the host DNA with subsequent replication. The virus then remains in a latent state in the transformed B-lymphocytes, with no assembly or production of mature virus particles. One or two events may subsequently occur. The EBV genome may remain in a latent state in a small number of B-lymphocytes, which express EBNA or LYDMA and may circulate indefinitely. This latent state may occur after any primary EBV infection. Reactivation infection occurs when these latently infected cells reenter the lytic-synthesis cycle. Alternatively, a transforming event as a cytogenetic change occurs in the latently infected cells, resulting in the subsequent overgrowth of an autonomous cell clone resulting in a malignancy as Burkitt's lymphoma, nasopharyngeal carcinoma, or PTLD. The malignant transformed cells carry EBV genomic copies in a latent state and express several markers including LYDMA, EBNA, and EMA. Kline [10] proposed a three-step hypothesis for the evaluation of Burkitt's lymphoma from cells latently infected with EBV. In the first step, initiation and immortalization of the preneoplastic B-lymphocytes by EBV occur, with these cells capable of continued division. Next, promotion of B-lymphocyte division and possible interference with normal differentiation of long-lived latent preneoplastic B-lymphocytes occur with chronic antigenic stimulation. Lastly, there is selective emergence of a single clone with a highly specific cytogenetic abnormality as the t(8;14) translocation.

Unique features of EBV are important in the pathogenesis of these infections. This virus is not T-cell dependent, and thus on its own may stimulate B-cells which are programmed to produce immunoglobulin. Only one virus particle per cell is needed to cause transformation and immortalization of these target B-lymphocytes. This results in the development of EBNA-positive permanent lymphoblastoid cell lines in vitro. The in vivo correlate is the establishment of a permanent carrier state in which small numbers of latently infected B-cells which express LYDMA and/or EBNA circulate in seropositive individuals.

EBV is ubiquitous. In immunocompetent patients oropharyngeal shedding of EBV occurs in approximately 17% of seropositive patients. However, in renal transplant recipients up to 87% of patients demonstrate oropharyngeal shedding of EBV within the first year after transplant [11]. Between 10% and 50% of these patients demonstrate a significant increase in EBV antibody titers following transplantation. The oropharyngeal epithelial cells are the most likely source of the infectious transmissible virus, with infection of these cells resulting in subsequent B-lymphocyte infection.

The humoral immune responses to EBV are as follows:

- Current primary infection
  - ☐ Early appearance anti-VCA IgG, later decreased
  - ☐ Increased anti-VCA IgG
  - ☐ Transient increase in anti-D (diffuse EA component)
  - ☐ Absence of anti-EBNA during acute infection, later increase and persists
- Reactivation infection
  - ☐ Absence of anti-VCA IgM
  - ☐ Fourfold or greater increase in anti-VCA IgG
  - ☐ Preexistence of anti-EBNA

- Past primary infection
  - [ ] Absence of anti-VCA IgM
  - [ ] Unchanging anti-VCA IgG titers
  - [ ] Absence of anti-EA
  - [ ] Unchanging anti-EBNA
- Posttransplant lymphoproliferative disorders
  - [ ] High anti-VCA IgG titers
  - [ ] Anti-EA titers variable
  - [ ] Evidence of reactivated infection or primary infection

While these are the characteristic immunologic responses with various EBV infections, one must be aware that antibody responses may be abnormal in immunocompromised individuals such as organ transplant recipients. In addition to the humoral responses, cellular immune responses to EBV infection may exist. EBV-specific cytotoxic T-lymphocytes have been detected in the peripheral blood of patients with infectious mononucleosis. Theses cells may be the most important factor controlling EBV-induced B-cell proliferation. Impairment of this T-cell response is associated with uncontrolled B-cell proliferation. In addition, natural killer (NK) cells may prevent EBV reactivation infection by destroying virus-infected cells as they leave the latent phase to enter the replicative or lytic cycle. However, NK activity may be depressed in organ transplant recipients. Antibody-dependent cell-mediated cytotoxicity may also be operative in patients with Burkitt's lymphoma, nasopharyngeal carcinoma, and PTLD.

Further evidence of the role of EBV in PTLD has been demonstrated with molecular diagnostic techniques. In DNA hybridization studies EBNA and EBV genomes have been found in tumor tissue [12]. In examination of endonuclease restriction patterns of EBV genomic termini, EBV-determined clonal changes have been found in tissue samples from patients with PTLD [13]. Latent membrane protein and EBV nuclear protein 2 have been detected in B-lymphocytes of immunocompromised patients with EBV-induced lymphoproliferative disease [14]. These proteins are expressed typically in B-lymphocytes undergoing in vitro proliferation in response to transformation by EBV. In another series of 28 patients with PTLD, EBV-virus infected lymphoid cells were identified by in situ hybridization techniques in 26 of the 28 patients [15]. Most recently, expression of the EBER-1 gene was examined in a series of 24 patients with PTLD [16]. This gene, which codes for a small messenger RNA, is normally expressed during latent EBV infection. In 17 patients (71%) the EBER-1 gene was demonstrated in the mononuclear cells. At autopsy EBER-1 positive cells were identified within the lymphoproliferative lesions. Further study in this area will be of interest to determine whether EBER-1 gene expression may be used in the early identification of patients with PTLD.

The influence of the immunosuppressive regimen on the incidence of subsequent malignancies in organ transplant recipients has been examined. The impact of cyclosporine has been studied in several series [17-21]. Penn and Brunson [17] and Penn [18] found the overall incidence of posttransplant malignancies in patients receiving cyclosporine to be comparable to that seen in patients receiving conventional immunosuppressive therapy of azathioprine with or without cyclophosphamide, prednisone, or antilymphocyte globulin. However, the cyclosporine-treated patients developed more PTLD than the conventionally treated patients, and these disorders occurred at a shorter interval after transplant in the cyclosporine group. These findings and the differences in clinical presentation of the PTLD are summarized in Table 1. An increased frequency of PTLD in patients treated with cyclosporine-containing regimens was likewise found in series from other institutions [19, 20]. However, a series from our institution found both the overall frequency of malignancies and of PTLD to be no greater in patients who received cyclosporine-containing regimens [21]. In the latter series the interval from transplant to diagnosis of the PTLD was comparable in both groups. Thus from these trials it is not clear whether the use of cyclosporine for chronic immunosuppressive therapy results in an increased incidence of PTLD, or has no effect on the frequency of this complication.

Turning to a newer immunosuppressive agent, OKT3, an increased incidence of PTLD was noted in a series of cardiac transplant patients who received this drug for immunosuppressive therapy [22]. Nine of 79 patients (11.4%) receiving OKT3 developed PTLD, compared to only one of 75 patients (1.3%) who did not receive OKT3 for immunosuppressive therapy. The cumulative dose of OKT3 was also significant. Among those receiving a cumulative dose of 75 mg or less only 6% developed PTLD, compared to 36% of those who received a cumulative dose of more than 75 mg of OKT3. While these are results from a single institution, the increased incidence of PTLD in patients in this series receiving OKT3 is disturbing and warrants evaluation in future clinical trials.

Table 1: Immunosuppressive regimen and subsequent posttransplant lymphoproliferative disorders (from [17, 18])

	Conventional immunosuppressive therapy	Cyclosporine
Lymphomas	12%	29%
Time from transplant to diagnosis (months)		
Mean	45	12
Range	1 - 196.5	1 - 160
Extranodal disease	78%	52%
Small bowel involvement	12%	22%
CNS involvement	39%	14%

Presentation

Pathologic Characteristics

A variety of histologic, immunologic, and cytogenetic findings may be present in patients with PTLD. A wide spectrum in the morphology of PTLD exists, ranging from benign polyclonal hyperplastic processes to monoclonal malignant lymphomas [23, 24]. Only a minority of cases fit criteria of the International Working Formulation for the classification of non-Hodgkin's lymphomas [25]. The term "polymorphic lymphoma" has been used to describe the lesions, defined as a proliferation of cells with varied morphology, including immunoblasts, plasmacytoid lymphocytes, plasma cells, and large atypical lymphoid cells with angulated and cleaved nuclei. Geographic areas of necrosis may be present. In contrast, lesions of polymorphic hyperplasia lack atypia, have a predominance of the plasmacytoid cell component, and necrosis, if present, is of the single cell type.

These disorders may be polyclonal or monoclonal. In polyclonal lesions the appearance of clonality as determined by cytogenetic changes is believed to result in the evolution to a monoclonal process.

With regard to immunophenotype, the vast majority of PTLD are of a B-cell immunophenotype [26]. However, T-cell lymphomas which contain EBV DNA have been described in patients with chronic EBV infections [27]. In our series two patients had a PTLD of a T-cell immunophenotype. The result of EBV hybridization studies performed in one of these patients was negative. Posttransplant T-cell lymphoproliferative processes may have a different etiology, clinical course, and outcome than the B-cell processes.

Cytogenetic studies of PTLD are limited. In a series of 30 patients with EBV-associated lymphoproliferative diseases, cytogenetic abnormalities were noted in five [28]. Four patients with low frequency cytogenetic abnormalities were observed for a median of 2 years and remained disease-free. The fifth patient was disease-free after chemotherapy. In another series recurring cytogenetic abnormalities were found in 9 of 15 patients [29]. These abnormalities were divided into four groups: (a) t(8;14) or t(8;22), (b) trisomy 11, (c) trisomy 9, and (d) other translocations involving 14q32 or 22q11. The number of patients in these series is too small to attempt correlation of specific cytogenetic abnormalities with variables of clinical presentation and outcome.

Clinical Characteristics

Time from Transplantation to Diagnosis of PTLD. The possibility has been examined that the time from transplantation to the onset of a PTLD has an influence on the subsequent clinical disease patterns. In series of 19 patients Hanto et al. [30, 31] described two groups with divergent clinical characteristics. Eight patients (mean age of 23 years) presented with an infectious mononucleosis-type syndrome 9 months after transplantation, with fever, pharyngitis, and lymphadenopathy. Disease was widespread at presentation. Response to acyclovir therapy was seen in this group, which had a mortality rate of 50%. In comparison, 11 patients with a mean age of 48 years presented with localized solid tumor masses 6 years (mean) after transplantation. Disease at presentation was commonly localized but extranodal. Response to acyclovir was uncommon, and the mortality rate was high (91%). These patients, in addition to subsequent cases identified at our institution, were included in a recent series [32]. No clearcut differences were seen in clinical presentation or outcome of patients diagnosed with a PTLD less than 1 year after transplant compared to those diagnosed more than 1 year after transplant. In a preliminary report of a series of postcardiac transplant lymphoproliferative disorders Swinnen et al. [33] described two types of clinical presentation. Six patients presented within 4 months of transplantation with a PTLD. These patients generally had a polyclonal immunophenotype and had stage IV disease. Only one of six patients achieved a complete response to therapy, and the mortality rate was 83%. In contrast, 11 patients presented at a median time of 11 months after transplant. The majority of these patients presented with stage IV disease but generally had a monoclonal immunophenotype. While only 2 patients achieved a complete response to therapy, mortality in this group was 36%. Additional studies in larger series of patients with PTLD will be of interest to determine whether trends in disease presentation and outcome are related to the time of disease onset after transplantation.

Clinical Presentation and Sites of Disease. Patients with PTLD present with a wide variety of clinical findings. These disorders may complicate the course of both pediatric and adult patients. The clinical characteristics of the 26 patients from our series of PTLD are summarized in Table 2 [32]. At presentation, disease may be localized (stages I, II) or extensive (stages III, IV). Disease occurring in sites such as the central nervous system, lung, bowel, kidney, soft tissues, and skin is quite common. Central nervous system and pulmonary involvement were common in our series, although involvement in these two sites was generally independent of each other. Central nervous system involvement was manifest by solitary intracranial lesions, with no patients having lymphomatous meningitis. In contrast to the widespread extranodal involvement, bone marrow involvement was quite uncommon in these patients.

Table 2: Clinical characteristics of posttransplant lymphoproliferative disorders ($n=26$; from [32])

Age (years)	
Median	42
Range	6 - 68
Sex (male/female)	12/14
Type of transplant	
Kidney	21 (81%)
Heart, heart lung	4 (15%)
Liver	1 (4%)
Living donor	14 (54%)
Cadaveric	12 (46%)
Disease stage	
I	9 (35%)
II	4 (15%)
III	6 (23%)
IV	7 (27%)
Disease sites	
Extralymphoreticular	12 (46%)
Lymphoreticular	5 (19 %)
Both sites	9 (35%)
Marrow involvement	3 (14%)
CNS involvement	7 (27%)
Lung involvement	6 (23%)
Lactate dehydrogenase (IU/l)	
Median	510
Range	164 - 2840

Approaches to Therapy

At the time of diagnosis of PTLD immunosuppressive therapy is commonly decreased or discontinued as the first step in therapy. Anecdotal cases of disease regression with reduced immunosuppression have been reported. Further therapeutic strategies vary, depending on whether the patients present with localized or extensive disease.

In patients with localized disease surgical extirpation may be used when applicable. Patients presenting with localized central nervous system or gastrointestinal tract disease may be candidates for this approach. In addition, involved field radiation therapy may be employed in several settings. This may be used adjuvantly in the postoperative setting, in the treatment of intracranial mass lesions, or to achieve local control in other disease sites. The ability to attain local control in this patients is prognostic for a favorable long-term outcome.

In cases of extensive disease, the development of effective antiviral drugs over the past 2 decades has made these agents available for the therapy of patients with PTLD [32, 34]. Acyclovir, which act by inhibiting EBV DNA replication in virus-producing cell lines, is the most common antiviral drug used in this setting. An initial 2- to 6-week course of high-dose parenteral therapy is employed, with doses ranging of 5-15 mg/kg given intravenously every 8-12 h. Patients need to be closely observed for evidence of response or disease progression over this period. If no response is seen after this initial course, alternative therapies must be considered. Of the 14 patients in our series who received high-dose parenteral acyclovir after an initial reduction in immunosuppressive therapy, four responded [32]. In our series, as also noted in prior reports, patients with histologic lesions of polymorphic hyperplasia and/or polyclonal disorders are most likely to respond to acyclovir. Ganciclovir, administered in a dose of 3 mg/kg given every 12-24 h, has also been utilized in a limited fashion in the care of these patients [35]. Additional antiviral drugs which show preliminary in vitro evidence of activity against EBV include foscarnet and HPMPC. The role of these drugs in the therapy of patients with PTLD is yet to be determined.

Experience with combination chemotherapy in the care of patients with PTLD is limited but appears to be much less successful than in patients with conventional non-Hodgkin's lymphomas. Anthracycline-based regimens such as cyclophosphamide, doxorubicin, vincristine, prednisone [36] or variants have been used with limited success in these patients [32, 37, 38]. Complete responses, including some patients with long-term disease-free survival, have been reported only anecdotally in these series. More intensive chemotherapy regimens such as cyclophosphamide, doxorubicin, etoposide, cytosine arabinoside, bleomycin, vincristine, methotrexate, leucovorin, and prednisone have been used in a limited number of patients [33, 39]. Five of seven patients with postcardiac transplant lymphoproliferative disorders achieved a response to this regimen [33]. However, myelosuppression with neutropenic sepsis was a complication in this series.

Infusional chemotherapy regimens offer a potentially attractive alternative to the standard multidrug regimens [32]. The infusional regimens may be less myelosuppressive than bolus therapy and may also overcome intrinsic resistance of the tumor cells. Myelosuppression, due not only to chemotherapy but also to underlying marrow suppression from prior immunosuppressive therapy, remains a significant problem in the treatment of these patients. Prospective therapeutic trials of infusional regimens such as cyclophosphamide, doxorubicin, vincristine, prednisone, and etoposide are underway.

Because of the poor response to conventional therapies in these patients alternative therapeutic approaches have been devised. Interferon-α has been used in the therapy of a small number of patients with EBV-associated lymphoproliferative disorders which developed either following bone marrow transplantation or in the course of an underlying immunodeficiency disorder [6, 40, 41]. The mechanism of action of interferon-α is not clear but may be related to a direct antiviral effect or antiproliferative effect on the B-lymphocytes infected with EBV, or it may alter the host immune response by other mechanisms that are not yet clearly defined. High-dose intravenous immunoglobulin has also been used alone or in conjunction with interferon therapy. Anti-B-cell monoclonal antibodies (anti-CD21 and anti-CD24) have also been used in the therapy of these disorders [42, 43]. Responses have occurred in patients with oligoclonal B-cell proliferations but not in those with monoclonal B-cell proliferations. Lastly, low doses of interleukin-2 have been shown to prevent the development of EBV-associated lymphoproliferative disorders in the SCID-human mouse model [44]. The applicability of this approach in humans awaits further study.

The optimal approach to the diagnosis and therapy of patients with PTLD is not clear. New developments in molecular diagnostic techniques hold promise for methods of earlier detection. If these methods can be devised, efforts directed at prophylaxis in this group of patients will be needed. The use of new immunosuppressive regimens in these patients will need to be accompanied by examination of complications as the frequency of posttransplant malignancies. Lastly, the best approach to therapy of these patients is not known. With the poor response rate seen with most therapies and the infrequent long-term survival after diagnosis of a PTLD, new therapeutic approaches need to be devised. Agents as new antiviral drugs, monoclonal antibodies, and immunomodulary agents such as interferons and interleukins may hold promise in improving the outcome of these patients.

References

1. Starzl TE (1968) Discussion of Murray JE, Wilson RE, Tilney NL et al. Five year's experience in renal transplantation with immunosuppressive drugs: survival, function, complications, and the role of lymphocyte depletion by thoracic duct fistula. Ann Surg 168: 416-435
2. Penn I, Hammond W, Brettschneider L et al. (1969) Malignant lymphomas in transplantation patients. Transplant Proc 1: 106-112
3. Dummer JS, Bound LM, Singh C, Atchinson RW, Kapadia SB, Ho M (1984) Epstein-Barr virus-induced lymphoma in a cardiac transplant patient. Am J Med 77: 179-184
4. Starzl TE, Nalesnik MA, Porter KA et al. (1984) Reversibility of lymphomas and lymphoproliferative lesions developing under cyclosporine-steroid therapy. Lancet 1: 583-587
5. Shapiro RS, Gross T, Haake R, Ramsay N, McGlave P, Kersey J, Filipovich AH (1992) Epstein-Barr virus (EBV) associated B cell lymphoproliferative disorders (BLPD) following bone marrow transplantation (BMT) (Abstr). Blood 80: 138a
6. Shapiro RS, McClain K, Frizzera G, Gajl-Peczalska KJ, Kersey JH, Blazar BR, Arthur DC, Patton DF, Greenberg JS, Burke B, Ramsay NKC, McGlave P, Filipovich AH (1988) Epstein-Barr virus associated B cell lymphoproliferative disorders following bone marrow transplantation. Blood 71: 1234-1243
7. Joncas JH, Russo P, Brochu P, Simard P, Brisebois J, Dube J, Marton D, Leclerc JM, Hune H, Rivard GE (1991) Epstein-Barr virus polymorphic B-cell lymphoma associated with leukemia and with congenital immunodeficiencies. J Clin Oncol 8: 378-384
8. Hanto DW, Frizzera G, Purtilo DT, Sakamoto K, Sullivan JL, Saemundsen AK, Klein G, Simmons RL, Najarian JS (1981) Clinical spectrum of lymphoproliferative disorders in renal transplant recipients and evidence for the role of Epstein-Barr virus. Cancer Res 41: 4253-4261

9. Hanto DW, Frizzera G, Gajl-Peczalska KJ, Simmons RL (1985) Epstein-Barr virus, immunodeficiency, and B cell lymphoproliferation. Transplantation 39: 461-472
10. Klein G (1979) Lymphoma development in mice and humans: diversity of initiation is followed by convergent cytogenetic evolution. Proc Natl Acad Sci USA 76: 2442-2446
11. Chang RS, Lewis JP, Reynolds RD, Sullivan MJ, Neuman J (1978) Oropharyngeal excretion of Epstein-Barr virus by patients with lymphoproliferative disorders and by recipients of renal homografts. Ann Intern Med 88: 34-40
12. Ho M, Miller G, Atchinson RW, Breinig MK, Dummer JS, Andiman W, Starzl TE, Eastman R, Griffith BP, Hardesty RL, Bahnson HT, Hakala TR, Rosenthal JT (1985) Epstein-Barr virus infections and DNA hybridization studies in post-transplant lymphoma and lymphoproliferative lesions: the role of primary infection. J Infect Dis 152: 876-886
13. Patton DF, Wilkowski CW, Hanson CA, Shapiro R, Gajl-Peczalska KJ, Filipovich AH, McClain KL (1990) Epstein-Barr virus-determined clonality in post-transplant lymphoproliferative disease. Transplantation 49: 1080-1084
14. Young L, Alfieri C, Hennesey K, Evans H, O'Hara C, Anderson KC, Ritz J, Shapiro RS, Rickinson A, Kieff E, Cohen JI (1989) Expression of Epstein-Barr virus transformation-associated genes in tissues of patients with EBV lymphoproliferative disease. N Engl J Med 321: 1080-1085
15. Berg LC, Copenhaver CM, Morrison VA, Gruber SA, Dunn DL, Gajl-Peczalska K, Strickler JG (1992) B-cell lymphoproliferative disorders in solid-organ transplant recipients: Detection of Epstein-Barr virus by in situ hybridization. Hum Pathol 23:159-163
16. Randhawa PS, Jaffe R, Demetris AJ, Nalesnik M, Starzl TE, Chen YY, Weis LM (1992) Expression of Epstein-Barr virus-encoded small RNA (by the EBER-1 gene) in liver specimens from transplant recipients with post-transplantation lymphoproliferative disease. N Engl J Med 327: 1710-1714
17. Penn I, Brunson ME (1988) Cancers after cyclosporine therapy. Transplant Proc 20 (Suppl 3): 885-892
18. Penn I (1987) Cancers following cyclosporine therapy. Transplantation 43: 32-35
19. Wilkinson AH, Smith JL, Hunsicker LG, Tobacman J, Kapelanski DP, Johnson M, Wright FH, Behrendt DM, Corry RJ (1989) Increased frequency of post-transplant lymphomas in patients treated with cyclosporine, azathioprine, and prednisone. Transplantation 47: 293-296
20. Smith JL, Wilkinson AH, Hunsicker LG, Tobacman J, Kapelanski DP, Johnson M, Wright FH, Behrendt DM, Corry RJ (1989) Increased frequency of post-transplant lymphomas in patients treated with cyclosporine, azathioprine, and prednisone. Transplant Proc 21: 3199-3200
21. Gruber SA, Skjei KL, Sothern RB, Robinson L, Tzardis P, Moss A, Gillingham K, Canafax DM, Matas AJ, Dunn DL (1991) Cancer development in renal allograft recipients treated with conventional and cyclosporine immunosuppression. Transplant Proc 23: 1104-1105
22. Swinnen LJ, Constanzo-Nordin MK, Fisher SG, O'Sullivan EJ, Johnson MR, Heroux AL, Dizikes GJ, Pifarre R, Fischer RI (1990) Increased incidence of lymphoproliferative disorder after immunosuppression with the monoclonal antibody OKT3 in cardiac transplant recipients. N Engl J Med 323: 1723-1728
23. Frizzera G (1987) The clinico-pathological expressions of Epstein-Barr virus infection in lymphoid tissues. Virchows arch [B] 53: 1-12
24. Frizzera G, Hanto DW, Gajl-Peczalska KJ, Rosai J, McKenna RW, Sibley RK, Holahan KP, Lindquist LL (1981) Polymorphic diffuse B-cell hyperplasias and lymphomas in renal transplant recipients, Cancer Res 41: 4262-4279

25. Non-Hodgkin's Lymphoma Pathologic Classification Project (1982) National Cancer Institute sponsored study of classification of non-Hodgkin's lymphoma. Summary and description of a working formulation for clinical usage. Cancer 49: 2112-2135
26. Gajl-Peczalska KJ, Bloomfield CD, Frizzera G, Kersey JH, LeBien TW (1982) Diversity of phenotypes of non-Hodgkin's malignant lymphomas. In:Vitetta E, Fox FC (eds.) B and T cell tumors, biological and clinical aspects. Academic, New York, UCLA Symp Mol Cell Biol 24: 63-67
27 Jones JF, Shurin S, Abramowsky C, Tubbs RR, Sciotto CG, Wahl R, Sands J, Gottman D, Katz BZ, Sklar J (1988) T-cell lymphomas containing Epstein-Barr viral DNA in patients with chronic Epstein-Barr virus infections. N Engl J Med 318: 733-741
28. Vose JM, Harrington D, Sanger W, Speaks S, Bierman PJ, Armitage JO, Purtilo D (1989) Cytogenetic abnormalities in Epstein-Barr virus (EBV) associated lymphoproliferative diseases (LPD) do not always signify lymphoma (Abstr). Proc Am Soc Clin Oncol 88: 252
29. Liebowitz D, Anastasi J, Thangavelu M, Hagos F, Marcus B, Swinnen L, McKeithan T, Vardiman JW, LeBeau MM, Olopade OI (1992) B-cell lymphoproliferative disorders following organ transplantation: clinicopathological, cytogenetic, and virologic characterization (Abstr). Blood 80 (Suppl) 1: 39a
30. Hanto DW, Gajl-Peczalska KJ, Frizzera G, Arthur DC, Balfour HH Jr, McClain K, Simmons RL, Najarian JS (1983) Epstein-Barr virus (Epstein-Barr virus) induced polyclonal and monoclonal B-cell lymphoproliferative diseases occurring after renal transplantation. Ann Surg 198: 356-369
31. Hanto DW, Sakamoto K, Purtilo DT, Simmons RL, Najarian JS (1981) The Epstein-Barr virus in the pathogenesis of post-transplant lymphoproliferative disorders. Surgery 90: 204-213
32. Morrison VA, Dunn DL, Manivel JC, Gajl-Peczalska KJ, Peterson BA (1994) Therapy and outcome of post-transplant lymphomas. Am J Med 97: 14-24
33. Swinnen LJ, Constanzo-Nordin MR, Fisher RI (1992) Pro MACE-CytaBOM induces durable complete remissions in post cardiac transplant lymphoma (Abstr) Proc Am Soc Clin Oncol 11: 318
34. Hanto DW, Frizzera G, Gajl-Peczalska KJ, Sakamoto K, Purtilo DT, Balfour HH Jr, Simmons RL, Najarian JS (1982) Epstein-Barr virus-induced B-cell lymphoma after renal transplantation. N Engl J Med 306: 913-918
35. Pirsch JD, Stratta RJ, Sollinger HW, Hafez GR, D'Alessandro AM, Kalayoglu M, Belzer FO (1989) Treatment of severe Epstein-Barr virus-induced lymphoproliferative syndrome with ganciclovir: two cases after solid organ transplantation. Am J Med 86: 241-244
36. McKelvey EM, Gottlieb JA, Wilson HE et al. (1976) Hydroxydaunomycin (Adriamycin) combination chemotherapy in malignant lymphoma. Cancer 38: 1484-1493
37. Robertson L, Rice L, Riggs S, White M, Young J, Frazier O (1990) Lymphomas after cardiac transplantation: Houston experience and successful therapy (Abstr). Blood 76 (Suppl 1): 369a
38. Manning KR, Powell BL, Peacock JE, Miller HS, Hackshaw BT (1991) Effective combination chemotherapy for high-grade non-Hodgkin's lymphoma after cardiac transplant (Abstr). Blood 78 (Suppl 1): 468a
39. Lien YH, Schröter GPJ R III, Robinson WA (1991) Complete remission and possible immune tolerance after multidrug combination chemotherapy for cyclosporine-related lymphoma in a renal transplant recipient with acute pancreatitis. Transplantation 52: 739-742
40. Shapiro RS, Chauvenet A, McGuire W, Pearson A, Craft AW, McGlave P, Filipovich A (1988) Treatment of B-cell lymphoproliferative disorders with interferon alfa and intravenous gamma globulin. N Engl J Med 318: 1334

41. Shapiro RS (1990) Epstein-Barr virus-associated B-cell lymphoproliferative disorders in immunodeficiency: meeting the challenge. J Clin Oncol 8: 371-373
42. Blanche S, Le Deist F, Veber F, Lenoir G, Fischer AM, Brochier J, Boucheix C, Delaage M, Griscelli C, Fischer A (1988) Treatment of severe Epstein-Barr virus-induced polyclonal B-lymphocyte proliferation of anti-B-cell monoclonal antibodies. Ann Intern Med 108: 199-203
43. Fischer A, Blanche S, Le Bidois J, Bordigoni P, Garnier JL, Niaudet P, Morinet F, Le Deist F, Fischer AM, Griscelli C, Hirn M (1991) Anti-B-cell monoclonal antibodies in the treatment of severe B-cell lymphoproliferative syndrome following bone marrow and organ transplantation. N Engl J Med 324: 1451-1456
44. Baiocchi RA, Caligiuri MA (1993) Low dose IL-2 prevents the development of Epstein-Barr virus-associated lymphoproliferative disorder in the SCID-human mouse (Abstr). Blood 82 Suppl 1: 385a

Impact of Selective Decontamination of the Digestive Tract for Infecion Prophylaxis in Orthotopic Liver Transplantation: Incidence and Outcome of Infections Within 90 Days After Transplantation

F. Stöblen, G. Blumhardt, W.-O. Bechstein, P. Neuhaus

Introduction

At the beginning of the 1980s selective decontamination of the digestive tract (SDD) was introduced as a regimen to reduce colonization of the oropharynx and gastrointestinal tract with aerobic gram-negative micro-organisms, since these are thought to be the endogenous sources of severe nosocomial infections in intensive care units [16]. Published data on SDD may be summarized as follows: (a) SDD significantly eradicates the colonization of the oropharynx and upper gastrointestinal tract with aerobic gram-negative microorgansisms, (b) nosocomial infections by aerobic gram-negative bacilli are significantly reduced, (c) the influence of SDD on mortality rates is not yet established [7].

The initial trials to evaluate the effectiveness of SDD were performed by Stoutenbeek and his group. SDD was shown to reduce the occurrence of nosocomial infections in intensive care patients. Initial trials in transplant patients were performed once SDD was established as an effective method in intensive care settings [4, 18, 19]. Summarizing the experiences of these groups, a remarkable reduction in severe infectious complication was detected. The combination of SDD with systemic short-term parenteral antibiotics was shown to be more effective, especially in cases of infections acquired prior hospital [1, 8].

In patients after orthotopic liver transplantation (OLT) infectious complications are still a major cause of or contributing factor to morbidity and mortality [6] (Grauhan et al., 1994, submitted). Progress in immunosuppression may result in higher risk for infection by more potent immunosuppressive agents. Therefore efforts to reduce incidence and outcome of infection after OLT are of tremendous importance [10, 14]. In transplant patients several factors influence the occurrence of infection. Specific supportive therapy is necessary to reduce the risk of infection [3]. Especially the perioperative period is decisive for infectious complications in the intensive care course [14]. The impact of SDD on infectious complications after OLT has been evaluated in a few trials [2, 9, 19]. No consensus on the value of SDD in OLT patients has yet been established. In intensive care patients a European Consensus Conference in 1991 on this topic showed a reduction in the risk of nosocomial pneumonias, but no impact on mortality was revealed by routine use of SDD [5].

Material and Methods

A total of 400 OLTs were performed in 366 patients from September 1988 to 21 June 1993 at our department; 34 were second or third transplantations. The preoperative diagnoses are listed in Table 1. Surgery was performed in the standard manner, with side-to-side instead of end-to-end bile duct anastomosis [11] and veno-venous bypass. Immunosuppression used different study protocols with standard quadruple therapy with antithymocyte globulin or quadruple therapy with interleukin-2 (IL-2) receptor antagonist instead of ATG or FK 506 with prednisolone. Rejection therapy was performed with steroid boli, OKT3 or conversion to FK 506. Infection prophylaxis consisted of the following regimens:

1. SDD is initiated with active donor search for the patient and continued 21 days after OLT in an uneventful course of the patient. SDD is used as a oral suspension with 100 mg colistin, 80 mg tobramycin and 500 mg amphotericin B four times daily.
2. Systemic antibiotic prophylaxis for 48 h perioperatively is administered with 4 x 1 g cefotaxime, 3 x 40 mg tobramycin, and 2 x 500 mg metronidazole.
3. Supportive perioperative managment: early extubation, pulmonary oriented fluid restriction and early enteral feeding.
4. Ciprofloxacin (2 x 250 mg/day) is administered with the start of active donor search for prophylaxis of legionnaires disease. Cotrimoxazole (3 x 480 mg/week) is prescribed after OLT up to 2 weeks after discharge for prevention of *Pneumocystis carinii* pneumonia.

Parenteral adminstration of imipenem and vancomycin is prescribed in severe infections without immediate knowledge of the causing micro-organisms. Ciprofloxacin is used in presumed cholangitis. If micro-organisms causing the infection are identified, appropriate antibiotic treatment is administered to the patient. The patients are checked daily for any signs of infection. A direct and aggressive approach to diagnosis and treatment is used in presumed infection. The definition of infection is as follows [15]: (a) cholangitis: fever and positive bile cultures and either elevated cholestatic parameters or histological features of cholangitis in liver biopsy specimens; (b) urinary tract infection: typical clinical sign of urinary infection and positive urine cultures with more than 100 000 micro-organisms; (c) sepsis: positive blood cultures and three symptoms of a severe general infection (body temperature over 38.5C; positive shock index, leucocytosis or leucopenia); (d) pneumonia: new onset of respiratory symptoms, new infiltratres on chest X-rays, clinical signs of infection, and positive specimens of bronchoalveolar lavage or sputum.

The data of the patients were collected prospectively in our liver transplant database.

Table 1: Indications for 400 liver transplantations

Diagnosis	n
Hepatitis B cirrhosis	83
Cryptogenic cirrhosis	13
Alcoholic cirrhosis	63
Non-A/Non-B cirrhosis	77
Primary biliary cirrhosis	34
Primary sclerosing cholangitis	22
Secondary sclerosing cholangitis	5
Wilson's disease	6
Autoimmune cirrhosis	9
Budd-Chiari syndrome	6
Acute liver failure	25
α_1-Antitrypsin deficiency	2
Porphyria	3
Hemochromatosis	3
Polycystic liver disease	5
Bile duct carcinoma	9
Carcinoid metastasis	1
Retransplantation	34

Results

The actuarial 1-year patient survival was 91% at the present 317 of 366 patients are alive (87%). Survival 90 days after OLT was 97% (356/366); within this period six patients died with or due to infectious complications (Table 2). The 30-day patient survival rate was 99% (361/366); within this time three patients died due to infectious complications. The infections in 400 OLTs are listed in Table 3. The most common infection was urinary tract infection, followed by cholangitis and pneumonia. With regard to pneumonia the most frequently encountered micro-organism was CMV, followed by *Legionella* and *Enterococcus*. On the other hand, *Enterococcus* was the most prevalent bacillus concerning cholangitis and also for urinary tract infections. Peritonitis and sepsis occurred rarely with a variety of micro-organisms isolated.

For the first 206 OLTs we have previously reviewed gastrointestinal colonization and bacterial resistance to antibioitics [15]. Concerning the oropharynx, all potentially pathogenic gram-negative micro-organisms were eradicated 1 week after OLT; in the third week only two patients had newly detected gram-negative micro-organisms. Colonization with enterococci and coagulase-negative staphylococci was greatly increased by this time. Rectal colonization presented comparable results. No development of antibiotic resistance of gram-negative micro-organisms was found. Only coagulase-negative staphylococci were found to be increasingly resistant to imipenem, and enterococci were found to be increasingly resistant to ciprofloxacin over time. These micro-organisms are not influenced or eradicated by SDD and may therefore be selected by additional parenteral antibiotics used at our Department.

Table 2: Cause of death in 366 patients within 90 days after OLT

Patient no.	Diagnosis	Death day after OLT	Cause of death
1	Non-A/non-B	33	Mycormycosis
2	Acute liver failure	33	*Aspergillus*
3	Hemochromatosis	20	Cardiac arrest
4	Alcoholic Cirr	16	*Pneumocystis carinii* pneumonia
5	Primary biliary cirrhosis	14	*Legionella*
6	Non-A/non-B	38	Hypoxia
7	Primary biliary cirrhosis	82	Cytomegalovirus
8	Klatskin-carcinoma	13	Bleeding
9	Primary biliary cirrhosis	58	Hypoxia
10	Acute liver failure	24	Cytomegalovirus

Discussion

The most critical period of life-threatening infections after OLT is the time from immediately after surgery until 90 days later. During this time technical problems, high immunosuppression, and postoperative intensive care problems lead to a high risk for infection. Reducing the technical complications by improved and standardized operative procedures decreased the incidence of infections related to surgery. Especially the infections related to biliary anastomotic problems were less common and less severe in our patient group. The main reason for this is the side-to-side anastomosis of the bile duct [12]. This anastomosis is associated with less frequent stenosis and consequently less frequent cholangitis. An additional benefit of this anastomosis technique is the better blood supply due to the vascular anatomy of the common bile duct.

The average onset of urinary tract infections at out clinic is on the 10th day after OLT. The main cause of this is an indwelling bladder catheter after OLT. The bacillus spectrum in this study clearly displays the effect of SDD. In the past year we have experienced an unexplained increase in early *Pseudomonas* urinary infections (average, 7th day). The incidence of sepsis and perotonitis is low in our patients. Only two patients in each group experienced an infection with gram-negative microorganisms in spite of SDD. There were 41 pneumonias occurring during the first 90 days after OLT. We observed only one *Pseudomonas* pneumonia. The fungal pneumonias all occurred before our Department changed location from an old to a new hospital. The difference in occurrence of *Aspergillus* pneumonia is significantly different for the location side (Grauhan 1994, submitted). This shows the contributing factors of the overall hospital environment. All deaths caused by infections were due to *Pneumonias*, and this confirms the great importance of life-threatening pneumonias in patients after OLT for morbidity and mortality. A good perioperative patient managment including early extubation, fluid restriction, ventilation training, and early enteral feeding have a positive impact on patients at this time prone to disease.

In addition to the eradicating of gram-negative and fungal micro-organisms, one must consider whether SDD has a direct binding effect on endotoxin or reduces by pretransplant application the amount of gram-negative bacilli and therefore the quantity of endotoxins and thus has a beneficial effect during the anhepatic phase of OLT. After clamping the portal vein, endotoxins are prone to harm the ischemically damaged graft. Thus initial nonfunctioning of the graft in our patients was less than 2%, which compares remarkably well with other experiences. Possible reasons for this are the technique of harvesting, routine use of aprotinin, and dismissing the first blood after reperfusion and SDD.

The effect of SDD on the incidence and outcome after OLT requires further evaluation. Summarizing our experience with the routine use of SDD in patients after OLT, we think that SDD is one piece of the puzzle to reducing early post-OLT mortality due to infections.

Table 3: Infections after OLT with routine SDD

Micro-organism	Incidence	Day after OLT (mean)
Pneumonia	41	21
Aspergillus	4	31
Mucor	1	18
Legionella	6	13
Enterococcus	6	18
Pseudomonas	1	13
Pneumocystis carinii	4	26
Staphylococcus coag. neg.	4	5
Cytomegalovirus	15	34
Cholangitis	47	19
Enterococcus	33	18
Enterobacter	3	45
Staphylococcus coag. neg.	4	12
Acinetobacter	1	23
Pseudomonas	4	9
Candida	1	47
Klebsiella	1	5
Urinary tract infection	57	19
Candida albicans	1	21
Enterococcus	34	10
Escherichia coli	3	16
Proteus	2	33
Pseudomonas	16	7
Staphylococcus	1	5
Sepsis	16	46
Enterococcus	2	22
Pseudomonas	2	21
Staphylococcus coag. neg.	4	62
Mucor	1	18
Candida	2	38
Streptococcus viridans	1	15
Aspergillus	4	73
Peritonitis	8	8
Pseudomonas	2	15
Enterococcus	2	14
Staphylococcus coag. neg.	2	6
No bacillus detected	2	7

References

1. Alcock SR (1990) Short-term parenteral antibiotics used as a supplement to SDD regimens. Infection 18 Suppl 1: 14-17
2. Badger IL, Crosby HA, Kong KL, Baker JP, Hutchings P, Elliott TSJ, McMaster P, Bion JF, Buckels JAC (1991) Is selective decontamination of the digestive tract beneficial in liver transplant patients? Interim results of a prospective, randomized trial. Transplant Proc 23: 1460-1461
3. Bechstein WO, Wiens M, Raakow R, Keck H, Blumhardt G, Neuhaus P (1993) Spezielle unterstützende Therapie (Ernährung, Infektionsbekämpfung, Intensivtherapie) in der Transplantationsmedizin. Zentralbl Chir 118: 477-481
4. Bonatti H, Bäsmüller C, Königsrainer A, Vogel W, Margreiter R (1991) Unsere Erfahrungen mit der Infektionsprophylaxe und -therapie nach 53 Lebertranplantationen. Langenbecks Arch Chir 376: 133-138
5. European Consensus Conference in Intensive Care and Emergency Medicine (1992) Selective digestive decontamination in intensive care unit patients. Intensive Care Med 18: 182-188
6. Kusne S, Dummer JS, Singh N, Iwatsuki S, Makowka L, Esquivel C, Tzakis AG, Starzl TE, Ho M (1988) Infections after liver transplantation. Medicine 67: 132-143
7. Lawin P, van Saene HKF, Stoutenbeek CP (1991) Welcome and Introduction of the Satellite Symposium "Prevention of Infection in Intensive Care." 16th International Congress of Chemotherapy, June 1989, Jerusalem/Israel. Infection 18 Suppl 1
8. Ledingham IM, Alcock SR, Eastaway AT, McDonald JC, McKay IC, Ramsay G (1988) Triple regimen of selective decontamination of the digestive tract, systemic cefotaxime, and microbiological surveillance for prevention of aquired infection in intensive care. Lancet 1: 785-790
9. Mora NP, Husberg BS, Gonwa TA, Goldstein R, Klintmalm GB (1992) The impact of the different infections on the outcome of liver transplantation. A study of 150 patients. Transpl Int 5 Suppl 1: 209-210
10. Neuhaus P (1991) Infektionsprophylaxe bei Lebertransplantation. Langenbecks Arch Chir 376: 131-132
11. Neuhaus P, Neuhaus R, Pichlmayr R, Vonnahme F (1982) An alternative technique of biliary reconstruction after liver transplantation. Res Exp Med 180: 239-242
12. Neuhaus P, Blumhardt G, Bechstein WO, Steffen R, Platz KP, Keck H (1994) Technique and results of biliary reconstruction using side-to-side choledochocholedochostomy in 300 orthotopic liver transplants. Ann Surg (in press)
13. Rocha LA, Martin MJ, Pita J, Seco C, Margusino L, Villanueva R, Duran MT (1992) Prevention of nosocomial infection in critically ill patients by selective decontamination of the digestive tract. Intensive Care Med 18: 398-404
14. Roissant R, Raakow R, Lewandowski K, Slama K, Steffen R, Lütgebrune R, Neuhaus P, Falke K (1991) Strategy for prevention of infection after orthotopic liver transplantation. Transplant Proc 23: 1965-1966
15. Steffen R, Reinhartz O, Blumhardt G, Bechstein WO, Raakow R, Langrehr JM, Roissant R, Slama K, Neuhaus P (1994) Bacterial and fungal colonization and infections using oral selective decontamination in orthotopic liver transplantations. Transplant Int 7: 101-108
16. Stoutenbeek CP, Saene van HKF (1990) How to improve infection prevention by selective decontamination of the digestive tract. Infection 18 Suppl 1: 10-13

17. Van Saene HKF, Stoutenbeek CP, Gilbertson AA (1990) Review of available trials of selective decontamination of the digestive tract (SDD). Infection 18 Suppl 1: 5-9
18. Wiesner RH (1980) The incidence of gram-negative bacterial and fungal infections in liver transplant patients treated with selective decontamination. Infection 18 Suppl 1: 19-21
19. Wiesner RH, Hermans PE, Rakela J, Washington II JA, Perkins JD, DiCecco S, Krom R (1988) Selective bowel decontamination to decrease gram-negative aerobic bacterial and candida colonization and prevent infection after orthotopic liver transplantation. Transplantation 45: 570-574

Section 10:

*Design, Methodology and Interpretation of
Clinical Trials in Shock and Sepsis*

Causality of Disease - the Problems of Animal Studies and Clinical Results

A.E. Baue

Introduction

This conference has brought together many investigators, scientists and clinicians who have made immense contributions to our understanding of injury, inflammation and infection. Our understanding of what happens to a biologic organism after trauma, with the development of infection and the necessary but often excessive inflammatory process is increasing rapidly. In this wonderful world of cytokines, mediators, receptors, adhesion molecules and growth factors our scientific knowledge exceeds our ability to do much about it in patients.

Magic Bullets?

The search continues for a magic bullet to help critically ill patients, but a series of less than successful clinical trials of agents that showed great promise in animal studies raise questions about such trials [1-5]. The goal sought is for mortality to be greatest in the placebo group (Fig. 1). Experimental evidence in animals and human volunteers for concepts, mechanisms and treatment of injury or illness can be substantial, persuasive and exciting. However, the positive effects of potential therapy suggested by such excellent animal and clinical research may be difficult to demonstrate in sick patients. Clinical evidence for efficacy of new treatments can be difficult to prove, because clinical situations, in spite of the importance of the biologic phenomena are so variable and complex. In addition, there is redundancy and overlap of mediators and the problem of timing. A major cause of this dilemma is not ill conceived clinical trials or poorly developed hypotheses. The clinical trials have been well thought through and diligently pursued. The hypotheses upon which they are based are exciting. Rather, the problem is due to a matter of the cause or causability of human disease, the *causa vera* or "specific cause" as described by Stehbens [6].

Many of the recent clinical trials of monoclonal antibodies (MAbs) and other agents have been carried out on an intensive care unit (ICU) population with sepsis, infections, the sepsis syndrome or any one of a number of different diseases. A MAb to endotoxin would seem to be effective on a disease which produces endotoxin and at a time when endotoxin is actively causing trouble. Here again, endotoxin is a manifestation of the disease and not its cause. The cause is an infection with endotoxin containing gram-negative organisms. Antibiotics which kill or halt these bacteria will cure the disease. An endotoxin MAb would only, under the best of circumstances, control some of the manifestations of the disease. A summary of some of the recent trials is shown in Table 1. There are other clinical trials which will very likely be reviewed at this meeting. There are a number of reasons why these trials and these agents, which showed so much promise in the animal laboratory, have not yielded a break through in clinical care. Some of these reasons are shown as follows:

1. Causality of diseases - many different and complex diseases being treated
2. Redundancy and overlap of mediators
3. No one factor is the lethal activator
4. Timing of treatment
5. Problem of modulation of an essential biologic function - inflammation
6. Immune deficiency or immune excess

I would like to focus attention on one of these reasons, which I think is most important for our present and future considerations, and that is the matter of causality of disease.

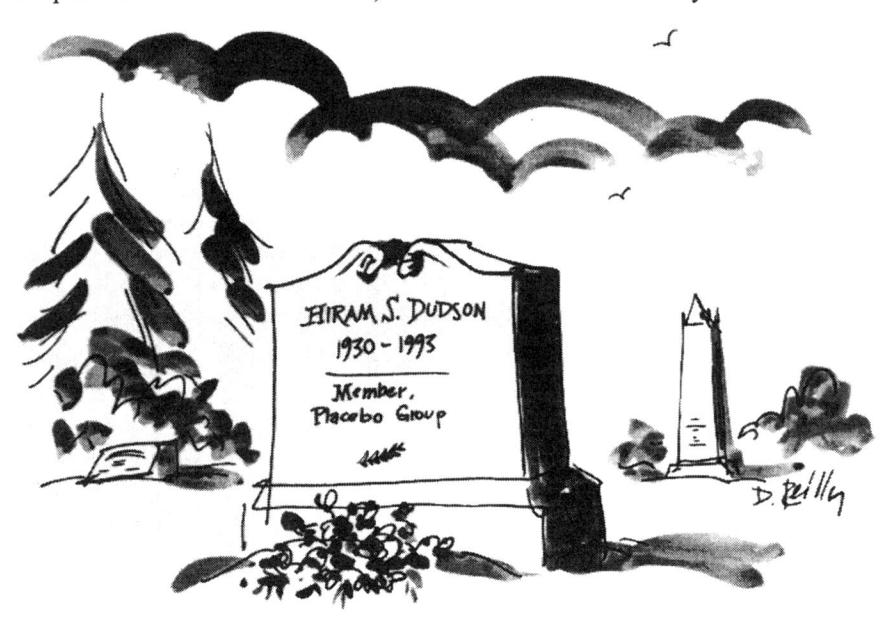

Fig. 1: The ultimate fate of the placebo group in a positive study (adapted from D. Reilly, The New Yorker Magazine)

Causality of Disease

William Stehbens, a pathologist at the Wellington School of Medicine in New Zealand, has written extensively about this, particularly as it relates to atherosclerosis. He has stated that, when prevention or treatment is based upon the *causa vera* or the specific cause of a disease, then extinction of a disease is possible, as in the case of smallpox [7, 8]. Only elimination of the cause will eradicate or cure the disease. Thus treatment of a disease, when based on symptoms or clinical manifestations is at best palliative and nonspecific. Thus basic to disease prevention and management is the concept of specific disease entities. Cause can in no way logically entail the effects, and cause must be both necessary and sufficient. It is, therefore, unjustifiable to refer to ameliorating factors as curative factors.

Table 1: Magic Bullets?

HA-1A (centoxin)	No benefits in total group
	Retrospective subgroup analysis - ↑survival
J5	
Initial study	No benefit overall
	Benefit with gram-negative sepsis
Later study	No benefit in high risk group (Gm−)
	↑ mortality with gram-positive infection
IL-1ra	No overall benefits
	Subgroup analysis indicates a new study
Anti-TNF-MAb	Phase II trial
	No benefits

An example of this would be influenza, where the cause is the influenza virus, and the only specific treatment is prevention by flu shots. The manifestations of the disease, however, are fever, chills, malaise, muscle aches and pains, nausea, vomiting and diarrhea amongst other things. The treatment for these manifestations is palliative at best and includes aspirin, nonsteroidal anti-inflammatory agents, Lo-Motil, Kaopectate and bed rest. Treatment of the manifestations may make us feel better until the disease runs its course. Stehbens further points out that epidemiologic "causes" encompass contributing, modifying, predisposing, aggravating and conditional factors, but they are not causes. He recognizes that this does not minimize the role of secondary factors that can be quite important. Stehbens goes on to say that it is essential to differentiate between specific diseases and those abnormalities that represent: (1) a class of disorders, (2) complications common to many diseases and (3) merely symptoms, signs, a physical state or laboratory findings. In our zeal to bring molecular biology into the ICU and into therapeutic regimens for our sick patients, we have tended to focus on the complications and on too many diseases. We have identified a class of disorders and sometimes set up studies based upon symptoms, signs, a physical state or laboratory findings, rather than the cause of the disease.

MOF, MODS and SIRS Are Not Diseases

In our world of injured, operated, infected, and inflamed patients there are many diseases. Multiple organ failure (MOF) is not one of them. MOF is not a disease or even a syndrome. It is the final common pathway for a great number of diseases, each of which has a cause. A syndrome is defined in Blakiston's Gould Medical Dictionary, 3rd Edn as "a group of symptoms and signs which, when considered together, characterize a disease or lesion". When I helped to develop the concept of MOF in 1975, I described MOF as a syndrome of the 1970s [9]. I believe now, in retrospect, that it was a disservice to call MOF a syndrome, because it suggested that we can lump all of these problems together. McCormick believes that a "multi-causal etiology" is a euphemism for ignorance or a synonym for unknown etiology" [10]. Admission to an ICU is not a disease, nor is an APACHE score of 30, sepsis, the sepsis syndrome or an injury severity score of 26 or a consensus conference definition of a human state. This dilemma is as follows: How do you treat?

    An ISS of 26
    An APACHE III score of 30
    SIRS
    MOF
    The sepsis syndrome
    A consensus conference definition of a human state

These entities cannot be treated. Patients with these characteristics can only be supported. The modern ICU has been an exciting development which has increased the possibilities of survival for many patients. It has led to an exciting new discipline and superspecialty in medicine in which many basic specialties share interests. Thus, for example, the Society of Critical Care Medicine and the American College of Chest Physicians (and surgeons), among other professional organizations interested in the critically ill, have made a number of contributions. There has been sharing of information and interests, joint studies and new information, but, in addition, there has been the development of a common terminology for diseases and clinical problems. This produces a complication of not getting at the cause of the diseases. Thus the investigators who carried out the interesting studies on potential magic bullets began as "lumpers" who carried out prospective randomized blinded placebo-controlled clinical trials of agents on an ICU population with characteristics of being in trouble from a number of illnesses such as sepsis or the sepsis syndrome. It is not surprising that many are getting negative results. These investigators are fast becoming "splitters" to define subgroups at higher risk for death, believing that such an approach will produce positive results. It certainly will if a disease is identified and the treatment is specific for that disease. Being at high risk for death is not a disease. I remind the reader of the questions and statements made by Beale and Bihari [11] stating that "the search for a unifying mechanism for MOF (enhanced by the chance of effective therapy) has been intense." Beal and Cerra [12] said that "the cause of the systemic inflammatory response system/multi-organ dysfunction syndrome (SIRS/MODS) is complex and not fully understood, but multiple mediators and stimulated macrophages likely are important components" and, finally, Frank Cerra in 1992 [13] in a discussion said "What is MOF? I wish I knew. A lot of people in this room have done a lot of work, and I think we know a lot about what it is not, but what it is remains elusive and needs a lot more research." Certainly, with more research, we will learn more about the problems of organ failure - single and multiple, progressive and interrelated. However, I think it is time to go back to the specific diseases that lead to MOF rather than focusing on trying to determine what MOF is. I do not think we can lump together all of the various processes shown in Table 2.

Clinical Investigative Dissociation

Much of the present exciting research is about the mediators and manifestations of injury, operations, ischemia and infections. In such circumstances, it may be difficult to dissect out and identify clinically a single factor or mediator as the most important clinical variable that may be measured and treated or controlled. All biologic processes require a level of activity that can be hazardous in excess but dangerous if decreased or eliminated, whether it be blood pressure, heart rate, respiration, gut function, tumor necrosis factor (TNF), interleukin-1

(IL-1), endothelium-derived relaxing factor (EDRF or nitric oxide), prostacyclin, thromboxane or the adherence molecules (ELAMs) or messenger RNA (mRNA). There is no doubt about the effects of various mediators of inflammation on human volunteers and in animal studies. Endotoxin, TNF and IL-1 infusions produce many of the clinical effects of infection and injury [14]. As described by Michie and Wilmore, TNF has fulfilled Koch's postulates for producing many of the symptoms for gram-negative infections [14]. There are many other mediators and in excess they produce tissue damage and/or remote organ damage which has been called a modern "horror autotoxicus" [15]. However, an inflammatory response is necessary for survival and healing after injury. There are also many feedback loops or control mechanisms that modulate the inflammatory response. The question then is, can we fool mother nature?

Many potential therapeutic agents that have statistically significant protective value in experi-

Table 2: Lumping or splitting

All infections: G+, G-, fungus, etc.
Medical patients with
Sepsis
Pneumonia
UTIs
Other
Trauma patients with or without sepsis
Low cardiac output: ischemia, gangrene
Peritonitis
Abdominal injury
Neoplastic diseases
Transplants

mental animals may never have demonstrable or positive effects in multi-system injured, operated upon or septic patients. There are many reasons for this. Most biologic processes have built in redundancies or overlaps in function. A carefully prepared animal experimental model can allow a single pertubation that can be measured and may influence survival or other vital processes. An LD_{50} (a lethal dose or effect in 50% of the animals) preparation may be influenced significantly by a small change. As shown in Fig. 2, tipping the balance may produce a significant change in mortality in the animals that may never be demonstrable clinically [16]. Such an experimental demonstration may be clinically insignificant in patients where the prospective randomized double-blinded placebo-controlled clinical trial is standard. Historic controls are unacceptable no matter how comparable they seem, because critical care gradually improves over time. This has been called "critical care creep." Normal healthy animals are used in animal experiments. They are anesthetized and instrumented. There is usually a single pertubation such as endotoxin infusion, cecal ligation and puncture and other noxious insults. The various experimental models to produce sepsis in animals are listed as follows:

    LPS - injection
    E. coli injection - i.v. or i.p.
    Cecal ligation and puncture
    Fecal pellet implantation
    Staphylococcus aureus injection
    TNF injection
    Implantation of human feces

THERAPEUTIC SIGNIFICANCE

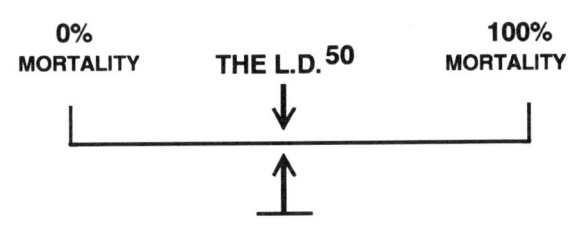

```
      0%                              100%
   MORTALITY      THE L.D.50       MORTALITY
      |_____↓_____|
                       ↑
```

Fig. 2: The balanced animal study

There is no common model used by all. A few experimental preparations use a combination of trauma and infection. Before or after the insult, there is an intervention, short term measurements are made of organ function, mediators, receptors, etc. with survival measured usually at 24 h, occasionally as long as 1 week. By and large, intensive care is not provided for the animals. Most initial human experiments are carried out in normal young human volunteers. They are awake, they are instrumented, and a single pertubation such as an infusion of a bolus or continuous infusion of a low level, nonlethal dose of a substance such as endotoxin is carried out. Symptoms, organ function and mediators are recorded and measured with observations for a period as long as 3 days. These animal and clinical studies are important in demonstrating mechanisms and mediators of disease. However, they may not be able to produce positive clinical facts in complex sick patients. Some of these studies overwhelm the animals or are acute in human volunteers, so that there is not time for the natural protective processes of the biologic response to develop. The problems with mediator blockade, for example, are as follows:

1. Redundancy - overlap
2. No single factor is the answer
3. Therappy ideally before or at the time of insult (like steroids)
4. IL-6 high in those that die but infusion of IL-6 does not harm
5. Many different diseases lumped together

Presently, the problems of trying to demonstrate the importance of various biologic phenomena in injured and septic patients are examples. These include bacterial translocation [17, 18], stress ulcer prophylaxis leading to overgrowth of bacteria in the gastrointestinal tract [19], selective decontamination of the gut [20], stiff and defective red cells [21], hypertonic solutions [22], prostaglandin E_1 [23, 24], recombinant superoxide dismutase [25] and many others.

A Historic Reference

Historically, one can remember many interesting studies and proposals, where the excitement from animal studies eventually dissipated in the face of clinical uncertainty. Many of these were simply impractical in man, despite considerable evidence and years of work in experimental laboratories. Such was true with the dextrans and, particularly, with low molecular weight dextran, which was proposed as an anti-sludging agent [26, 27]. Where is it now? THAM or TRIS-hydroxymethoaminomethane, an intracellular buffer, was initially thought to be important, because it would help with cellular acidosis. However, it never came into clinical usefulness [26]. Despite extensive studies, 2,3 diphosphoglycerate, an important factor in the affinity of hemoglobin for oxygen, has never been clinically useful [28]. Some years ago, the α-adrenergic blocking agent phenoxybenzamine (Dibenzyline) was studied extensively for the treatment of shock because it was believed that prolonged stimulation with catecholamines was deleterious. In spite of these extensive animal studies, this drug was never approved for use in patients with shock and when evaluated clinically, was found to be deleterious [29]. Steroids for the treatment of septic shock are based upon their use in experimental models, where they were given before at the time of endotoxin or gram-negative organism infusions. Only carefully controlled clinical trials stopped such use of steroids [30]. The same was true with the use of steroids for head injuries [31].

In comparison, the use of surfactant in newborn infants with respiratory distress is effective, because the clinical problem is a deficiency of surfactant [32]. It is not surprising, therefore, that surfactant has not been very helpful in the adult respiratory distress syndrome (ARDS) [33].

Biologic Conundrums

Certainly, the biologic response to injury and an overwhelming inflammatory response from tissue necrosis, ischemia or infection can overwhelm an individual. However, these mediators and other factors are also necessary for survival. The biologic conundrum, puzzle or riddle is simply that inflammation (mediators) is necessary for survival but too much inflammation may be lethal. Therefore, how can we block or modulate a necessary but excessive activity? There are a number of examples where studies contradict each other. Thus the harmful effects of a mediator can be demonstrated in one experiment but the necessity for that mediator demonstrated in another experimental preparation. One example of such a conundrum is what Bruce et al. [34] have found in germ-free rats with hemorrhagic shock. Germ-free animals have better survival after hemorrhagic shock, however, complement depletion is greater, IL-6 levels are higher, IL-1 levels are higher and there are negative blood cultures [35]. Thus, if the inflammatory response is thought to be deleterious when excessive, why is it that germ-free animals have such high levels of mediator or cytokine responses to simple hemorrhage [36]? Another example is with TNF. Infusion of TNF produces shock, toxicity and symptoms of infection. A monoclonal antibody to TNF protects against the infusion of endotoxin [14]. However, the TNF-MAb does not protect against peritonitis in animals [37] and it increases lethality in the cecal ligation and puncture model of peritonitis [38]. In patients, the TNF-MAb was tolerated, but mortality was not changed [5]. There is another example with endotoxin. Endotoxin resistant mice (C3H/Hej mice) are TNF deficient. They have improved survival from hemorrhagic shock, however, they have a much higher mortality after cecal ligation and puncture [39]. On the other hand, endotoxin-sensitive mice (C3H/Hen) had no better survival from shock with TNF-MAb pretreatment, and they had a lower mortality after cecal ligation and puncture. Also, endotoxin tolerance does not prevent the elevation of inflammatory mediators (TNF, IL-1, IL-6) after cecal ligation and puncture [40]. There are also species specificities in mediators and responses which make comparison of therapeutic regimens in animals difficult. Many other biologic conundrums could be cited such as these which indicate the complexities of these biologic processes.

Options for the Future for Therapy

Retrospective subgroup analyses suggested improvement and better survival in some of the mediator blockade studies. Thus prospective subgroup studies may be very worthwhile. The problem will be identifying those specific diseases at the time of admission, to the hospital, to the emergency department or to the ICU. In Table 3 I have listed various diseases that may have to be separated in future prospective trials. This has the hazard, of course, of splitting large populations into smaller groups, and the necessity then for a longer period of trial and smaller numbers of patients. It may be difficult to lump all trauma patients together. Blunt trauma producing long bone and pelvic fractures will differ considerably from penetrating trauma with colon perforation and peritonitis. So it is with infection. Urinary tract infections differ significantly from peritonitis, empyema and other problems. Voerman et al. noted that the endocrine and metabolic responses observed in trauma patients do not occur in medical patients with severe sepsis [41]. Thus I recognize the dilemma and the complexities. I have nothing but praise for those who have participated in these clinical studies. They are difficult, and I compliment those who have worked so hard to do them. Knaus et al. [42] have acknowledged this problem by saying, "First the number of cases needed within well-defined diagnostic categories that would be capable of demonstrating a consistent and unique weighting scheme disease by disease, would require a data base substantially larger than the 17,440 patients contained within the current APACHE III file." He also observed that fewer than half of the septic patients in their database had fever or leukocytosis, both of which are considered as necessary signs for sepsis.

Table 3: Diseases

Trauma	Blunt
	With vital organ injury
	Long bone and pelvic fractures
	Later infection
	Penetrating
	With colon perforation
	Lung and cardiac injury
	Major hepatic trauma
	Later infection
Trauma	Operative
	Cardiopulmonary bypass, heart
	Large bowel
	Transplantation
	Major organ resection
Infection	Urinary tract
	Wound
	Pneumonia
	Hepatitis
	Peritonitis
	Empyema
	Lung abscess
	Abdominal wall
	Fungemia
Inflammation	Pancreatitis
	Toxic megacolon
	Regional enteritis
Organ disease	Heart: myocardiopathy
	MIs
	Cirrhosis
	Renal failure
	COPD

MI, myocardial infarction; COPD, chronic obstructive pulmonary disease

Will all of the excitement about the mediators of inflammation, infection or injury be of great interest but go for naught in treatment? Greater precision in therapy rather than treating all comers will be necessary. There is the problem of specific therapy for non-specific disease or nonspecific therapy for a number of different and specific diseases. I believe that stimulation of natural defenses or control mechanisms of inflammation, replacement of lost or decreased host factors and better understanding of the interrelationships and mechanisms of inflammation will contribute to therapy. Growth factors and other things to stimulate healing and immunomodulation to control infection may reap great benefits [15]. A single magic bullet for complex and diverse diseases is not very likely to appear.

References

1. Ziegler EJ, Fischer C, Sprung C et al. (1991) The HA-1A Sepsis Study Group. Treatment of gram-negative bacteremia septic shock with HA-1A human monoclonal antibody against endotoxin. N Engl J Med 324: 429-436
2. Greenman RL, Schein RMH, Martin MA et al. (1991) A controlled clinical trial of E5 murine monoclonal antibody to endotoxin in the treatment of gram-negative sepsis. JAMA 266: 1097-1102
3. Bone RC (1993) Monoclonal antibodies to tumor necrosis factor in sepsis: help or harm? Crit Care Med 21: 311-312
4. Fisher CJ, Slotman GJ, Opal SM et al. (1993) Human recombinant interleukin-1 receptor antagonist (IL-1ra) in the treatment of patients with sepsis syndrome. Circ Shock 1: 42
5. Fisher CJ, Opal SM, Dhainault JF et al. (1993) Influence of an anti-tumor necrosis factor monoclonal antibody on cytokine levels in patients with sepsis. Crit Care Med 21: 318-327
6. Stehbens WE (1992) Causality in medical science with particular reference to heart disease and atherosclerosis. Perspect Biol Med 36: 97-119
7. Stehbens WE (1985) The concept of cause in disease. J Chronic Dis 38: 947-950
8. Stehbens WE (1990) Basic precepts and the lipid hypothesis of atherosclerosis. Medical Hypotheses 31: 105-113
9. Baue AE (1975) Multiple, progressive or sequential systems failure. Arch Surg 110: 779-781
10. McCormick J (1988) The multifactorial aetiology of coronary heart disease. A dangerous delusion. Perspect Biol Med 32: 103-108
11. Beale R, Bihari DJ (1993) Multiple organ failure: the pilgrim's progress. Crit Care Med 21: 51-53
12. Beal AL, Cerra FB (1994) Multiple organ failure syndrome in the 1990's. JAMA 271: 226-233
13. Cerra FB (1992) Closing discussion. Arch Surg 127: 169
14. Michie HR, Wilmore DW (1990) Sepsis, signals and surgical sequelae: a hypothesis. Arch Surg 125: 531-536
15. Baue AE (1992) The horror autotoxicus and multiple organ failure. Arch Surg 172: 1451-1462
16. Baue AE (1983) Keynote address: shock, research and therapy in the 1980's. Adv Shock Res 9: 1-16
17. Brathwaite CEM, Ross SE, Nagele R et al. (1993) Translocation occurs in humans after traumatic injury: evidence using immunofluorescence. J Trauma 34: 586-590
18. Munster AM, Smith-Meek M, Dickerson C, Winchurch RA (1993) Translocation - an incidental phenomenon or true pathology? Ann Surg 218: 321-327
19. Tryba M (1991) Sucralfate versus antacids H_2 antagonists for stress ulcer prophylaxis: a meta-analysis on efficacy and pneumonia rate. Crit Care Med 19: 942-949

20. Van Saene HKF, Stouthenbeek CC, Scoller JK (1993) Selective decontamination of the digestive tract in the intensive care unit: current status and future prospects. Crit Care Med 20: 691-703
21. Machiedo GW, Powell RJ, Rush BF Jr et al. (1989) The incidence of decreased red blood cell deformability in sepsis and the association with oxygen free radical damage in multiple-system organ failure. Arch Surg 124: 1386-1389
22. Vassar MJ, Perry CA, Holcroft JW (1993) Prehospital resuscitation of hypotensive trauma patients with 7.5% Nacl versus 7.5% NaCl with added dextran: a controlled trial. J Trauma 34: 622-633
23. Bone RC, Slotman G, Maunder R et al. (1989) Randomized double-blind multicenter study of prostaglandin E_1 in patients with the adult respiratory distress syndrome. Chest 96: 114-119
24. Slotman GJ, Kerstein MD, Bone RC (1992) The effects of prostaglandin E_1 on non-pulmonary organ function during clinical acute respiratory failure. J Trauma 32: 480-489
25. Marzi I, Bühren V, Schüttelar A, Trentz O (1992) First experiences with recombinant superoxide dismutase therapy in polytraumatized patients. In: Faist E, Meakins J, Schildberg SW (eds). Host defense dysfunction in trauma, shock and critical care. Springer, Berlin, Heidelberg, New York
26. Baue AE (1968) Recent developments in the study and treatment of shock. Surg Gynecol Obstet 127: 849-878
27. Mailloux L, Swartz CD, Capizzi R et al. (1967) Acute renal failure after administration of low-molecular weight dextran. N Engl J Med 277: 1114-1118
28. Miller LD, Oski FA, Diaco JF et al. (1970) The affinity of hemoglobin for oxygen: its control and in vivo significance. Surgery 68: 187-195
29. Eckenhoff JE, Cooperman LH (1965) The clinical application of phenoxybenzamine in shock in vasoconstrictive states. Surg Gynecol Obstet 121: 484
30. Bone RC, Fisher CJ Jr, Clemmer TP et al. (1987) A controlled clinical trial of high-dose methylprednisolone in the treatment of severe sepsis and septic shock. N Engl J Med 317: 653-658
31. Saul TG, Ducker TB, Saleman N, Carro E (1981) Steroids in severe head injury: a prospective randomized clinical trial. J Neurosurg 54: 596-600
32. Liechty EA, Donovan E, Purohit D et al. (1991) Reduction of neonatal mortality after multiple doses of bovine surfactant in low birth weight neonates with respiratory distress syndrome. Pediatrics 88: 19-28
33. Horbar JD, Soll RF, Sutherland EJM et al. (1989) A multi-center randomized placebo-controlled trial of surfactant therapy for respiratory distress syndrome. N Engl J Med 320: 959-965
34. Bruce CJ, Rush BF Jr, Ferraro FJ, Murphy TF, Hsieh JT, Machiedo GW (1992) The effect of the germ-free state on survival followed hemorrhagic shock. A study in germ-free and germ-bearing rats. Surg Forum 43: 47-51
35. Bruce CJ, Rush BF Jr, Felsen D et al. (1993) The impact of bacteria on the inflammatory mediator profile during hemorrhagic shock. Crit Care Med 21: A158
36. Bruce C, Rush BF Jr, Felsen D et al. (1992) Inflammatory mediator profiles differ in germ-free (GF) and germ-bearing (GB) rate during hemorrhagic shock (HS). Circ Shock 37: 19
37. Eskandari MK, Bolgos G, Miller C, Nguyen DT, DeForge LE, Remick DG (1992) Anti-tumor necrosis factor antibody therapy fails to prevent lethality after cecal ligation and puncture or endotoxemia. J Immunol 148: 2724-2730
38. Echtenacher B, Falk W, Männel DN, Krammer PH (1990) Requirement of endogenous tumor necrosis factor cachectin for recovery from experimental peritonitis. J Immunol 145: 3762-3766

39. McMasters KM, Peyton J, Cheadle WG (1994) Endotoxin (LPS) resistant C3H/HeJ mice are not resistant to cecal ligation and puncture despite absence of TNF production. Arch Surg (in press)
40. Ayala A, Kisala JM, Felt JA, Perrin MM, Chaudry IH (1992) Does endotoxin tolerance prevent the release of inflammatory monokines (interleukin 1, interleukin 6, or tumor necrosis factor) during sepsis? Arch Surg 127: 191-197
41. Voerman HJ, Groenevald J, de Boer H et al. (1993) Time course and variability of the endocrine and metabolic response to severe sepsis. Surgery 114: 951-959
42. Knaus WA, Sun X, Nystrom PO, Wagner DP (1992) Evaluation of definitions for sepsis. Chest 101: 1656-1662

Comparison of Criteria for Early Sepsis Classification (Elebute Score, SIRS) in Postcardiac Surgical Patients

G. Pilz, S. Kääb, E. Kreuzer, K. Werdan

Introduction

Sepsis and septic shock still constitute a major cause of intensive care unit (ICU) mortality [17]. Therefore, both standardized sepsis definitions for clinical research purposes and practicable parameters for predicting the risk at an early stage of developing septic complications in the individual patient are of considerable importance.

Given the difficulty encountered with the diagnosis of and the estimation of severity based solely on clinical judgment, various criteria have been proposed. One approach is the introduction of scoring systems, such as the Elebute score [4]. This score, which was established for surgical patients, divides the response to sepsis into four categories: local effects, temperature response, systemic effects, and laboratory data. Grundmann et al. showed that an Elebute score of ≥ 12 was highly indicative and specific for the definition of postoperative sepsis in general surgical patients ($n = 300$) [6]. Other definitions of sepsis have used a combination of routinely available single parameters [1, 18, 25]. In the most recent attempt to standardize the terminology has defined criteria for the new term "systemic inflammatory response syndrome (SIRS)." [2].

In the specific case of patients who have undergone cardiac surgery, there is a high incidence of postoperative infection, which is associated with considerable morbidity and mortality [16]. This predisposition mainly results from the intraoperative use of extracorporeal circulation (ECC) and the sequelae [5, 7, 8]. In addition, the underlying cardiac impairment [15] limits the capacity for postoperative circulatory compensation [22]. In this patient population, however, the early identification of patients at risk of developing sepsis and verification of the diagnosis of sepsis using the above-mentioned criteria may be hampered by nonspecific alterations of the parameters due to ECC, leading to sepsis-like changes in the early postoperative course [8, 23]. With regard to the definition of SIRS in general, its specificity for sepsis is still under discussion [21].

In the present study, therefore, we evaluated whether the Elebute score and the SIRS criteria were applicable to the classification of clinically defined (see "Methods") sepsis and sepsis-related outcome in patients who have undergone cardiac surgery. Conceptually, this represents the comparison of a quantitative grading for sepsis (Elebute score) with a primary categorical definition (SIRS).

Patients and Methods

Since the publication of the SIRS definition, we have retrospectively calculated the SIRS criteria for a previously monitored patient population (for details, see [19]). This population consisted entirely of patients undergoing elective openheart surgery (excluding transplantation) during a 4-month period at the Department of Cardiac Surgery, Grosshadern Hospital, University of Munich, Germany, who fulfilled the following criteria: (1) preoperative informed consent; (2) need - based on clinical judgment - for invasive hemodynamic monitoring until the second postoperative day; (3) postoperative course longer than 24 h.
The monitoring within this observational study included daily prospective assessment of scoring systems such as the Elebute and APACHE II [10] score. The immediate postoperative data were recorded on the evening of the operative day ("day 0"). This monitoring was continued in all surviving patients for at least 3 postoperative days (in patients with a longer stay: until ICU discharge). The scoring systems were assessed as originally described (for minor modifications, see [18]). Mortality was determined on ICU discharge. To assess the presence of "clinically defined sepsis and sepsis-related outcome (mortality)," charts were reviewed by both the operating cardiac surgeon and the ICU physician in charge prior to evaluation of the score-based classification. For this clinical diagnosis of "sepsis," both reviewing physicians had to agree on the presence of strong evidence for sepsis based on clinical judgment. For statistical analysis, see [19].

Results

Study Population

During the observation period, 110 patients fulfilled the inclusion criteria and were monitored within the study. The type of cardiac operation performed was: aortocoronary bypass grafting (64%), valve operations (26%) and combined procedures and miscellaneous (10%). Mortality in the study population was 12/110 (11%) and - according to clinical judgment - was mainly due to sepsis. Thus, clinically defined sepsis (see "Methods") was present in 9 out of the 12 nonsurviving patients prior to death.

Comparison of Elebute Score and SIRS for Evaluation of Clinically Defined Sepsis and Mortality in Cardiac Surgery Patients

Both the Elebute score and SIRS showed a significant correlation with parameters reflecting the general and sepsis-related severity of the patients' postoperative clinical course (Table 1). In comparison to SIRS, the Elebute score correlations were better for all the parameters tested (Table 1). Evaluation of the optimal classification criterion for the mainly sepsis-related outcome (see above) in this population gave maximal Youden indices [24] of 0.87 for the Elebute score (best criterion, score ≥ 12 on ≥ 2 days; accuracy, 94%) compared to 0.42 for SIRS (best criterion, SIRS definition fulfilled on ≥ 3 days; accuracy, 67%). Accordingly, the Elebute score ROC curve areas for both overall and (clinically defined) sepsis-related prognostic evaluation were significantly larger than for SIRS (Fig. 1). This higher overall accuracy of the Elebute score was primarily due to a more valid assessment on the first and second postoperative days, when SIRS still displayed a high false-positive classification rate (> 45%, see Fig. 2).

Table 1: Correlation of Elebute score and SIRS with parameters reflecting the clinical postoperative course of postcardiac surgical patients ($n = 515$ patient days; all $p < 0.0001$).

Clonical parameter	Correlation with sepsis score	
	Elebute score	SIRS status
Mortality	0.59	0.32
Microbiological findings[a] (numner)	0.44	0.29
ICU treatment (days)	0.51	0.32
Mechanical ventilation (days)	0.54	0.32
Vasopressor requirement (days)	0.59	0.33
Antibiotic therapy (days)	0.36	0.26

[a]Positive microbiological cultures from various sites.

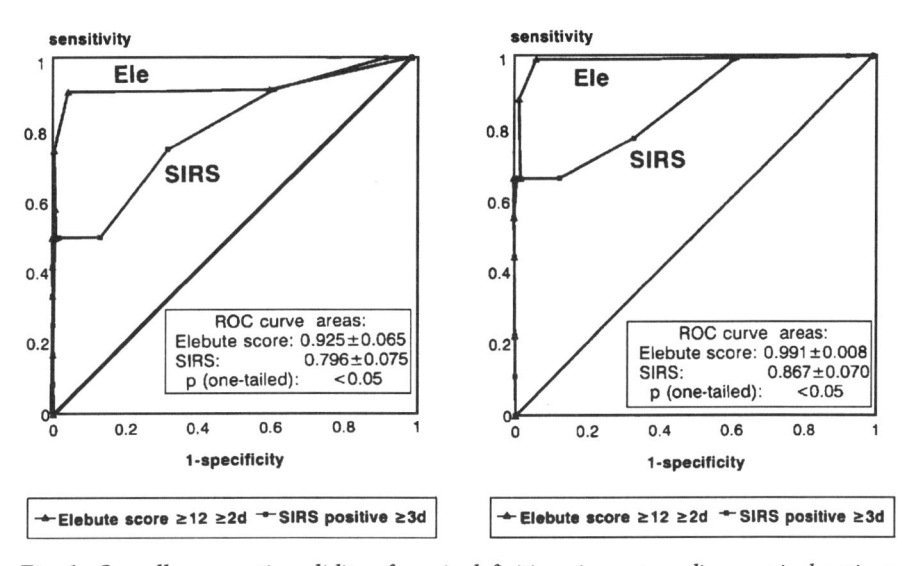

Fig. 1: Overall prognostic validity of sepsis definitions in post cardiac surgical patients (n=110). Comparison of Elebute score and SIRS. Left panel, overall mortality; right panel, clinically defined (see "Methods") sepsis-related mortality. d, days. [From 21]

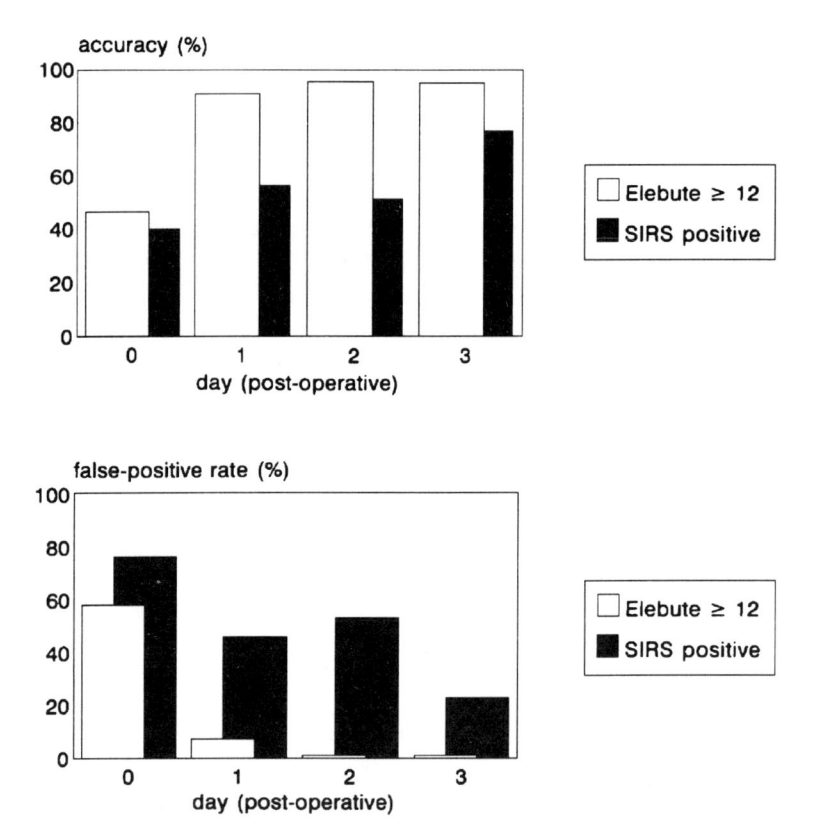

Fig. 2: Prognostic validity of sepsis definitions in post cardiac surgical patients (n = 110) during the early postoperative course: accuracy (top) and false-positive classification rate (bottom). [From 21].

Definition of Postoperative Sepsis in Cardiac Surgery Patients by Elebute Score

According to these results, in the present study the Elebute score seemed suitable as a parameter for classification of sepsis. It allowed a clear separation of the study population into two groups: one group ($n = 94$) with an uneventful postoperative course (mortality 1%, unrelated to sepsis) and another group ($n = 16$) with "septic complications," associated with a significantly ($p < 0.0001$) worse prognosis (mortality 69%, mainly due to sepsis, see above). Likewise, the postoperative course of patients with sepsis as defined by the Elebute score was significantly worse with regard to the duration of ICU treatment, mechanical ventilation, vasopressor support, antibiotic treatment, and number of microbiological findings (Table 2).

Regarding preoperative patient characteristics, there were no significant differences between patients with and without postoperative septic complications in age and preoperative values for LVSWI, CI, and SVR (Table 2). Septic complications occurred more frequently in women. Patients with postoperative septic complications showed significantly higher preoperative values for the NYHA functional class and for the pulmonary capillary wedge pressure (PCWP). The duration of ECC was significantly longer in patients who later became septic (Table 2).

Table 2: Perioperative patient data according to the presence of septic complications.

Parameter	"No septic complication" (n = 94)	"Septic complication" (n = 16)	p
Preoperative data (day - 1)			
Age (years)	58.4 ± 1.1	61.0 ± 2.3	NS
Sex (m/f)	76 / 18	8 / 8	<0.05
NYHA classification[a]	2.3 ± 0.6	3.3 ± 0.5	<0.0001
LWSWI (g · m/m^2 BSA)	43.8 ± 1.2	38.5 ± 4.1	NS
CI (l/min · m^2 BSA)	2.5 ± 0.7	2.6 ± 0.2	NS
SVR (dyn · cm^{-5} · s)	1271 ± 42	1406 ± 104	NS
PCWP (mmHg)	10.7 ± 0.6	20.6 ± 1.8	<0.0001
Operation			
ECC duration	74.4 ± 2.6	111.3 ± 14.9	<0.05
Postoperative course			
ICU treatment (days)	2.9 ± 0.1	7.3 ± 1.6	<0.05
Mechanical ventilation (days)	1.1 ± 0.0	6.8 ± 1.7	<0.0001
Vasopressor support (days)[b]	0.9 ± 0.1	5.9 ± 1.3	<0.0001
Antibiotic treatment (days)	3.1 ± 0.1	8.0 ± 1.6	<0.0001
Microbiological findings (sum)[c]	0.1 ± 0.0	2.1 ± 0.8	<0.0001

[a]New York Heart Association functional class.
[b]Exceeding dopamine in "renal" dosage.
[c]Positive microbiological cultures from various sites.

Discussion

SIRS Criteria in Postcardiac Surgery Patients

Recently, the definition of systemic inflammatory response syndrome (SIRS) has been proposed by a consensus conference to be applied to patients with sepsis and its sequelae [2]. Evaluating this definition, Knaus et al. [12] showed that SIRS was superior to the traditional definition of sepsis syndrome [1] regarding its sensitivity for identifying the 519 patients with a clinically defined primary diagnosis of sepsis out of the APACHE III score patient database [11] (sensitivity 97% vs. 59%). However, as pointed out elsewhere [21], the question of its specificity for sepsis has not been definitively answered. Thus, it has been proposed that the SIRS definition must be used only with a precise clinical diagnosis [13].

When applied to our study population with its non-sepsis-specific alterations in the early postoperative course, the SIRS criteria displayed a low specificity (i.e., high false-positive classification rate) for clinically defined sepsis-related mortality during the first postoperative days (Fig. 2). Since about half of the patients with SIRS during this period had an uneventful further clinical course and ultimately survived (Fig. 2), patient assessment solely on the base of SIRS would have led to a misclassification in half of the cases. Even though the more stringent definition of at least 3 days with SIRS fulfilled reduced the misclassification rate to 1/3 (see "Results"), application of such an inclusion criterion for sepsis therapy trials might result in a considerable delay in the onset of treatment. Thus, the use of the SIRS definition per se did not seem to allow a sufficiently reliable classification of septic complications in the early postoperative course of our cardiac surgical patients. Whether the combination of SIRS with a patient-specific risk score [13] will improve classification accuracy in this patient population, will have to be determined.

Validation of the Elebute Score for Cardiac Surgery Patients

In the present study, the definition of postoperative sepsis after general surgery by the Elebute score criterion ≥ 12 [6] was validated for cardiac surgery patients in an extended form (see below). This is of importance, since ECC use during cardiac surgery leads to nonspecific alterations (abnormal bleeding, fever) in the early postoperative course [8, 23]. Expectedly, within the total study population (n = 110, including 94 nonseptic patients) the mean number of days per patient with an Elebute score ≥ 12 was 1.4 ± 0.2, providing evidence for a lack of specificity of Grundmann et al.'s traditional definition in cardiac surgery patients in the very early postoperative course. However, the resulting false positive classification rate was virtually restricted to the evening of the operation day ("day 0") and dropped markedly on the morning of the following day to values < 10% (Fig. 2). Accordingly, starting with the first postoperative day, its daily classification accuracy exceeded 90% (Fig. 2). Thus, extending the criterion "Elebute score ≥ 12" to ≥ 2 days proved to adequately increase specificity for clinically defined sepsis-related outcome in this patient population. This definition proved to correlate well with parameters reflecting either disease or sepsis severity, such as the incidence of infections, MOF severity, duration of ICU treatment and, most importantly, overall mortality and particularly death due to clinically defined sepsis (see increase of the ROC curve area for the latter, Fig. 1).

This Elebute score criterion differs from that used by Dominioni et al. (score ≥ 20 [3]) for immunoglobulin sepsis therapy, because our study aimed at the early diagnosis of developing septic complications, while the former trial was designed to include severely septic patients with a bad prognosis.

Despite its diagnostic accuracy being confirmed in the present study, the use of Elebute scoring for routine sepsis monitoring is limited. It does not seem practicable to measure daily all variables required over a potentially longer period, and some of the parameters are not immediately available (for details, see [18]). Therefore, as presented in detail elsewhere [14, 20], we have subsequently investigated and validated an APACHE II score-based approach that allowed an early routine prospective risk stratification for the imminent development of septic complications, which has already been used with the intention to treat [20].

Conclusion

In the early postoperative course after cardiac surgery, the SIRS definition displayed a lower specificity (high false-positive classification rate) for subsequent clinically defined sepsis-related mortality as opposed to a high classification accuracy achieved by the Elebute sepsis score (best criterion: score ≥ 12 on ≥ 2 days). These results indicate that the validity of quantitative sepsis grading was superior to that of a categorical definition in this patients population.

Acknowledgement

This presentation contains results from a recently published original paper [19].

References

1. Bone RC, Fisher CJ, Clemmer TP, Slotman GJ, Metz CA, Balk RA, and The Methylprednisolone Severe Sepsis Study Group (1989) Sepsis syndrome: a valid clinical entity. Crit Care Med 17: 389-393
2. Bone RC, Balk RA, Cerra FB, Dellinger RP, Fein AM, Knaus WA, Schein RMH, Sibbald WJ (1992) Definitions for sepsis and organ failure and guidelines for the use of innovative therapies in sepsis. Chest 101: 1644-1655
3. Dominioni L, Dionigi R, Zanello M, Chiaranda M, Dionigi R, Acquarolo A, Ballabio A, Sguotti C (1991) Effects of high-dose IgG on survival of surgical patients with sepsis scores of 20 or greater. Arch Surg 126: 236-240
4. Elebute EA, Stoner HB (1983) The grading of sepsis. Br J Surg 70: 29-31
5. Eskola J, Salo M, Viljanen MK, Ruuskanen O (1984) Impaired B lymphocyte function during open heart surgery. Effects of anaesthesia and surgery. Br J Anaesth 56: 333-338
6. Grundmann R, Kipping N, Wesoly C (1988) Der "Sepsisscore" von Elebute und Stoner zur Definition der postoperativen Sepsis auf der Intensivstation. Intensivmed 25: 268-273
7. Kharazmi A, Andersen LW, Baek L, Valerius NH, Laub M, Rasmussen JP (1989) Endotoxemia and enhanced generation of oxygen radicals by neutrophils from patients undergoing cardiopulmonary bypass. J Thorac Cardiovasc Surg 98: 381-385
8. Kirklin JK, Westaby S, Blackstone EH, Kirklin JW, Chenoweth DE, Pacifico AD (1983) Complement and the damaging effects of cardiopulmonary bypass. J Thorac Cardiovasc Surg 86: 845-857
10. Knaus WA, Draper EA, Wagner DP, Zimmerman JE (1985) APACHE II: A severity of disease classification system. Crit Care Med 13: 818-829
11. Knaus WA, Wagner DP, Draper EA, Zimmerman JE, Bergner M, Bastos PG, Sirio CA, Murphy DJ, Lotring T, Damiano A, Harrell FE (1991) The APACHE III prognostic system. Risk prediction of hospital mortality for critically ill hospitalized adults. Chest 100: 1619-1636
12. Knaus WA, Sun X, Nystrom PO, Wagner DP (1992) Evaluation of definitions for sepsis. Chest 101: 1656-1662
13. Knaus WA, Sun X, Wagner DP (1994) Evaluation of definitions for sepsis (Letter to the editor). Chest 105: 970-971
14. Kreuzer E, Kääb S, Pilz G, Werdan K (1992) Early prediction of septic complications after cardiac surgery by APACHE II score. Eur J Cardiothorac Surg 6: 524-527
15. Marsh HM, Abel MD (1989) Postoperative management of adult cardiac surgical patients. In: Tarhan S (ed.) Cardiovascular anesthesia and postoperative care. 2nd Edn. Year Book Medical Publishers, Chicago, pp. 609-630
16. Miholic J, Hudec M, Domanig E, Hiertz H, Klepetko W, Lackner F, Wolner E (1985) Risk factors for severe bacterial infections after valve replacement and aortocoronary bypass operations: analysis of 246 cases by logistic regression. Ann Thorac Surg 40: 224-228

17. Parrillo JE, Parker MM, Natanson C, Suffredini AF, Danner RL, Cunnion RE, Ognibene FP (1990) Septic shock in humans - advances in the understanding of pathogenesis, cardiovascular dysfunction, and therapy. Ann Intern Med 113: 227-242
18. Pilz G, Gurniak T, Bujdoso O, Werdan K (1991) A BASIC program for calculation of APACHE II and Elebute scores and sepsis evaluation in intensive care medicine. Comput Biol Med 21: 143-159
19. Pilz G, Kääb S, Kreuzer E, Werdan K (1994) Evaluation of definitions and parameters for sepsis assessment in patients after cardiac surgery. Infection 22: 8-17
20. Pilz G, Kreuzer E, Kääb S, Appel R, Werdan K (1994) Early sepsis treatment with immunoglobulins in score-identified high-risk cardiac surgery patients. Chest 105: 76-82
21. Pilz G, McGinn P, Werdan K (1994) Evaluation of definitions for sepsis (Letter to the editor). Chest 105: 970
22. Shoemaker WC, Kram HB, Appel PL (1990) Therapy of shock based on pathophysiology, monitoring, and outcome prediction. Crit Care Med 18: S19-S25
23. Wilson APR, Treasure T, Grüneberg RN, Sturridge MF, Burridge J (1988) Should the temperature chart influence management in cardiac operations? J Thorac Cardiovasc Surg 96: 518-523
24. Youden WJ (1950) Index for rating diagnostic tests. Cancer 3: 32-35
25. Ziegler EJ, Fisher CJ, Sprung CL, Straube RC, Sadoff JC, Foulke GE, Wortel CH, Fink MP, Dellinger RP, Teng NNH, Allen IE, Berger HJ, Knatterud GL, LoBuglio AF, Smith CR, and The HA-1A Sepsis Study Group (1991) Treatment of gram-negative bacteremia and septic shock with HA-1A human monoclonal antibody against endotoxin. N Engl J Med 324: 429-436

Consensus-Assisted Development of a Study Protocol for Sepsis: Discussion Forum, Protocol Chart and a Formalized Method for Clinical Algorithms

W. Lorenz, H. Sitter, F. Weitzel

Introduction

In the recent years of exploding recombinant technology and critical evaluation of new agents for the treatment and prophylaxis of sepsis, even experts find it difficult to stay abreast of the almost endless possibilities provided by basic research and industry. Bone [2] prepared a comprehensive list of mediators and drugs against their actions which are all suitable for entry into randomized trials to assess effectiveness at saving life (Table 1). However, even for single drugs there is too much choice, not to mention the exponential growth of possibilities if only two or three are combined with each other or with the present "standard" treatment of respiratory support, various types of apparatus, and drugs to improve the function of physiological systems and antibiotics. In sharp contrast to all this choice, there have been virtually no trials which have established a positive influence of drugs on the mortality rate of patients with sepsis [14, 27]. Antibiotics may sometimes prove to be the exception, as the meta-analysis of the SDD Trialists Collaboration Group in Milan, Italy, has demonstrated this year [22]. However, this study has also been criticized for its unsatisfactory sensitivity analysis (Goris, this congress).

Factors Responsible for the Present Failure of Sepsis Trials

1. Despite the many useful recommendations from the Shock Society [26] and other organizations, there are still many animal experiments that are not convincingly clinically relevant. The main reason for this is not that the pathophysiological or cell-biological parameters are inappropriate, but that the experimental conditions do not include antibiotics and/or operative procedures in many cases. The models lack the complexity which is typical for the clinical situation of sepsis [24], for instance when only single microbes are used or single organ dysfunction and failure is produced in genetically defined and

Table 1: New treatments for sepsis [2]

Monoclonal antibodies to	Neutrophil inhibitors
Endotoxin	Pentoxifylline
Exotoxin	Adenosine
Tumor necrosis factor alpha	Dapsone
Interleukin 1	Antioxidants
Phospholipase A_2	Heavy metal chelators
Complement fragment $C5_a$	Oxygen radical scavengers
Adhesion molecules	Protease inhibitors
Contact factors	Modulators of coagulation
Receptor antagonists to	Antithrombin III
Tumor necrosis factor alpha	Protein C
Interleukin 1	Thrombomodulin
Platelet activating factor	Hirudin
Thromboxane A_2	$alpha_1$-Antitrypsin Pittsburgh
Bradykinin	Aprotinin
Prostaglandins	Soybean trypsin inhibitor
Prostaglandin E_2	Plasminogen activators
Prostaglandin I_2	Other
Other inhibitors of inflammation	Gut decontamination
C1 inhibitor	Antihistamines
MX-1 (a C5 blocker)	Naloxone
Arachidonic acid inhibitors	Thyroid-releasing hormone
Cyclooxygenase pathway (e.g., ibuprofen)	Glucagon
Thromboxane synthetase (e.g., imidazole)	Surfactant
Lipoxygenase pathway (e.g., diethylcarbamazine)	Extracorporeal membrane oxygenation
	Calcium channel blockers
Specific leukotriene inhibitors	Growth factors
	Growth hormone

deficient rodents. Reductionism is thought to be the wrong direction if it does not represent the complexity at the different scientific levels [23]. Hence, much of molecular biology is of use for increasing our knowledge, but not for demonstrating effectiveness of therapy.

2. A new treatment such as the antiendotoxin monoclonal antibody HA/1A may produce either beneficial of harmful effects depending on the status of the mediator network or the cytokine network [25, 27, 28]. Hence subgroups must be defined with more accuracy than in the present trials, but the first requirement is to explain and test which subgroups should be used and what they should be compared with.

3. The question of the correct time to intervene with treatment - either as prophylaxis or as therapy - is not answered by the experimenter's decision, but by the clinical choices and needs. Usually prophylaxis leads to better-defined patient-related and situation-related entry criteria into the study than therapy, but the clinical problem may demand treatment instead of prophylaxis.

4. Randomized trials to investigate sepsis are very complex. There may be too many conditions for the patients' entry into the study, the course of the sepsis syndrome and the underlying disease and especially for the numerous types of interventions. A sophisticated design of the randomized trials can solve such problems [15], including independent

observers who assess and evaluate the treatment performed by their colleagues responsible for the patients. However, the time required for operations [15] is short compared with the day and night work over several weeks in intensive care units. Hence the observation of clinicians in sepsis trials is a further tedious procedure in the assessment of what clinicians, nurses and technicians really do [4] if they support septic patients by the "human factor" during sepsis treatment.
5. Basic errors can be made in designing, conducting and analyzing sepsis trials such as the definition of patient entry criteria into the study based on bacteriology, which is inadequate in many cases, and is considered unreliable for the sepsis syndrome even if it is positive. Very often there are no simple solutions as to the methodology of a certain trial, but a way must be found to reconcile the aims and requirements of a team of pathophysiologists (cell biologists, molecular biologists), of statisticians and decision-makers and of clinicians, who are usually highly ranked on the Dreyfus scale of expertise [10]. There is no necessity to bow to ego of a single, dominating person in a team. This last statement is critical for consensus conferences because fascinating experts can always manipulate the opinion of a very heterogenous jury - as in a town council meeting [17].
6. Finally, however, it has not yet been emphasized enough that sophisticated, very specialized conditions in randomized trials need to be transformed into the clinical routine of intensive care units to allow for the generalization of the results. This is an increasingly difficult task for doctors since clinicians' methods and routines need to be standardized in the future, not only in the treatments.

Special Recommendations to Overcome the Failure of Sepsis Trials

These are philosophical and general thoughts, but also include special recommendations from expert groups and medical societies on overcoming current frustrating situations in sepsis trials. The problem for clinical trialists is how to transform these recommendations into practical concepts and acceptable trial design. A successful protocol is required which is capable of being carried out with dropout rates of less than 10%, low observer variation, good data quality and faster than previously considered possible. Only significant results are of use (accepting the alternative hypothesis), because insignificant results will not lead to application of the drug tested. However, in modern trials a significant result is no longer only acceptable for the whole study sample, but also has to be shown in subgroups [14] and - as a new condition - also after regression modeling with a whole battery of patient and treatment covariables [1]. Finally - and this is a relatively new condition - the study sample and the management conditions must be representative of the septic patient population and of the local and general health care system of a reasonable number of physicians - at least as many as required to be profitable to the suppliers.

Our cautious answer to many of these problems and our method of proceeding is the concept of a Consensus-Assisted Development of a Study Protocol on Sepsis [15]. This concept can possibly be best understood if a time schema is presented as a protocol chart [20] (Fig. 1). Clinical trials on sepsis are very complex and need time for protocol development. However, because the number of drugs and devices available for such trials is growing exponentially, the whole process of cell culture and animal experimentation (Fig. 1, top), clinical phase I and II trials, protocol development, buildup of the organizational structure of the multicenter trial and standardization of diagnostic and treatment approaches in the ICU among different centers has to be shortened by a temporal overlapping of the individual phases.

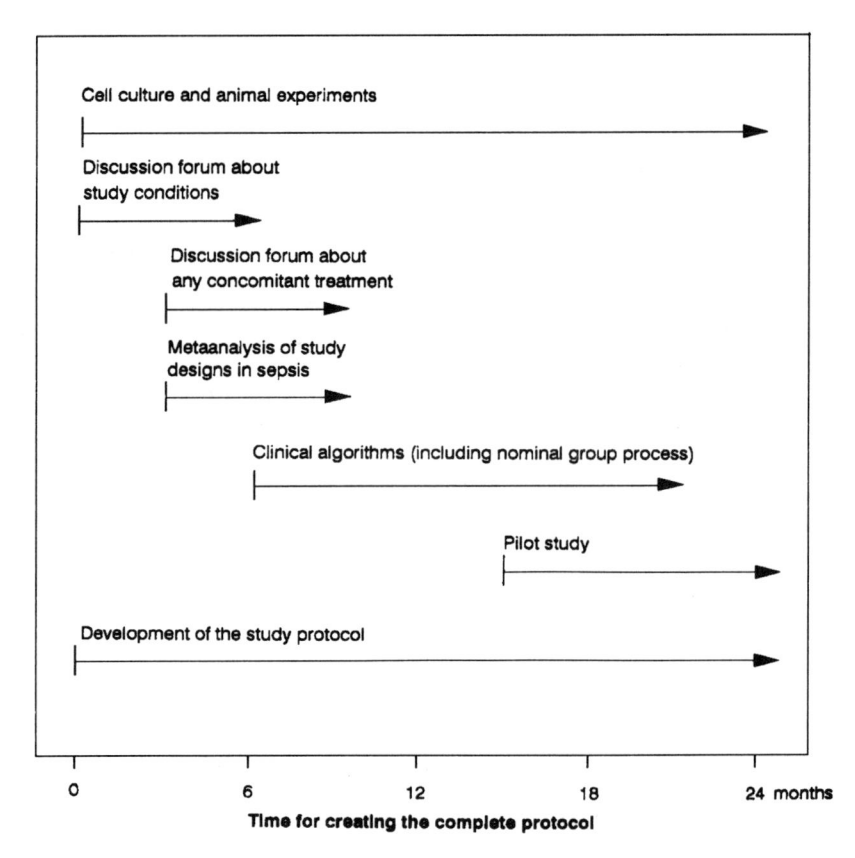

Fig. 1: Time schema for consensus-assisted development of a study protocol for sepsis

Protocol development should start after the first successful animal experiments [24] that show effectiveness. It should not be delayed until exhaustive evidence is obtained for a dose-dependent cost benefit from animal models and near-complete explanations of the pathomechanisms. Work on the cellular and molecular biology should continue during protocol development as shown in the top line of Fig. 1 and should involve members of the study team. Trials on the immunotherapy of sepsis should not be designed without the inclusion of cell or molecular biologists in the study group.

The second feature of this concept is a published discussion forum based on the opinions of eight to ten expert groups in this field about a published study protocol [19]. Why should it be published? Because after the conduct and publication of the trial results the pre- and post-trial arguments can be compared and can be related to any post-trial criticism [12]. Why should it be a discussion forum of eight to ten expert groups? Because agreement and disagreement of leading people can be considered by the trialists before the trial runs into analysis of conduct or data. Why should it be a published study protocol? Because all the very thoughtful and clever experts should be enforced not to talk, but to advise in detail what they would like to do differently in a given protocol.

We have recently completed the first discussion forum as outlined in Fig. 1: the trial protocol [19] and the forum have been published in *Theoretical Surgery* [14]. The discussion forum included 14 contributions from experts from various disciplines, in surgery and anesthesiology as well as specialists in intensive care medicine (Table 2). The titles are shortened from the original contributors to make the table readable. But most important was not the number or the general excellence of the participants in the discussion forum, but the content of each article in response to the original study protocol [19].

Table 2: Discussion forum - methodology of clinical trials in sepsis [14]

Lorenz et al.	Introduction...
Solomkin	Sepsis as a descriptor...
Seifert	Immunological aspects of i.v. gammaglobulin...
Reemst et al.	Scoring systems
Knaus et al.	Individual patient risk assessment...
Ohmann, Quick	Computerized information system...
Balk, Bone	Methodological issues in the design...
Schein	The role of planned reoperations...
Margolis	Clinical algorithms in sepsis trials...
Peduzzi, Shatney	Design of clinical trials in sepsis...
Wyatt	Insights from cancer trials...
Koller et al.	Double-blind controlled trials...
Evans	Organizational problems...
Neugebauer	Multicenter trials in sepsis...
Lorenz et al.	Consensus-assisted development of study protocol on sepsis...

Invitation to the discussion forum was a request to criticize (Table 3). It was therefore not surprising that there were more arguments against than in favor. The two exceptions were participants No. 5 (Ohmann) and No. 8 (Margolis). Margolis [16] welcomed the development of clinical algorithms in the Pilz study [19], which is also a major component of the concept of a Consensus-Assisted Protocol Development [15]. However, both the group in Munich who developed the study design [19] and the readers of the discussion forum will recognize that several arguments were raised repeatedly while others were unique from the special field of expertise or were controversial among the experts. Three examples of clusters of arguments were: (1) the selection of the target population which did not represent precisely enough patients with bacterial infections. (2) Bias was suspected if the study groups did not adhere to the intention-to-treat rule [18]. (3) There was no clear, unequivocal handling of the ethically demanded interim analysis by an external monitoring group. We as the readers of the results of the discussion forum are all convinced that the study group in Munich will carefully consider these arguments to reach a consensus whereas they will proceed unpredictably in controversial issues.

One recent example of how an intention-to-treat analysis changes an impressive difference in mortality (44%) into a negligible difference is the trial of antithrombin III concentrates in septic shock conducted by Fourrier et al. [9].

A third further element of consensus finding is qualitative meta-analysis, e.g., that of ten study designs of well-known sepsis trials, including the Ziegler trial [28], the Fisher trial [8], the Bone trial [3], the VA study on methylprednisolone [11] and a series of others. This consensus is mostly technical, but the trial makers will find their way through the heterogeneity of trial conditions which make a comparison of these trials often impossible.

Table 3: Number of arguments for and against features of the Pilz study design. No. 1 = Solomkin

Participant	Number of arguments proposed	
	Pro	Contra
1	1	6
2	1	8
3	1	8
4	5	10
5	2	1
6	3	11
7	1	5
8	1	0
9	2	9
10	2	9
11	0	7
12	1	10
13	0	7
	1 (0-5)	8 (0-11)

Clinical Algorithms for the Management of Patients with Sepsis in a Multicenter Trial

The most important process of consensus finding in the concept of Consensus-Assisted Development of a Study Protocol in Sepsis is the development of clinical algorithms for the management of patients with sepsis by the participants of the multicenter trial. Terms or definitions are very often used today without precise and sufficient knowledge of the methodology for which the definitions were primarily designed by experts in the field. Hence it is necessary first to clarify the definitions with which clinical algorithm maps may become confused:

1. Clinical algorithm maps are not identical to recommendations of a consensus conference. They are the result of a defined psychological procedure (so-called DelBecque technique and Delphi technique) among a group of about 10-20 participants who in sepsis trials are identical to the participants of the multicenter trial.
2. Clinical algorithm maps can be used as standardized clinical guidelines which meet criteria according to the Institute of Medicine in Washington such as reliability (repeatability by a series of users in defined, modeled clinical cases), validity and clarity. They do not, therefore, correspond to the usually verbalized practice guidelines of many medical societies.
3. Clinical algorithm maps are, however, similar to the computerized critical care protocols developed by East et al. [6] for their study on "Extracorporal CO_2 Removal for ARDS." This trial, however, contains far too many rules, which were not developed by a nominal group process.
4. Clinical algorithm maps do not correspond to management procedures such as those published by Edwards [7], because these flow charts do not use If/Then logic and are not the result of a consensus procedure.

5. Clinical algorithms are not identical to flow charts per se because flow charts are just a form and do not imply a certain procedure of consensus for their generation.
6. Finally, clinical algorithms are not just a mathematical technique as used in informatics. We have not yet developed clinical algorithms for management of sepsis because the development of consensus for the trial is still underway and is not yet complete (Fig. 1). However, to give an example of successful development of consensus of an algorithm, we present our data on cholecystectomy (Fig. 2) [13]. This algorithm starts with symptomatic gallstone disease (which is already provocative), describes the choice of pathways between stones in the biliary tract and no stones in this part of the biliary tract and proceeds to the choice of several types of treatment. Finally a decision needs to be made.

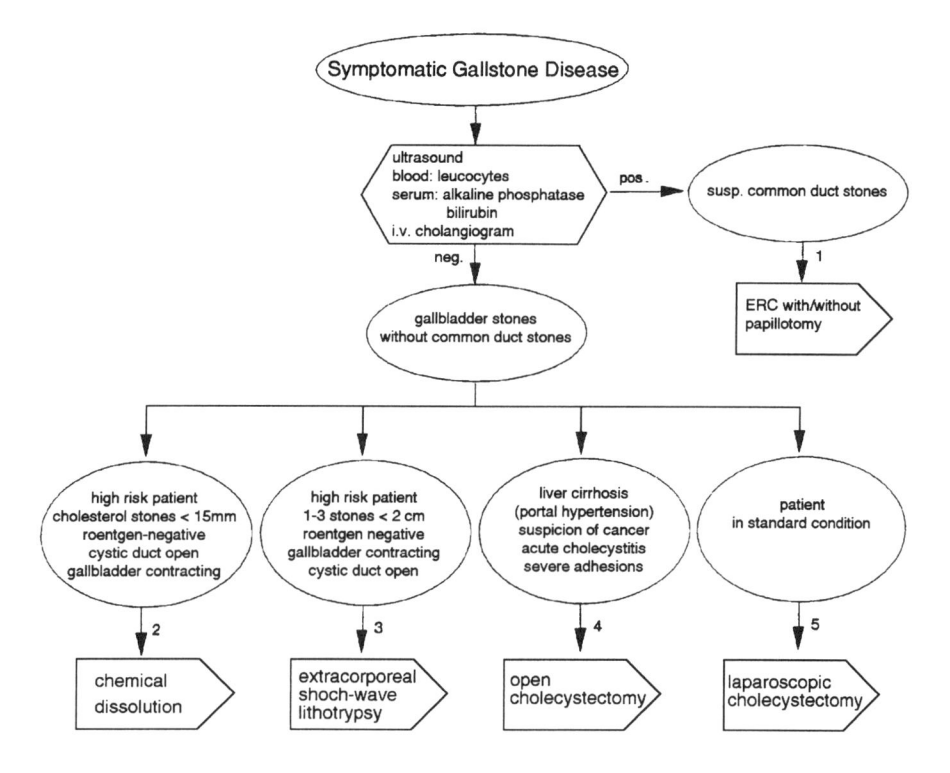

Fig. 2: Clinical algorithm. Question 8 in the conference: Do you agree to these treatment strategies for symptomatic cholelithiasis? Panel (n = 7): 5, yes, 2 with reservations, 0 no. General audience (n = 62): 8 yes, 39 with reservations, 15 no (from [21])

Clinical algorithm maps should not be complicated and should not contain too many steps. They use formalized boxes for entrance, for yes/no decisions, for findings or statements and for tasks. They are also the result of a formalized group process between the restricted number of members, in our case those of the participants of a multicenter trial.

637

Conclusions

1. Controlled clinical trials in patients with sepsis are very complex and most likely to fail.
2. The concept of Consensus-Assisted Development of a Study Protocol on Sepsis has been created to overcome the present difficulties.
3. This concept includes discussion fora, meta-analysis of trial protocols and clinical algorithm maps as elements which have been established by consensus-finding methods.
4. The first steps in this procedure were found to be successful and satisfactory for the participants. Further steps are now in the process of being implemented.

References

1. *Altmann DG, Dorè CJ (1990) Randomisation and baseline comparisons in clinical trials. Lancet 335: 149-153*
2. *Bone RC (1991) A critical evaluation of new agents for the treatment of sepsis. JAMA 266: 1686-1691*
3. *Bone RC, Fisher CJ, Clemmer TP, Slotman GJ, Metz CA, Balk RA (1987) A controlled clinical trial of high-dose methylprednisolone in the treatment of severe sepsis and septic shock. N Engl J Med 317: 653-658*
4. *Christensen C, Cottrell JJ, Murakami J, Mackesy ME, Fetzer B, Elstein AS (1993) Forecasting survival in the medicinal intensive care unit: a comparison of clinical prognoses with formal estimates. Methods Med 32: 302-308*
5. *Cross AS, Opal SM, Sadoff JC, Gemski P (1993) Choice of bacteremia in animal models of sepsis. Infect Immun 61: 2741-2747*
6. *East TD, Morris AH, Wallace CJ, Clemmer TP, Orme JF, Weaver LK, Henderson S, Sittig DF (1992) A strategy for development of computerized critical care decision support systems. Int J Clin Monit Comput 8: 263-269*
7. *Edwards JD (1993) Management of septic shock. Br Med J 306: 1661-1664*
8. *Fisher CJ, Slotman GJ, Opal SM, Pribble JP, Bone RC, Emmanuel G, Bloedow DC, Catalano MA, the IL-1RA Sepsis Syndrome Study Group (1994) Initial evaluation of human recombinant interleukin-1 receptor antagonist in the treatment of sepsis syndrome: a randomized, open-label, placebo-controlled multicenter trial. Crit Care Med 22: 12-21*
9. *Fourrier F, Chopin C, Huart J-J, Runge I, Caron C, Goudemand J (1993) Double-blind, placebo-controlled trial of antithrombin III concentrates in septic shock with disseminated intravascular coagulation. Chest 104: 882-888*
10. *Hilden J (1991) Intuition and other soft modes of thought in surgery. Theor Surg 6: 89-94*
11. *Hinshaw L, Peduzzi P, Young E, Sprung C, Shatney C, Sheagren J, Wilson M, Haakenson C (1987) Effect of high-dose glucocorticoid therapy on mortality in patients with clinical signs of systemic sepsis. N Engl J Med 317: 659-665*
12. *Hobsley M, Moss J, Levi R, Clarke RSJ, Fisher MMcD, Watkins J (1988) Discussion forum about a protocol of a controlled clinical trial: induction of anesthesia and perioperative risk. Theor Surg 3: 55-77*
13. *Lorenz W (1993) Clinical trials in sepsis and septic shock: a scrutiny of methodology. Theor Surg 8: 59-60*

14. Lorenz W, Neugebauer E, Pilz G, Werdan K, Lorenz M (1994) Introduction to the discussion forum. Theor Surg 9: 10-11
15. Lorenz W, Duda D, Dick W, Sitter H, Doenicke A, Black A, Weber D, Menke H, Stinner B, Junginger T, Rothmund M, Ohmann C, Immich H, Healy MJR, the Trial Group Mainz/Marburg (1994) The incidence and clinical importance of perioperative histamine release: the effects of volume loading and antihistaminics after induction of anaesthesia. Lancet 343: 933-940
16. Margolis CZ (1994) Clinical algorithms in sepsis trials. Theor Surg 9: 43-44
17. Mullan F, Jacoby I (1985) The town meeting of technology. The maturation of consensus conference. JAMA 254: 168-172
18. Peto R, Pike MC, Armitage P, Breslow NE, Cox DR, Howard SV, Mantel N, McPherson K, Peto J, Smith PG (1976) Design and analysis of randomized clinical trials requiring prolonged observation of each patient. I. Introduction and design. Br J Cancer 34: 585-612
19. Pilz G, Fateh-Moghadam S, Viell B, Bujdoso O, Döring G, Marget W, Neumann R, Werdan K (1993) Supplemental immunoglobulin therapy in sepsis and septic shock - comparison of mortality under treatment with polyvalent i.v. immunoglobulin versus placebo. Protocol of a multicenter, randomized, prospective, double-blind trial. Theor Surg 8: 61-83
20. Pliskin JS (1988) Medical strategies, clinical algorithms, protocol charts and decision analysis: some definitions and implications for surgical care. Theor Surg 2: 199-203
21. Schröder D, Bockhorn H, Beger HG, Lorenz W (1992) Treatment of cholelithiasis - the first consensus conference of the CAS on defining surgical standards. 12th Meeting of the Permanent Working Party on Clinical Studies (CAS) of the German Surgical Society, 15-16 November 1991 in Frankfurt/Main, Federal Republic of Germany. Theor Surg 7: 206-211
22. SDD Trialists' Collaborative Group (1993) Meta-analysis of randomized controlled trials of selective decontamination of the digestive tract. Brit Med J 307: 525-532
23. Velanovich V (1994) The box-counting method of fractal analysis for complex biological shapes, illustrated with reference to wound healing. Theor Surg 9: 68-71
24. Lorenz W, Reimund K-P, Weitzel F, Celik I, Kurnatowski M, Schneider C, Mannheim W, Heiske A, Neumann K, Sitter H, Rothmund M (1994) G-CSF prophylaxis before operation protects against lethal consequences of postoperative peritonitis. Surgery 116: 925-934
25. Wenzel RP (1992) Anti-endotoxin monoclonal antibodies - a second look. N Engl J Med 326: 1151-1153
26. Wichterman KA, Baue AE, Chaudry IH (1980) Sepsis and septic shock - a review of laboratory models and proposal. J Surg Res 29: 189-201
27. Zanetti G, Glauser M-P, Baumgartner J-D (1983) Anti-endotoxin antibodies and other inhibitors of endotoxin. New Horizons 1: 110-119
28. Ziegler EJ, Fisher CJ, Sprung CL, Straube RC, Sadoff JC, Foulke GE, Wortel CH, Fink MP, Dellinger RP, Teng NNH, Allen IE, Berger HJ, Knatterud GL, LoBuglio AF, Smith CR, HA-1A Sepsis Study Group (1991) Treatment of gram-negative bacteremia and septic shock with HA-1A human monoclonal antibody against endotoxin. N Engl J Med 324: 429-436

Threats to Double-Blinding in Sepsis Trials: Role of Expectancies Toward Treatment Outcome

M. Koller, W. Lorenz

Introduction

Sepsis is considered to be a major clinical problem, with a high incidence (half a million cases in the United States/year), a high mortality rate (35%), and high costs for care (US $ 5-10 billion annually) [4, 30]. There are a number of treatment regimens available, but there is no agreement concerning their relative merits. To date, there is no generally accepted standardized sepsis treatment, and the decision for one or the other treatment strategy depends primarily on the "attitude" prevailing in the hospital. Hence, there is an urgent need for clinical studies investigating this problem to provide necessary data that allow for rational treatment decisions.
However, sepsis trials are very difficult to perform. Medical and logistic obstacles, such as the inhomogenity of the patient sample or the difficulties in standardizing the treatment regimens, have been discussed in detail in the discussion forum on sepsis trials recently published in Theoretical Surgery [19].
The focus of this contribution is a particular methodological issue: Can the ideal of double-blindness be achieved in the case of sepsis trials? This question is interesting since researchers are rash in characterizing their studies as "double-blind, placebo-controlled, randomized, and prospective" [24, p 75]. Whereas the latter three characteristics mainly depend on the proper organization of a study [9], we will argue that there are a number of obstacles in implementing double-blindness [20, 22] that become especially apparent in studies on complex clinical problems, such as sepsis.

Criteria of Good Clinical Studies

The ultimate goal of any scientific study is to establish a cause-effect relationship [7]. In everyday life cause-effect relationships are usually highly visible [8]. For instance, one drinks a glass of water and is no longer thirsty; thus, water is subsequently considered as thirst quenching.

Unfortunately, things are much more complicated in a clinical context. One is faced with a multivariate environment. To give an example, the recovery of a patient may have many potential causes:
1. The good constitution of the patient
2. Successful operation of the immune system
3. Good nurse care
4. Family support
5. Motivation
6. Or the real effect of a given medication.

A good study has to be designed so that the real effect of the medication can be disentangled from the other possible causes [26]. There are a variety of reasons, however, why controlled clinical trials have failed in the past. The following list of potential shortcomings is adopted from Lorenz [17]:
1. Relevant existing information has been neglected
2. Clinically unimportant end points have been selected
3. Known prognostic factors have been omitted
4. Clinical pharmacology has been ignored
5. Methods of assessment have been imprecise
6. Follow-up has been incomplete
7. Medical audit and quality control have been lacking or poor

Double-blindness was not mentioned in this list. Indeed, certain clinical trials (particularly in surgery) cannot be performed in a double-blind manner, since surgeons are certainly aware of the treatment being performed [16]. In most other clinical trials double-blindness has not been checked (the study by Lorenz et al. being an exception [18]). Therefore, it is timely to analyze the issue of double-blindness in more detail.

Double-Blindness: Concept and Violations

Double-blindness means that neither the subjects nor the investigators know the identity of the intervention assignment. In other words, no one involved in the actual conduct of the study knows whether the patient receives the verum or the placebo [29]. On a conceptual level, double-blindness means that expectancies concerning treatment outcome are approximately equal across subjects and do not differ systematically between the various intervention groups (because group identity is not known).

Thus, double-blindness is always in danger when in the course of the study differential expectancies concerning treatment outcome arise, and when these expectancies are systematically different in the different treatment groups [5].

Unfortunately, sepsis treatment has certain characteristics that might give rise to such differential expectancies.

Sepsis treatment is multifaceted. It includes volume substitution, intubation, parenteral feeding, antibiotics, etc. These different concomitant treatment options are highly visible and may serve as cues upon which to base expectancies concerning treatment outcome and assignment.

Sepsis treatment is time consuming. It may last for weeks or even months, involving a close contact between physician and patient. Inevitably, speculations concerning group assignment will arise that are either fed by the necessity to provide concomitant treatment options (see above), and/or in turn determine the decision to do so.

To be more concrete, the following scenario describes what may happen in the course of the treatment of a single patient.
1. The primary medication does not work.
2. Enhanced concomitant treatment is proceeded with.
3. The physician speculates that the patient is in the placebo condition.
4. Since the placebo condition is associated with a bad prognosis, patient care declines.
5. Eventually, the outcome is poor.

If this emergence of negative outcome expectancies is systematically more pronounced in the placebo group, the design is no longer double-blind. The poor outcome of the placebo group is confounded with negative expectancies. The effect of the verum (which may truly be there) is largely overestimated.

The Power of Expectancies

One may doubt whether expectancies really constitute a methodological problem of considerable magnitude. The following examples illustrate the manner in which researchers' expectancies influence study and treatment outcomes, and determine treatment decisions.

Rosenthal [25] performed an impressive research project in order to demonstrate the influence of experimenters in the behavioral sciences on the performance of particular subjects.

The basic research paradigm can be described as follows: Experimenters (i.e., the individuals who actually conducted the study and had close contact with the research subjects) were led to believe that one group of subjects was intelligent (as indicated by scores in a previous intelligence test), whereas the other group was not. Later, subjects had to work on a mathematical problem. It turned out that the "intelligent" subjects performed better on this problem than the "unintelligent" ones. Dozens of studies have replicated this so-called experimenter expectancy effect. This effect was even found in studies utilizing animals as subjects, and in real-life classroom settings.

A nice example for the researcher expectancy effect in a clinical context is provided by a study on the efficacy of analgesic drugs in dental extraction [12]. Clinicians knew that there were two groups of patients: In one group patients received either a placebo or a narcotic antagonist; in other words, no effective pain relief was administered. In a second group of patients effective pain management was possible for some patients, who were randomly administered a narcotic analgesic instead of a placebo. An interesting effect occurred when comparing pain measures in the placebo groups of the first and second groups of patients: Pain was significantly weaker in this second placebo group, suggesting that clinicians' knowledge of the range of possible treatments made the difference.

Well-known and highly clinically relevant is the placebo effect [13, 31], which refers to both researchers' and patients' expectancies concerning favorable treatment outcome. A broad definition "includes any improvements in a patient not specifically due to a particular ingredient in a treatment" [2, 11]. The size of the placebo effect varies largely from study to study, and has been reported to range from 0% to 100%. The placebo effect is most accentuated in conditions such as head pain, rheumatism, or sea sickness, and is lowest in sleeping disorders, schizophrenia, and multiple sclerosis [28]. Furthermore, in the case of a particular medical problem, namely peptic ulcer, considerable geographical differences have been found: The placebo effect was most pronounced in Lausanne, Zürich, and Oslo (60% and more), and weakest in London and Glasgow (20%) [3]. It is commonly accepted as a rule of thumb that placebo effects account for a third of patients' recoveries [29]. However, recent research suggests that the placebo effect is twice as strong as expected. Particularly in conditions of mild or medium severity, and in a clinical setting where an enthusiastic doctor is treating a trusting patient, placebos produce positive results in two thirds of patients [11].

The exact mechanisms underlying researcher expectancy effects and placebo effects are yet not fully understood. It has been hypothesized that these effects are mediated by expectancy-oriented subtle changes in communication, mode of thinking, and subsequent behaviors [25, 27]). However, expectancies may influence behavior not only in subtle, but also in overt ways, as recent research in clinical decision making suggests. Murray et al. [23] investigated how the prediction of outcome influences management in neurosurgical patients. The study included more than 1000 patients with severe head injuries in four British neurosurgical units. In one phase of the study, the patient prognosis was routinely estimated using a specially adapted computer program for clinical purposes. Accordingly, patients' probable outcome was characterized as poor (dead or vegetative), moderate (severe disability), or good (moderate disability or good recovery). When comparing this routine prediction phase with patient management in phases where prediction was not routinely established, dramatic changes in patient management became apparent: routine prediction increased intensity of care for patients with a good prognostic outcome (osmotics, intubation, intracranial-pressure monitoring). At the same time, there was a decrease of 39% in the average frequency of the use of these modes of intensive management in patients with the worst prognosis. In other words, once physicians were alerted to possible outcomes, these expectancies largely determined their decisions for either or not providing certain aspects of patient care. Comparable results have been reported by Knaus et al. [15], showing that prognostic estimates lead to stopping active treatment for patients with three or more organ failures.

Coming to Terms with Expectancy Effects: Recommendations for an Improved Study Design in Sepsis Trials

How can we cope with this state of affairs? Should we abandon the ideal of double-blindness or give up clinical studies in sepsis research at all? There is certainly no need for regression toward scientific pessimism. Rather, one should take up the challenge and consider means of strengthening study designs:

1. Above all, include an assessment of expectancies toward treatment outcome. In the conduct of a sepsis trial, physicians should indicate their estimates of patients' chances of survival on a regular basis at fixed intervals. The exact format of these rating scales should be designed in collaboration with the physicians to reflect clinical reality, and clinicians' mental representation of probabilities [14, 21] (e.g., in terms of percentages or in terms of labels such as "highly likely/highly unlikely").
2. One also should measure physicians' general optimism/pessimism at the very beginning of the study, since this attitude may moderate incoming information related to patients' condition, and subsequent decisions [6].
3. It is absolutely essential to keep track of concomitant treatments. Both the treatment options chosen and the motives for doing so should be recorded. What were the specific clinical circumstances that led the physician to start concomitant treatment X at time Y?

4. Furthermore, it is necessary to establish clear rules for documenting complications. Whether a given symptom is interpreted as a complication and, hence, properly documented may well be moderated by physicians' expectancies concerning patients' treatment assignment and survival.

Analyzing the data by means of appropriate regression models [1] will determine the manner in which various factors such as expectancies, chronic optimism/pessimism, the reporting of complications, and concomitant treatment options are related to treatment outcome.

Conclusions

This contribution has attempted to alert the reader to the following points:
1. Expectancies toward treatment outcome may affect treatment decisions and outcome per se.
2. Controlling for expectancies are one step toward an improved study design.

Even when data analyses of an appropriately designed sepsis trial will yield no expectancy effects, we are left with the rewarding feeling that we have thought about this possibility. Our confidence in the data rises. Additionally, we have a major asset against other potential critics: a thought-through design, controlling for a methodological problem that may do considerable harm to the interpretation of study results.

References

1. Aiken LS, West SG (1991) Multiple regression: testing and interpreting interactions. Sage, Newbury Park
2. Beecher HK (1961) Surgery as placebo. JAMA 176: 1102-1107
3. Blum AL, Seiwert JR, Halter F (1987) Ulkustherapie mit Cimetidine. Dtsch Med Wochenschr 103: 135-139
4. Bone RC (1991) A critical evaluation of new agents for the treatment of sepsis. JAMA 266: 1686-1691
5. Byngton RP, Curb JD, Mattson ME (1985) Assessment of double-blindness at the conclusion of the beta-blocker heart attack trial. JAMA 253: 1733/1736
6. Christensen C, Cotrell JJ, Murakami J, Mackesy ME, Fetzer B, Elstein AS (1993) Forecasting survival in the medical intensive care unit: a comparison of clinical prognoses with formal estimates. Methods Inf Med 32: 302-308
7. Cook TD, Campbell DT (1979) Quasi-experimentation. Houghton Mifflin, Boston
8. Eimer M (1987) Konzepte von Kausalität. Huber, Bern
9. Evans M (1993) Organisational problems peculiar to multicentre trials. Theor Surg 9: 57-59
10. Friedman LM, Furberg CD, DeMets DL (1982) Fundamentals of clinical trials. Wright, Boston
11. Goleman D (1993) Placebo effect is shown to be twice as powerful as expected. New York Times, August 17, pp. 6-9
12. Gracely RH, Dubner R, Deeter WR, Wolskee PJ (1985) Clinicians' expectations influence placebo analgesia. Lancet 1: 43-43
13. Hippius H, Überla K, Laakmann G, Hasford J (eds.) (1986) Das Placebo-Problem. Fischer, Stuttgart

14. Higginbotham HN, West SG, Forsyth DR (1988) Psychotherapy and behavior change. Pergamon, New York
15. Knaus WA, Rauss A, Alperovitch A, le Gall JR, Loirat P, Patois E, Marcus SE, the French Multicentric Group of ICU Research (1990) Do objective estimates of chances for survival influence decisions to withhold or withdraw treatment? Med Decis Making 10: 163-171
16. Kramer MS (1988) Clinical epidemiology and biostatistics. Springer, Berlin, Heidelberg, New York
17. Lorenz W (1982) Attitudes to controlled clinical trials. Lancet 1: 1460-1461
18. Lorenz W, Duda D, Dick W, Sitter H, Doenicke A, Black A, Weber D, Menke H, Stinner B, Junginger T, Rothmund M, Ohmann C, Healey MJR, the Trial Group Mainz/Marburg (1994) Incidence and clinical importance of perioperative histamine release: randomised study of volume loading and antihistamines after induction of anaesthesia. Lancet 343: 933-940
19. Lorenz W, Neugebauer E, Pilz G, Werdan K, Lorenz M (1994) Methodology of clinical trials in sepsis - introduction. Theor Surg 9: 10-11
20. Margraf J, Ehlers A, Roth WT, Clark DB, Sheikh J, Agras WS, Taylor CB (1991) How "blind" are double-blind studies? J Consult Clin Psychol 59: 184-187
21. Mazur DJ, Hickam DH (1993) Patient interpretations of terms connoting low probabilities when communicating about surgical risk. Theor Surg 8: 143-145
22. Modestin J, Hodel J (1977) Wie blind ist ein Doppelblindversuch wirklich? Int Pharmacopsych 12: 129-136
23. Murray LS, Teasdale GM, Murray GD, Jannett B, Miller JD, Pickard JD, Shaw MDM, Achilles J, Bailey S, Jones P, Kelly D, Lacey J (1993) Does prediction of outcome alter patients management? Lancet 341: 1487-1491
24. Pilz G, Fateh-Moghadam S, Viell B, Bujdoso O, Döring G, Marget W, Neumann R, Werdan K (1993) Supplemental immunoglobulin therapy in sepsis and septic shock - comparison of mortality under treatment with polyvalent i.v. immunoglobulin versus placebo. Protocol of a multicenter, randomized, prospective, double-blind trial. Theor Surg 8: 61-83
25. Rosenthal R (1966) Experimenter effects in behavioral research. Appleton Century Crofts, New York
26. Rosenthal R (1985) Designing, analyzing, interpreting, and summarizing placebo studies. In: White L, Tursky B, Shwartz GE (eds.) Placebo. Guilford, New York, pp. 110-136
27. Ross M, Olson JM (1981) An expectancy attribution model of the effects of placebo. Psychol Rev 88: 408-437
28. Turnheim K (1987) Plazebo als unspezifischer Behandlungsfaktor. Wien Klin Wochenschr 99: 705-710
29. Walach H (1992) Wissenschaftliche homöopatische Arzneimittelprüfung. Haug, Heidelberg
30. Wenzel RP (1992) Anti-endotoxin monoclonal antibodies - a second look. N Engl J Med 326: 1151-1153
31. White L, Tursky B, Schwartz GE (eds.) (1985) Placebo. Guilford, New York

Clinical Algorithms in Sepsis Trials

C.Z. Margolis

Some Misconceptions Regarding Clinical Algorithms

Before commenting on the use of clinical algorithms in sepsis trials, I would like to review four concepts that are frequently misunderstood [1]. First, an algorithm, clinical or not, is frequently thought of, mistakenly, as a flow chart. A flow chart, however, is only one format of presenting an algorithm. The algorithm itself is a concept: a step-by-step approach for solving a problem that usually involves conditional logic. By extension, a clinical algorithm is a step-by-step approach to solving a clinical problem. What then is a flow chart? A flow chart is a graphic format for depicting a process that involves linked, sequential events over time. Flow charts may therefore depict the flow of historical events (historical flow charts), the flow of physical events (the coagulation cascade) or the flow of dependent decisions, such as the decision tree or the clinical algorithm. It follows that an algorithm may not be depicted as a flow chart, and a flow chart may not depict an algorithm.

Second, a misconception closely related to equating algorithms with flow charts is that prose descriptions of algorithms (e.g. the section of a general surgery text that describes the approach to the management of primary peritonitis) are not algorithms. However, since algorithm is a fundamental concept, like the concept of numbers, algorithms, like numbers, can be presented in a variety of forms, including prose, lists of instructions or flow charts. A review of the approach to managing a clinical problem, a clinical protocol and a bedside discussion on how to manage a clinical problem all describe clinical algorithms.

The third misconception is that all algorithms are mathematical, or, in more precise terms, that all algorithms process a finite input to a finite output. Most mathematical or computer algorithms (a computer program is an algorithm usually presented in a list format) process finite inputs to finite outputs. For example, addition algorithms add a set of numbers to yield a sum. However, there is another sort of algorithm, the practical algorithm, that processes a somewhat fuzzy problem situation to a not entirely predictable solution. Such algorithms, which might for example deal with car repair, classifying types of plants, or managing primary peritonitis, require human judgement. They reduce uncertainty, but do not eliminate it.

A fourth, related misconception is that a clinical algorithm is a mechanistic, rigid procedure that forces the clinician to diagnose and treat the patient according to certain rules, no matter what. This would be true of a mathematical algorithm. Since, however, a clinical algorithm is a practical algorithm that, like an expert system, must be used with expert judgement, it is characterized by purposely fuzzy definitions and by the necessity to decide at each step in the algorithm whether or not it applies to the patient.

Use of Clinical Algorithms in Sepsis Management

Keeping in mind the concepts I have attempted to explain, there are a number of uses for different types of clinical algorithms (CAs) that can help to manage patients with sepsis.

First, the diagnosis of sepsis and estimation of its severity will be made more accurate using sharp clinical criteria and well-defined clinical scores, such as the APACHE II and Elebute scores [2]. Although these tools are perhaps not immediately recognizable as simple CAs, they are by definition stepwise procedures for diagnosing and assessing severity. One of the first published CAs in the English language literature was a diagnostic one used by Tuddenham [3] to train radiology technicians to diagnose barium enemas. Since Tuddenham's study, which had a diagnostic accuracy of over 80%, all published, validated diagnostic CAs known to us have had high diagnostic accuracy (over 80%).

Second, a CA developed using the state-of-the-art, standard techniques proposed by the Society for Medical Decision Making [4] would describe the overall diagnostic and therapeutic approach to the patient with surgical sepsis and would include annotations and references that justify or discuss specific decisions. Such a carefully constructed CA is an excellent method for teaching and learning to manage patient problems and for defining which clinical decisions are rational and which reflect clinical custom. Customary but unproven decisions approaches should be justified by data collection or controlled clinical trials that provide a basis for rational decision making [1]. A standard CA can also be converted to one or more protocol charts or can be incorporated into an electronic patient record for directly guiding patient management [1, 5].

Third, the deterministic protocol of a study to determine IVIG effectiveness is itself a CA, as can be seen in Fig. 7 of Pilz et al.'s [2] proposal. Presumably, experienced clinicians and scientists reviewed a sepsis management algorithm, whether it was actually drawn or was implicit in their clinical approach to sepsis. They found the management decisions not buttressed by experimental evidence, and designed a research CA for determining which therapy to use. This clinical research application of CA technology is also an example of validating the effect of a management CA on outcome. Validation is a little practiced but necessary final step in proposing CAs for use as practice guidelines. Just as one validates a diagnostic CA by comparing its diagnostic accuracy to a gold standard, so also should one validate a clinical management CA by demonstrating its positive effect on outcome.

References

1. Margolis CZ (1988) Solving common pediatric problems: an algorithm approach. Solomon, New York, pp. 5-14
2. Pilz G, Fateh-Moghadam S, Viell B, Bujdoso O, Doring G, Marget W, Neumann R, Werdan K (1993) Supplemental immunoglobulin therapy in sepsis and septic shock - comparison of mortality under treatment with polyvalent i.v. immunoglobulin versus placebo. Protocol of a multicenter, randomized, prospective, double-blind trial. Theor Surg 8: 61-83

3. Society for Medical Decision Making Committee on Standardization of Clinical Algorithms (1992) Proposal for clinical algorithm standards. Med Decis Making 12: 149-154
4. Tuddenham WJ (1968) The use of logical flow charts as an aid in teaching roentgen diagnosis. AJR 102: 797-803
5. Warshawsky S, Noi E, Boehm D, Goldfarb D, Urkin J, Margolis C (1993) CLINIC - a computerized medical record system for use in primary health care setting - a descriptive study. In: Reichert A, Sadan BA, Bengtsson S, Bryant J, Piccolo U (eds.) MIE 93: 11th international congress of the European Federation for Medical Informatics. Freund, London, pp. 608-610

Organisational Problems Peculiar to Multicentre Trials

M. Evans

Few people would deny that medical treatment is more effective today than it was 100 or more years ago. Some of the advances came about in the form of spectacular discoveries by original thinkers and the acceptance of these advances was rapid. The only comparison that was necessary was with what happened to patients before the new treatments were introduced. Nobody was likely to question the improvement brought about by the introduction of general anaesthesia, asepsis, or antibiotics. Nowadays, however, new techniques and new drugs have less striking benefits, and the proof that they are beneficial rests with properly conducted randomised controlled clinical trials. Any other form of clinical research is much more likely to introduce bias.

In Britain the Medical Research Council set up a Therapeutic Trials Committee in 1931. It did little work of any value and many of the trials of new drugs did not even include control groups. The turning point in clinical therapeutic research was in 1946 when the Medical Research Council commissioned Bradford Hill to conduct a multicentre evaluation of the value of streptomycin in pulmonary tuberculosis. Its value in miliary tuberculosis was in no doubt, but the drug was in short supply and the government wanted to make sure that it would work for pulmonary disease as well.

The streptomycin trial was remarkably well designed, considering that it was the first randomised clinical trial. It recruited 107 patients in seven hospitals and departed from traditional methods in four ways. Firstly, eligibility of patients and controls was strictly defined by clinical and radiological criteria. Secondly, eligible patients were reported to a central office where the next numbered envelope was opened and the randomised instructions to "streptomycin" or "control" were given to the participating doctor. Thirdly, evaluation of the outcome of treatment was made by observers who were kept in ignorance of whether the patient had had streptomycin or not. Finally, the trial considered ethical matters but came down in favour of a policy which is now entirely unacceptable. The report stated that: "Patients were not told before admission that they were to get special treatment. Control patients did not know throughout their stay in hospital that they were control patients in a special study... It was important for the success of the trial that the details of the control scheme should remain completely confidential... this information was not made public throughout the 15 months of trial" [7].

Surgeons lagged behind physicians and oncologists in carrying out randomised trials. It was not until 14 years after the streptomycin trial that the first surgical trial was organised by Goligher et al. [5]. In two hospitals (Leeds and York) three operations for duodenal ulcer were compared but there is no mention in the published paper that patients were told that their operation was decided by chance.

The number of randomised controlled trials in surgery gradually increased, but problems arose. Twenty years ago it was comparatively easy to organise a randomised controlled trial, but gradually ethical, legal, and bureaucratic constraints have built up to such an extent that one of the leading proponents of clinical trials has written a convincing argument in favour of their replacement in certain circumstances by "accurate honest audit" [9]. The skeleton rules for the organisation of controlled trials in sepsis are well known [3]; multicentre trials, however, require different emphasis. The more people who are involved in the organisation and administration of a trial, the more necessary it is that the principles as well as the practice should be spelt out in simple and unequivocal terms.

Philosophy

There is one fundamental condition that must be fulfilled before a randomised controlled trial may be conducted: no investigator taking part should hold an opinion about the efficacy of the treatment(s) being tested. He must accept the null hypothesis that the regimen being tested is neither better nor worse than the one that is already being used. If any investigator believes that the experimental regimen is better (or worse) than his current standard treatment (or the treatment laid down by the organiser as the control treatment) it is unethical for him to take part in a trial. This principle is rarely stated, but it underpins the ethical conduct of these trials and should be an integral part of every protocol.

Terminology and Definitions

Before any group of people can work together they must all understand what they mean by particular terms. For example, "sepsis" and "septic shock" mean different things to different people. Microbiologists in particular like to give the name "sepsis" to any process resulting in the production of pus, whereas to surgeons and those in charge of intensive care units sepsis means a systemic inflammatory response, usually but not necessarily to infection. "Wound infection", "peritonitis", "pneumonia", and "deep abscess" are among other conditions that require consensus agreement. For example, one clinician may define a wound infection as the discharge of pus from the wound, whereas another will classify it microbiologically, and another may countenance only total breakdown of the suture line. Is peritonitis to be graded by the Mannheim Peritonitis Index - as I am sure it will be in some centres, but not in others? What are the criteria for diagnosing pneumonia in patients, many of whom will be on ventilators?

Standardisation of Laboratory Results

It should go without saying that all laboratory tests must be reported in the same manner - either Système Internationale (SI) or traditional units. If SI units are to be used there is no excuse for measuring sodium and potassium in mmol/l and creatinine in mg/dl. Packed cell volume should be given instead of haematocrit, and the number of white cells should be given as $\times 10^9/l$.

There should also be some unified quality assessment among laboratories. It is not sufficient merely to obtain a list of reference ranges (there is no such thing as a "normal" value) from each laboratory; the reference range will differ depending on the method of measurement. The correct way is for the coordinating laboratory to send quality control samples to be tested in each participating laboratory at regular intervals to make sure that they are all working within the same narrow band of error, otherwise inaccuracies will occur. Ideally there should also be a steering committee which is responsible for the auditing of the quality control data.

Exclusions

One of the most difficult problems to tackle in any multicentre study - not just in randomised controlled trials - is the exclusion (deliberate or otherwise) of eligible patients. This was dealt with in the St Mary's Large Bowel Cancer Project (an audit of 4572 patients operated on for large bowel cancer by 94 surgeons in 23 hospitals in the United Kingdom) by employing a coordinator who travelled round to each centre every six months and examined admission registers, operating theatre books, and pathological records to make sure that every eligible patient was recorded.

A multicentre trial that was severely criticised for the enormous number of eligible patients that were excluded was the comparison of extracranial-intracranial bypass with conservative treatment for inoperable extracranial arterial obstruction; it was eventually admitted that 50%-70% of patients who should have been randomised had not been [1]. The result was that the conclusion of the trial (that the operation conferred no benefit) was severely criticised by the proponents of the operation, who claimed that it is beneficial to some patients. The implication is that many patients had chosen operation and had therefore been excluded from randomisation.

Another trial that fell into the same trap was the National Surgical Adjuvant Breast Project trial of regimens for the treatment of breast cancer [4]; 2163 patients were recruited from 89 specialist centres in 7 years, which is a mean of roughly three patients/centre per year. A further 320 patients were then "excluded" for various reasons (including refusal to take part in a trial and refusal to accept the treatment to which they were randomised), and so the results of only 1843 were available for analysis. We are not told how the 320 (or any of the other excluded patients) were treated; nor are we told what became of them.

The results of trials that do not include all eligible patients are not generalisable to all patients with the disease being studied. This makes them seriously defective. Of course it does not mean that the conclusions that the trialists came to are wrong; merely that they were not shown to be right.

Withdrawals

There will always be withdrawal of eligible patients after randomisation and before the end of the specified period of study in any trial - and particularly in trials of sepsis and septic shock in which between a third and a half of the patients are likely to die. It is therefore imperative that every patient who was randomised and, for whatever reason, did not complete the study period should be documented as assiduously as those who did. Their results should be analysed and published as a separate group within the trial, because they are essential to the overall picture.

Interventions Other Than Those Specified in the Protocol

The more interventions that are used at the discretion of the participating doctors in addition to the one being tested, the less convincing the results of the trial. In the treatment of sepsis and septic shock, for example, the number of additional treatments that may affect the outcome and which the participants may use is considerable. These might include total parenteral nutrition, additional antibiotics, peritoneal lavage, etappenlavage, and - more generally - the quality of care in a particular intensive care unit, which should all be taken into account. If the effort is not made there is a possibility that quite by chance there may be a subgroup that is large enough to make the outcome of the two treatments being tested significantly different.

One way of dealing with this problem is by stratifying the randomisation - for example, patients with Gram-negative sepsis could be randomised separately from those with Gram-positive sepsis, medical patients separately from surgical ones, and patients whose sepsis developed postoperatively from those who presented with sepsis. That would at least mean that equal numbers within each subgroup were allotted to the experimental and placebo arms of the trial.

Informed Consent

Before patients or relatives can give "informed" consent they must understand what they are being told, and communication is made more difficult by fear of operations, of anaesthesia, and of the unknown. The depersonalisation implicit in the atmosphere of a hospital, and particularly an intensive care unit, will only add to the confusion, as will the inadvertent intimidation of being surrounded by people in strange uniforms and masks. Edwards [2] emphasised the need for simplicity, lack of jargon, and the use of everyday words.

Kitching [6] reviewed the standard of English used in leaflets giving information to patients about drugs and quoted a review that showed that the educational standard of a second-year college student was needed to understand the explanations about the effects of ten of the most commonly prescribed drugs in the United States.

We are left with a paradox: on the one hand the legal niceties may have been satisfied, but on the other hand few patients will have even the vaguest idea of what is happening to them.

Interim Analyses

There is nothing intrinsically wrong with interim analyses; indeed, some say that they are ethically desirable as long as they are done by somebody impartial who does not report the results of the analyses to the investigators. The disclosure of a difference, even if it is not significant, could bias participants in favour of or against the treatment being tested. The only occasions on which disclosure is not only acceptable but obligatory are: firstly if evidence emerges that harm is being done to patients in one arm of the trial and, secondly, if one of the treatments is shown to be highly significantly better than the other (for example, some might accept $p < 0.01$ in a two-tailed test). The reason for this is that the more interim analyses that are done, the more likelihood there is of a type I error (false rejection of the null hypothesis). With ten interim analyses of one end point, there is a 20% chance of reaching $p < 0.05$ even if the null hypothesis is true [8].

Conclusion

The organisation of a multicentre trial is not a task to be undertaken lightly, and however well it is done there will always be people ready and willing to criticise. But "Nothing will come of nothing" (Shakespeare, King Lear), and it is only by organising trials and audits and learning from our mistakes that we can possibly answer even the simplest question.

References

1. Dudley HAF (1987) Extracranial-intercranial bypass, one; clinical trials, nil. *BMJ 294: 1501-1502*
2. Edwards M (1991) Communicating with patients. *Medical Audit News 1: 69-70*
3. Evans M, Pollock AV (1985) A score system for evaluating random control clinical trials of prophylaxis of abdominal surgical wound infection. *Br J Surg 72: 256-260*
4. Fisher B, Bauer M, Margolese R, Poisson R, Pilch Y, Redmond C, Fisher E, Wolmark N, Deutsch M, Montague E, Saffer E, Wickerham L, Lerner H, Glass A, Shibata H, Deckers P, Ketcham A, Oishi R, Russell I (1985) Five-year results of a randomized clinical trial comparing total mastectomy and segmental mastectomy with or without radiation in the treatment of breast cancer. *N Engl J Med 312:665-673*
5. Goligher JC, Pulvertaft CN, Walkinson G (1964) Controlled trial of vagotomy and gastroenterostomy, vagotomy and antrectomy, and subtotal gastrectomy in elective treatment of duodenal ulcer. Interim report. *BMJ 1: 455-460*
6. Kitching JB (1990) Patient information leaflets - the state of the art. *J R Soc Med 83: 298-306*
7. Medical Research Council (1948) Streptomycin treatment of pulmonary tuberculosis. *BMJ 2: 76669-782*
8. Pocock SJ, Hughes MD, Lee RJ (1987) Statistical problems in the reporting of clinical trials. A survey of three medical journals. *N Engl J Med 317: 426-432*
9. Pollock AV (1993) Surgical evaluation at the crossroads. *Br J Surg 80: 964-966*

End Point Selection, Sample Size, Interim Monitoring, and Final Data Analysis in Multicenter Clinical Trials in Sepsis

C.H. Shatney, P. Peduzzi

End Point Selection

Clinical studies are prodigious undertakings, and problems are common throughout the design and conduct of such projects. Trials in patients with sepsis not only have the same hurdles as other clinical studies but also have unique difficulties. Foremost, sepsis is a multifaceted entity with several potential initial manifestations. In addition, it is now known that the "sepsis syndrome" frequently occurs in the absence of serious infection [1], which is why this term has been replaced by "systemic inflammatory response syndrome" [2]. These circumstances can create problems both in targeting the population for study and in selecting appropriate and clinically relevant end points to assess treatment. Hence, numerous primary and secondary outcome indicators have been utilized in sepsis studies to evaluate the efficacy of therapy. Some of these end points are good, and others pose difficulties.

The best treatment response to assess - and the one most commonly used as a primary end point - is mortality. The reason mortality is an ideal end point is that it can be positively ascertained in an unbiased manner. However, if the trial is not designed properly, bias can be introduced into even this seemingly definitive outcome indicator and can lead to spurious results. One such situation occurs when the follow-up period is not the same for all the patients. For example, survival to hospital discharge is a potentially biased point, because not all patients with a given disease process will have the same length of hospitalization. Not only do medical problems cause variations in hospital stay, but there is also considerable physician subjectivity in the duration of hospitalization for patients with similar circumstances [3]. Furthermore, deaths occurring after hospital discharge may not be included in the final data analysis, due to either loss of patients to follow-up or the fact that such deaths are not "counted," because they occurred after the patient completed the trial (at hospital discharge). This latter phenomenon was clearly demonstrated in studies of surgical wound infection, wherein it was shown that the infection rate is substantially higher if patients are followed for 30 days postoperatively, rather than until hospital discharge [4]. To avoid such potential bias in sepsis trials, it is essential that mortality occurring during a certain time interval after patient entry into a study be the variable that is measured, rather than in-hospital mortality.

A second problem that commonly occurs when mortality is used as an end point is the attempt to classify death as due to sepsis or some other cause, so-called "attributable mortality." There are various reasons why this practice could introduce bias into a study. First, all deaths cannot be classified with certainty as being related or unrelated to sepsis. More importantly, from a patient safety standpoint, the use of attributable mortality as a response indicator creates a situation whereby detrimental effects of treatment on mortality can be overlooked, particularly in the group classified as dying from causes other than sepsis. For these reasons, all-cause mortality is the most appropriate and clinically relevant end point in clinical trials of sepsis. In addition to avoiding the pitfalls already mentioned, all-cause mortality accounts for the potential impact of preexisting conditions on outcome. To further enhance the validity of all-cause mortality as an outcome indicator, it is essential to standardize all aspects of patient care as much as possible - something that is still not routinely done in sepsis trials [5, 6].

For responses other than mortality, it is desirable to blind their assessment regarding treatment assignment, preferably using a double-blind trial design. When such a design is not possible, classification of outcome should be made by an independent committee or laboratory that determines outcome without knowledge of treatment assignment. This procedure is particularly important for outcomes that are subjective in nature, such as quality of life and ability to return to work. For outcomes based on a change in a particular measurement, it is advantageous to have all measurements performed at a central facility to standardize their determination and reduce variability.

Recent sepsis trials have also included numerous secondary objectives, in addition to the primary response indicator. For example, it is common for studies to assess the incidence and resolution of organ failure. While these are appropriate end points, provided the sample size is sufficient, problems have occurred in this area regarding acceptable definitions of both the presence and resolution of organ failure, as well as the inclusion of patients in such analyses who have an element of organ failure at baseline [6, 7]. Similar difficulties have occurred when the incidence and resolution of "septic shock" have been used as outcome indicators. Another secondary end point that can pose problems is analysis of the duration of ICU stay. As with the duration of hospitalization, the length of time a patient spends in an ICU is somewhat physician dependent. Therefore, this end point is not unbiased, but, rather, has a fair amount of potential subjectivity. To eliminate additional bias with the use of ICU stay as an end point, the study design must account for the fact that some patients will die in the ICU. Such deaths will obviously influence the results and can lead to spurious conclusions if proper analysis is not performed.

Sample Size

The inability of many trials to demonstrate a treatment difference (effect) can often be attributed to inadequate sample size. Insufficient sample size reduces the power of a study, its ability to detect significant treatment effects when they are present [8]. This problem occurs primarily because the observed event rates and treatment effects are usually lower than those hypothesized during the design of the trial. A large number of protocol deviants (dropouts, noncompliers, etc.) can also have an adverse effect on the power of a study. To control for these problems, trials should be designed conservatively, that is, by calculating sample size to detect moderate treatment effects using lower than expected event rates. Sample size is also adjusted upwards to account for the potential loss of power due to protocol deviants. Although most well-designed trials adhere to these basic principles, sample size determination is still a "guesstimate".

Recent trials of gram-negative sepsis [9-11] have had special problems, because the target groups of patients could not be identified with 100% certainty at the time of enrollment. This situation has occurred because of the need to treat patients early in the disease, often before culture results are available. Consequently, it has been necessary to include all patients with signs of sepsis in these studies. In some of these trials, treatment was possibly beneficial for certain subsets of patients with gram-negative infections, but not for the other patients enrolled in the study. The validity of many of these subgroup analyses is questionable, however, as was amply demonstrated by the HA-1A clinical trials [12]. Since the majority of patients in these studies did not have gram-negative sepsis, there was no overall benefit of treatment, and the products were not approved for use in patients. Some physicians might argue that it is unethical to withhold beneficial therapy from patients (certain subgroups with gram-negative sepsis). However, the clinical reality of the situation is that, at the present time, such patients cannot be identified before the treatment needs to be given [13]. Since most of the drugs evaluated recently are expensive, and might exert detrimental effects in patients without gram-negative infection [9, 12], the practical and ethical position is not to administer them to patients with sepsis.

In gram-negative sepsis trials the sample size required to demonstrate an overall treatment effect is highly dependent on the prevalence of the target infection among enrolled patients, as well as the observed treatment effect in both the target and nontarget groups. Table 1 displays sample size requirements to detect a significant difference in outcome between control and treated groups for a variety of prevalence and event rates, assuming type I and II error rates of 5% and 20%, respectively [14]. As shown in Table 1, sample size must be increased markedly as the prevalence rate decreases, even when treatment is highly beneficial in the target subgroup, and not harmful in the nontarget subgroup (same outcome rate as in control group). For example, a sample size of 110 patients is required to detect a 50% reduction with treatment in the event (outcome) rate, from 50% to 25%, when all patients have the target infection (100% prevalence). When only 25% of patients have the target infection, and treatment is not harmful in nontarget patients, the sample size increases to 1590 patients; the overall reduction with treatment in the event rate among the entire study population decreases from 50% to 12%, because 75% of enrolled patients derive no benefit from the therapy. The effect on sample size is even more dramatic when treatment may be harmful in nontarget patients (Table 1). If treatment is detrimental to the nontarget group by increasing the event rate by 10% (from 50% to 55%), the required sample size increases to 13 600 patients, and the overall reduction in the event rate by treatment is only 5%. The findings are even more striking for a 30% event rate in control subjects and a 33% treatment effect (20% outcome rate in treated target group), rates usually seen in clinical practice. Thus, to demonstrate the overall benefit of treatment large numbers of patients are needed when the prevalence of the target group is low, even if treatment is highly effective in the target population.

Table 1: Influence of prevalence of target population on sample size requirements

Prevalence of target group (%)	Outcome rate (%) in control group [a]	Outcome rate (%) with treatment			Overall study treatment effect (% reduction)	Sample size required
		Target group	Nontarget group	Combined		
100	50	25	NA[b]	25	50	110
75	50	25	50	31	37	230
50	50	25	50	38	25	530
25	50	25	50	44	12	1590
75	50	25	55	33	35	250
50	50	25	55	40	20	770
25	50	25	55	48	5	13 600
100	30	20	NA[b]	20	33	580
75	30	20	30	23	25	1080
50	30	20	30	25	17	2500
25	30	20	30	28	8	10 300
75	30	20	32	23	23	1240
50	30	20	32	26	13	3950
25	30	20	32	29	3	65 300

[a] Outcome rates for control patients, with and without target infection, are assumed to be equal
[b] NA, not applicable, since all patients have target disease at entry (100% prevalence)

Clearly, the design of sepsis trials will become more efficient (lower sample size requirement) when expedient procedures are developed to permit the identification of the infecting organisms at the onset of the disease process. In the absence of such techniques, the prevalence of the target population among patients eligible to be enrolled remains an important determinant of effective trial design. Some physicians might argue that the overall treatment effect is inconsequential, and that the important effect is the one in the target subgroup - as long as treatment is not harmful in the nontarget population. However, since all eligible patients must be treated in order to evaluate the desired effect in the target subgroup, the overall effect is of primary importance because the benefits of treatment must outweigh the risks. Thus, the only proper evaluation is the one based on all patients who receive therapy. This consideration becomes particularly important when the prevalence of the target population is low. For example, in the Department of Veterans Affairs Gram-Negative Sepsis Trial of Steroid Therapy [9] there was a 75% reduction in mortality with steroid treatment in the small subgroup of 51 patients with gram-negative bacteremia. For the remaining 172 patients in the study, administration of steroids increased the mortality rate by 25%, yielding only a 5% reduction in overall mortality with steroid therapy.

Interim Monitoring and Final Data Analysis

All well-designed clinical trials evaluate the accumulating data periodically for ethical and safety reasons. In an experimental study it is unethical to administer a harmful treatment to patients, or to withhold beneficial therapy. For these reasons, statistical methods have been developed to control for multiple looks at the data and preserve the overall type I error [15-18]. Such a system must be established before a trial is initiated, to preserve the integrity of the study.

There is often a tendency to exclude protocol deviants (losses to follow-up, noncompliers, etc.) from the final efficacy analysis. The only unbiased data analysis, however, is the one which includes all randomized patients according to original treatment assignment, i.e., intent-to-treat analysis [19, 20]. This method is optimal because it avoids selection bias, assures balance among treatment groups of both measured and unmeasured factors, and guarantees the validity of most statistical tests, that is, gives valid p-values. Methods of analysis that exclude randomized patients, for whatever reason, are potentially biased and should not be used. There are some procedures, however, that can be utilized, in conjunction with the intent-to-treat analysis, to examine the impact of noncompliance on the estimation of the treatment effects [21-23].

In the majority of the sepsis trials conducted to date, the primary focus has been on evaluating the influence of treatment in patients with gram-negative infections, not the overall effect. In fact, most of the published reports of these studies have concentrated on the findings in the gram-negative patients. However, since all patients with sepsis have to be treated to achieve these results, the primary analysis should be intent-to-treat analysis, particularly since the prevalence of gram-negative sepsis is fairly low. Separate evaluations of patients with and without gram-negative sepsis constitute subgroup analyses that should be evaluated at more stringent type I error levels to appropriately control for the multiplicity of comparisons.

As a basic principle, data analysis should be consistent with the design of the study. Thus, trials that use a randomized design should be analyzed as randomized. From both the clinician's and the patient's perspective, this is also the relevant analysis.

Acknowledgement

Dr. Peduzzi's contribution to this research was supported by the Department of Veterans Affairs Cooperative Studies Program of the Veterans Health Services and Research Administration.

References

1. Shatney CH (1992) Steroids and multiple organ failure: the case for steroid use. In: Fry DE (ed.) Multiple system organ failure. Mosby-Year Book, St Louis, pp. 345-352
2. Beal AL, Cerra FB (1994) Multiple organ failure syndrome in the 1990s. Systemic inflammatory response and organ dysfunction. JAMA 271: 226-233
3. Boulanger BR, McLellan BA, Sharkey PW et al. (1993) A comparison between a Canadian regional trauma unit and an American level I trauma center. J Trauma 35: 261-266

4. Condon RE, Schulte WJ, Malangoni MA et al. (1983) Effectiveness of a surgical wound surveillance program. Arch Surg 118: 303-307
5. Pilz G, Fateh-Moghadam S, Viell B et al. (1993) Supplemental immunoglobulin therapy in sepsis and septic shock - comparison of mortality under treatment with polyvalent i.v. immunoglobulin versus placebo. Theor Surg 8: 61-83
6. Warren HS, Danner RL, Munford RS (1992) Anti-endotoxin monoclonal antibodies. N Engl J Med 326: 1153-1157
7. Peduzzi P, Shatney CH (1994) Design of clinical trials in sepsis - critique of the Pilz et al. trial of supplemental immunoglobulin therapy in sepsis and septic shock. Theor Surg 9: 45-47
8. Sheps S (1993) Sample size and power. J Invest Surg 6: 469-475
9. The Veterans Administration Systemic Sepsis Cooperative Study Group (1987) Effect of high-dose glucocorticoid therapy on mortality in patients with clinical signs of systemic sepsis. N Engl J Med 317: 659-665
10. Ziegler E, Fischer CJ, Sprung CL et al., the HA-1A Sepsis Study Group (1991) Treatment of gram-negative bacteremia and septic shock with HA-1A human monoclonal antibody against endotoxin - a randomized, double-blind, placebo-controlled trial. N Engl J Med 324: 429-436
11. Greenman RL, Schein RMH, Martin MA et al., the XOMA Sepsis Study Group (1991) A controlled clinical trial of E5 murine monoclonal IgM antibody to endotoxin in the treatment of gram-negative sepsis. JAMA 266: 1097-1102
12. Luce JM (1993) Introduction of new technology into critical care practice: a history of HA-1A human monoclonal antibody against endotoxin. Crit Care Med 21: 1233-1241
13. Wenzel RP (1992) Anti-endotoxin monoclonal antibodies - a second look. N Engl J Med 326: 1151-1153
14. Lachin J (1981) Introduction to sample size determination and power analysis for clinical trials. Controlled Clin Trials 2: 93-113
15. Lan KKG, DeMets DL (1983) Discrete sequential boundaries for clinical trials. Biometrika 70: 659-663
16. Lan KKG, Wittes J (1988) The B-value: a tool for monitoring data. Biometrics 44: 579-585
17. O'Brien PC, Flemming TR (1979) A multiple testing procedure for clinical trials. Biometrics 35: 549-556
18. Pocock SJ (1977) Group sequential methods in the design and analysis of clinical trials. Biometrika 64: 191-199
19. The Coronary Drug Project Research Group (1980) Influence of adherence to treatment and response of cholesterol on mortality in the coronary drug project. N Engl J Med 303: 1038-1041
20. Peduzzi P, Wittes J, Detre K, Holford H (1993) Analyses as randomized and the problem of nonadherence: an example from the Veterans Affairs randomized trials of coronary artery bypass surgery. Stat Med 12: 1185-1195
21. Lagakos SW, Lim LL-Y, Robins JM (1990) Adjusting for early treatment termination in comparative clinical trials. Stat Med 9: 1417-1424
22. Efron B, Feldman D (1991) Compliance as an explanatory variable in clinical trials (with comment and rejoinder). J Am Stat Assoc 86: 9-26
23. Sommer A, Zeger SL (1991) On estimating efficacy from clinical trials. Controlled Clin Trials 10: 45-52

Contributors

Barber, A. E., M. D., Department of Surgery/Texas Tech University, Health Services Center, 3601 Fourth Street, Lubbock, TX 79430, USA

Baas, J., M. D., Department of Surgery, Ruprecht Karls University, Im Neuenheimer Feld 110, 69112 Heidelberg, Germany

Baue, A. E., M. D., Prof., Department of Surgery, University Health Sciences, Center, 3635 Vista Avenue at Grand Boulevard, St. Louis, MO 63110-0250, USA

Boekstegers, P., M. D., Medical Clinic I, Ludwig Maximilian University, Grosshadern, Marchioninistr. 15, 81377 Munich, Germany

Bohuon, C., M. D., Prof., Institute Gustave-Roussy, 39 Rue Camille Desmoulins, 94805 Villejuif Cedex, France

Brinkmann, A., M. D., Departments of Anaesthesiology, University Clinic, 89075 Ulm, Germany

Büchler, M. W., M. D., Department of Visceral and Transplantation Surgery, University Hospital, Freiburgstr. 80, 3010 Berne, Switzerland

Catania, A., M. D., 1st Medical Clinic, University, 20122 Milan, Italy

Cervós-Navarro, J., M. D., Institute of Neuropathology, University-Clinic, Hindenburgdamm 30, 12200 Berlin, Germany

Closa, D., M. D., Molecular Pathology Unit., C.I.D., CSIC, J. Girona 18-26, 08034 Barcelona, Spain

Deitch, E. A., M. D., UMD-New Jersey Medical School, University Heights, 185 S. Orange Avenue/Suite G-506, Newark, NJ 07103-2714, USA

Denz, H., M. D., Andreas-Hofer-Str. 4, 6020 Innsbruck, Austria

Dimmeler, S., M. D., Department of Surgery, Biochemical and Experimental Division, University, Ostmerheimer Str. 200, 51109 Cologne, Germany

Dunn, D. L., M. D., Ph. D., Department of Surgery, University of Minnesota, Phillips-Wangensteen Bldg., 516 Delware Street S. E., Minneapolis, MN 55455, USA

Dwenger, A., M. D., Biochemical Division, Medical School, Konstanty-Gutschow-Str. 8, 30625 Hannover, Germany

Einsele, H., M. D., Department of Internal Medicine II, Eberhard-Karl University, Otfried-Müller-Straße 10, 72076 Tübingen, Germany

Etheredge, E. E., M. D., Department of Surgery, Tulane University School of Medicine, New Orleans, LA 70112, USA

Evans, M., M. D., Scarborough Hospital, Scarborough, North Yorkshire YO12 6QL, UK

Farthmann, E. H., M. D., Clinic of Surgery, University, Hugstetterstr. 55, 79106 Freiburg, Germany

Fry, D. E., M. D., Prof., Department of Surgery, University of New Mexico School of Medicine, Albuquerque, NM 87131, USA

Fuchs, D., M. D., Institute for Medical Chemistry and Biochemistry, University, Fritz-Pregl-Str. 3, 6020 Innsbruck, Austria

Függer, R., M. D., Department of Surgery, University, Währinger Gürtel 18-20, 1090 Wien, Austria

Gaitzsch, A., M. D., 2. Department of Surgery, University, Ostmerheimer Str. 200, 51109 Cologne, Germany

Gawaz, M., M. D., I. Medical Clinic, Rechts der Isar, Technical University, Ismaninger Str. 22, 81675 Munich, Germany

Gerlach, H., M. D., Clinic of Anaesthesiology and Critical Care Medicine, UKRV, Humboldt University, Augustenburger Platz 1, 13353 Berlin, Germany

Grotz, M., M. D., Department of Traumatology, Medical School, Konstanty-Guschow-Str.8, 30625 Hannover, Germany

Hase, T., M. D., Department of Emergency Medicine, Shiga University of Medical Science, Seta, Tsukinowa-cho, Otsu 520-21, Japan

Hirata, K., M. D., Ph. D., Department of Surgery (Section I), Medical University, West-16, South-1, Chuo-ku, Sapporo 060, Japan

Horn, J. K., M. D., Department of Surgery, General Hospital, 1001 Potrero Avenue, San Francisco, CA 94110, USA

Hunsicker, A., M. D., Department of Surgery, University, Friedrich-Löffler-Str. 23, 17489 Greifswald, Germany

Kinneart, P., M. D., Biomedical Research Laboratory, Faculty of Medicine, University, 808 Route de Lennik, 1070 Brussels, Belgium

Koch, T., M. D., Department of Anaesthesiology and Critical Care, Clinic Mannheim, Theodor-Kutzer-Ufer, 68167 Mannheim, Germany

Koller, M., M. D., Institute of Theoretical Surgery, Philipps University, Baldingerstr., 35043 Marburg/Lahn, Germany

Köhl, J., M. D., Institute of Medical Microbiology, Medical School, Konstanty-Gutschow-Str. 8, 30625 Hannover, Germany

Kopprasch, S., M. D., Department of Internal Medicine III, Medical Faculty, Technical University, Fetscherstr. 74, 01307 Dresden, Germany

Lasson, A., M. D., Department of Surgery, Malmö General Hospital, 21401 Malmö, Sweden

Le Gall, J. R., M. D., Prof., Intensive Care Unit., St. Louis Hospital, 1 avenue Claude Vellefaux, 75010 Paris, France

Lehmann, U., M. D., Surgical Clinic, Medical School, Konstanty-Gutschow-Str. 8, 30625 Hannover, Germany

Lorenz, W., M. D., Prof., Institute of Theoretical Surgery, Centre of Operative Medicine I, Philipps University, Baldingerstr., 35043 Marburg/Lahn, Germany

Margolis, C., M. D., Prof., Faculty of Health Sciences, Ben-Gurion University of the Negev, PO Box 653, Beerh Sheva 84105, Israel

Marshall, J., M. D., General Hospital, Eaton North 9-234, 200 Elizabeth Street, Toronto/Ontario, M5G 2C4, Canada

Michalopoulos, A., M. D., Surgical Intensive Care, Onassis Cardiac Surgery Center, 356 Syngrou Avenue, 17674 Athens, Greece

Miyashita, M., M. D., First Department of Surgery, Nippon Medical School, 1-1-5 Sendagi, Bunkyo-ku, Tokyo 113, Japan

Moch, D., M. D., Division for Surgical Research, University, 89073 Ulm, Germany

Moore, E. E., M. D., Department of Surgery, Denver General Hospital, 777 Bannock Street, Denver, CO 80204, USA

Morrison, V. A., M. D., Medicine Service, Veterans Affairs Medical Center, Sections of Hematology/Oncology and Infectious Disease, Minneapolis, MN 55455, USA

Neugebauer, E.A., M.D., Ph.D., Department of Surgery, Biochemical and Experimental Division, University, Ostmerheimer Str. 200, 51109 Cologne, Germany

Niederau, C., M. D., Prof., Department of Medicine, Gastroenterology, Department of General Surgery, Heinrich-Heine-University, Moorenstr. 5, 40225 Düsseldorf, Germany

Novitsky, T. J., Ph. D., Associates of Cape Cod. Inc., 704 Main Street, Falmouth, Ma 02540, USA

Ogawa, M., M. D., Department of Surgery II, University Medical School, Honjo 1-1-1, Kumamoto 860, Japan

Pape, H.-C., M. D., Department of Trauma Surgery, Medical School, Konstanty-Gutschow-Str. 8, 30625 Hannover, Germany

Pierrakakis, S., M. D., Department of Surgery, Sismanoglion General Hospital, 17674 Athens, Greece

Pilz, G., M. D., Department of Medicine I, Ludwig Maximilian University, Grosshadern, Marchioninistr. 15, 811377 Munich, Germany

Pincemail, J., M. D., Department of Cardiovascular Surgery, University of Liège CHU Hospital, B35 Sart Tilman, 4000 Liège, Belgium

Pruitt, B. A., M. D., U.S. Army Institute of Surgical Research, Brooke Army Medical Center, Fort Sam Houston, TX 78234-6315, USA

Rabinovici, R., M. D., Department of Surgery, Jefferson Medical College, 1025 Walnut Street, Philadelphia, PA 19107-5083, USA

Reimund, K.-P., M. D., Department of General Surgery, Centre of Operative Medicine I, Philipps University, Baldingerstr., 35043 Marburg/Lahn, Germany

Rodrick, M. L., M. D., Brigham and Women's Hospital, Department of Surgery, 75 Francis Street, Boston, MA 02115, USA

Rossaint, R., M.D. Ph.D., Clinic of Anaesthesiology, UKRV, Humboldt University, Augustenburger Platz 1, 13353 Berlin, Germany

Rotstein, O. D., M. D., Toronto Hospital, 200 Elizabeth St EN #9-236, Toronto, Ontario M5G 2C4, Canada

Rowlands, B. J., M. D., Department of Surgery, Institute of Clinical Science, Grosvenor Road, Belfast BT12 6BJ, Northern Ireland, UK

Sakamoto, K., M. D., Department of Surgery II, University Medical School, Kumamoto 860, Japan

Schilling, J., M. D., Institute of Social and Preventive, Medicine, Sumatrastr. 30, 8006 Zurich, Switzerland

Schweinfest, C. W., Ph. D., Medical University of South Carolina, Hollings Cancer Center, 171 Ashley Avenue, Charleston, SC 29425, USA

Sganga, G., M. D., Department of Surgery, Catholic University and National Research Council, Center for the Study of the Pathophysiology of Shock, Rome, Italy

Shatney, C. H., M. D., Division of General Surgery, Santa Clara Valley Medical Center, 751 South Bascom Avenue, San Jose, CA 95128, USA

Shelby, J., M. D., Department of Surgery, University Medical Center, Salt Lake City, Utah 84132, USA

Siegel, J. H., M. D., Departments of Surgery and of Anatomy, Cell Biology and Injury Sciences, New Jersey Medical School, Newark, NJ 07103-2406, USA

Slotman, G. J., M. D., Three Cooper Plaza, Suite 411, Camden, NJ 08103, USA

Stöblen, F., M. D., Central Institute of Radiology, University, Hufelandstr. 55, 45122 Essen, Germany

Stüber, F., M. D., Clinic for Anaesthesiology and Critical Care, Christian Albrecht University, Arnold-Heller-Str. 7, 24105 Kiel, Germany

Tilz, G. P., M. D., Clinical Immunology Unit., Karl Franzens University, Auenbrugger Platz 15, 8036 Graz, Austria

Vincent, J. L., M. D., Prof., Department of Intensive Care, Erasme University Hospital, Route de Lennik 808, 1070 Brussels, Belgium

Wacha, H. M.D., Prof., Department of Surgery, Hospital Holy Ghost, Langestr. 2-4, 60311 Frankfurt am Main, Germany

Watson, D. K., Ph. D., Medical University of South Carolina, Hollings Cancer Center, 171 Ashley Avenue, Charleston, SC 29425, USA

Weimar, W., M. D., Departments of Internal Medicine and, Cardiology, University Hospital Rotterdam-Dijkzigt, Dr. Molewaterplein 40, 3015 GD Rotterdam, The Netherlands

Wolf, Ch.-F., M. D., Institute of Clinical Chemistry, University, Robert-Koch-Str. 8, 89081 Ulm, Germany

Index

-!-

6-keto-PGF1α 272-273, 275, 359, 419

-A-

activated neutrophils 37, 132, 531
activated oxygen species 203
acute-phase response 183, 192, 248-249, 256, 351, 528
acute edematous pancreatitis (AEP) 543
acute necrotizing pancreatitis (ANP) 543
acute pancreatitis 37, 40, 196-197, 249, 332, 333, 335, 336, 510-515, 517-521, 523-534, 537, 538, 542-551, 554, 556-560, 562-564, 601
acute respiratory distress syndrome (ARDS) 102, 183, 363, 429
adhesion molecules 131, 133, 248, 254, 341, 342, 386, 464-466, 612
adult respiratory distress syndrome (ARDS) 58, 301, 400, 403, 406, 417, 434, 437, 444, 618
albumin 62, 134, 192, 193, 230, 249, 284, 309, 395, 396, 398, 419, 426, 519, 532, 539, 589
aldosterone 273, 275, 276
allogeneic bone marrow transplantation 566, 568, 570
α-MSH 400
α-tocopherol 259, 348, 350, 532, 538
alveolar-arterial oxygen tension difference (AaDO2) 407
alveolar macrophages 393, 394, 396, 399, 408, 409, 416, 506, 572
animal models 44, 46, 110, 120, 122, 133, 175, 203, 251, 275, 289, 307, 319, 330, 386, 391, 400, 493, 494, 546, 634, 638
anti-CMV hyperimmunoglobulin 587, 591
anti-PGI2 antibody 366- 368
antibiotics 20, 42, 43, 55, 67, 171, 245, 265, 309, 344, 351, 358, 494, 502, 517, 525, 527, 553, 563, 573, 579, 584, 603, 605, 608, 613, 631, 641, 649, 652
antioxidants 209, 214, 259, 344, 346, 347-352, 508, 532

665

antioxidant selenium 543
antithrombin III 192, 193, 442, 635, 638
APACHE 53, 104, 107, 112, 184, 338, 339, 343, 348, 467, 468, 470, 471-476, 478-480, 483, 511, 523, 524, 527, 528, 530, 552, 556, 615, 619, 624, 627-630, 647
APACHE II score 184, 338, 339, 348, 472, 475, 476, 480, 552, 556, 628, 629
arachidonic acid 91, 138, 142, 248, 250, 253, 255, 417, 418, 490, 534
arginine 128, 248, 256, 319, 323, 427, 432, 434-436, 529
Aspergillus 568, 570, 575, 579-583, 585, 606
attributable mortality 655
autologous marrow transplant 566

-B-

bacteremia 36, 37, 39, 40, 43, 47, 57, 74, 75, 111, 133, 168, 169, 172, 174, 178, 181, 189, 246, 250, 252, 255, 291, 292, 305, 344, 365-368, 370, 425, 453, 458, 503, 549, 554, 567, 620, 630, 638, 639, 657, 659
bacterial-enterocyte interactions 121, 129, 130
bacterial/endotoxin translocation 132
bacterial endotoxin lipopolysaccharide (LPS) 386
bacterial overgrowth 120
bacterial pathogens 130
bacterial peritonitis 36, 170, 448, 449, 457
bacterial sepsis 159, 174, 180, 181, 417
bacterial translocation 104, 118, 120-126, 128, 130, 133, 136, 141, 297, 316, 317, 319, 322, 323, 617
bacterial viability 124
Bacteroides fragilis 448-456, 460, 465
base modification 203
β-carotene 259
biliary obstruction 291, 317-319, 321-324, 539, 542, 554
biogenic amines 244, 246
biopterin 146, 485-488, 490-492
blood-brain barrier 84, 97, 159, 357
blood transfusions 302, 305, 582, 588
bone marrow 262, 377, 380, 403, 494, 502, 566-571, 587, 592, 597, 599, 602
bovine serum albumin (BSA) 230, 284, 309

brain edema 84, 86-88, 92, 94, 97, 98
burn injury 252, 255, 265, 268, 291, 316
burn patients 120, 158, 249-253, 255, 264, 283, 483
burn wound 302, 503

-C-

c-fos 240, 356
C-reactive protein (CRP) 62, 64, 183, 187, 192, 259, 475, 501, 512, 529
C1-esterase inhibitor 192, 193
calcitonin 158
Candida 49, 176, 434, 436, 457, 567, 568, 570, 573, 575, 579, 580-586, 609
cardiac surgery 338, 343, 429, 433, 437, 623, 624, 626, 628-630
cardiovascular failure 78, 99, 521, 552
causality of disease 77, 612, 613
cDNA 215-221, 223, 224, 226-233, 236, 238, 240-242, 393
cell-mediated immunity 144, 149, 150, 154, 252, 317-319, 569
cellular hypoxia 39, 74, 106, 112
central nervous system 26, 27, 32, 80, 84, 97, 208, 212, 249, 350, 353, 356-358, 581, 582, 588, 597, 598
cerebral blood flow 86, 98
cerebral capillaries 84
chemotaxins 162
chloramphenicol 237
cholestasis 201, 322, 324, 370, 371, 383, 542
chronic 20, 28, 41, 49, 53, 62, 77, 93, 104, 113, 148, 149, 153, 249, 282, 283, 324, 338, 370, 383, 427, 431, 440, 457, 459, 475, 476, 483, 511, 526, 527, 537, 538, 554, 567, 569-574, 577, 592, 593, 595, 596, 601, 620, 644
chronic antigen stimulation 592
ciprofloxacin 604, 605
circulatory inadequacy 41
circulatory shock 99, 101-103, 347, 348, 352, 369, 528
clinical algorithms 635-637, 639, 646-648
clinical trials 46, 47, 55, 56, 71, 77, 78, 80, 99, 350, 386, 493, 502, 503, 513, 517, 543, 595, 612, 613, 615, 618, 633, 638, 639, 641, 644, 645, 647, 649, 650, 653-656, 658, 659

clotting cascade 162

CMV prophylaxis 574, 587

coenzyme Q10 259, 348

collagen 93, 94, 192, 268, 271, 382, 462, 569

complement 36-38, 40, 94, 133, 152, 162, 163, 168-170, 180, 246, 249, 250, 261, 282, 283, 285, 286, 291, 300, 304, 315, 316, 331, 368, 393, 394, 399, 400, 435, 451, 463, 466-468, 513, 516, 520, 525, 529, 548-550, 563, 574, 618, 629

complement system 162, 331, 548

contamination of pancreatic necrosis 525, 551, 556, 563

corticosteroids 250, 253, 260, 261, 573, 585

cortisol 246, 269, 273, 276, 309, 310, 314, 315, 519

crosslinked hemoglobin 213

cyclooxygenase 40, 48, 246, 272, 276, 290, 302, 315, 364, 417, 420, 424, 537

cyclooxygenase blocker 417

cyclosporine 577, 584, 585, 588, 594, 595, 599-601

cytokine production 253, 261, 262, 264, 285-287, 289, 300, 310, 314, 315, 393

cytokines 62, 64, 110, 113, 115, 124, 144-146, 151, 157, 159, 161, 162, 178, 179, 186, 187, 189, 215, 244, 248-250, 253, 254, 256, 257, 265, 266, 268, 277, 279, 285, 286, 289, 302, 305, 307, 309, 310, 314, 319, 322, 323, 324, 332, 333, 335-337, 376, 382, 386, 391, 393, 394, 400, 407, 411, 412, 415, 416, 434, 464, 466, 467, 472, 493, 494, 501-503, 512, 513, 522-524, 526, 537, 612

cytomegalovirus 147, 153, 218, 567, 568, 570, 571, 574, 576, 577, 579, 587, 591

-D-

deferoxamine (DFO) 504

definitions of MOF 23, 74

dexamethasone 261, 376

dimethindene 279

dinitrofluorobenzene (DNFB) 265

DNA scission 203

dopamine 101, 104, 273, 552, 553

-E-

eicosanoid 72, 138, 203, 244, 369, 485

Elebute score   338, 339, 623, 624, 625, 626, 628

endothelium   84, 91, 93, 133, 203, 261, 285, 342, 377, 387, 391, 416, 427, 431-433, 455, 464, 507, 616

endothelium-derived relaxing factor (EDRF)   427

endotoxemia   36, 39, 40, 43, 46, 49, 111, 113, 171, 174, 175, 178-181, 203, 210, 212, 250, 255, 280, 305, 344, 353, 356, 357, 365, 370, 383, 400, 401, 485, 488, 490, 508, 550, 621, 629

endotoxin   36-40, 42, 43, 48, 49, 57, 76, 80, 94, 111-114, 118-120, 124, 130, 132, 134, 136, 142, 158, 161, 169, 171-182, 186, 210, 246, 250, 253, 255, 256, 261, 278-281, 283, 290, 291, 300-302, 304, 305, 307-310, 314-319, 321-326, 330, 353, 354, 356, 369, 370, 383, 386, 393-395, 399, 401, 420, 436, 453, 458, 470, 475, 483, 485-488, 490, 491, 492, 501-508, 606, 612, 613, 616-618, 620, 622, 630, 639, 645, 659

endotoxin shock   39, 40, 48, 80, 94, 114, 169, 210, 256, 280, 369

enteral nutrition   62, 323, 554

Enterococcus fecalis   448, 456

epinephrine   273, 275, 276, 309

Epstein-Barr virus   147, 153, 575, 592, 599-602

Escherichia coli   40, 130, 131, 178, 218, 226, 232, 242, 289, 297, 300, 307-309, 321, 326, 369, 395, 448-456, 458, 460, 463, 465, 466, 485, 486, 517, 558, 567, 573, 616

esophagectomy   257, 407, 411

excessive fluid resuscitation   21

extracorporeal circulation   418, 441, 445, 589, 623

extracorporeal lung support   437, 440, 442, 443

-F-

Fc receptors   284, 286

fibrinogen receptor activity   341, 342

free radical production   203, 207-212, 214, 350, 532, 537

fungal infections   566, 567, 570, 575, 579-586, 609

-G-

GCSF   256-258, 260

glucan   176

glutamine   208, 213, 265, 308, 309, 496

grading of sepsis 55, 342, 471, 483, 629
graft-versus-host disease (GvHD) 566
gram-negative sepsis 40, 177, 180-182, 485, 490, 491, 506, 620, 652, 656-659
granulocyte-colony stimulating factor (G-CSF) 256, 494, 503
growth hormone 248, 250
gut ischemia/reperfusion 132, 134, 142

-H-

HA-1A 40, 182, 503, 620, 630, 639, 656, 659
heart failure 41, 62, 101, 102, 407
hemorrhagic shock 32, 98, 115, 116, 118, 119, 133, 134, 141, 184, 199, 296, 297, 300-306, 325, 330, 347, 352, 395, 618, 621
hepatic dysfunction 40, 115, 552, 554, 556
hepatic function 116, 119, 199
hepatic parenchymal cell 370
hepatic reserve 115
histamine 245, 246, 248, 254, 255, 277-281, 417, 420, 464, 513, 639, 645
histamine antagonists 281
hormones 42, 186, 244, 250, 263, 269, 276, 425, 527
host defenses 120, 448, 450, 456-460, 502, 579
human volunteer endotoxin studies 307
humoral mediators 256, 344
hydroxyethyl starch 418
hypoxia 39, 74, 86, 90, 92, 97, 105-107, 109, 110, 112, 255, 305, 330, 331, 346, 356, 358, 383, 412-416, 428, 525, 527

-I-

Ibuprofen 272, 273, 276, 304, 307, 310, 314, 359, 360, 363, 364, 369
ICP 84, 87, 88, 92
ICU 30, 44, 46, 51, 55, 56, 57, 62, 66, 78, 80, 132, 133, 163, 164, 168, 189, 348, 350, 480, 481, 528, 551, 552, 554, 558, 559, 572, 612, 614, 615, 618, 623, 624, 626, 628, 633, 645, 655
IgG 268, 283, 284, 286, 354, 574, 588, 589, 593, 594, 629
IgM 40, 268, 574, 588, 593, 594, 659

immune complexes 152, 282-284, 286, 287, 289-292
immune dysfunction 282, 294, 303
immune responsiveness 314
immunoglobulin 177, 268, 271, 283, 284, 309, 418, 420, 465, 570, 571, 587-589, 591-593, 599, 628, 639, 645, 647, 659
immunoglobulin M 177
immunomodulation 294, 303, 319, 570, 620
immunoregulation 151, 154, 269
immunoregulatory neurohormone 268
immunosuppressive therapy 566, 573, 584, 592, 594, 595, 598
improved study design 643, 644
infection after OLT 603
inflammatory cascade 38, 132, 134, 294, 303
inflammatory mediators 249, 253, 319, 336, 386, 393, 462, 485, 490, 491, 513, 526, 534, 543, 618
inflammatory reactions 162, 400, 465, 466, 496
inhaled NO 427-430
intensive care 21, 22, 28, 30-32, 41, 44, 48, 49, 51, 58, 61, 62, 66, 76, 80, 104,132, 161-163, 179, 192, 213, 290, 305, 338, 343, 347, 348, 351, 369, 431, 436, 444, 445, 459, 473, 482-483, 511, 517, 522-524, 551, 554, 555, 558, 559, 561, 603, 604, 606, 608, 612, 617, 621, 623, 630, 633, 635, 638, 644, 650, 652
intent-to-treat analysis 658
interferon-γ (IFN-γ) 264, 485
interferon-gamma 144, 149, 150
interleukin (IL-1) 391
interleukin-1β (IL-1β) 250, 253, 256, 309, 310, 314, 332, 400, 410
interleukin-1 receptor antagonist 40, 46, 48, 114, 253, 305, 620, 638
interleukin-6 (IL-6) 62, 67, 107, 110, 112, 118, 119, 159, 161, 162, 169, 183, 184, 186-188, 189, 248-250, 253, 254, 256, 257, 259-261, 264-269, 271, 300-302, 304, 319, 323, 332, 371, 376, 383, 391, 393, 400, 435, 410, 471, 493, 501, 528, 573, 576, 617, 618
interleukin-8 (IL-8) 161, 248, 253, 254, 256, 257, 261, 301, 319, 391, 393, 407, 408, 410, 411, 463, 464
intestinal barrier function 120, 121
intestinal mucosa 120, 134
intraabdominal infections 448, 453, 491

intravascular platelet aggregation 366
ions 21, 92, 244, 346, 415, 532
irreversible platelet degranulation 338
ischemia/hypoxia 412
ischemia reperfusion 203, 207
Ito cells (fat-storing cells) 382

-K-

kinetics of drug metabolites 199
kinins 244, 463, 516, 548
Koch-Dale analysis 246
Kupffer cells 318, 319, 322, 323, 371, 376, 382, 383, 568

-L-

leukotrienes 248, 425, 464
lidocaine 199
limulus amebocyte lysate (LAL) test 171, 179
lipid peroxidation 203, 204, 208, 256, 347, 350-352, 504-508, 532, 533, 537
lipopolysaccharide-binding protein 286
liver blood flow 36-38, 115
liver dysfunction 199, 257, 554
liver failure 23, 32, 330, 441
lung failure 99, 330, 395, 398
lung transplantation 214, 572-578, 583, 586
lymphoproliferative disorders 592, 594, 596, 598-602

-M-

malignant infections 579
mammalian host 456
mechanisms of MSOF 32
mediator response 62, 248
mediators of septic shock 244-247
MEGX test 199, 200, 202

melatonin   249, 250, 263-271

membrane glycoproteins   128, 338, 339, 341

meningitis   88, 158, 159, 164, 178, 581, 597

mesenteric traction   272, 273, 275, 276, 359, 360, 363, 364

metabolism   35, 36, 39, 47, 65, 84, 98, 104-106, 110-113, 124, 162, 249, 250, 254, 270, 295, 307, 315, 346, 360, 413, 415, 417, 424, 428, 450, 454, 455, 485, 508, 537

methylprednisolone   48, 57, 80, 104, 257, 621, 629, 635, 638

microbial synergy   448-450, 454

microcirculatory arrest   36, 343

microvascular blood flow   99, 297, 306, 369

molecular biological approach   215

molecular dissection   158

monitoring   21, 44, 98, 144, 169, 196, 291, 303, 330, 395, 439, 441, 467, 468, 470-472, 491, 492, 514, 515, 523, 528, 543, 551, 553-556, 574, 576, 588, 624, 628, 630, 635, 643, 654, 658, 659

MSOF 23, 473

multicentre trials   644, 649, 650

multiple organ failure (MOF)   20-24, 27-31, 39, 44, 47-49, 73, 74, 80, 81, 102-104, 110, 120, 130, 132, 141, 183, 186, 192, 199, 202, 244, 254, 256-260, 283, 294, 301, 303, 323, 325, 326, 330, 331, 333, 336, 338, 339, 341, 342, 346, 347, 349, 353, 369, 395, 396, 398, 399, 412, 416, 467, 470-472, 482, 484, 485, 493, 517, 520, 521, 523, 548, 549, 551, 554, 556, 614, 615, 620, 628, 658

multiple trauma   30, 40, 41, 62, 199, 202, 325, 330, 331, 344, 395, 403

-N-

necrotizing pancreatitis and organ complications   558

neopterin   144-150, 152-157, 250-255, 305, 485, 490-492

neuropeptide α-melanocyte stimulating hormone   400

neuropeptides   262, 269

neutrophil(s)   36-38, 40, 72, 128, 129, 132, 133, 142, 162, 169, 248, 284, 290, 300, 304, 316, 319, 323, 332, 333, 336, 337, 346, 351, 391, 393, 395, 396, 398-402, 405, 407-412, 416, 417, 450-452, 454, 455, 460, 464, 466, 501, 508, 516, 526, 531, 534, 567, 569, 629

neutrophil count   410, 411, 501, 567

neutrophil depletion   401

neutrophil elastase   336, 408, 410
neutrophil inhibition   451
new treatments   612, 649
nitric oxide (NO)   256, 427, 434
nitric oxide synthase inhibitors   434, 436
norepinephrine   101, 273, 275, 519, 552
nosocomial pneumonias   604
NOx   259, 260
nutrition   25, 44, 62, 323, 344, 350, 554, 581, 652

-O-

obstructive jaundice   283, 317, 319-324, 542
OKT3   581, 587, 595, 600, 604
one-hit model   133
operative therapy of necrotizing pancreatitis   559
organ damage   77, 294, 300, 301, 303, 330, 616
organ failure   20-23, 27-32, 35-40, 44, 47-49, 57, 71, 72-74, 78, 80, 81, 99, 102-104, 110, 120, 130, 132, 133, 139, 141, 169, 183, 186, 191, 192, 197, 199, 202, 244, 250, 253, 254, 256, 261, 283, 294, 323, 325, 330-333, 336, 338, 339, 341, 343, 346, 347, 351, 353, 368, 369, 395, 398, 399, 411, 412, 416, 420, 470, 472, 473, 475, 481-485, 491, 493, 502, 525, 548, 549, 551, 553-556, 558, 566, 614, 615, 620, 621, 629, 655, 658
outcome   33, 44, 45, 47, 50, 51, 56, 58-62, 66, 88, 93, 98, 104, 107, 111, 162, 168-170, 175, 177, 186, 229, 244, 253, 304, 323, 349, 350, 352, 395, 424, 439, 443, 444, 449, 457, 468, 470-473, 475, 478-485, 491, 495, 510-514, 520-524, 528, 530, 551, 552, 554, 556, 576, 596, 598, 599, 601, 603, 607, 608, 624, 628, 630, 640-645, 647, 649, 652, 654-656
oxidative damage   213, 344, 346-348, 513, 538
oxidative stress   150, 204, 211, 259, 344, 352, 506
oxygen consumption   35, 58, 105, 106, 110, 111, 133, 141, 330, 366-369, 376, 439, 553
oxygen delivery   30, 35, 36, 50, 104-106, 109-113, 248, 366, 367, 369, 552, 553
oxygen free-radicals   146, 147
oxygen free radicals   147, 207, 246, 345, 351, 352, 531, 532, 534, 537, 538

-P-

parenteral nutrition 44, 344, 554, 581, 652

passive immunization 40, 49, 113, 503, 587, 591

pathophysiological and therapeutic studies of MOF 395

pentoxifylline 415, 416

peptides 158, 160, 177, 232, 238, 244, 402, 454, 463, 526, 528

peritoneal cavity 27, 300, 449, 450, 452, 453, 456-464, 466, 494, 557

peritonitis scoring 473

phagocytic function 317, 318, 539

phagocytosis 284-287, 322, 452, 454, 457-459, 542, 572

phospholipase A2 138, 142, 485, 486, 491, 492, 512, 515, 525, 529, 535, 538, 564

physiologic hyperspace 59, 64

physiologic state classification 58, 62, 64, 66, 71

pit cell 380, 383

plasma endotoxin 136, 178, 181, 310, 322, 353, 354, 356, 505

plasma proteins 192, 196, 203, 249, 398, 412, 441

platelet-activating factor (PAF) 133, 138, 248, 386, 417

polymorphonuclear leukocyte elastase (PMN-E) 332

polyunsaturated lipids 208

prediction of outcome 58, 66, 475, 530, 556, 643, 645

predictive efficacy 52

predict sepsis in advance 187

probabilities of survival 59

probability models 51

procalcitonin 158, 160, 161

procollagen III peptide 193, 197

prodrome to MSOF 32

proinflammatory anaphylatoxins 162

prophylaxis 493, 494, 496, 498, 502, 503, 506, 554, 566, 569-571, 573-575, 577-579, 583, 584, 586, 587, 591, 599, 603, 604, 617, 620, 631, 632, 639, 653

prostacyclin (PGI2) 272, 359, 364, 369, 429

prostaglandins 98, 170, 248, 290, 307, 319, 323, 324, 360, 364, 368, 369, 371, 419, 464, 502, 513, 514, 534, 537

Pseudomonas aeruginosa 302, 417-420, 424-426, 434, 436, 503, 567

pulmonary graft recipients 572

pulmonary hilar stripping 572

pulmonary hypertension 102, 364, 368, 369, 420, 427-429, 431-433, 436, 572
pulmonary impairment 403
pulmonary oxygenation 407, 429
pulmonary shunt 359, 360, 363, 364, 434-436
pulmonary vascular resistance 359, 365, 428

-Q-

quantitative liver function 115, 118

-R-

rabbit polyclonal anti-BSA IgG 284
Ranson score 549, 551
reactive oxygen intermediates 37-39, 162
reactive oxygen metabolites (ROM) 504
reamed femoral nailing 403
remote organ failure 22, 23, 29, 48, 473, 482
renal failure 21-23, 25-27, 32, 33, 77, 257, 301, 317, 323, 324, 342, 353, 511, 514, 515, 523-525, 543, 552, 553, 621
renin 186, 246, 273, 275, 276, 515, 526
respiratory failure 21, 22, 29, 365, 366, 368, 369, 437, 438, 444, 445, 515, 517, 553, 621
reticuloendothelial system 383, 458, 517, 539, 542

-S-

sample size determination 656, 659
scores 56, 57, 74, 78, 107, 112, 175, 343, 347, 470, 471, 473, 478, 480-483, 511, 519, 523, 552, 629, 630, 642, 647
scoring systems 23, 57, 338, 339, 467, 468, 472, 475, 480, 483, 511, 512, 523, 524, 530, 551, 556, 623, 624
screening and sequencing of genes 215, 229
secondary peritonitis 467, 468, 471
selective decontamination 584, 586, 603, 608, 609, 617, 621, 639

sepsis 21, 22, 26, 27, 29, 30, 31, 35, 37, 39-44, 46-51, 55-58, 62, 67, 71, 72, 74-78, 80, 81, 94, 97, 101-107, 109-115, 141, 158-165, 168-170, 174, 175, 177-184, 186-189, 191, 200, 203, 210, 244, 246, 248-251, 253, 255, 260, 261, 271, 281-283, 290-292, 294, 297, 301, 303-305, 317, 319, 323, 331, 335, 337-339, 341-344, 346-349, 351-353, 357, 365-371, 382, 386, 393, 394, 399, 417, 424, 441, 453, 458, 459, 467, 470-473, 475, 483, 485,490-494, 501-508, 512, 513, 517, 521, 523-525, 543, 552, 553, 556, 559, 564, 567, 570, 581-583, 598, 604-606, 612, 615, 616, 619-641, 643-647, 650-652, 654-659

sepsis model 74, 335, 337

sepsis therapy 628

sepsis trial 188, 631, 633, 635, 636, 639, 640, 643, 644, 646, 655, 657, 658

septic response 32, 35-39, 41-45, 47, 74, 283, 472

septic shock 29, 30, 34, 40, 47-49, 55, 57, 74, 75, 80, 94, 102, 104, 111-113, 115, 168, 174, 175, 177-181, 186, 191, 210, 213, 244-247, 255, 277-280, 282, 289-291, 301, 315, 343, 344, 365, 366, 368, 369, 389, 393, 400, 401, 411, 412, 415, 427, 432, 434-436, 458, 483, 488, 491, 492, 503, 507, 529, 549, 556, 567, 618, 620, 621, 623, 630, 635, 638, 639, 645, 647, 650, 652, 655, 659

serum bilirubin values 199

serum lactate 105, 109

severe trauma 325, 330, 395, 399, 553

shock 21, 27, 29, 30, 32, 34-36, 39-41, 47-49, 55, 57, 58, 62, 71, 72, 74, 75, 76, 80, 93, 94, 98, 99, 101-104, 106, 111-116, 118, 119, 130, 131, 133, 134, 139, 141, 142, 168, 169, 174, 175, 177-181, 183, 184, 186, 191, 199, 203, 210, 213-216, 244-247, 254-256, 261, 277-282, 289-291, 294-297, 300-306, 315, 325, 330, 331, 343, 344, 346-349, 351-353, 365, 366, 368, 369, 383, 389, 393-395, 399-401, 411, 412, 415, 420, 427, 432, 434-436, 445, 453, 458, 466, 475, 483, 485, 488, 491, 492, 503, 504, 507, 508, 510, 513, 514, 521, 523, 528, 529, 549, 553, 556, 558, 567, 604, 617, 618, 620, 621, 623, 630, 631, 635, 638, 639, 645, 647, 650, 652, 655, 659

simplified acute physiology score (SAPS II) 51, 57

sinusoidal lining cell 370

skeletal muscle pO2 106, 107, 110, 112

solid-organ transplants 579

soluble CD14 287, 289

soluble interleukin-2 receptor assay 151

soluble TNF receptors 154-156, 183, 186, 301, 501

soluble tumor necrosis factor receptors 150, 155, 157

splanchnic hypoperfusion 132, 139

stage of immune function 151
stress-induced gene expression 215
stroma-free hemoglobin 181
superior mesenteric artery (SMA occlusion) 353
superoxide anion (O2-) 259
surgical trauma 62, 192, 193, 196, 197, 256, 276, 315, 347, 411
sympathetic overactivity 41
systemic inflammation 38, 46, 132, 133, 250, 252, 253, 400, 401
systemic inflammatory response syndrome 43, 45, 55, 74, 75, 133, 183, 245, 249, 256, 365, 467, 493, 512, 548, 549, 551, 623, 627, 654

-T-

T-lymphocytes 144, 145, 490, 594
thrombin 139, 142, 459
thromboxane 98, 142, 248, 342, 367-369, 371, 419, 420, 424, 428, 514, 537, 616
tissue damage 88, 248, 249, 256, 260, 294, 330, 346, 365, 415, 504, 507, 531, 535, 616
tissue factor 452
TNF receptors (TNF-R) 155
toxins 42, 43, 175, 209, 244, 245, 246, 317, 548, 549
transplantation 28, 118, 148, 163, 203, 209, 210, 213, 214, 282, 291, 295, 304, 494, 502, 566-579, 581-588, 590-593, 596, 599-603, 608, 609, 624
trauma 20-22, 30, 39, 40-42, 48, 49, 58, 59, 61, 62, 64-66, 71, 72, 77, 80, 81, 84, 87, 88, 91, 92, 94, 97, 98, 103, 104, 112, 115, 119, 120, 130, 132, 133, 138, 139, 141, 142, 158, 179, 187-189, 192, 193, 196, 197, 199-203, 215, 253-256, 262, 269, 271, 276, 278, 290, 294, 297, 301-306, 315-317, 319, 323, 325, 330, 331, 335-337, 344, 346, 347, 349-352, 395, 398, 399, 403, 406, 410, 411, 443, 448, 483, 491, 512, 553, 612, 617, 619-621, 658
tumor necrosis factor (TNF) 37, 40, 62, 115, 155, 159, 162, 187, 210, 244, 246, 248-250, 252-254, 289, 300, 301, 304, 309, 310, 314, 319, 332, 335, 337, 371, 382, 383, 387, 389-391, 393, 394, 400, 410, 412-416, 435, 464, 465, 471, 475, 485, 492-496, 498, 501, 502, 513, 615, 616, 618, 622
two-hit model 132, 133

-U-

unreamed femoral nailing 403, 406

-V-

vascular resistance 35, 37, 101-104, 109, 275, 330, 359, 365, 412, 418, 420, 424, 428, 435, 515
vasopressin 246, 273, 275, 276

-W-

wound healing 248, 317, 639

-Z-

zymosan-activated plasma (ZAP) 325, 326